CLINICAL ENDOCRINOLOGY

SAFFRON WHITEHEAD

Professor of Endocrine Physiology, St George's University of London, UK

JOHN MIELL

Consultant Endocrinologist, Lewisham Healthcare NHS Trust, London, UK

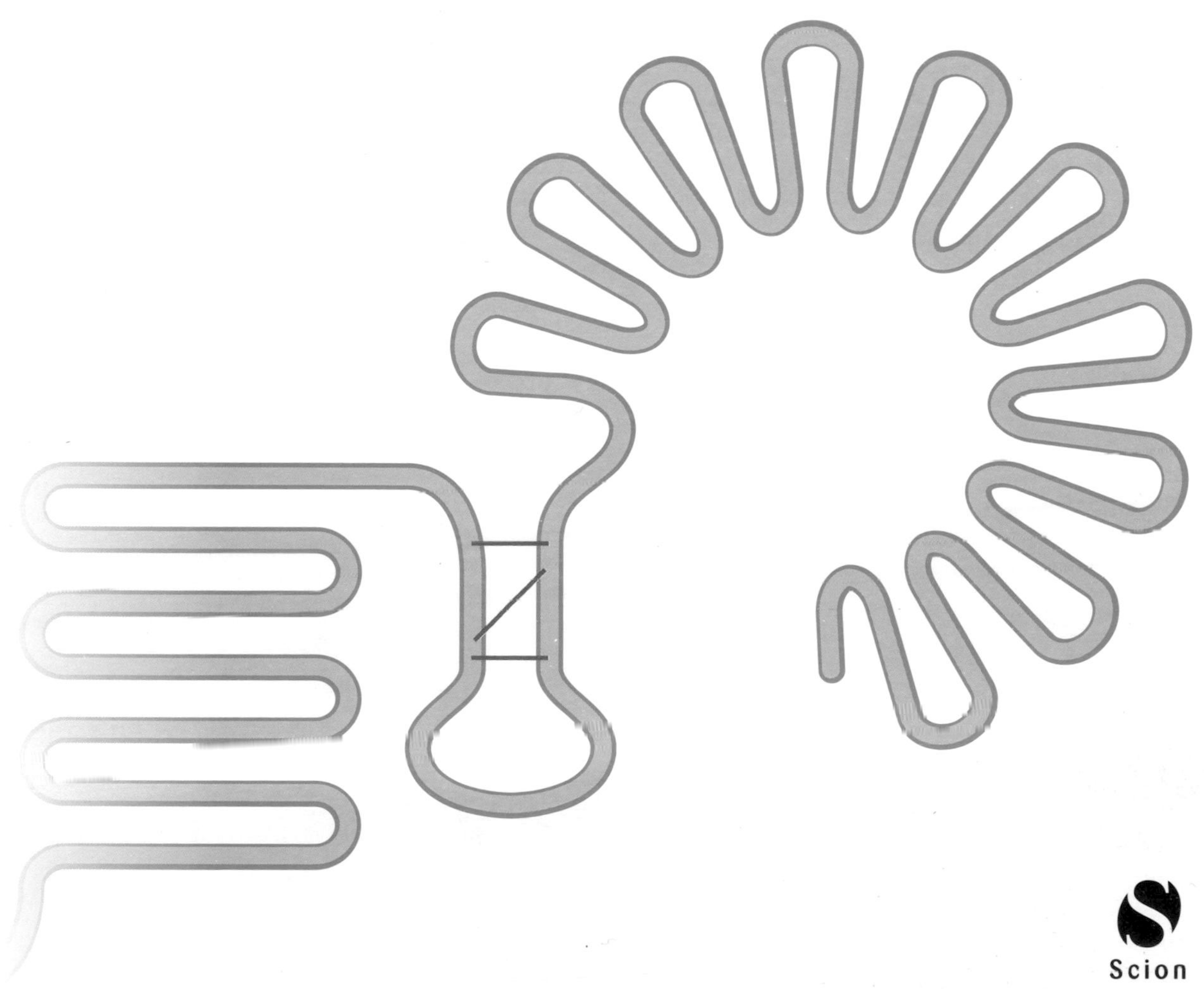

Scion

First published 2013

A CIP catalogue record for this book is available from the British Library.

ISBN 978 1 904842 85 9

Scion Publishing Limited
The Old Hayloft, Vantage Business Park, Bloxham Road, Banbury OX16 9UX, UK
www.scionpublishing.com

Important Note from the Publisher
The information contained within this book was obtained by Scion Publishing Limited from sources believed by us to be reliable. However, while every effort has been made to ensure its accuracy, no responsibility for loss or injury whatsoever occasioned to any person acting or refraining from action as a result of information contained herein can be accepted by the authors or publishers.

Readers are reminded that medicine is a constantly evolving science and while the authors and publishers have ensured that all dosages, applications, and practices are based on current indications, there may be specific practices which differ between communities. You should always follow the guidelines laid down by the manufacturers of specific products and the relevant authorities in the country in which you are practicing.

Although every effort has been made to ensure that all owners of copyright material have been acknowledged in this publication, we would be pleased to acknowledge in subsequent reprints or editions any omissions brought to our attention.

Page and cover design by amdesign, www.amdesigner.co.uk
Illustrations by Matthew McClements at Blink Studio Ltd, www.blink.biz
Typeset by Phoenix Photosetting, Chatham, Kent, UK
Printed in India by Imprint Digital Limited.

Contents

Abbreviations xiv
Preface xvii
Acknowledgements xviii
How to use this book xix

Chapter 1 – Principles of endocrinology and diagnosis of endocrine disorders

1.1 Introduction 1
1.2 Major endocrine glands 2
Case 1.1 3
1.3 Chemical classification of hormones 3
1.3.1 Protein and peptide hormones 3
1.3.2 Steroid hormones 4
1.3.3 Amino acid derived hormones 7
1.4 Synthesis and secretion of hormones 7
1.4.1 Protein and peptide hormones 7
1.4.2 Steroid hormones 10
1.4.3 Endocrine disorders related to aberrant hormone synthesis 13
1.5 How do hormones deliver their messages to target cells? 14
1.5.1 Protein and peptide hormones 14
1.5.2 Endocrine disorders associated with mutations in cell surface receptors 15
1.5.3 Steroid and thyroid hormones 19
1.6 Hormone binding, receptor regulation, and disease 21
1.7 Control of hormone secretions 23
Case 1.1 24
1.8 Autoimmunity and endocrine disorders 24
1.9 Diagnosing endocrine disorders 27
1.9.1 Measuring hormone levels 27
1.9.2 Diagnosing endocrine disorders with hormone measurements and dynamic tests of endocrine function 30
Case 1.1 31
Case 1.1 33
1.9.3 Imaging modalities for the endocrine system 34
Case 1.1 46
1.10 Further reading 46
Useful websites 47
1.11 Self-assessment questions 47

Chapter 2 – The pituitary gland

2.1 Introduction 49
2.2 Anatomy and embryology 51
- 2.2.1 Anatomy 51
- 2.2.2 Embryology 53
- 2.2.3 Craniopharyngioma 55

2.3 Basic physiology of growth hormone 58

Case 2.1 58
- 2.3.1 Actions of growth hormone 59
- 2.3.2 Synthesis and secretion of GH 60

2.4 Excess growth hormone – acromegaly 61
- 2.4.1 Symptoms and signs of acromegaly 63
- 2.4.2 Investigation and management of acromegaly 65

Case 2.1 70

2.5 Growth hormone deficiency 71
- 2.5.1 Childhood growth hormone deficiency 71
- 2.5.2 Investigation and management of childhood GHD 73
- 2.5.3 Adult growth hormone deficiency 73

2.6 Basic physiology of prolactin 75

Case 2.2 76
- 2.6.1 Synthesis, action, and control of prolactin secretion 76

2.7 Hyperprolactinemia 77
- 2.7.1 Prolactinomas 79

Case 2.2 84

2.8 Trophic hormones of the anterior pituitary gland – ACTH and the glycoprotein hormones 84
2.9 Basic physiology of oxytocin and vasopressin 85
- 2.9.1 Oxytocin 85
- 2.9.2 Vasopressin 86

2.10 Disorders related to vasopressin secretion and action 88
- 2.10.1 Diabetes insipidus 88
- 2.10.2 Hyponatremia and the syndrome of inappropriate antidiuretic hormone secretion 91
- 2.10.3 Adipsia 94

2.11 Hypopituitarism 95

Case 2.3 95
- 2.11.1 Causes of hypopituitarism 97
- 2.11.2 Treatment of hypopituitarism 101

Case 2.3 101

2.12 Non-functioning pituitary adenomas 102
- 2.12.1 Clinical signs and symptoms 102
- 2.12.2 Treatment 102

2.13 Further reading 103
2.14 Self-assessment questions 103

Chapter 3 – The thyroid gland

3.1 Introduction 107
3.2 Anatomy and embryology 108
3.2.1 Anatomy 108
3.2.2 Embryology 109
3.3 Hyperthyroidism 110
Case 3.1 110
Case 3.2 111
3.4 Basic physiology 111
3.4.1 Thyroid hormones and their actions 111
3.4.2 How do thyroid hormones exert their cellular effects? 113
3.4.3 Synthesis and release of thyroid hormones and mechanisms of control 115
3.4.4 Transport, peripheral metabolism, and excretion of thyroid hormones 118
3.4.5 TSH and the control of thyroid hormone synthesis and secretion 119
3.5 Hyperthyroidism 122
3.5.1 Graves disease 123
3.5.2 Diagnosis of hyperthyroidism – biochemical measurements of thyroid hormone status 125
Case 3.1 127
3.5.3 Other causes of primary hyperthyroidism 127
Case 3.1 128
Case 3.2 129
Case 3.3 130
3.5.4 Thyrotoxicosis associated with structural (nodular) thyroid disease 131
Case 3.4 132
3.5.5 Hyperthyroidism in pregnancy 134
Case 3.5 134
Case 3.5 135
3.5.6 Treatment of hyperthyroidism 136
3.6 Hypothyroidism 141
Case 3.6 142
3.6.1 Autoimmune hypothyroidism 142
Case 3.7 143
3.6.2 Other causes of primary hypothyroidism 144
3.6.3 Central (secondary) hypothyroidism and resistance to thyroid hormone 144
Case 3.7 145
3.6.4 Symptoms and treatment of hypothyroidism 145
3.7 Fetal, neonatal, and childhood hypothyroidism 146

Case 3.6 147

Case 3.7 148

3.8 Structural thyroid disease and thyroid cancer 148

Case 3.8 148

3.8.1 Thyroid nodules 149
3.8.2 Investigation of thyroid nodules 149
3.8.3 Thyroid cancer 151

3.9 Abnormal thyroid function test results 155

Case 3.8 157

3.10 Further reading 158
3.11 Self-assessment questions 158

Chapter 4 – Endocrine control of calcium and phosphate

4.1 Introduction 161
4.2 Turnover of calcium and phosphate 163
4.3 Anatomy and embryology of the parathyroid glands 164
4.3.1 Anatomy of the parathyroid glands 164
4.3.2 Embryology of the parathyroid glands 165
4.4 Basic physiology 165

Case 4.1 165

4.4.1 Actions of parathyroid hormone 166
4.4.2 Synthesis and control of parathyroid hormone secretion 171
4.4.3 The calcium sensing receptor 171
4.4.4 Actions of vitamin D 172
4.4.5 Synthesis, transport, and metabolism of vitamin D 173
4.4.6 Fibroblast growth factor 23 176
4.4.7 Calcitonin, PTH-related peptide, and other hormones in calcium homeostasis 177
4.4.8 Integrated calcium and phosphate homeostasis 179

Case 4.2 179

4.5 Hypercalcemia 181

Case 4.1 and 4.2 182

4.5.1 Primary hyperparathyroidism 182
4.5.2 Secondary and tertiary hyperparathyroidism 184
4.5.3 Other causes of hypercalcemia 186

Case 4.2 187

4.5.4 Treatment of hypercalcemia 188
4.5.5 Treatment of primary hyperparathyroidism 189

Case 4.1 190

Case 4.2 191

4.6 Hypocalcemia 191

Case 4.3 191

4.6.1 Hypoparathyroidism 192

Case 4.3 195
4.6.2 Pseudohypoparathyroidism 195
4.6.3 Vitamin D deficiency 197
Case 4.4 199
Case 4.4 200
4.7 Metabolic bone disease 201
4.7.1 Osteoporosis 202
4.7.2 Paget disease of bone 205
4.8 Further reading 209
4.9 Self-assessment questions 210

Chapter 5 – The endocrine pancreas

5.1 Introduction 213
5.2 Anatomy and embryology of the pancreas 214
5.2.1 Anatomy 214
5.2.2 Embryology 215
Case 5.1 215
Case 5.2 216
5.3 Basic physiology 217
5.3.1 Actions of hormones secreted by pancreatic islets 217
5.3.2 Overview of glucose, amino acid, and fat metabolism 217
5.3.3 Actions of insulin and glucagon on liver, muscle, and adipose tissue metabolism 222
5.3.4 Insulin: glucagon secretion and integrated metabolism 223
5.3.5 Synthesis, release, and metabolism of insulin secretion 225
5.3.6 How does insulin exert its cellular effects? 227
5.3.7 Synthesis, release, and metabolism of glucagon 229
5.3.8 How does glucagon exert its cellular effects? 231
5.4 Diabetes mellitus 231
5.5 Type 1 diabetes mellitus 232
5.5.1 Etiology of type 1 diabetes mellitus 232
5.5.2 Metabolic disturbances in type 1 diabetes mellitus 234
5.5.3 Management of type 1 diabetes mellitus 237
Case 5.1 240
5.6 Type 2 diabetes mellitus 241
5.6.1 Management of type 2 diabetes mellitus 241
Case 5.2 245
5.7 Rarer forms of diabetes mellitus 246
Case 5.3 246
Case 5.3 247
5.8 Diabetic complications 248
5.8.1 Common diabetic complications resulting from macro- and microvascular disease 249
5.8.2 Preventing diabetic complications 254

5.9 Hypoglycemia 254
Case 5.4 254
5.9.1 Physiological responses to hypoglycemia 256
5.9.2 Classification and causes of hypoglycemia 257
Case 5.4 260
5.9.3 Hypoglycemia related to endogenous hyperinsulinism 261
5.10 Further reading 261
5.11 Self-assessment questions 262

Chapter 6 – The adrenal glands

6.1 Introduction – adrenal cortex and medulla 265
6.2 Embryology and development of functional zonation of the adrenal glands 267
6.2.1 Steroid synthesis in the adrenal glands 269
6.3 Basic science 270
6.3.1 Glucocorticoids and their actions 270
6.3.2 How do glucocorticoids exert their cellular effects? 273
6.3.3 Transport and metabolism of glucocorticoids 276
6.3.4 Availability of cortisol at the glucocorticoid receptor and its metabolism 277
6.3.5 Adrenal androgens 278
6.3.6 CRH, ACTH, and the control of glucocorticoid and androgen production 281
6.3.7 Feedback control of glucocorticoids 283
6.4 Excess glucocorticoids – Cushing syndrome 284
Case 6.1 284
Case 6.2 284
6.4.1 Causes of Cushing syndrome 285
6.4.2 Diagnosis of Cushing syndrome 287
Case 6.1 292
Case 6.2 293
6.4.3 Treatment of Cushing syndrome 293
6.5 Adrenocortical cancer 296
6.5.1 Epidemiology 296
6.5.2 Clinical presentation 296
6.5.3 Histopathology and staging of adrenocortical tumors 297
6.5.4 Diagnosis of adrenocortical tumors 297
6.5.5 Treatment of ACC and prognosis 300
6.5.6 Adrenal incidentalomas 300
6.6 Adrenal insufficiency – Addison disease and other causes 305
6.6.1 Causes of adrenal insufficiency 305
Case 6.3 306
6.6.2 Symptoms and signs of adrenal insufficiency – chronic and acute 308
6.6.3 Diagnosis of adrenal insufficiency 309

6.6.4 Determining the etiology of adrenal insufficiency 310
6.6.5 Treatment of adrenal insufficiency – adrenal crisis and long-term treatment 311
Case 6.3 **311**
6.7 More basic physiology **312**
6.7.1 Aldosterone and its actions 312
6.7.2 Control of aldosterone secretion 315
6.7.3 Integrated endocrine control of salt and water balance 316
6.8 Primary aldosteronism **316**
Case 6.4 **317**
6.8.1 Clinical features of PA 317
6.8.2 Etiology of PA 317
6.8.3 Diagnosis of PA 318
6.8.4 Management of PA 319
Case 6.4 **319**
6.9 Excess adrenal androgens – congenital adrenal hyperplasia **320**
Case 6.5 **320**
Case 6.5 **324**
6.10 The adrenal medulla and pheochromocytoma **324**
6.10.1 Actions of catecholamines 325
6.10.2 Pheochromocytomas 326
Case 6.6 **326**
Case 6.6 **331**
6.11 Further reading **331**
Useful websites 332
6.12 Self-assessment questions **332**

Chapter 7 – The gonads

7.1 Introduction – hormones of gonadal control **335**
7.2 Sexual determination and differentiation **336**
Case 7.1 **336**
7.2.1 Development of the gonads and internal reproductive tracts 336
7.2.2 Sexual development of the external genitalia 341
7.2.3 Androgen insensitivity syndromes 342
Case 7.1 **343**
7.2.4 Steroid production in the fetal and neonatal gonads 343
7.3 Puberty **345**
Case 7.2 **345**
7.3.1 Hormonal changes during puberty – adrenarche and gonadarche 346
7.3.2 Onset of puberty and consonance 348
7.3.3 Precocious puberty, precocious pseudopuberty, and delayed puberty 350

7.4 Turner syndrome 356
Case 7.2 359
7.5 Testicular function and its control 359
7.5.1 Anatomy of the testis 359
Case 7.3 360
7.5.2 Functions of the testis 361
7.5.3 Spermatogenesis 364
7.5.4 Erection and ejaculation 365
7.5.5 Causes of male infertility 367
7.5.6 Klinefelter syndrome 368
Case 7.3 370
7.6 Ovarian function and its control 371
Case 7.4 371
7.6.1 Anatomy of the ovary 371
7.6.2 Functions of the ovary 372
7.6.3 Oogenesis and folliculogenesis 374
7.6.4 The menstrual cycle and its disorders 376
7.6.5 Amenorrhea 381
Case 7.4 382
7.6.6 Polycystic ovary syndrome 382
Case 7.5 383
Case 7.5 388
7.7 Premature ovarian failure and the menopause 388
7.7.1 Premature ovarian failure 388
Case 7.6 389
Case 7.6 394
7.7.2 The menopause 395
7.8 Further reading 395
Useful websites 396
7.9 Self-assessment questions 396

Chapter 8 – Endocrinology beyond the 'classical' endocrine glands

8.1 Introduction 399
8.2 The pineal gland and biological rhythms 400
8.2.1 Melatonin 402
8.3 Basic science – the endocrinology of fat 404
Case 8.1 404
8.3.1 Development of adipose tissue and obesity 405
8.3.2 Hormones from adipose tissue 406
8.3.3 Obesity, adipose tissue macrophages, and inflammatory cytokines 410
Case 8.1 412

8.4 The endocrinology of the gut and gastroenteropancreatic tumors 412
8.4.1 Carcinoid tumors and carcinoid syndrome 417
Case 8.2 417
8.4.2 Other GEP-NETs: tumors of the pancreas/islets 421
Case 8.2 425
8.5 Multiple endocrine neoplasia 426
Case 8.3 426
8.5.1 MEN-1 426
8.5.2 MEN-2 429
Case 8.3 431
Case 8.4 431
8.6 Hormones secreted by the cardiovascular system, kidney, and bone 432
8.6.1 Hormones of the cardiovascular system 432
Case 8.4 436
8.6.2 Hormones of the kidney 437
8.6.3 Hormones released from bone 439
8.7 Further reading 440
8.8 Self-assessment questions 441

Appendix 1 – Answers to self-assessment questions 443

Appendix 2 – Reference ranges in endocrinology 449

Index 453

Abbreviations

3β-HSD	3β-hydroxysteroid dehydrogenase
ACC	adrenocortical cancer
ACE	angiotensin-converting enzyme
ACTH	adrenocorticotropic hormone
ADH	antidiuretic hormone
AIS	androgen insensitivity syndrome
ALS	acid-labile subunit
AME	apparent mineralocorticoid excess
AMH	anti-Müllerian hormone
AMPK	AMP-activated protein kinase
ANP	atrial natriuretic peptide
APA	aldosterone-producing adenoma
APC	antigen presenting cell
APS	autoimmune polyendocrine syndrome
AVP	arginine vasopressin
bd	twice a day
BMD	bone mineral density
BNP	B-type natriuretic peptide
CAH	congenital adrenal hyperplasia
CaSR	calcium-sensing receptor
CBG	corticosteroid-binding globulin
CCK	cholecystokinin
CDGP	constitutional delay of growth and puberty
CKD	chronic kidney disease
CNP	C-type natriuretic peptide
COC	combined (estrogen and progestogen) oral contraceptive
CRH	corticotropin releasing hormone
CT	computed tomography
DKA	diabetic ketoacidosis
DDAVP	1-deamino-8-D-arginine vasopressin (desmopressin)
DEXA	dual-energy X-ray absorptiometry
DHEA	dehydroepiandrosterone
DI	diabetes insipidus
DOPA	dihydroxyphenylalanine
DPP-4	dipeptidyl peptidase-4
ELISA	enzyme-linked immunosorbent assay
ESR	erythrocyte sedimentation rate
FFA	free fatty acid
FGF	fibroblast growth factor
FHH	familial hypocalciuric hypercalcemia
FNA	fine needle aspiration

FSH	follicle stimulating hormone
GC/MS	gas chromatography/mass spectroscopy
GEP-NET	gastroenteropancreatic neuroendocrine tumor
GH	growth hormone
GHD	growth hormone deficiency
GHRH	growth hormone releasing hormone
GIP	gastric inhibitory peptide
GLP-1	glucagon-like peptide 1
GMCSF	granulocyte monocyte colony stimulating factor
GnRH	gonadotropin releasing hormone
GPCR	G-protein coupled receptor
GRA	glucocorticoid remediable aldosteronism
GRE	glucocorticoid response element
hCG	human chorionic gonadotropin
hGR	human glucocorticoid receptor
HHS	hyperosmolar hyperglycemic state
5-HIAA	5-hydroxy indole acetic acid
HLA	human leukocyte antigen
HONK	hyperosmolar non-ketotic coma
HPT-JT	hyperparathyroidism jaw tumor
HRE	hormone response element
HRT	hormone replacement therapy
hsp	heat shock protein
HU	Hounsfield Unit
IDDM	insulin-dependent diabetes mellitus
IGF-1	insulin-like growth factor-1
IGTT	oral glucose tolerance test
[^{123}I]-MIBG	^{123}iodine-metaiodobenzylguanidine
IR	insulin receptor
IST	insulin stress test
IV	intravenous
IVC	inferior vena cava
LDL	low density lipoprotein
LFTs	liver function tests
LH	luteinizing hormone
MDIs	multiple daily injections
MEN	multiple endocrine neoplasia
MHC	major histocompatibility complex
MRI	magnetic resonance imaging
MSH	melanocyte stimulating hormone
MTC	medullary thyroid carcinoma
NAT	*N*-acetyltransferase
NEFA	non-esterified fatty acid
NFPA	non-functioning pituitary adenomas
NICE	National Institute for Health and Clinical Excellence
od	once daily
OXM	oxyntomodulin
PA	primary aldosteronism

PCOS	polycystic ovary syndrome
PET	positron emission tomography
PHP	pseudohypoparathyroidism
POF	premature ovarian failure
POMC	pro-opiomelanocortin
POP	progestogen only pill
PPAR	peroxisome proliferator-activated receptor
PRA	plasma renin activity
PRLR	prolactin receptor
PTH	parathyroid hormone
PTHrP	parathyroid hormone-related peptide
RANK	receptor of activation of nuclear factor kappa
RAS	renin–angiotensin system
SCN	suprachiasmatic nucleus
SERM	selective estrogen receptor modulator
SHBG	sex hormone binding globulin
SIADH	syndrome of inappropriate ADH secretion
SPECT	single photon emission computed tomography
SRIF	somatostatin release-inhibiting factor
SSTR	somatostatin receptor
T1DM	type 1 diabetes mellitus
T2DM	type 2 diabetes mellitus
TAG	triacylglycerol
TBG	thyroxine-binding globulin
tds	three times a day
TGF-β	transforming growth factor β
THE	tetrahydrocortisone
THF	tetrahydrocortisol
TLR	toll receptor
TNF-α	tumor necrosis factor-α
TSH	thyroid stimulating hormone
UAH	unilateral adrenal hyperplasia
U&Es	urea and electrolytes
VDBP	vitamin D binding protein
VDR	vitamin D receptor
VLDL	very low density lipoprotein
VP	vasopressin

Preface

Endocrinology is one of the more scientific specialties in medicine based on sound principles of protocol-driven investigation and management, underpinned by evidence. Despite this, endocrinologists must also use a degree of artistry – complex hormonal abnormalities can be challenging to diagnose and manage effectively and with compassion. This book is the result of a collaboration between a basic scientist (SW) and a practicing clinical endocrinologist (JM), both of whom have a background in medical education and a passion for the subject. The aim was to create a book that realistically unites a sound knowledge of basic science principles with a case-based approach to clinical management of patients with endocrinopathy. Hopefully the result is an integration of physiology and biochemistry with real-life pathology illustrated by clinical cases – all of which are completely genuine.

The book is aimed primarily at undergraduate medical and biomedical science students, but we have added boxes of additional material (outlined in purple) that take it beyond that level and make it suitable for students pursuing specialist study modules, and for qualified doctors hoping to pursue a career in endocrinology. It is therefore ideal for use by Specialist Trainees in the UK and to Residents in the USA who need to refresh their memories of basic principles. It is also a useful reference book for all those in allied medical healthcare specialties interested in endocrinology. By its very nature, endocrinology is a rapidly advancing field but we have tried to include completely up to date scientific, diagnostic, and therapeutic information wherever possible within the scope of a textbook such as this.

Following a general introduction, the subject material is divided into chapters focusing on each of the major endocrine organs, with a final chapter covering endocrinology beyond the classical glands, including the adipocyte. Although not rigidly based on any particular curriculum (but structured around the GMC guidelines in the UK and the ACGME requirements in the USA) we feel that the book covers the information needed to be competent in endocrinology whether at undergraduate or early postgraduate level.

We hope you enjoy the book.

Saffron Whitehead and John Miell
London, July 2012

Acknowledgements

We are extraordinarily grateful to the medical students of King's College London who gave advice at the outset of the book, particularly to Charissa Hu and Sindu Yoharajan. As for junior doctors, the 'two Michaels' (Miles and Michail) helped with aspects of the calcium chapter, and various registrars from the London rotation in endocrinology have contributed ideas and suggestions: Anna White, Christine Leong, Cynthia Mohandas and, above all, a great friend and colleague Omar Mustafa. We sincerely thank the Cellular Pathology Department at St George's Hospital for allowing us to reproduce photographs from their Pathology Museum archives and especially Caroline Findlayson and Carol Shiels for their help in accessing the material. We would also like to thank Alan Johnstone, Debbie Baines, Suman Rice and Helen Mason for useful discussions and casting a critical eye over sections of the book during its preparation.

We acknowledge the valuable feedback on the proofs from Romesh Khardori at Eastern Virginia Medical School and Uzma Khan at University of Missouri School of Medicine.

We hope that we have correctly and accurately acknowledged any source or illustrative material that was not our own, but if we have failed anywhere please contact us.

We thank Matthew McClements of Blink Studio Ltd for turning our rough drawings into the polished artworks you see here.

Finally, we would like to thank Jonathan Ray of Scion Publishing Ltd for his encouragement, good humour and, above all, patience.

How to use this book

Basic principles of endocrinology and assessment of endocrine disorders are covered in Chapter 1 and this gives readers an overall understanding of the discipline. The following six chapters address the endocrinology of our six classical endocrine glands, namely the pituitary gland, thyroid gland, parathyroid gland (and vitamin D), the adrenal gland, and the gonads. Each of these chapters opens with basic anatomy, embryology, and physiology as a basis for understanding endocrine diseases and their treatments, which are covered in the second half of each chapter. The final chapter goes beyond the classical endocrine glands and addresses the endocrine function of adipose tissue, bone, the cardiovascular system, and the kidney. Within each chapter there are:

- *Learning points* – summarizing what the chapter should enable the student to achieve.
- *Case studies* – all chapters have case studies which are not only used to illustrate the importance of understanding the physiology of the endocrine system but in understanding the etiology of endocrine disorders and their treatments. All cases are genuine.
- *Boxes* – the light blue boxes provide information on material related to the text, such as basic physiology, causes of endocrine disorders, and clinical features. The purple boxes provide more advanced content that is more appropriate for students specializing in endocrinology, such as residents and specialist trainees, or for final year biomedical science students and postgraduate students who need to be introduced to the latest scientific and clinical developments in the field.
- *Clinical sections* – these provide a level of clinical detail that builds on the science-based introduction and shows readers the causes of endocrine disorders, their clinical features, and their treatments.
- *Further reading* – recent review articles from the primary literature to help readers access additional information for more detailed study.
- *Self-assessment questions* – these include single best answer questions (SBAs), typically used in medical education assessment, and two short answer questions (SAQs) based on clinical cases so that students can check that they have understood and mastered the material, and how a diagnosis can be made from clinical facts.

CASE 1.1 | 3 | 24 | 31 | 33 | 46

- Woman of 62 years with 4 month history of polyuria and polydipsia
- Poor appetite and weight loss of 6 kg
- Normal fasting blood sugar, slightly raised creatinine and raised calcium
- ? Hypercalcemia

For example: A 62 year old woman was referred by her family doctor with a 4 month history of polyuria and polydipsia associated with fatigue, mental 'fogginess', and constipation. Her appetite had been poor for several months and this was associated with a weight loss of about 6 kg (13 lb). On close questioning she admitted to a long history of non-specific symptoms including general malaise and aches and pains. She had no significant past medical history and denied any family history of note. Initial investigations had revealed:

- fasting blood sugar 4.5 mmol/L (NR 3.5–6.1)
- creatinine: 110 μmol/L (NR 53–106)
- total calcium: 3.4 mmol/L (NR 2.2–2.58)

Other blood tests (including albumin, globulins, full blood count, and film) were all normal. This is clearly a case of hypercalcemia, but what is causing it and what is the explanation of her symptoms?

Case studies are used to illustrate the importance of understanding normal function of the endocrine system so that abnormalities and their potential causes can be recognized and understood. Thus there is a clinical case near the beginning of each chapter or each main section within a chapter. After a description of the basic physiology the case is developed so that readers may begin to understand why and how different endocrine disorders arise, their clinical features, how they are best investigated, and what the treatment options are. The follow-up to these cases is thus embedded in the clinical sections of each chapter. For those students who are following a science course they may not want to delve too deeply into the clinical aspects, although for all science subjects it is important to appreciate the practical applications of these studies.

The book is not intended as a diagnostic manual and so does not aim to describe every disorder. However, the cases and the clinical content do highlight the major endocrinopathies you are likely to come across and the very rare causes of endocrine disorders are generally listed in tables that give the spectrum of different etiologies of a particular endocrine abnormality. Finally, attention has been paid to the incidence/prevalence of all the major endocrine disorders so that students understand which disorders are very common, those that are less common, and those that are relatively rare.

CHAPTER 01 Principles of endocrinology and diagnosis of endocrine disorders

After working through this chapter you should be able to:

- Identify the major endocrine glands and the different types of hormones they secrete
- Outline the synthesis of hormones and their different signaling mechanisms at target cells
- Understand that endocrine disorders can arise from abnormal hormone synthesis and receptor mechanisms
- Know the importance of negative feedback control in the endocrine system and its importance in diagnosing endocrine disorders
- Understand the significance of autoimmunity in endocrine disorders
- Know the basic principles of diagnosing endocrine disorders

1.1 Introduction

The nervous system and the endocrine system are two communicating systems in the body which co ordinate bodily functions and help maintain a relatively constant internal environment (homeostasis). They also allow us to react and respond to wide variations in the external environment. The nervous system uses the frequency and pattern of electrical impulses generated by activated neurons to communicate, whereas the endocrine system communicates using hormones (chemical signals), each of which has a unique chemical structure that is recognized by specific receptors on target cells.

ENDOCRINE
Hormones released by an endocrine cell into the general circulation and acting on distant target sites

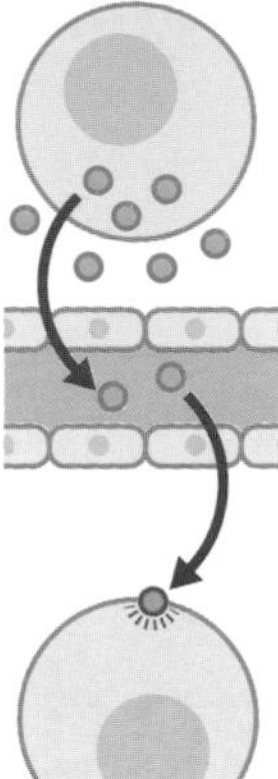

PARACRINE
Hormones released by an endocrine cell which act locally on adjacent cells

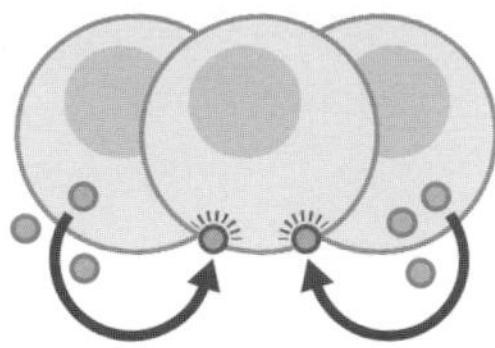

AUTOCRINE
Hormones released by a cell which act back on the same cell

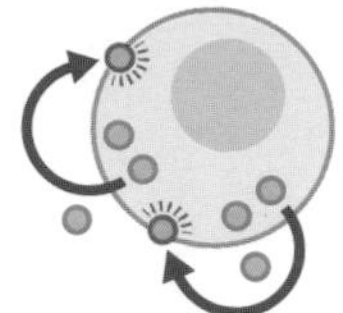

INTRACRINE
Conversion of an inactive hormone to an active hormone that acts within that cell

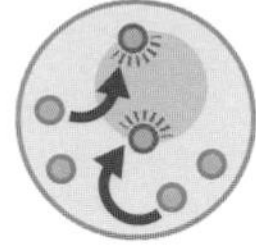

Figure 1.1. Signaling mechanisms in the endocrine system.

The chemical signals of the endocrine system may be simple molecules such as modified amino acids or fatty acids, or they may be more complex peptides and proteins, or molecules derived from cholesterol (steroids). There are four different signaling mechanisms used by the endocrine system to communicate (see *Figure 1.1*):

- in the 'classical' *endocrine* system groups of specialized cells (endocrine organs) secrete hormones into the general circulation where they are transported to their target cells
- in *paracrine* signaling the hormones only act locally; they are released into the extracellular fluid and reach adjacent or nearby target cells by diffusion
- in *autocrine* signaling a cell releases a chemical (usually a growth factor/ hormone) which acts back on the same cell
- in *intracrine* signaling a precursor hormone is taken up from the circulation and is converted into an active hormone that acts within the same cell.

This chapter covers the basics of endocrinology outlining the major endocrine glands, hormone synthesis, how hormones act on their target cells, the factors that regulate the synthesis and secretion of hormones and, finally, clinical approaches that are used to diagnose endocrine disorders, which at times, is not always that simple – as *Case 1.1* shows. This is a case of excess secretions of thyroid hormones (hyperthyroidism) which stimulates an increase in metabolic rate. This case will be followed throughout the chapter to illustrate why it is important to understand the regulation of hormone secretions, the biochemical measurement of hormone levels, dynamic tests of endocrine function and the importance of imaging in the diagnosis of endocrine disorders.

1.2 Major endocrine glands

Three of the classical peripheral endocrine glands (see *Table 1.1*) are controlled by hormone secretions from the brain and pituitary gland (together called the hypothalamic–pituitary axis):

CASE 1.1 | 3 | 24 | 31 | 33 | 46

- 28 year old woman with increased metabolic rate and a palpable goiter
- Abnormal TFTs

A 28 year old woman presented to her primary care physician with a relatively long history of tremor, palpitation, weight loss and increased frequency of bowel habit. Her periods had become less frequent and lighter. She was also concerned that her friends had commented on a swelling in her neck, although she herself had not noticed this and it was not causing any symptoms associated with neck compression (difficulty in swallowing or stridor, for example). She had never been pregnant and was not using the oral contraceptive. She had no relevant previous medical history and close questioning revealed no family history of note – particularly no history of thyroid problems or other endocrine disorders. The primary care physician was struck by the symptoms suggestive of an increase in metabolic rate (weight loss, voracious appetite, tachycardia and palpitations) and felt this might be due to thyroid overactivity, particularly given the presence of a thyroid swelling (goiter) that was clearly palpable on examination. He ordered some basic blood tests which revealed a normal full blood count, normal urea and electrolytes and liver function and normal inflammatory markers (C-reactive protein and erythrocyte sedimentation rate (ESR)). However, the thyroid function tests were indeed abnormal:

- free (unbound) T_4 34 pmol/L (NR 10–20)
- free T_3 11 pmol/L (NR 2.5–6.2)
- TSH 4.1 mIU/L (NR 0.4–4.2)

The primary care physician found these investigations a little difficult to interpret and sought an endocrine specialist opinion.

- the thyroid gland which secretes thyroid hormones
- the adrenal cortex which secretes steroid hormones
- the gonads (testes and ovaries) which secrete steroid hormones.

The adrenal medulla secretes the catecholamines (including epinephrine/adrenaline and nor-epinephrine/nor-adrenaline and these secretions are mainly under control of the sympathetic nervous system. Two other peripheral endocrine organs are the endocrine pancreas and the parathyroid glands which, instead of being controlled by hormone secretions from the hypothalamic–pituitary axis, are controlled by blood sugar levels and circulating concentrations of calcium, respectively.

Several other organs and tissues are now also considered to be peripheral endocrine organs because they secrete hormones into the general circulation; these include the heart, the kidneys, adipose tissue, and the gastrointestinal tract (see *Chapter 8*). Additionally, there is the thymus gland which is important in immune function and the pineal gland which is involved in circadian rhythms of the body (see *Table 1.1*).

1.3 Chemical classification of hormones

1.3.1 Protein and peptide hormones

The majority of hormones are peptides or proteins (*Table 1.2*) with a large diversity in size, ranging from just three amino acids to nearly 200 amino acids. Some are

Table 1.1. Endocrine glands and their major secretions

Gland	Secretions
Peripheral glands controlled by the hypothalamic–pituitary axis	
Thyroid gland	Thyroxine (T_4) and triiodothyronine (T_3), calcitonin
Adrenal cortex	Cortisol, aldosterone, androgens
Testes	Testosterone
Ovaries	Estradiol, progesterone
Pituitary gland	
Anterior lobe	Thyroid stimulating hormone (TSH), adrenocorticotropic hormone (ACTH), luteinizing hormone (LH), follicle stimulating hormone (FSH), growth hormone (GH), prolactin (PRL)
Posterior lobe	Vasopressin (VP) / antidiuretic hormone (ADH), oxytocin
Intermediate lobe cells	Melanocyte stimulating hormone
Hypothalamus	Thyroid releasing hormone (TRH), corticotropin releasing hormone (CRH), gonadotropin releasing hormone (GnRH), growth hormone releasing hormone (GHRH), somatostatin, dopamine
Glands not under direct control of the hypothalamic–pituitary axis	
Pancreas	Insulin, glucagon
Parathyroid glands	Parathyroid hormone (PTH)
Pineal gland	Melatonin
Adrenal medulla	Epinephrine (adrenaline), nor-epinephrine (nor-adrenaline)
Other organs with endocrine functions	
Heart and blood vessels	Atrial natriuretic peptide (ANP), endothelins, nitric oxide
Kidney	Erythropoietin (EPO), renin (enzyme) stimulating aldosterone production in adrenal cortex via activation of angiotensin, synthesis of the active form of vitamin D
Adipose tissue	Leptin, adiponectin, resistin, conversion of androgens to estrogens
Bone	Fibroblast growth factor 23, osteocalcin

straight chain molecules whilst others are folded or made up of two subunits created by disulfide bonds between two cysteine residues in the amino acid chain(s) (*Figure 1.2*).

1.3.2 Steroid hormones

The second major group of hormones are all derived from cholesterol and are called the steroid hormones (*Figure 1.2*). These hormones are generally released by the adrenal glands, testes and ovaries, although biologically active steroids may also

Table 1.2. Classification of the major human hormones by chemical structure

Hormones	Amino acid or fatty acid derived	Peptide/protein	Steroid
Hypothalamic hormones		Thyrotropin releasing hormone (TRH) Corticotropin releasing hormone (CRH) Gonadotropin releasing hormone (GnRH) Growth hormone releasing hormone (GHRH) Somatostatin Prolactin releasing factor (PRF) Dopamine Arginine vasopressin	
Anterior pituitary hormones		Thyroid stimulating hormone (TSH) Adrenocorticotropic hormone (ACTH) Luteinizing hormone (LH) Follicle stimulating hormone (FSH) Somatotropin/growth hormone (GH) Prolactin (PRL) Melanocyte stimulating hormone (MSH)	
Posterior pituitary hormones		Oxylocin Arginine vasopressin	
Thyroid hormones	Thyroxine (T_4) Triiodothyronine (T_3)	TSH	
Pancreatic hormones		Insulin Glucagon Somatostatin Pancreatic polypeptide	
Calcium regulating hormones		Parathyroid (PTH) Calcitonin (CT) Parathyroid hormone-related peptide (PTHrp)	1,25-dihydroxy vitamin D
Hormones of the adrenal cortex		Adrenocorticotropic hormone	Cortisol Androgens Aldosterone
Adrenal medullary hormones	Epinephrine Nor-epinephrine		
Male reproductive hormones		Luteinizing hormone (LH) Follicle stimulating hormone (FSH) Inhibin	Testosterone Dihydrotestosterone Estrogens
Female reproductive hormones		Follicle stimulating hormone (FSH) Luteinizing hormone (LH) Prolactin Inhibin Oxytocin Human chorionic gonadotropin (hCG) Human chorionic somatotropin	Estradiol Progesterone Androgens

Table 1.2. **Continued**

Hormones	Amino acid or fatty acid derived	Peptide/protein	Steroid
Cardiovascular hormones	Nitric oxide	Atrial natriuretic peptide (ANP) Endothelins	
Pineal hormones	Melatonin Serotonin		
Growth factors or cytokines		Insulin-like growth factors (IGFs) Epidermal growth factor (EGF) Interleukins (ILs) Tumor necrosis factor (TNF)-α	
Eicosanoids	Prostaglandins Thrombosane Prostacyclin Leukotrienes Lipoxins		

Note that this list is not intended to be comprehensive

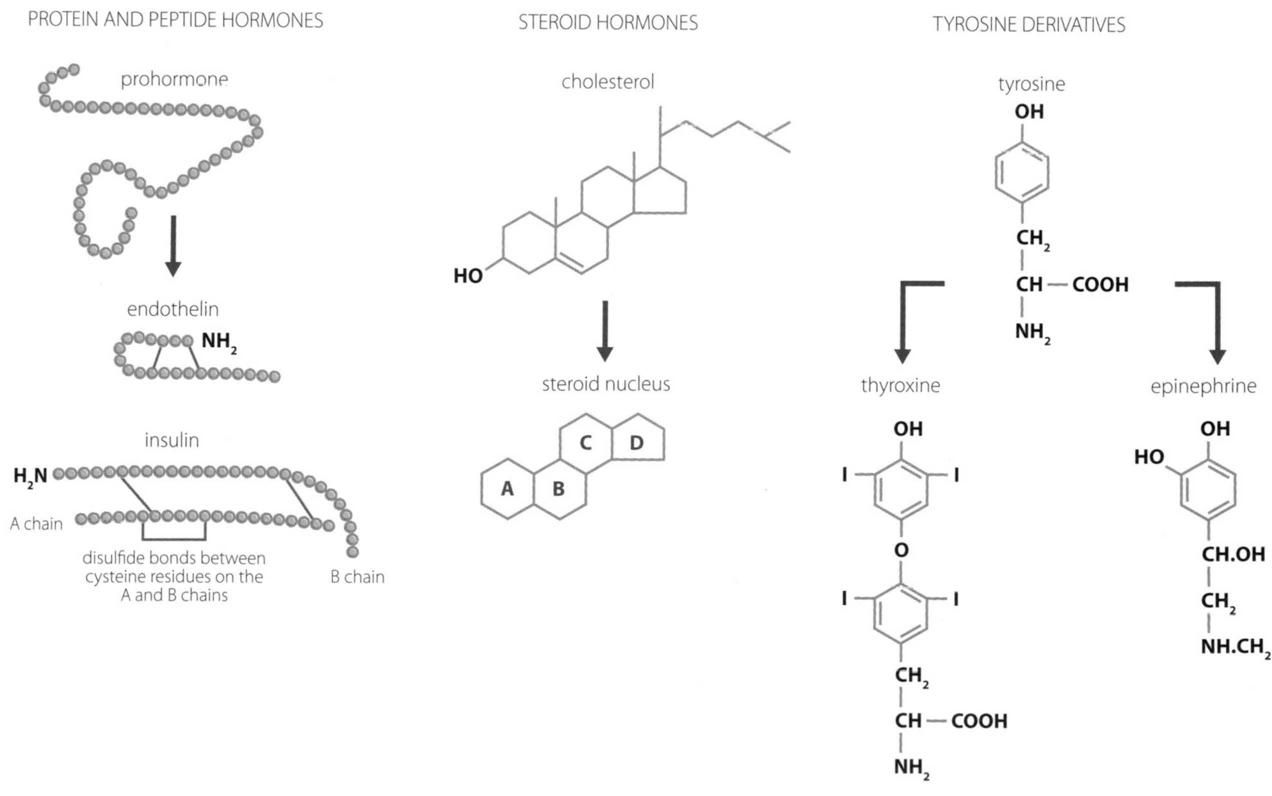

Figure 1.2. Chemical structure of hormones.
Other hormones include those derived from tryptophan (serotonin and melatonin) and those derived from fatty acids (eicosanoids).

be synthesized from circulating precursors by other tissues including the placenta, adipose tissue, brain, skin and liver. The active form of vitamin D (synthesized between skin, liver, and kidney) is also a steroid hormone.

1.3.3 Amino acid derived hormones

The catecholamines released by the adrenal medulla are made from a single amino acid, tyrosine, whilst melatonin secreted by the pineal gland is a single amino acid derived from tryptophan. Interestingly, the thyroid hormones are made up of two tyrosine molecules which become iodinated, but their transport, half-lives, and receptors are more similar to steroid hormones than to the catecholamines epinephrine (adrenaline) and nor-epinephrine (nor-adrenaline) (*Table 1.3*)

Table 1.3. **The differences in the circulating half-life, transport in the circulation and the type of receptors used according to the different chemical structures of hormones**

Hormone	Circulating half-life ($T_{1/2}$)	Transport in circulation	Receptors
Protein and peptide hormones	Minutes	Largely free, some bound to binding proteins	Cell surface receptors
Tyrosine derivatives			
Catecholamines	Seconds	Free in circulation	Cell surface receptors
Thyroid hormones	Hours	Bound to plasma proteins	Mainly nuclear receptors
Steroids; cholesterol derivatives	Hours/days	Bound to plasma proteins	Mainly nuclear receptors
Fatty acid derivatives	Minutes	Free in circulation	Cell surface receptors

Finally, there are hormones derived from fatty acids such as arachidonic acid and other small molecules such as nitric oxide derived from citrulline, but these tend to act locally in a paracrine function rather than being released into the general circulation.

1.4 Synthesis and secretion of hormones

1.4.1 Protein and peptide hormones

Protein and peptide hormones are encoded in genes and their synthesis requires:

- transcription of the gene
- post-transcriptional modifications
- translation
- post-translational modifications prior to secretion.

The genetic code of the gene is determined by the sequence of nucleotides, each of which consists of a 5 carbon sugar (deoxyribose) attached to one of four organic bases: adenine (A), guanine (G), thymidine (T), or cytidine (C). The purine bases, A and G, can form complementary pairs with the pyrimidine bases T and C, respectively, and this allows formation of the double-stranded, helical formation of DNA. The DNA in each chromosome is organized into nucleosomes which comprise about 180 double-stranded nucleotides curled around eight histone proteins; each nucleosome is linked by stretches of about 30 nucleotides. Further coiling of the nucleosomes to a higher order forms the chromosomes.

Transcription occurs when a transcription factor binds to a promoter region of the DNA. This then attracts a complex of co-regulatory proteins which will open up the coiled DNA by acetylation of the histone proteins. Downstream (in the 3′ direction) from the promoter region is the 'start site' for the synthesis of ribonucleic acid (RNA) which contains sequences that bind transcription complexes and RNA polymerase II. The RNA polymerase moves along the single strand of DNA and assembles an RNA transcript with a sequence of the nucleotides and bases which is complementary to the DNA. The RNA differs in structure from DNA: it has ribose instead of deoxyribose as its sugar and uridine instead of thymidine as one of its pyrimidine bases.

The transcribed strand of the RNA is called precursor messenger RNA and it contains both coding sequences (exons) and non-coding sequences (introns). Prior to their transport to the ribosomes on the rough endoplasmic reticulum, the introns are excised and the remaining exons are spliced together to form mature messenger RNA (mRNA) (see *Figure 1.3*). In some cases alternate splicing of the exons will produce different mRNAs that code for different proteins and so one or more protein hormones can be produced from a single gene.

Once exported from the nucleus a ribosome attaches to the mRNA (at the 5′ end) and moves along the mRNA until it encounters the AUG start codon. The

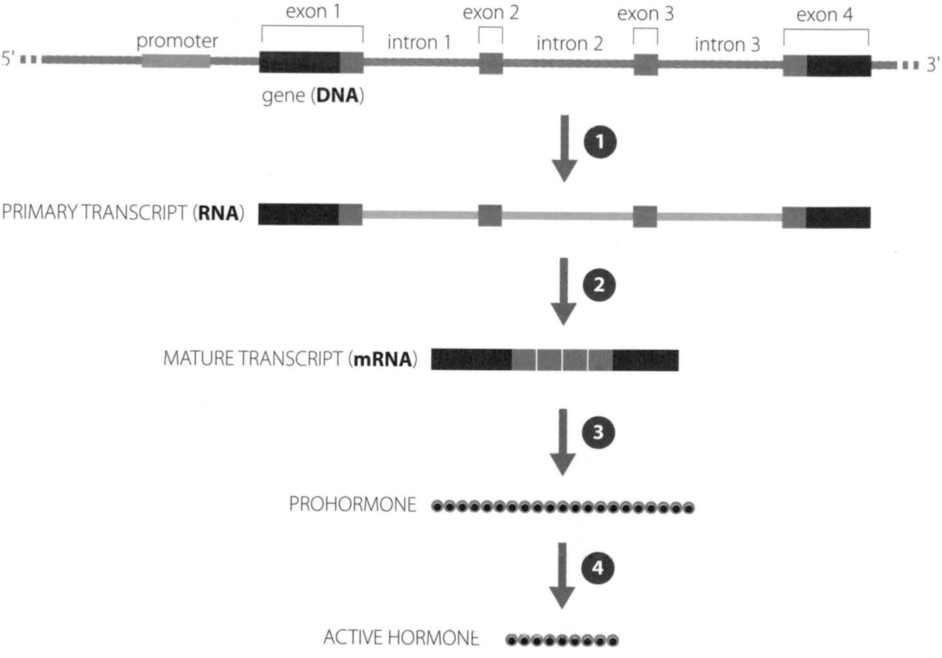

Figure 1.3. Synthesis of protein and peptide hormones.

[1] Transcription of the DNA sequence into RNA.

[2] Excision of sequences (introns) from the initial DNA transcript (splicing) and modifications of the 3′ and 5′ terminals.

[3] Translation of the mRNA into a large precursor protein, the prohormone.

[4] The prohormone is cleaved into fragments and this process, known as post-translational processing, occurs prior to secretion, mainly within the Golgi apparatus (see *Figure 1.4*).

ribosome slides along the mRNA, adding the appropriate amino acid to the growing polypeptide chain according to the codons of the mRNA. The amino acids are brought to the ribosome by small strands of transfer RNA (tRNA) which contain the complementary anti-codons to the codons on the mRNA (adenine binds to uridine and guanine to cytosine), and which are also charged with an amino acid. Ribosomal enzymes release the amino acid to be added to the growing chain of amino acids and the empty tRNA is shed. The cycle is repeated with elongation of the chain of amino acids until the ribosome reaches a stop codon, at which point the translation of the mRNA is complete. The ribosome falls off the mRNA and disassociates into its two subunits and the polypeptide is released.

Peptide and protein hormones need to be secreted from secretory granules so they must be synthesized within an intracellular membrane structure of the cell rather than being released from the ribosomes directly into the cytoplasm. Proteins destined for secretion therefore have a hydrophobic sequence of about 12–30 amino

(a)

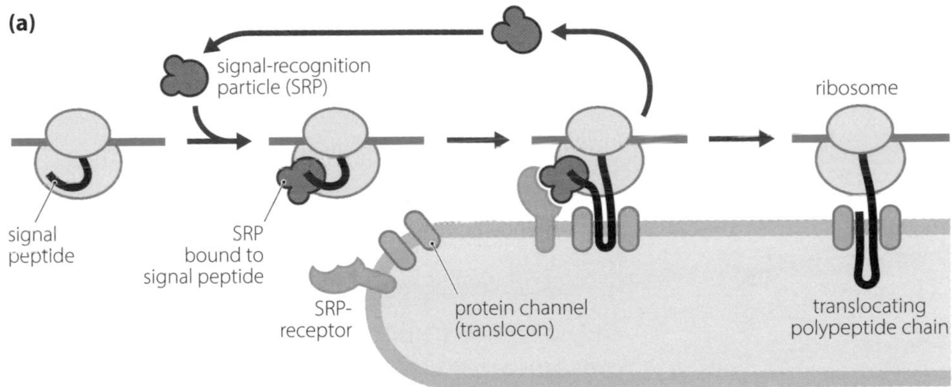

(b)

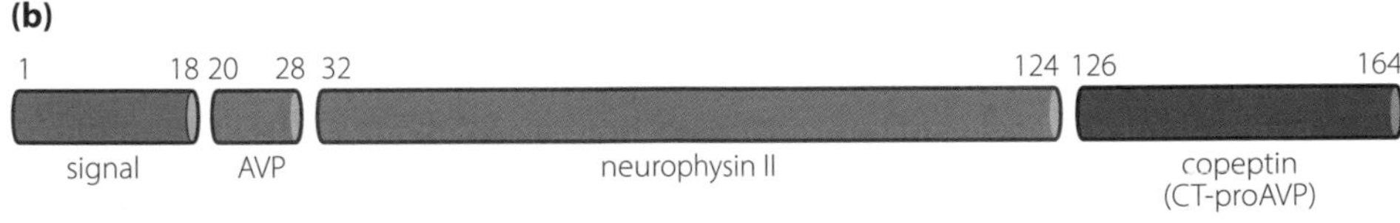

Figure 1.4. Synthesis of protein and peptide hormones within the endoplasmic reticulum and the process of post-translational modification.
(a) The initial amino acid sequence to be translated on the ribosome is the signal sequence that emerges from the ribosome and binds to a signal recognition particle (SRP). The SRP–ribosome complex then docks with the SRP receptor and protein channel (translocon). The SRP dissociates from the receptor and the polypeptide chain is translocated through the channel and into the lumen of the endoplasmic reticulum. As further synthesis of the growing polypeptide chain occurs, the polypeptide is directed through the translocon and into the lumen of the endoplasmic reticulum. The entire transcript of the mRNA is known as a pre-prohormone, but the signal sequence is usually cleaved off before the end of transcription. Newly synthesized polypeptide prohormones exit the endoplasmic reticulum in vesicles and then fuse with the Golgi apparatus; it is here that the large prohormone is cleaved into smaller peptides and biologically inactive fragments. The Golgi apparatus forms secretory granules in which the polypeptide hormones are stored and then secreted in response to a stimulus.
(b) The post-translational processing of arginine vasopressin (AVP) as an example. As described above, the whole mRNA transcript is known as a pre-prohormone. The signal sequence is cleaved off the pre-prohormone in the rough endoplasmic reticulum and the remaining 20–164 amino acid sequence, known as a prohormone, is further cleaved in the Golgi apparatus. Both the biologically active AVP and the other fragments (neurophysin II and copeptin) are packaged into secretory granules.

acids at their N-terminal ends. This is known as a signal sequence and is recognized by a signal recognition particle which then threads itself into the membrane of the endoplasmic reticulum. The signal sequence is internalized into the endoplasmic membrane and elongation of the amino acid chain continues within the endoplasmic reticulum. The signal sequence is usually cleaved off well before the entire protein has been synthesized (*Figure 1.4*).

The synthesis of protein and peptide hormones is somewhat wasteful in that large prohormones are made initially and these must be cleaved to form the active hormone prior to secretion. In the endoplasmic reticulum the prohormone may undergo disulfide bonding and in some cases glycosylation (addition of carbohydrate side chains). The partially processed protein is then entrapped in vesicles that bud off from the endoplasmic reticulum. These vesicles then fuse with the Golgi apparatus where further processing may take place. Finally the hormones, along with various enzymes, are packaged into immature secretory granules which bud off from the Golgi stacks. In these granules prohormones are then cleaved to leave the active hormone along with other biologically inactive fragments of the protein chain. Cleavage of prohormones can yield more than one biologically active fragment depending on the enzymes (hormone convertases) present in a particular gland, for example, the prohormone pro-opiomelanocortin and the prohormone of glucagon (see *Chapters 5* and *6*).

Protein and peptide hormones are stored deep in the cytoplasm of cells within their mature secretory granules, as are epinephrine and nor-epinephrine. In preparation for secretion a pool of readily releasable secretory granules exists which dock onto the cell membrane through partnering SNARE proteins on the vesicles (vSNARES) and on the cell membrane (target or tSNARES). In response to a stimulus and a consequent rise in intracellular calcium, there is a conformational change in the SNARE proteins such that fusion of the secretory granule membrane and cell membrane occurs and the contents of the granule are released.

1.4.2 Steroid hormones

The synthesis of steroid hormones does not require transcription of a gene, although this is required for the synthesis of steroidogenic enzymes, such as several specific cytochrome P_{450} enzymes (officially abbreviated to CYPs), hydroxysteroid dehydrogenases (HSDs) and steroid reductases.

There are four major families of lipid soluble steroid hormones: corticoids, progestins, androgens, and estrogens, which contain 21, 21, 19, and 18 carbon atoms respectively, hence the term C21, C19, C18 steroid. The precursor for all steroid hormones is cholesterol which is taken up into steroid-producing cells by low density lipoprotein receptors. The cholesterol can either be used directly for steroid synthesis or can be stored in lipid droplets and used subsequently after hydrolysis of the droplet (*Figure 1.5*).

Steroid hormone synthesis occurs by shuttling of steroid precursors between the mitochondria and smooth endoplasmic reticulum, with the first stage beginning in the mitochondria. Free intracellular cholesterol is transported from the outer to the inner mitochondrial membrane by a protein, steroidogenic acute regulatory protein (StAR). Within the mitochondria the cholesterol side chain cleavage enzyme, CYP11A (P_{450}scc), found in all steroidogenic tissues, snips off the side chain of C27

(a)

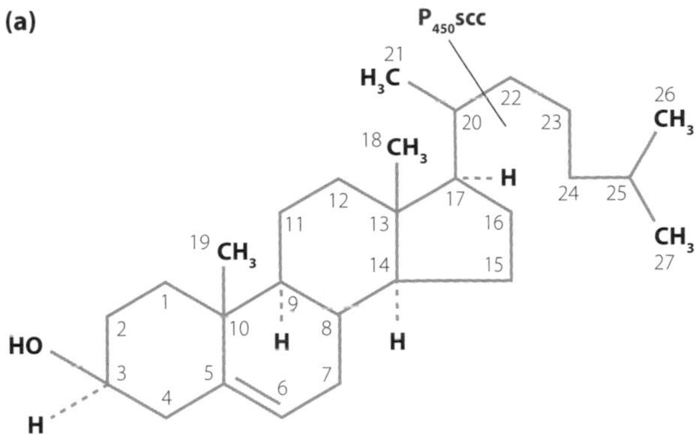

(b)

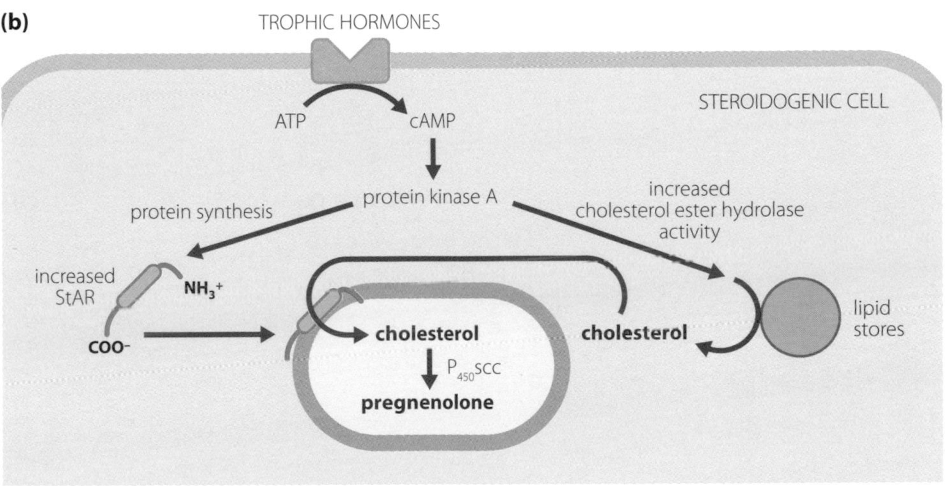

Figure 1.5. Control of steroid synthesis from cholesterol.

(a) The structure of cholesterol showing the numbering of carbon atoms and the site at which the cholesterol side chain cleavage enzyme (P_{450}scc) breaks off the side chain leaving a C21 steroid, pregnenolone. This is the first stage in the synthesis of all steroid hormones and occurs in the mitochondria.

(b) In response to a trophic hormone (e.g. ACTH, LH, FSH) cAMP is generated by the activation of adenyl cyclase which in turn activates protein kinase A. This stimulates the synthesis of StAR protein which transports cholesterol from the outer to the inner side of the mitochondrial membrane and helps to release stored cholesterol from lipid droplets. The production of StAR protein and the conversion of cholesterol to pregnenolone are the rate limiting steps in steroid synthesis.

cholesterol to form C21 pregnenolone (*Figure 1.5*). Pregnenolone is then converted to progesterone by 3β-hydroxysteroid dehydrogenase (3β-HSD), an enzyme that is found in both mitochondria and smooth endoplasmic reticulum. There are two isoenzymes of 3β-HSD:

- type 1 which is found in placenta and non steroidogenic tissues such as liver, kidney, and skin
- type 2 which is found in the classical steroidogenic glands, the adrenals, testes, and ovaries.

Pregnenolone and progesterone and the 17α-hydroxy derivatives form the precursors for all other steroid hormones (*Figure 1.6*).

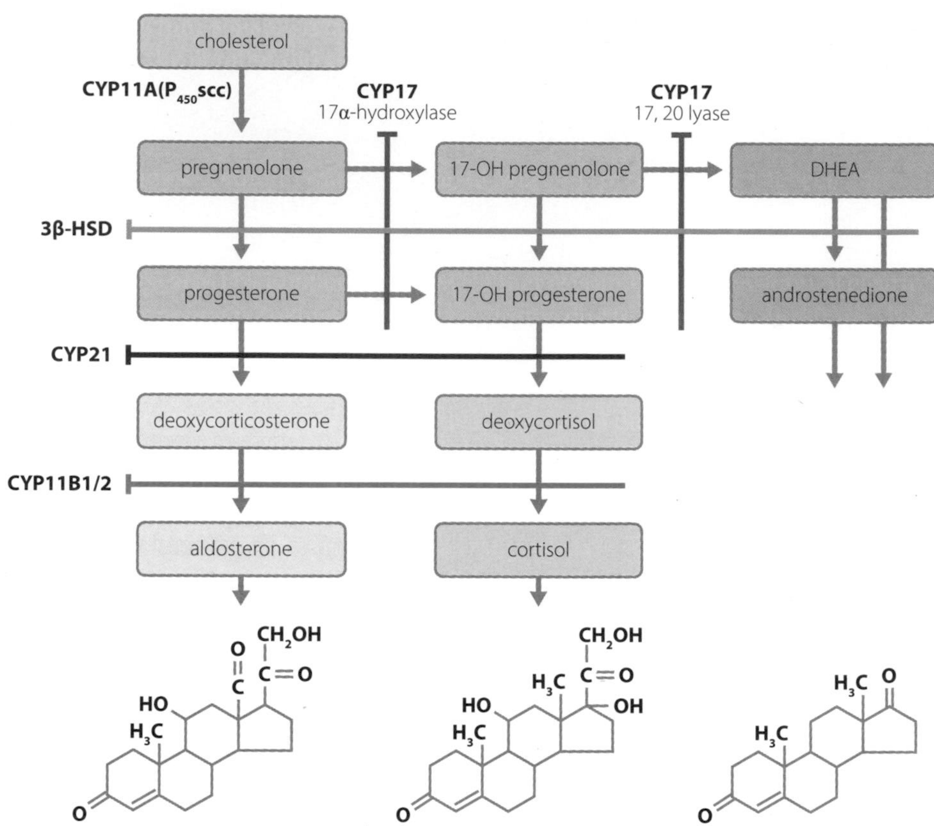

Figure 1.6. Outline of steroid hormone synthesis in the adrenal cortex.

In the adrenal glands adrenocorticotropic hormone (ACTH) controls the production of cortisol, via the cAMP-mediated protein kinase A pathway (*Figure 1.5*), whilst angiotensin and potassium selectively increase the synthesis of aldosterone. CYP21 (21-hydroxylase), which is present in the smooth endoplasmic reticulum and specific to the adrenal cortex, is responsible for the conversion of progesterone to 11-deoxycorticosterone (the aldosterone pathway) and of 17α-hydroxyprogesterone to 11-deoxycortisol (the cortisol pathway). Subsequently, 11-deoxycorticosterone is converted to aldosterone by CYP11B2 and 11-deoxycortisol converted to cortisol by CYP11B1. The weak androgens produced by the adrenal cortex, androstenedione and dehydroepiandrostenedione (DHEA), are formed by CYP17 which has both 17α-hydroxylase activity and 17,20 lyase activity. CYP17 is also found in the ovary and testis where it is essential for directing the synthesis of steroid hormone precursors towards the sex hormones, the androgens and estrogens. In the testis the weak androstenedione is converted to testosterone by 17β-hydroxysteroid dehydrogenase (17β-HSD), whilst in the ovary an additional enzyme, aromatase, is required to convert androgens to estrogens and these activities are controlled by the gonadotropins, luteinizing hormone (LH), and follicle stimulating hormone (FSH) (see *Chapter 7*). The synthesis of thyroid hormones, which is controlled by thyroid stimulating hormone (TSH) is outlined in *Chapter 3*.

Unlike protein and peptide hormones, once steroid hormones are synthesized they are released into the circulation and become bound to a plasma protein. This may be specific to the particular hormone or may be a general plasma protein such as albumin. Either way, more than 95% of circulating steroids are usually bound

Box 1.1 | Transport of steroid and thyroid hormones

An equilibrium exists between bound and free hormone.

$$H + BG \rightleftharpoons H.BG$$

$$K_{eq} = \frac{[H.BG]}{[H][BG]} \quad \frac{(H\ bound)}{(H\ free)}$$

$$[H] = [H.BG] \times \frac{1}{K_{eq}\,[BG]}$$

- Generally speaking over 95% of circulating steroid and thyroid hormones (H) are bound to their specific binding globulins (BG) and a smaller fraction to albumin.
- An equilibrium exists such that the equilibrium constant (K_{eq}) – a measure of affinity – is equal to the ratio of the bound hormone complex to the product of the free hormone and concentration of binding globulins.
- Only the free hormone can activate receptors, but binding of hormones to plasma proteins provides a reservoir of circulating hormones and delays their metabolism.
- Changes in the concentration of binding proteins alters total hormone concentration and free hormone concentration; it is more clinically relevant to measure free (i.e. active) hormone concentrations than total hormone concentrations (which is a measure of both bound and free hormone).

to plasma proteins, as are thyroid hormones, and this delays their metabolism and excretion and provides a source of circulating steroid hormones. The steroid hormones are inactive in the bound state but are able to interact with target specific receptors in their free state. When the concentration of free (unbound) circulating hormones becomes reduced through use, bound hormones are released into the free state because there is an equilibrium between bound and free hormones (*Box 1.1*).

1.4.3 Endocrine disorders related to aberrant hormone synthesis

There are rare endocrine disorders which are caused by mutations of genes coding for protein and peptide hormones, so that either a biologically inactive hormone is synthesized or the mutation results in defective post-translational processing of the pre-prohormone. In either case such mutations manifest pathophysiologically as a hormone deficiency. For example, mutations in the gene coding for the beta subunit of TSH cause hypothyroidism, whilst mutations in the gene coding for the beta subunit of FSH cause hypogonadism and infertility in both males and females. Mutations in the gene coding for insulin result in type 1 diabetes and that of parathyroid hormone in hypoparathyroidism and low blood calcium levels. There are numerous other examples and for all, knowing the function of the hormone, allows the outcome to be predicted.

Disordered steroid synthesis can result from mutations in the genes which encode enzymes of the steroidogenic pathways. Perhaps the best example is a mutation in the *CYP21* gene, which normally encodes CYP21 (the 21-hydroxylase enzyme) which is so important in the synthesis of aldosterone and cortisol (*Figure 1.6*). As a result of the mutation, CYP21 synthesis and activity is reduced or absent and the progesterone precursors of these pathways are shunted into the synthesis of androgens, resulting in excess androgen secretion. This is known as congenital adrenal hyperplasia (CAH) and causes loss of aldosterone and cortisol secretion, raised levels of ACTH (as a result of loss of negative feedback of cortisol) and masculinization of female fetuses (see *Chapter 6*). Rare cases of mutations in the gene encoding 3β-HSD have also been reported, resulting in a loss of all adrenal steroids including androgens. A further example is a mutation in the *CYP19* gene encoding aromatase, which normally catalyzes the conversion of androgens to estrogens. In females, reduced levels of aromatase can have profound effects causing virilization, pubertal failure, and cystic ovaries due to high levels of LH and FSH (a result of loss of negative feedback of estradiol). In males loss of aromatase leads to continual longitudinal growth because estrogens are important for epiphyseal closure. Many other mutations have been reported and, of course, the severity of steroid loss will depend on where in the synthetic pathway the mutation has occurred; thus a mutation in the gene for P_{450}scc, for example, leads to depletion of all steroid hormones.

1.5 How do hormones deliver their messages to target cells?

1.5.1 Protein and peptide hormones

Protein and peptide hormones, which are water soluble, cannot cross the phospholipid cell membrane. Thus their receptors in target cells are on the cell

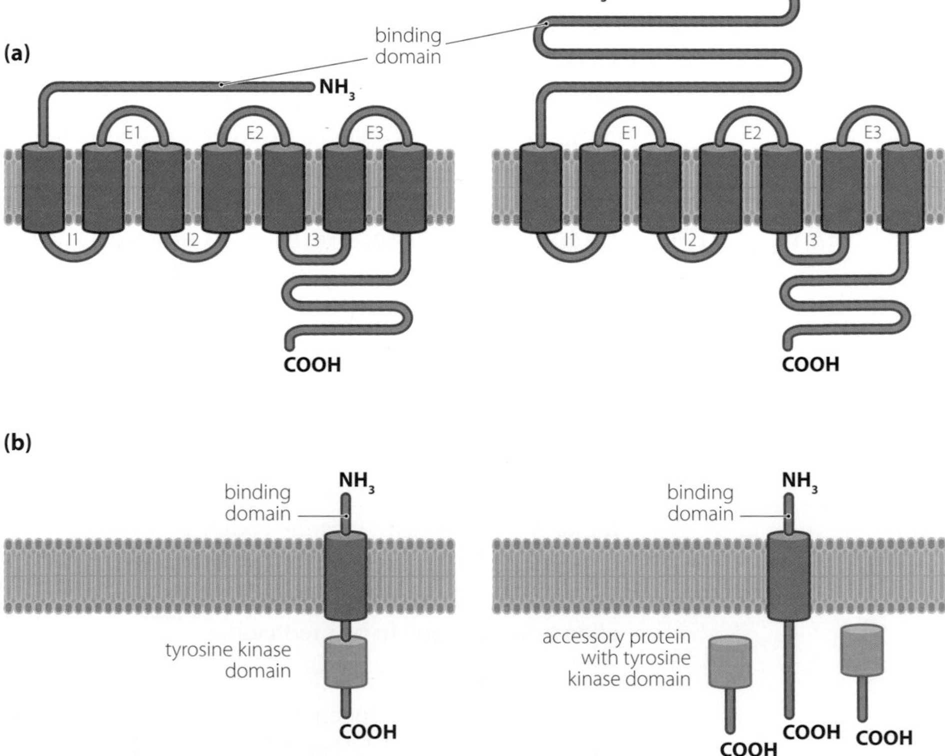

Figure 1.7. Cell surface receptors for protein and peptide hormones.
(a) The majority of protein and peptide hormones act via G-protein linked receptors which may have a short or long extracellular N-terminal domain. E1–3, extracellular loops; I1–3, intracellular loops.
(b) Some hormones such as growth factors and insulin act on receptors that have a tyrosine kinase domain in the intracellular portion of the receptor which is activated upon binding of the hormone. Other hormones, such as prolactin, growth hormone and cytokines act on receptors that are associated with a protein that has tyrosine kinase activity, such as the JAK/STAT signaling pathway (see *Figure 1.8e*).

membrane and have an extracellular domain which will recognize the hormone, a trans-membrane domain, and an intracellular domain that will transmit a signal stimulated by the hormone binding to the extracellular domain.

Many hormones act via G-protein coupled receptors (GPCRs). These have an extracellular N-terminal (NH_2) domain, a trans-membrane domain which contains 7-helical regions of amino acids with three external (E) and three internal (I) loops, and an intracellular carboxy-terminal (COOH) domain (*Figure 1.7*). Linked to this protein receptor is a G protein made up of three subunits, α, β, and γ. Once a hormone binds to the extracellular NH_2 terminal of the receptor, this activates the receptor which then activates the associated G protein by causing it to change conformation. The result of the conformation change is that the guanosine diphosphate bound to the α subunit is replaced by guanosine triphosphate, the α subunit disassociates from the β and γ subunits and activates an enzyme such as adenyl cyclase or phospholipase C in the cell membrane (*Figure 1.8a and b*). These enzymes then activate the production of a second messenger such as cAMP or the phosphoinositol signaling pathway. The subsequent generation of activated (phosphorylated) kinases may then phosphorylate and activate intracellular proteins (e.g. enzymes) or they may be translocated to the nucleus where they activate transcription factors and thus control gene activity.

The second group of receptors that are important in hormone signaling are the receptors that have inherent tyrosine kinase activity or are associated with proteins that have tyrosine kinase activity; some of the signaling pathways used by hormones which bind to these receptors are outlined in *Figure 1.8c–e*. In each of these cases, hormone binding to the receptor induces activation (phosphorylation) of tyrosine kinase which is either in the receptor itself or in an associated protein. Activation of these kinases then leads on to the phosphorylation of further kinases which, like GPCRs, activate intracellular proteins or gene transcription. The point to note is that intracellular signaling from receptor activation (hormone binding) to the cellular response is highly complex and involves a cascade of kinase phosphorylations and intermediary proteins, such as Ras proteins, Grb and SOS, which are important in signal transduction. To add to the complexity, there is convergence and divergence of different pathways such that one signaling pathway can modulate the activity of another one (*Figure 1.9*).

1.5.2 Endocrine disorders associated with mutations in cell surface receptors

The human genome may encode as many as 2000 different GPCRs and their importance in human physiology is reflected in the fact that over one-third of all prescription drugs bind to this sort of receptor. With respect to the endocrine system, a number of disorders have been linked to mutations either in the receptor itself or to mutations in the associated G protein. These mutations may either be inherited (familial) or arise spontaneously in a particular cell, in which case they are known as somatic mutations. These somatic mutations are the primary cause of human cancer. Either way such mutations may cause loss of function of either the receptor or the G protein and thus a hormone will be unable to activate a specific target cell. Other mutations may be activating mutations in which the receptor or G protein is constitutively active irrespective of hormone binding; this is described as a 'gain of function.'

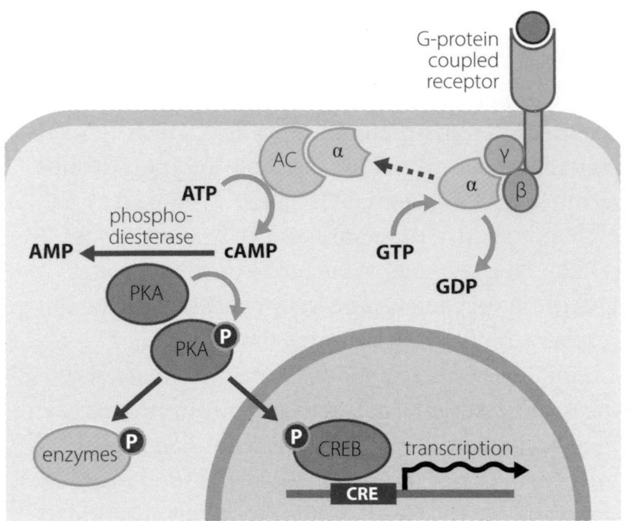
(a) Adenyl cyclase and cAMP signaling pathway
G-protein
coupled
receptor
AC
α
γ
α
β
ATP
phospho-
diesterase
AMP
cAMP
GTP
GDP
PKA
PKA
P
enzymes
P
P
CREB
transcription
CRE

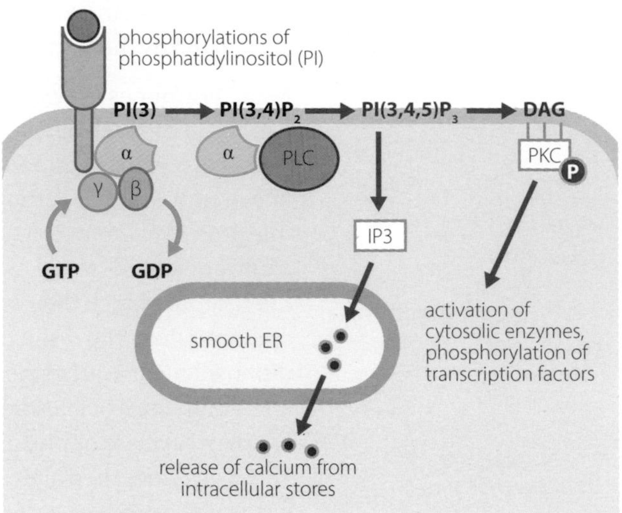
(b) Phosphoinositide signaling pathway
phosphorylations of
phosphatidylinositol (PI)
PI(3)
PI(3,4)P2
PI(3,4,5)P3
DAG
α
α
PLC
PKC
P
γ
β
GTP
GDP
IP3
smooth ER
activation of
cytosolic enzymes,
phosphorylation of
transcription factors
release of calcium from
intracellular stores

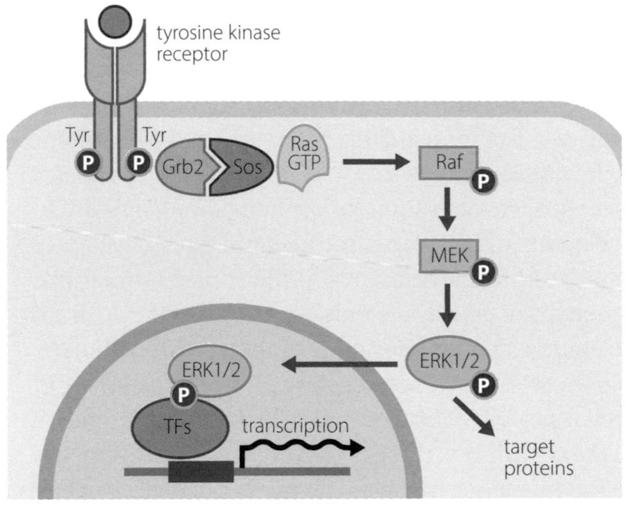
(c) Raf/MEK/ERK1/2 signaling pathway
tyrosine kinase
receptor
Tyr
Tyr
P
P
Grb2
Sos
Ras
GTP
Raf
P
MEK
P
ERK1/2
P
ERK1/2
P
TFs
transcription
target
proteins

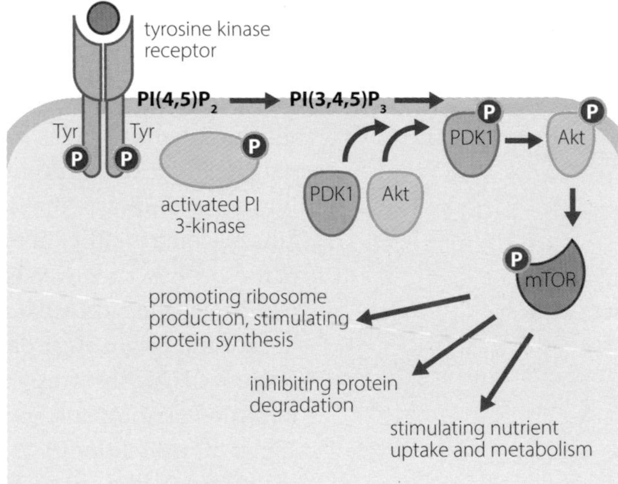
(d) Phosphatidylinositol kinase/AKT signaling pathway
tyrosine kinase
receptor
PI(4,5)P2
PI(3,4,5)P3
Tyr
Tyr
P
P
P
activated PI
3-kinase
PDK1
Akt
PDK1
Akt
P
P
P
mTOR
promoting ribosome
production, stimulating
protein synthesis
inhibiting protein
degradation
stimulating nutrient
uptake and metabolism

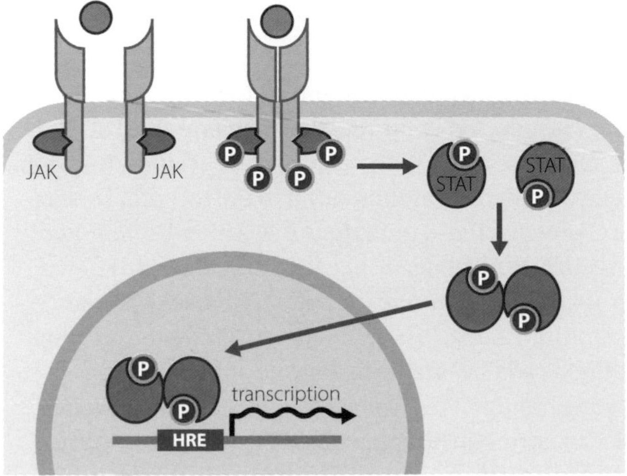
(e) JAK/STAT signaling pathway
JAK
JAK
P
P
P
P
P
STAT
STAT
P
P
P
P
P
transcription
HRE

Figure 1.8. Cell signaling pathways for protein and peptide hormones.
(a) Adenyl cyclase and cAMP signaling pathway. Binding of a hormone to its receptor activates the trimeric G protein with the release of the α subunit and activation of adenyl cyclase (AC), formation of cAMP and activation (phosphorylation) of protein kinase A (PKA). The PKA may activate cytoplasmic enzymes or enter the nucleus and activate transcription factors such as CREB (cAMP response element binding protein) which will bind to the cAMP response element (CRE) on DNA and initiate transcription.
(b) Phosphoinositide signaling pathway. A hormone activates a G protein which is coupled to phospholipase C (PLC). This initiates a series of phosphorylations of phosphoinositide (PI) resulting in the formation of inositol triphosphate (IP3) and activation of diacyl glycerol (DAG). IP3 raises intracellular calcium concentrations by releasing it from the smooth endoplasmic reticulum whilst DAG activates (phosphorylates) protein kinase C, which has similar effects to PKA (see above).
(c) The Raf/MEK/ERK1/2 signaling pathway. Hormones such as growth factors bind to receptors and, after their dimerization, the tyrosine kinase on the receptor is activated (phosphorylated). This initiates a series of phosphorylations on downstream kinases which may activate target proteins (enzymes) or transcription factors (TFs) in the nucleus. Raf, MEK, and ERK1/2 (extracellular regulated kinase) are all serine/threonine-selective protein kinases and are also known as mitogen-activated protein (MAP) kinases (K). Ras is a small monomeric G protein. Grb2 and Sos are adapter molecules in cell signaling.
(d) The phosphatidylinositol kinase/AKT signaling pathway. The phosphatidylinositol 3-kinases (PI3-kinases) are a family of enzymes involved in a wide range of cellular functions. They are activated by hormone binding to the receptor; PI 3 kinases phosphorylate phosphoinositides (PIs) – phosphatidylinositol 4,5-bisphosphate (PI(4,5)P2) and inositol (3,4,5) triphosphate (PI(3,4,5)P3) – which then activate Akt (also known as protein kinase B). One target of activated Akt is mTOR (mammalian target of rapamycin) which can have a variety of cellular actions as indicated. PI3-kinases may also be activated by GPCRs.
(e) The JAK/STAT signaling pathway. Growth hormone, prolactin, and cytokines act via the JAK (janus kinases)/STAT (signal transducers and activators of transcription) signaling pathway. JAK is a protein associated with a receptor and is activated (phosphorylated) upon hormone binding. The activated JAK phosphorylates STAT which will then move into the nucleus and activate transcription.

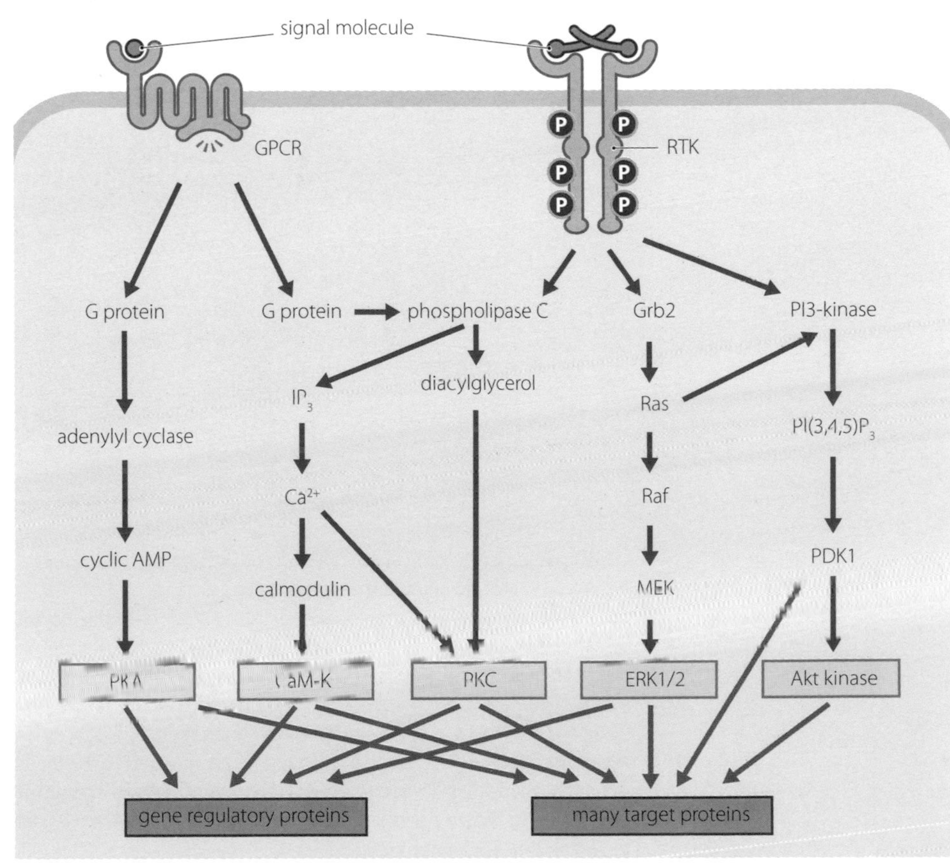

Figure 1.9. Convergence and divergence of cell signaling pathways.
This diagram illustrates how many cell signaling pathways can 'cross talk' with each other. Cell signaling is not a simple matter and this is how G-protein coupled hormone receptors (GPCRs) activate cell signaling pathways that can interact with those activated by the classical growth hormone tyrosine kinase receptors (RTK) via some of the pathways outlined in *Figure 1.8.*

Examples of endocrine disorders resulting from defective G-protein coupled receptors include:

- familial male precocious puberty resulting from an activating mutation in the LH receptor and thus uncontrolled secretion of testosterone, leading to testotoxicosis and early sexual development
- hyperthyroidism (thyroid adenoma) caused by a somatic activating mutation of the TSH receptor
- loss of function mutations in the FSH receptor causing hypergonadotropic hypogonadism and infertility.

Examples of endocrine disorders resulting from a defective G protein include:

- pseudohypoparathyroidism caused by loss of function of the parathyroid hormone receptor, resulting in hypocalcemia

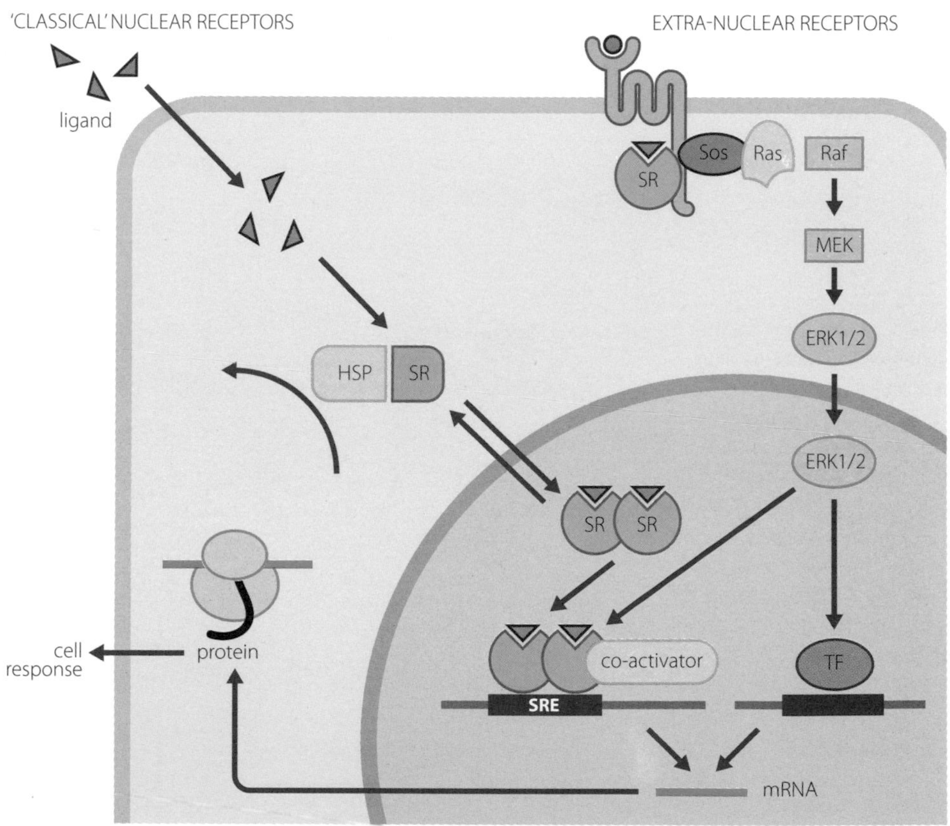

Figure 1.10. Steroid signaling at target cells.
Steroids are lipophilic and readily enter cells. Target cells have specialized steroid receptors (SRs) either in the cytoplasm or in the nucleus attached to DNA. Receptors in the cytoplasm are bound to heat shock proteins (HSP), and when a steroid binds to the receptor the HSP is released, two receptors dimerize and are then translocated to the nucleus where they bind to the steroid response element (SRE) on the DNA and initiate (or inhibit) transcription. It is now evident that steroids may also have receptors that are so-called 'extra-nuclear' as opposed to the classical 'nuclear receptors'. When activated by steroids, these extra-nuclear receptors may interact with other cell signaling pathways as outlined in *Figure 1.9* and these pathways may activate (phosphorylate) a transcription factor (TF) including a steroid receptor.

- McCune–Albright syndrome caused by an activating mutation resulting in autonomous endocrine function, and producing precocious puberty.

Inactivating mutations in genes coding for the tyrosine kinase group of receptors have also been reported and examples include mutations in the insulin receptor causing severe insulin resistance and in the GH receptor causing growth retardation. Constitutively active tyrosine kinase activity is associated with aberrant growth of cells and the development of certain tumors.

1.5.3 Steroid and thyroid hormones

Steroid hormones are lipophilic and readily cross cell membranes. They are thus capable of entering every cell in the body but they are only 'captured' by cells that contain specific receptors for a particular steroid hormone. These receptors are typically located intracellularly (not on the cell membrane) and either reside in the cytoplasm of the target cell attached to heat shock proteins, or in the nucleus attached to DNA (*Figure 1.10*). Binding of steroids to their receptors leads to dimerization of two receptors and, in the case of cytoplasmic receptors, release of heat shock proteins and translocation to the nucleus. Dimerized receptors then bind to the hormone response element (HRE) on DNA and initiate or inhibit gene transcription.

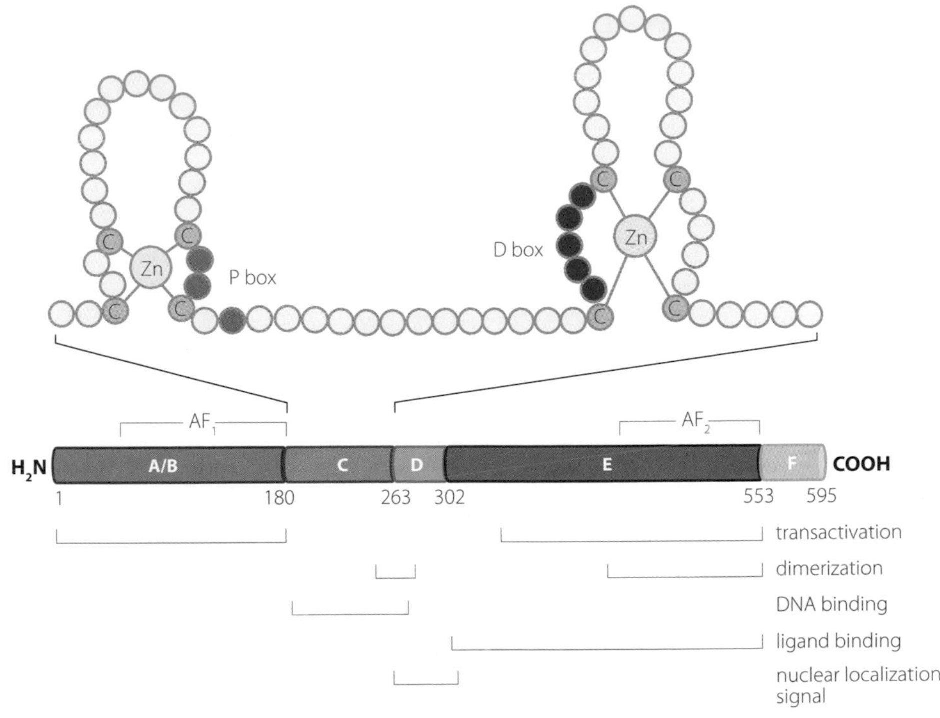

Figure 1.11. Basic structure of steroid receptors.
Steroid hormone receptors are transcription factors made up of distinct domains (A–F) with each domain having a different function. The C domain (enlarged) is highly conserved throughout all steroid hormone receptors and possesses two zinc fingers that slot into the double helix of the DNA. The P box of the C domain recognizes the nucleotide bases in the DNA and the D box is important for the dimerization and contact with the DNA phosphate backbone. The E domain is the ligand-binding domain and also the region where two receptors dimerize prior to DNA binding. The two activating function (AF) regions indicate the areas of the steroid receptor which attract co-regulators of gene transcription once the steroid receptor is activated.

Steroid hormone receptors belong to a large family of transcription factors and are typically made up of several domains (*Figure 1.11*). The N-terminal domains are denoted A/B and they have amino acid sequences that will attract large complexes of other proteins (co-regulators of gene transcription) upon steroid binding; such regions are known as activating factor (AF)-1. The C domain is the DNA-binding domain of the receptor which contains two zinc fingers that can slot into the helical structure of DNA. The D domain is the hinge region which alters the shape of the receptor upon hormone binding. The carboxy-terminal domain, E/F, is the region of the receptor to which the hormone binds. This domain also contains sequences of amino acids that can attract complexes of co-regulatory proteins, the AF-2 region (*Figure 1.11*).

One important action of co-regulatory proteins that attach to activated steroid hormone receptors is to open up or close the double helical structure of DNA that is wound round histone proteins. Thus the co-regulatory proteins attached to the activated steroid receptor will either have histone acetylation activity to open up the DNA and stimulate transcription, or histone deacetylation activity which will result in a closed DNA formation and inhibit further gene transcription. In addition, the co-regulatory proteins that control gene transcription will attract transcription complexes downstream of the bound steroid hormone receptors. This transcription machinery contains RNA polymerase that allows transcription of a single strand of DNA into complimentary RNA (*Figure 1.12*).

The classic way in which activated steroid receptors alter gene expression is through direct binding to a hormone response element on the DNA. It is now known,

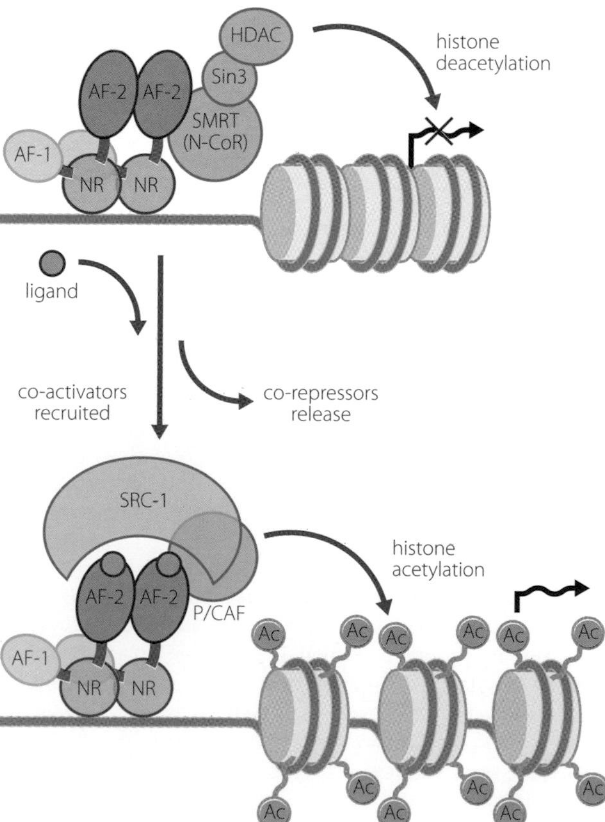

Figure 1.12. Activation of transcription by steroid hormones.
When there is no hormone binding the nuclear receptor (NR) is bound to complexes (called co-repressors, e.g. SMRT, Sin3) which have histone deacetylase activity and the chromatin remains closed. Upon binding of the ligand, the co-repressors are released and the AF-1 and AF-2 regions of the receptor attract co-activators (e.g. SRC-1) which have histone acetylation activity; this activity opens up the chromatin and allows transcription to occur.

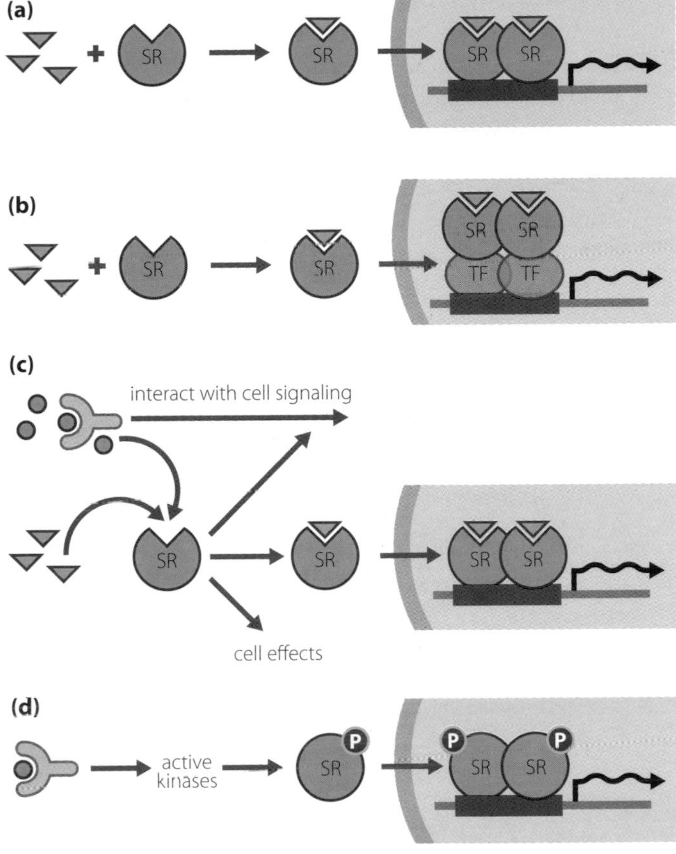

Figure 1.13. Different ways in which steroid receptors may be activated.
(a) Direct activation. Hormone binding activates the steroid receptor (SR) and initiates transcription.
(b) Tethered activation. Activated SRs may bind to transcription factors (TF) and initiate transcription.
(c) Non-genomic activation. Membrane-associated SRs may be activated by other signaling molecules, or vice versa, and induce gene transcription or other cellular effects.
(d) Growth factor activation. Growth factor (GF) signaling pathways may activate (phosphorylate) SRs.

however, that steroid hormone receptors may exert their effects in numerous other ways (*Figure 1.13*). Activated steroid receptors may not directly bind to DNA but may become tethered to and activate other transcription factors in the nucleus. Most steroid hormones also have rapid non-genomic effects on target cells and these are mediated by cell surface receptors, membrane-associated receptors or receptors in the cytoplasm. These receptors, when activated by steroid hormones, interact with various cell signaling pathways or may enter the nucleus and either bind a response element on the DNA or activate (phosphorylate) other transcription factors (tethered signaling). Finally, steroid receptors may be activated through a ligand-independent pathway in which the receptor becomes activated by a cell signaling kinase. Thus there is scope for considerable cross-talk between steroid receptor action and activation of cell signaling pathways by activated membrane receptors.

1.6 Hormone binding, receptor regulation, and disease

Interaction between hormones and their receptors depends on the number of receptors, the concentration of circulating hormone and the affinity of the hormone for the receptor. The latter is defined as the concentration of a hormone at which half the total number of receptors is occupied. The higher the affinity of a receptor, the lower the concentration of hormone required. Generally speaking, the affinity of a hormone receptor does not change and thus the biological response depends on the number of receptors and the concentration of hormone.

Usually less than 5% of hormone receptors are occupied at any one time and maximum biological responses are achieved when only a fraction of the total number of receptors are occupied. Thus it might be questioned why a small reduction in receptor number or a change in hormone concentration should make much difference to the overall biological response. This is governed by the law of mass action. If receptor numbers are reduced then the chances of a hormone binding to a receptor are decreased. Thus, a higher concentration of hormone is required to achieve the same receptor occupancy. A similar argument can be applied when hormone concentrations are reduced. Together these two parameters are important in determining the target cell's response to a hormone despite low occupancy of receptors.

Receptor regulation is an important part of endocrine function and this occurs through:

- increasing or decreasing receptor synthesis (up- or down-regulation of the number of receptors)
- uncoupling the receptor from the G protein (desensitization of the receptors)
- internalization of receptors, resulting in degradation by lysosomes or recycling back into the cell membrane.

These mechanisms are responsible for regulating the concentration of hormone receptors at the cell surface and the ability of the hormone ligand to activate cell signaling pathways.

Steroid receptor numbers are modulated by post-translational modification of the receptors and/or the synthesis of steroid receptors. Other pathways may either increase their degradation or prolong their life expectancy. If they become associated with a small protein, ubiquitin, this labels the receptor or its co-regulators for destruction (ubiquitination). Alternatively, they may become attached to a **s**mall **u**biquitin-related **mo**difier which attaches to proteins to prolong the life of a receptor or changes its location in the cell (**sumo**lyation). Thus post-translational modification of these receptors may stimulate or increase/decrease receptor numbers.

Regulation of receptors can induce resistance so that a greater concentration of hormone is required to induce any biological effect. For example, in type 2 diabetes mellitus (see *Chapter 5*), which is often associated with obesity, target cells become resistant to the action of insulin and this is thought to be due to defects in signal transduction rather than changes in the number of insulin receptors. Obesity itself is also associated with a resistance to leptin, the hormone secreted by adipose tissue that signals satiety to the brain (*Chapter 8*). Mutations of receptors can also cause resistance as described in *Section 1.5.2* and when a hormone is secreted in a high concentration for a prolonged period of time, this can cause down-regulation and desensitization of its own receptors. Indeed, receptor regulation plays an important role not only in endocrine disease but in normal function of endocrine target cells.

1.7 Control of hormone secretions

A fundamental process in the control of hormone secretions is negative feedback, such that the correct concentrations of circulating hormones can maintain homeostasis and regulate functions such as reproduction, growth and maintenance of nutrient supply. A negative feedback loop consists of several elements. First, the 'set point' that, in physical biological terms, is difficult to define; it is analogous to the setting of a thermostat on a domestic heating circuit. Then there are the controlling elements which regulate the controlled variable such as a specific hormone concentration or, for example, blood sugar levels. This is analogous to a heater on a domestic heating circuit. Finally, there are the sensors which detect the levels of a controlled variable. Any disparity between what the sensors detect and the set point is known as an error signal and this serves to correct the output to the controlling elements. So, for example, if a hormone concentration or blood sugar concentration rises above or falls below the set point then corrections will be made to rectify it back to a set point; just as a heater would be switched on or off if room temperature falls below or rises above the thermostat setting.

The thyroid gland, adrenal cortex and gonads are all controlled by hormones of the hypothalamic–pituitary axis and in these cases the controlled variable is the circulating concentration of hormones released by the peripheral endocrine glands

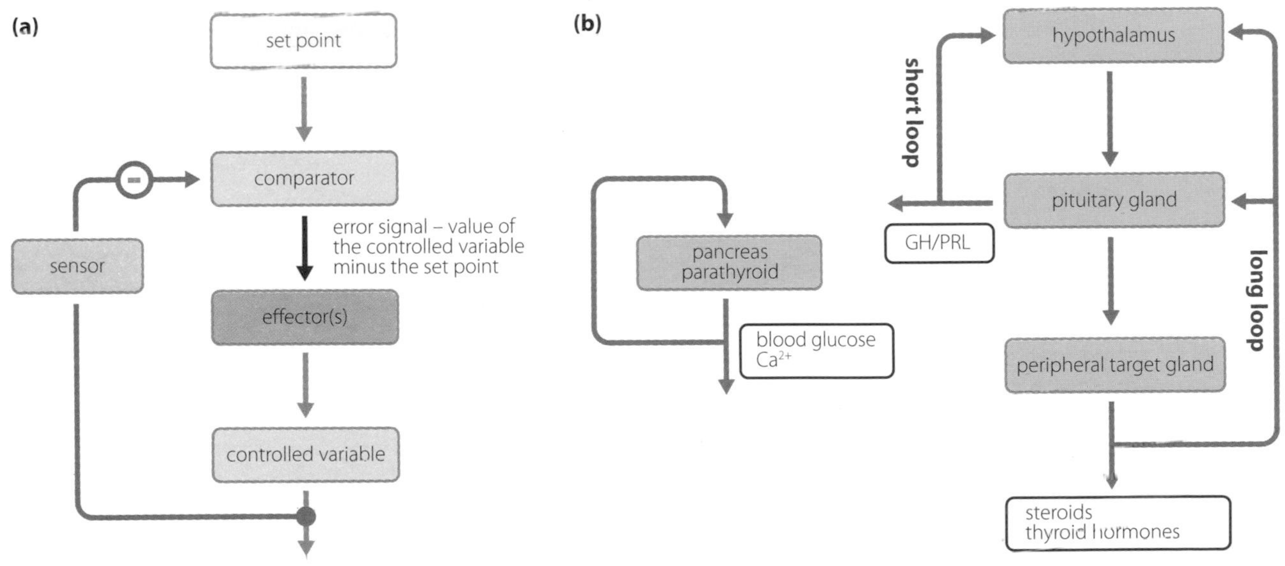

Figure 1.14. Negative feedback control in the endocrine system.
(a) Elements of a negative feedback loop are shown. Levels of a controlled variable (e.g. a hormone concentration) are sensed by a sensor which provides signals to a comparator that compares the level of a controlled variable to that of a set point. The difference between these two variables provides what is known as an error signal and this will either switch on effectors (if the controlled variable is lower than the set point) to raise the controlled variable, or vice versa if the level of the controlled variable is higher than the set point. A good analogy is the control of room temperature (a controlled variable) by the thermostat of a central heating system. In terms of regulating hormone secretions it is difficult to define what exactly is the comparator and the set point although the same principle applies. (b) In the endocrine system, the controlled variables are blood glucose and calcium, or the circulating concentrations of steroid and thyroid hormones. Growth hormone (GH) and prolactin (PRL) are also controlled variables, but as they have no specific peripheral endocrine target gland their secretions are controlled by a short loop feedback.

(*Figure 1.14*). Thus when the concentration of thyroid hormones or steroid hormones from the adrenal cortex or gonads rises, the brain and pituitary detect these variations and reduce production of the hormones that stimulate activity in these glands. The reverse occurs when circulating concentrations fall.

Two other major glands are the endocrine pancreas and the parathyroid glands, but their control does not directly involve the hypothalamic–pituitary axis. Instead, the controlled variables for hormone secretions from these glands are blood sugar concentrations (in the endocrine pancreas) and blood calcium levels (in the parathyroid glands). These controlled variables are detected by the glands themselves and they appropriately increase or decrease their hormone secretions (*Figure 1.14*).

CASE 1.1

3 24 31 33 46

- 28 year old woman with increased metabolic rate and a palpable goiter
- Abnormal TFTs

This patient had high levels of thyroid hormones and levels of TSH that were in the upper end of the normal range. In this case it appeared that the normal feedback of hormones had been impaired. In the light of elevated free thyroid hormone levels one would expect that pituitary TSH would be suppressed - indeed in most cases of significant thyroid overactivity, such as Graves autoimmune disease (*Chapter 3*), with elevated levels of free T_4 and free T_3 the TSH level would be undetectable. Common sense suggests that something has gone wrong, but what exactly? What are the possibilities?

- A problem with the assay, i.e. it is giving spurious results for some reason.
- A problem with the feedback mechanism. This could either be due to resistance of feedback (in this case some sort of resistance to thyroid hormone which is unable to 'tell' the pituitary to stop secreting TSH), or due to unregulated secretion of TSH at the pituitary itself, some sort of functional but unregulated adenoma of the pituitary, specifically producing TSH.

1.8 Autoimmunity and endocrine disorders

Autoimmunity is defined as an immune response against self-antigens as a result of the failure of self-tolerance. The main factors in the development of autoimmunity are the inheritance of susceptibility genes which may contribute to failure of self-tolerance and environmental triggers such as infections and other inflammatory stimuli that may activate self-reactive lymphocytes. Endocrine tissues appear more susceptible to autoimmunity than most other organs or tissues. So how does immunologic tolerance develop and why may failure of these processes lead to autoimmunity?

T and B lymphocytes originate from stem cells in bone marrow and, whilst B cells mature in the bone marrow itself, T cells mature in the thymus gland. The bone marrow and the thymus are known as the central or generative lymphoid organs, where the T and B lymphocytes become competent to respond to antigens in the peripheral or secondary lymphoid organs. These consist of the lymph nodes, spleen, and the mucosal and cutaneous immune systems which are organized to

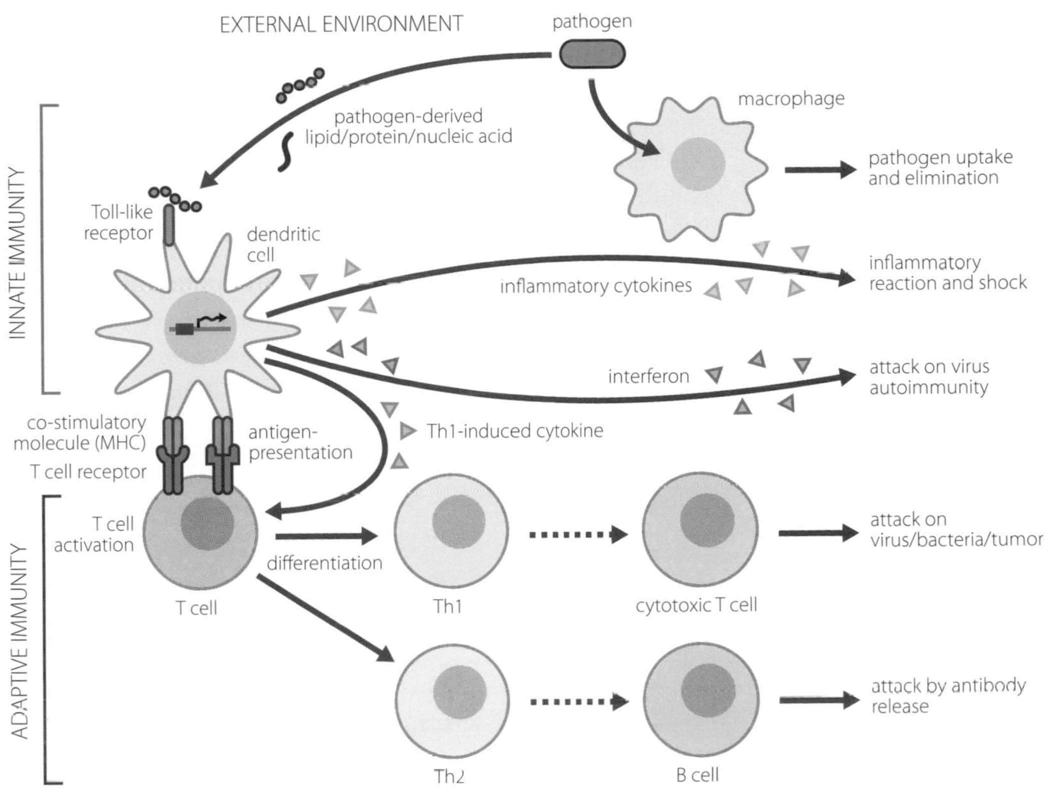

Figure 1.15. Innate and adaptive immunity.
The immune system is typically divided into innate and adaptive (acquired) immunity, although these distinctions are not mutually exclusive. Innate immunity refers to non-specific defense mechanisms that come into play within hours of a pathogen appearing in the body; essentially pathogen-derived antigens stimulate an acute inflammatory response. The pathogen-derived antigen is also presented to T cells which activate adaptive immunity; this takes longer to develop, is highly specific for antigens (including those associated with microbes), and shows memory that makes future responses against a specific antigen more efficient.

concentrate antigens and immune cells in a way that optimizes development of adaptive immunity (*Figure 1.15*).

The selection, proliferation and differentiation of T and B cells occurs in response to antigens which are recognized by these cells through specific receptors. T cells have specific receptors that respond to peptides that are presented to them by the major histocompatibility complex (MHC) molecules. In humans the MHC is referred to as human leukocyte antigen (HLA). MHC molecules are a set of glycoproteins encoded on chromosome 6 and whilst class I MHC is expressed on almost all nucleated cells, class II MHC is expressed on the surface of antigen presenting cells (APCs) such as cortical epithelial cells in the thymus and dendritic cells and macrophages in the periphery. The MHC genes that code for these glycoproteins are highly polymorphic in that there are many different alleles in different individuals in a population. B cells have membrane-bound antibodies on their surface and these antibodies are able to recognize shapes or conformations of specific macromolecules including proteins, lipids, carbohydrates and nucleic acids in addition to simple small chemical groups.

In the central lymphoid organs and in response to self-antigens, the naïve T and B cells are carefully selected because lymphocytes that recognize self-antigens undergo apoptosis (central tolerance). Cells that are not specific for self-antigens mature and become clones that move into the secondary or peripheral lymphoid organs. T cells in the thymus gland that recognize class I MHC complexes become $CD8^+$ lymphocytes; these are the cytotoxic T cells because they kill cells harboring intracellular microbes. Cells that recognize class II MHC complexes become $CD4^+$ lymphocytes; these are the helper T cells because they help B lymphocytes to produce antibodies and help phagocytes to destroy ingested microbes.

Selection against self-antigens (*Figure 1.16*) also occurs in peripheral lymphoid tissues when mature T cells recognize self-antigens leading to functional inactivation (anergy) or death. Mature B lymphocytes also become anergic when they encounter high concentrations of self-antigens and cannot again respond to that particular self-antigen. Thus both central and peripheral mechanisms to self-tolerance occur, but sometimes these mechanisms go wrong.

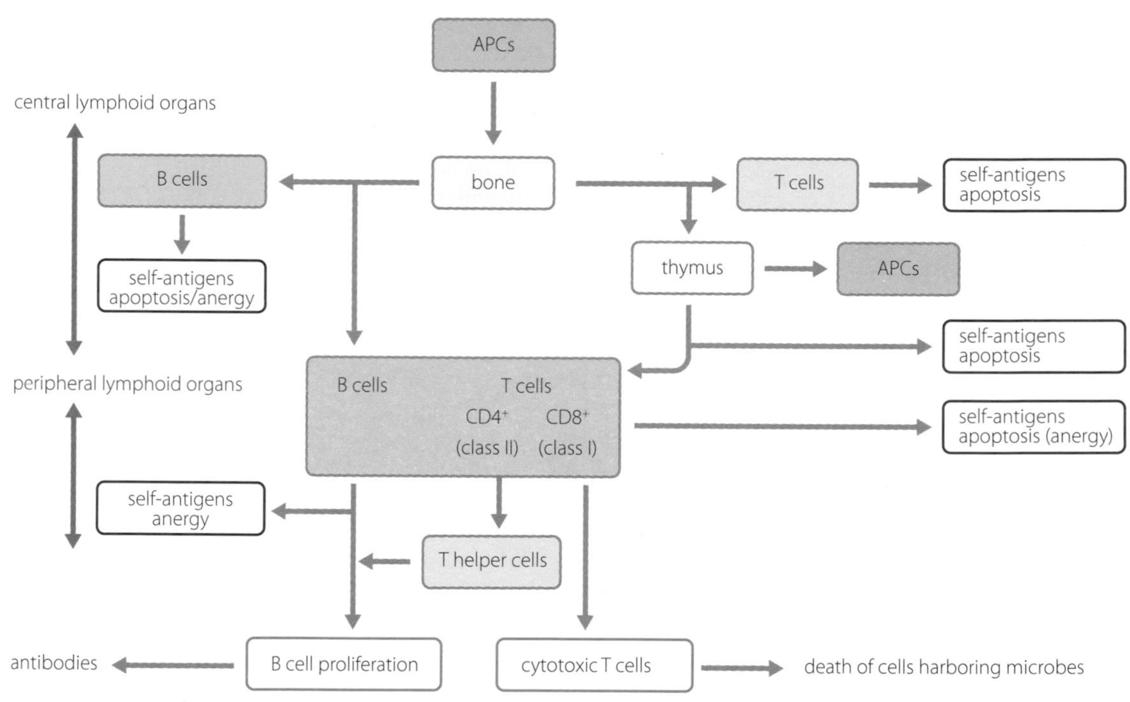

Figure 1.16. Autoimmunity.
A highly simplified diagram showing how the immune system selects against self-antigens. When immune cells recognize self-antigens they undergo apoptosis (cell death) or functional inactivation (anergy). An immune response against self-antigens occurs when these processes break down. APCs, antigen presenting cells.

Multiple genes predispose to autoimmune diseases and the most important of these are the highly polymorphic MHC/HLA genes which present antigens to the T lymphocytes. Thus the incidence of autoimmunity is higher in those individuals who inherit a particular HLA allele(s) and some of these have been identified. However, such inheritance does not necessarily lead to autoimmunity. That said, some non-MHC genes have also been identified which may cause defective elimination of self-reactive T and B lymphocytes. Infections by microbes may also promote autoimmunity in that an infection may 'break' T cell anergy to self-antigens and actually promote survival and activation of self-reactive T lymphocytes. Alternatively some infectious agents may produce antigens that are similar to and cross-react with self-antigens so that the microbial peptide may induce an immune response against self-antigens (molecular mimicry). Whatever the cause, there is still no clear explanation as to why autoimmune diseases are particularly prevalent in the endocrine system.

In fact, some of the most common endocrine disorders are a result of autoimmunity. Type 1 diabetes is caused by autoimmune destruction of the endocrine pancreas (see *Chapter 5*). Hashimoto disease is characterized by autoimmune destruction of the thyroid gland causing hypothyroidism. In contrast, Graves disease, which is a common cause of hyperthyroidism (thyrotoxicosis), is caused by autoimmune production of antibodies that activate the TSH receptors on the thyroid gland (see *Chapter 3*).

1.9 Diagnosing endocrine disorders

The two major diagnostic tools used for determining the etiology of endocrine disorders are biochemical measurements of hormones and various imaging techniques. Others include histological examination of biopsies taken from endocrine tissue and the assessment of hormone receptors by immunohistochemical techniques or receptor binding assays.

1.9.1 Measuring hormone levels

One of the earliest recorded assessments of 'hormone' levels is described in an ancient Egyptian papyrus whereby a woman would urinate on wheat and barley seeds and if they germinated then the woman was considered to be pregnant. If the barley seed germinated first then this would imply a male fetus, if the wheat was first then this would imply a female fetus. In the Middle Ages through to the seventeenth century the 'Pisse Prophets' of Europe claimed to be able to diagnose many different conditions, including pregnancy, by the colour of urine. Consequently another so-called pregnancy test was developed which involved mixing the urine of pregnant women with wine and seeing whether this changed the appearance of urine. Of course at this time hormones had not been discovered so there was no scientific basis to these tests.

By the late nineteenth century the idea of internal secretions was beginning to be accepted; in other words, chemical messengers that were released into the bloodstream and acted at distant targets, as opposed to messages that were sent by the nervous system. In 1902 William Bayliss and Ernest Starling discovered the gut hormone secretin and the science of endocrinology was effectively born. In 1905 Ernest Starling first introduced the word hormone (from the Greek word for 'excite' or 'arouse') for these chemical messengers.

The earliest ways of assessing hormone levels came from looking at whether or not a blood or urine sample could initiate a biological action; in other words a bioassay. For example, the first pregnancy test developed in the late 1920s was based on a bioassay which involved injecting women's urine into immature mice or rats and observing whether or not their ovaries were stimulated and they came into estrus. Subsequently this bioassay was modified and the South African clawed frog, *Xenopus laevis*, was used to detect pregnancy. Urine of pregnant women, when injected into the dorsal lymph sac, caused the frog to lay eggs within 12 hours. These assays were

Box 1.2 | Principles of radioimmunoassays

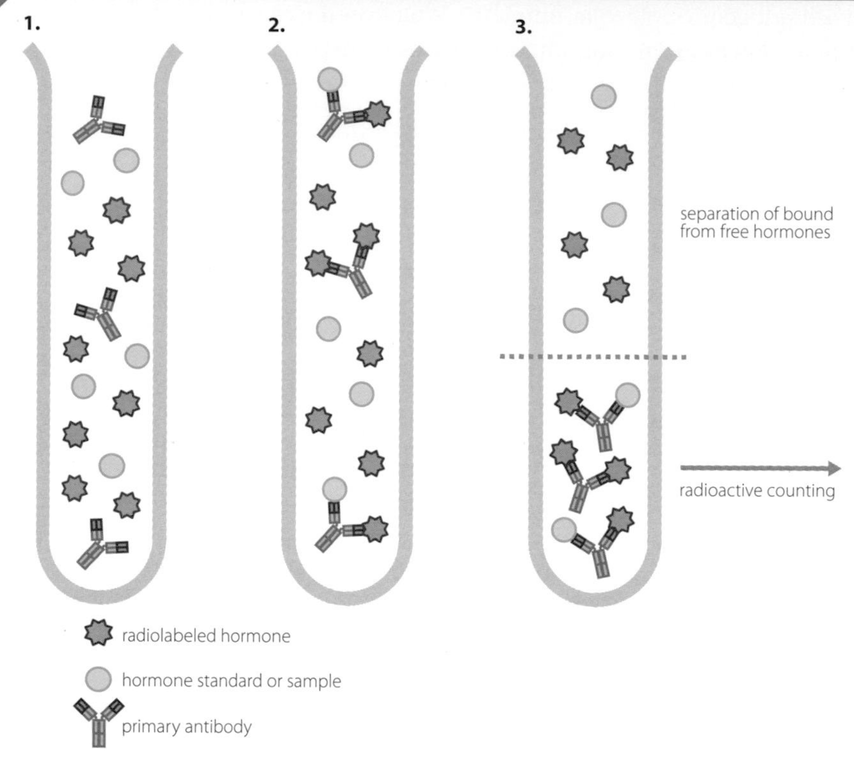

Box figure 1.1. A basic radioimmunoassay.

1. A primary antibody is incubated with a fixed concentration of a radiolabeled hormone and either a known concentration of an unlabeled hormone (hormone standard) or an unknown concentration of a hormone sample.
2. The hormone in the standard or sample will bind to the antibody competitively with the labeled hormone and so the lower the concentration of unlabeled hormone, the higher the amount of binding with the radiolabeled hormone, or vice versa.
3. The unbound hormone is then separated and the amount of bound radioactivity is measured.

A standard curve is then constructed (*Box figure 1.2*) and the concentration of the hormone in the unknown sample is then read off the curve as illustrated. In this example the counts per minute were 1200 and so the concentration of the hormone in the unknown sample was 2.5 x 10^{-7} mol/L.

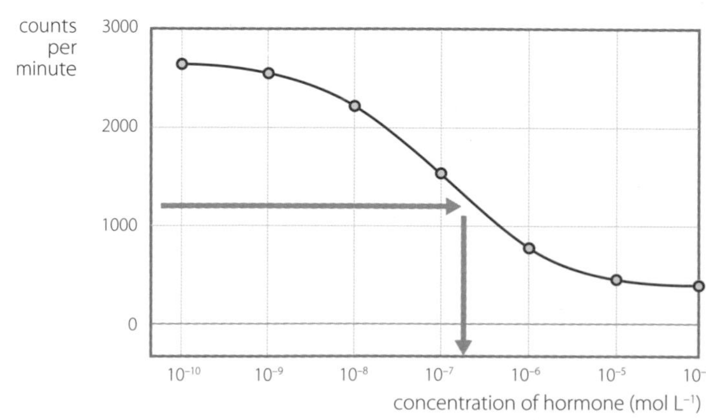

Box figure 1.2. Standard curve for a radioimmunoassay.

Box 1.3 | Principle of a typical ELISA

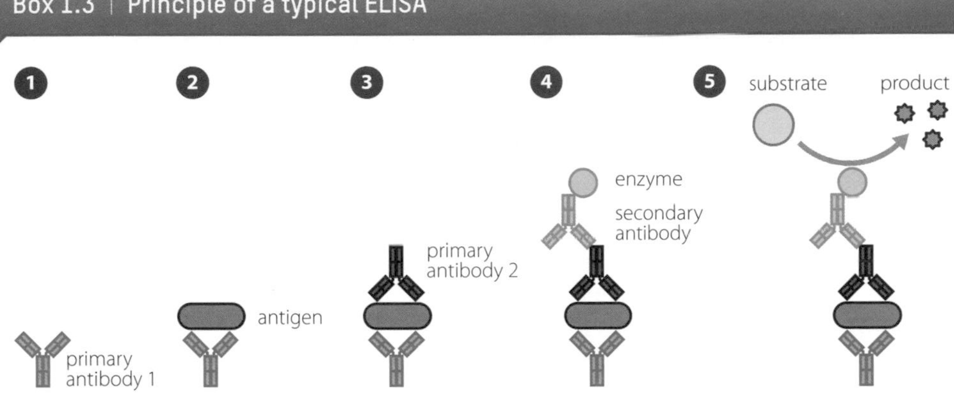

Box figure 1.3. A basic ELISA.

1. Wells are coated with a primary antibody to a particular antigen/hormone.
2. Standards of a known hormone concentration are added, or samples containing unknown concentrations of a hormone.
3. A second primary antibody is then added which recognizes amino acid sequences at the other end of an antigen (hormone) – a sandwich.
4. A secondary antibody is then added which combines with primary antibody 2. This antibody is labeled with an enzyme.
5. When a substrate is added the enzyme converts the substrate into a product that has fluorescence or color. The intensity is read on a plate reader and the fluorescence/color is directly proportional to the concentration of the hormone, as shown below. Concentrations of the unknown samples are read off the standard curve (*Box figure 1.4*).

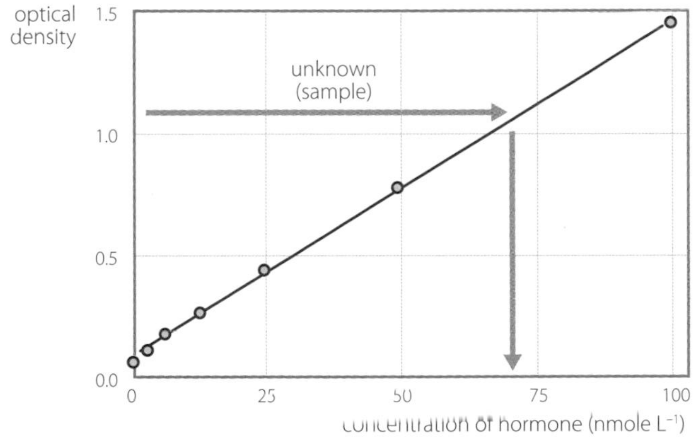

Box figure 1.4. Standard curve for an ELISA.

actually detecting human chorionic gonadotropin, secreted in high concentrations by the placenta in early pregnancy and which has identical actions to LH. Further bioassays were developed such as growth stimulation of the epiphysial cartilage plate of hypophysectomized rat's tibia by growth hormone (GH), the color change of frog's skin in response to melanocyte stimulating hormone (MSH), and *in vitro* testosterone secretion from Leydig cells by LH.

It was not until the 1960s that the first immunoassays were developed which, today, are the mainstay of biochemical testing for hormone secretions and diagnosis of endocrine disorders. All immunoassays are based on the ability of an antibody to bind to an antigen and, in the case of endocrinology, the antigen is the hormone. In essence they are competitive binding assays.

The earliest immunoassays were radioimmunoassays in which the hormone sample or standard (to create a standard curve) were incubated with a fixed amount of radiolabeled hormone and an antibody which would bind to an epitope on the specific hormone. The radiolabeled hormone competes with the hormone in the sample or standard. Thus if there were low levels of hormone in the samples or a low concentration of standard there would be greater binding of the radiolabeled hormone compared to the unlabeled hormone, and vice versa if concentrations of unlabeled hormone were high (*Box 1.2*). In most assays a second antibody is added that recognizes and binds to the first antibody to make a larger protein complex so that it is easier to separate the hormone bound to the antibody from the free hormone. The bound radiolabeled hormone is typically measured in a scintillation counter or a gamma counter.

The availability of monoclonal antibodies was important in the development of newer immunoassays with greater specificity and without the need for radiolabeled reagents. These assays, typically known as **e**nzyme-**l**inked **i**mmuno**s**orbent **a**ssays (ELISAs) are now widely used by both clinicians and researchers (*Box 1.3*). For small molecular weight hormones, such as steroid and thyroid hormones, that have only one, or at best a few, epitopes that can be recognized by an antibody, simple competitive ELISAs, using the same principle as the radioimmunoassay, were developed. Typically a primary antibody will be incubated with a hormone or standard along with a fixed amount of hormone conjugated with an enzyme. These compete for the antibody and, after removal of any unbound hormone, a substrate is added which changes color or fluoresces based on the amount of enzyme (conjugated to the hormone) that has been bound; the color change or fluorescence is read on a plate reader.

For protein and peptide hormones which have many more epitopes for antibody recognition, a sandwich ELISA is generally used (*Box 1.3*). In this assay a first primary antibody is attached to a solid phase (e.g. the surface of a well in a test plate) and this is used to capture the hormone in the standard or test sample. A second primary antibody is then added which will recognize a second epitope in the hormone structure. Finally, an enzyme-linked secondary antibody will be added that will bind to the second primary antibody and a substrate is added. Alternatively the second antibody can be labeled with a fluorescent marker and fluorescence intensity measured. In these assays the color change or fluorescence intensity are directly proportional to the concentration of the hormone. The advantage of these sandwich assays is that they can measure the active circulating hormone concentrations rather than peptide fragments that have been released from the gland or broken down in the circulation.

1.9.2 Diagnosing endocrine disorders with hormone measurements and dynamic tests of endocrine function

Hormone concentrations are usually measured in serum samples, but steroids such as cortisol can also be measured in urine or saliva samples. The over- or under-secretion of hormones from glands that are not controlled by hormones released by the hypothalamic–pituitary axis, i.e. the pancreas and parathyroid gland, can easily be identified by measuring the hormone concentration and its controlled variable, i.e. glucose or calcium. For example, high levels of insulin and its secreted C peptide

CASE 1.1 3 24 31 33 46

- 28 year old woman with increased metabolic rate and a palpable goiter
- Abnormal TFTs
- Check assay

The patient had high levels of free T_4 and free T_3 without suppression of TSH. Could the assay be incorrect? There are some situations where assays of thyroid hormones can be affected by circulating antibodies. These might be thyroid antibodies as part of the autoimmune process, 'heterophile' antibodies, e.g. human anti-mouse antibodies which affect the function of the 2-site assay or something like rheumatoid factor which can cause interference in the assay by aggregation of immunoglobulin.

The majority of the newer specific assays no longer suffer from significant interference but some still do. The patient's tests were repeated in two different assays and gave similar results. Furthermore, the symptoms of the patient were highly suggestive of excess thyroid hormone; normally spurious results due to assay interference come as a bit of a surprise in patients who are asymptomatic and without any obvious clinical features of thyroid hormone excess or deficiency.

along with low glucose levels (hypoglycemia) indicate an insulin-secreting tumor, whilst high levels of parathyroid hormone with high levels of circulating calcium indicate an adenoma of the parathyroid gland. Further investigations, such as imaging, would be required for a definitive diagnosis. In contrast, over- or under-secretion of hormones controlled by the hypothalamic–pituitary axis could indicate a defect either in the peripheral gland, the pituitary, or indeed the hypothalamus.

Measuring levels of hormones secreted by the thyroid gland, adrenal cortex, and gonads can show whether there is a deficiency or an excess of a particular hormone, but it will not provide any information as to the cause. In peripheral glands that are controlled by the hypothalamic–pituitary axis, measurement of the trophic hormone together with the hormone secreted by the peripheral gland will indicate whether or not the endocrine disorder is primary (i.e. in the peripheral gland) or secondary, resulting from a disorder of the pituitary gland. It is based on the negative feedback loop (*Figure 1.14*), for example:

- low TSH with high levels of free T_3/T_4 – primary hyperthyroidism
- high TSH levels with low levels of free T_3/T_4 – primary hypothyroidism
- high levels of TSH with high levels of free T_3/T_4 – secondary hyperthyroidism
- low levels of TSH and low levels of free T_3/T_4 – secondary or tertiary hypothyroidism.

In the last example the problem may not necessarily be caused by a pituitary deficiency, but could be due to a hypothalamic deficiency (tertiary deficiency) caused, for example, by a tumor or a head injury. Thus a further dynamic test of endocrine function, in this case a pituitary function test, would need to be undertaken and an example is given in *Figure 1.18*. The same principles may be applied to hormones secreted by the hypothalamic–pituitary adrenal axis and the gonadal axes, measuring trophic hormones together with the peripheral hormones to indicate the cause of an endocrinopathy, with further tests if a definitive diagnosis cannot be made.

The principle of dynamic tests of endocrine function is that if an over-secretion of a hormone is detected or suspected then a suppression test is used and in the case of under-secretion a stimulation test is used. *Figure 1.17* illustrates a suppression test for suspected acromegaly and a stimulation test for suspected GH deficiency. These tests are used for diagnosing GH disorders because obtaining a 'basal' level of GH is difficult: GH is secreted in discrete pulses during the day and levels are barely detectable between pulses and thus serial blood sampling would be required.

Other dynamic tests of endocrine function include:

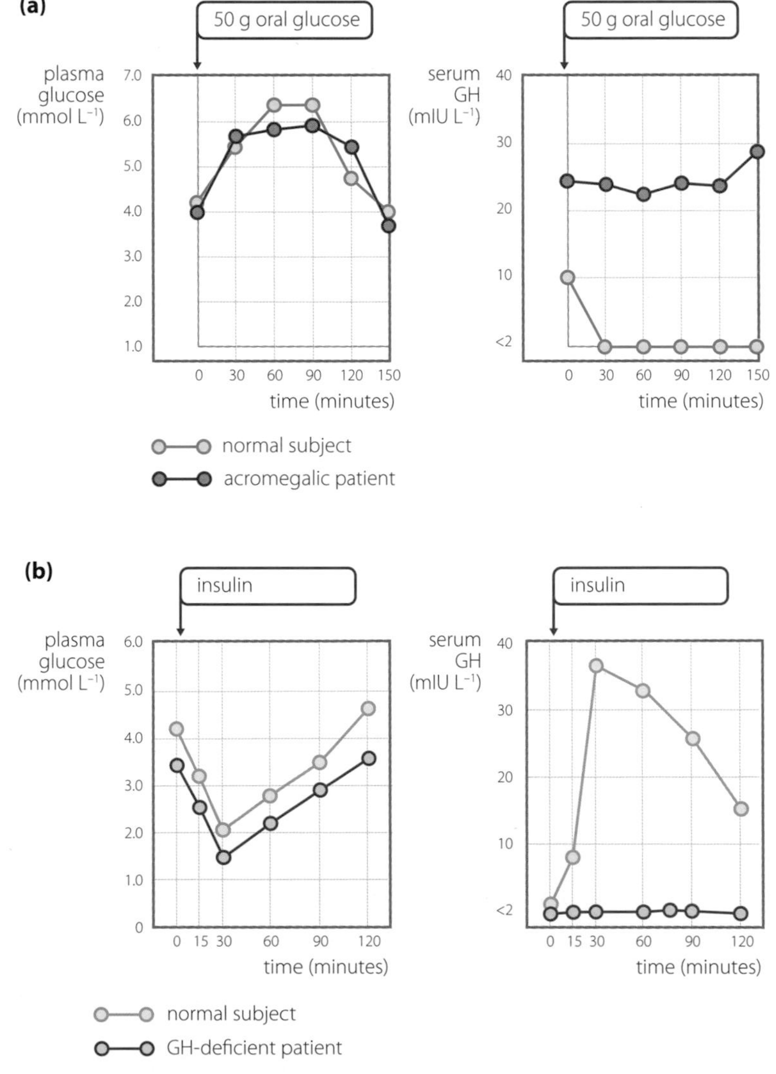

Figure 1.17. Dynamic tests of endocrine function: investigating growth hormone excess and deficiency. (a) An oral glucose load will initially increase plasma glucose concentrations until insulin acts to remove glucose from the circulation. The hyperglycemia will inhibit growth hormone (GH) secretion in normal subjects, but in those patients with acromegaly the excess GH from a pituitary adenoma will not be suppressed by the glucose load.
(b) An insulin stress test, where 0.15 units of insulin/kg weight are given in the fasted state, will lower plasma glucose levels. The hypoglycemia will stimulate GH secretion in normal subjects, but in patients with GH deficiency there will be little or no rise in serum GH levels.

- the low and high dose dexamethasone test for diagnosing the cause of excess cortisol secretion (see *Chapter 6*)
- the water deprivation test for investigating a deficiency or resistance to vasopressin secretion (see *Chapter 2*)
- a corticotropin releasing hormone (CRH) test (often called a pituitary function test) for investigating the cause of cortisol insufficiency (*Figure 1.18*; see also *Chapter 6*)
- an oral glucose tolerance test for investigating not only growth hormone deficiency (*Figure 1.17*), but also impaired glucose tolerance and diabetes (see *Chapter 5*).

CASE 1.1

3 24 31 33 46

- 28 year old woman with increased metabolic rate and a palpable goiter
- Abnormal TFTs
- Check assay
- Check response of pituitary to TRH – no response
- Check suppression of TSH with octreotide – TSH levels reduced
- Suspect pituitary adenoma – confirmation requires imaging

This patient presented to the endocrine clinic where the results were reviewed. It was clear that she had specific symptoms of thyroid overactivity with elevated thyroid hormone levels but no suppression of TSH. The possibilities remained of a resistance to thyroid hormone (negating normal negative feedback) or an autonomous unregulated production of TSH from the pituitary. The absence of a family history and the clear signs of thyroid overactivity made resistance to thyroid hormone less likely (*Chapter 3*). Would dynamic tests help?

If there was resistance to thyroid hormone, the ability of the pituitary to respond to a hypothalamic releasing factor (in this case TRH) should not be impaired, indeed it would normally be rather brisk. In contrast, if the thyrotrophs were autonomous there should be no ability to respond to TRH, resulting in a 'flat' curve. The patient underwent a TRH test with 200 µg of TRH being injected intravenously after a baseline sample for TSH. Samples at 20 min and 60 min post-injection were taken and these were identical to the baseline sample, showing no response. This supports the diagnosis of a TSH-secreting pituitary adenoma (a TSHoma) because it will autonomously secrete TSH in the absence of TRH. Further tests were undertaken. Some analytes are sensitive to thyroid hormone levels, e.g. sex hormone binding globulin (SHBG) which increases with raised thyroid hormone levels. In thyroid hormone resistance, therefore, levels of SHBG would be low, whereas if thyroid hormone sensitivity was not the case, levels of a thyroid hormone dependent protein should be high; this was indeed the case and this patient had a SHBG level of 215 nmol/L (NR 28–150).

Finally, many pituitary adenomas express somatostatin receptors (see *Chapter 2*). Somatostatin can inhibit autonomous production of hormones from pituitary adenomas, so the patient underwent a dynamic test of endocrine function; in this case a test dose of a short-acting somatostatin analog to see if the TSH could be suppressed; 100 µg of octreotide (a somatostatin analog) was injected intravenously and samples taken for TSH at 30 min, 60 min, and 3 h post-injection. The TSH dropped from a baseline of 4.4 mIU/L to a nadir of 2.3 mIU/L at 3 h. All these results pointed to a pituitary adenoma secreting TSH.

Imaging could confirm this suspected diagnosis.

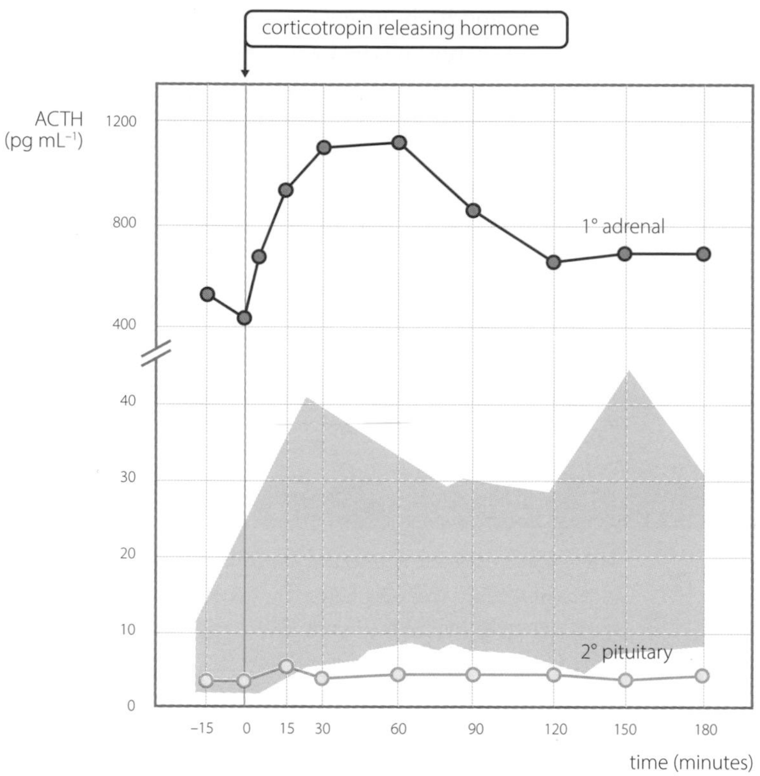

Figure 1.18. Pituitary function test to investigate the cause of cortisol deficiency.
A bolus injection of 100 µg of corticotropin-releasing hormone (CRH) is given and the ACTH response is measured. In normal subjects (shaded area) there will be a brisk ACTH response to exogenous CRH. If a patient has primary (red line) adrenocortical insufficiency the basal levels of ACTH will be high (loss of negative feedback) but there will be a good response to CRH. In secondary cortisol deficiency (green line), there is a loss of pituitary function, ACTH secretion is low and is not stimulated by an injection of CRH.

Further details of various tests will be found in the appropriate chapters, but it is important to note that hormone measurements may not always give a definitive diagnosis, but they will certainly indicate the etiology of different endocrinopathies. Imaging then plays an important role in reaching a definitive diagnosis.

1.9.3 Imaging modalities for the endocrine system

This section provides an overview of various imaging modalities that are used in the diagnosis (and management) of endocrine conditions; specific examples are given in the relevant sections of each subsequent chapter. In simple terms, imaging can give structural information (e.g. the use of ultrasound in the characterization of a thyroid nodule) or functional information (e.g. the uptake of nuclear medicine radionucleides by thyroid nodules (see *Chapter 3*)). Many different modalities might be used in the same patient to give differing pieces of information that are helpful in putting together the diagnostic jigsaw; an example of this is the use of MRI in the evaluation of a pituitary lesion followed by CT scanning (which is better at demonstrating calcification) if the lesion is thought to be calcium containing, e.g. a craniopharyngioma (see *Chapter 2*).

X-rays

X-rays generally have limited usefulness in the context of endocrine investigations. Historically, simple skull X-rays have been used to demonstrate enlargement of the bony sella turcica in pituitary disease (*Figure 1.19*) and in the context of acromegaly this may give further diagnostic clues (e.g. prognathism, interdental spacing). In the diagnosis of hyperparathyroidism, assessment is mainly biochemical with measurements of circulating levels of parathyroid hormone (see also *Chapter 4*), but

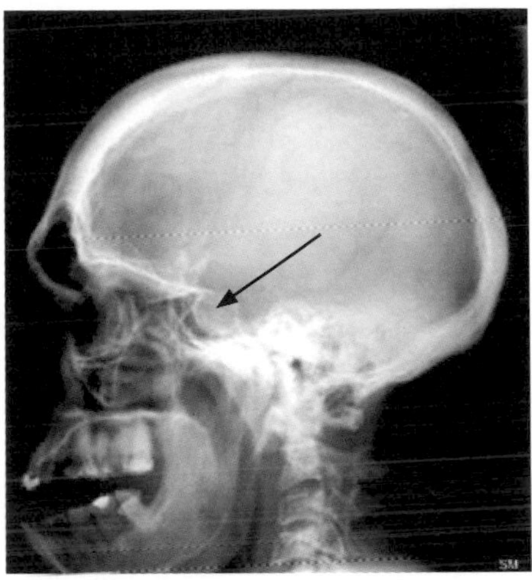

Figure 1.19. X-rays of the endocrine system: pituitary fossa.
Skull X-ray showing an enlarged sella turcica (arrow) suggesting an enlarged pituitary. Prognathism (enlargement of the lower mandible with impairment of the bite), increased interdental spacing and a generalized increased thickening of the bony skull can also be seen; features typically seen in acromegaly.

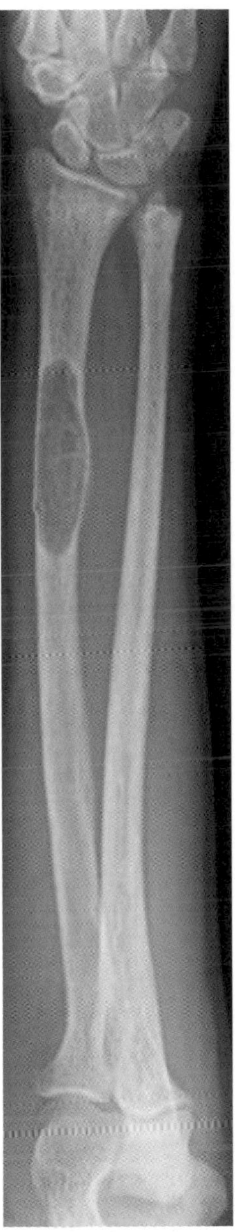

Figure 1.20. X-rays of the endocrine system: hyperparathyroidism and a 'brown tumor'.
'Brown tumor' of the distal radius, occurring as a result of excessive parathyroid hormone-induced osteoclastic activity. The term 'brown' refers to the hemosiderin deposition into the osteolytic cysts.

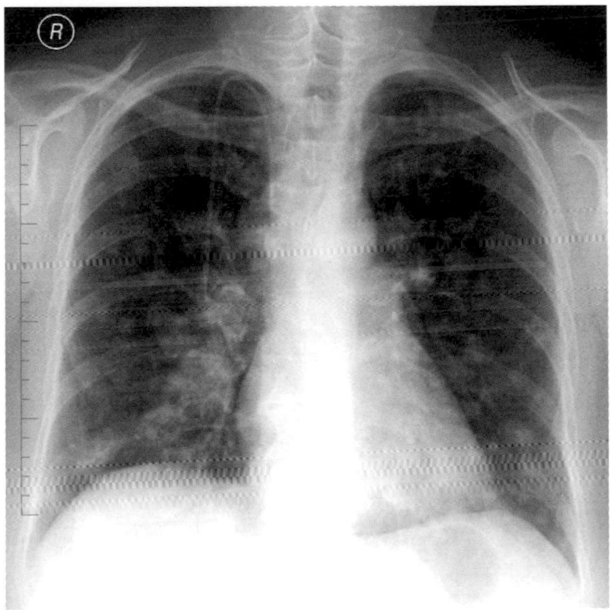

Figure 1.21. X-rays of the endocrine system: metastases of adrenocortical cancer.
Chest X-ray showing extensive pulmonary metastases from a primary adrenocortical cancer. Further images from the same patient are shown in *Figure 1.29*.

X-rays may still give some useful supporting evidence. For example, the presence of brown tumors (*Chapter 4*) is sometimes readily demonstrated on plain X-rays (*Figure 1.20*). Plain X-rays may also be helpful in assessing the extent of endocrine malignant disease, e.g. screening for lung metastases in endocrine cancers (*Figure 1.21* shows a chest X-ray demonstrating extensive pulmonary metastatic disease in a patient with adrenocortical cancer; see also *Chapter 4*). Other uses of X-rays include confirmation of certain clinical signs and in the estimation of bone age when considering endocrine-related disorders of maturation (*Figure 1.22*).

Ultrasound

Ultrasound is a safe and effective way of diagnosing and monitoring disease by using high frequency sound waves which can then be transduced to give images. It allows exact measurements of lesions and can distinguish between solid and cystic structures. Ultrasound involves no radiation exposure and has no side-effects. The main limitation is its use in very obese patients.

Ultrasound is particularly useful in thyroid disease, both in assessing thyroid nodules and guiding fine needle aspiration (FNA). Thyroid nodules may be solitary or may occur within a multinodular goiter. Nodules are frequently clinically obvious and noticed by the patient, relatives or healthcare professional, but they may occasionally be discovered as an incidental finding on other imaging modalities. Nodules in the thyroid gland can indicate malignancy (particularly in a euthyroid patient) and need to be assessed for size and features of malignancy (see *Chapter 3*). FNA can then be performed to provide histological information about the cell type. Ultrasound-guided FNA is particularly useful for small and posterior nodules and increases the chance of definitive FNA results.

Ultrasound is also useful in gynecological endocrinology. The diagnosis of PCOS (*Chapter 7*) requires two of three parameters to be present, one of which is structural polycystic ovaries on ultrasound scanning (*Figure 1.23*); transvaginal (internal)

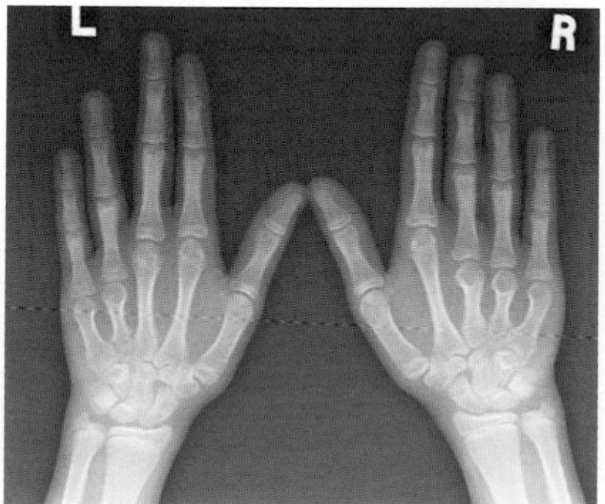

(a)

Figure 1.22. X-rays of the endocrine system: confirming clinical signs.
(a) X-rays of the hands may be useful in the confirmation of certain clinical signs, for example metacarpal shortening in gonadal dysgenesis. Here, X-rays of both hands show marked shortening of the 3rd–5th metacarpals on the right and the 4th and 5th metacarpal on the left in a patient with Turner syndrome (this may also be seen in pseudo- and pseudopseudohypoparathyroidism, see *Chapter 4*).

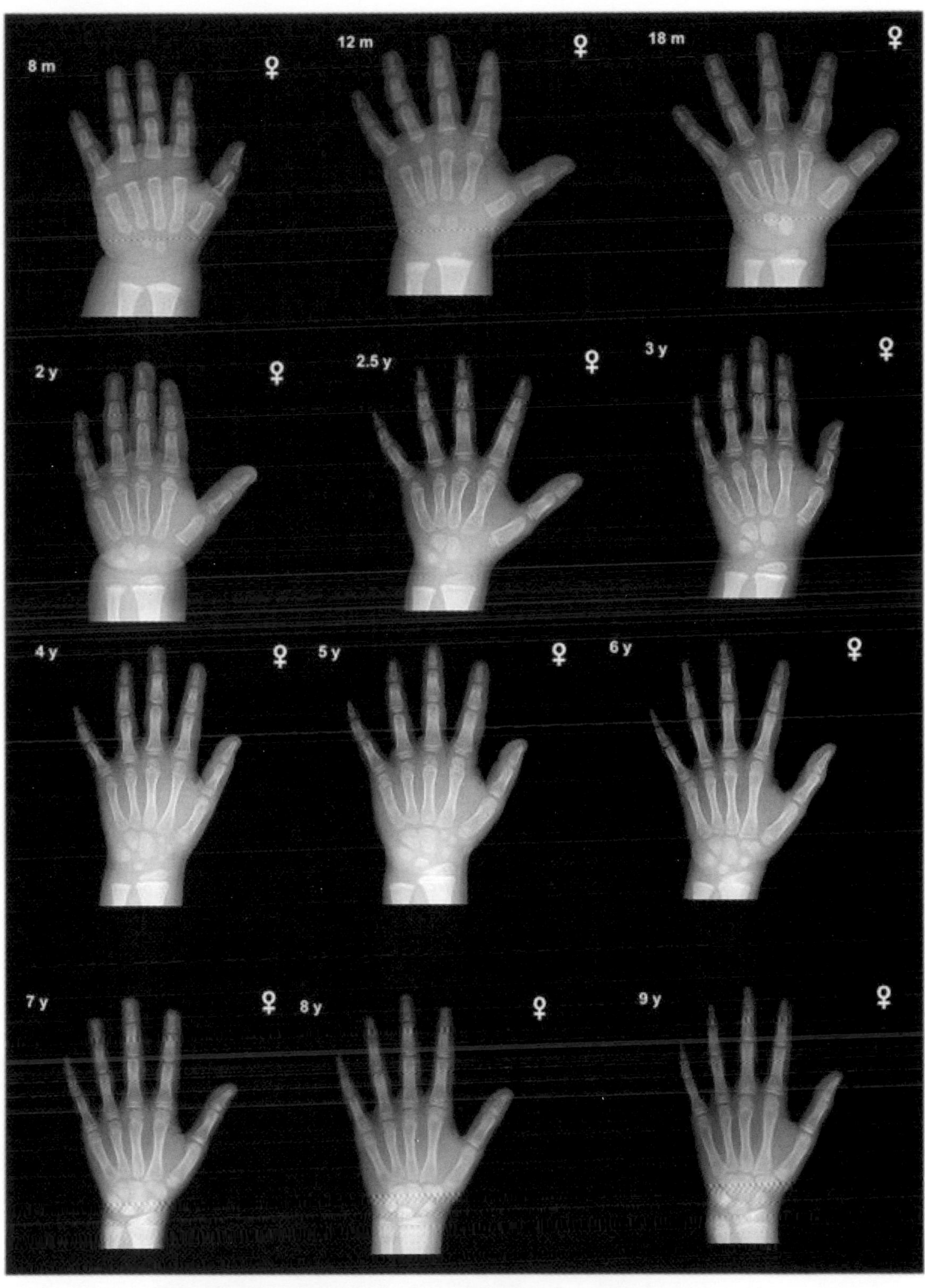

(b)

(b) In pediatric endocrinology, assessment of bone age by wrist X-rays may be extremely useful. Bone age often differs from chronological age and knowledge of advance or delay can be useful in management and diagnosis of conditions such as constitutional delayed puberty, precocious puberty, short stature, etc. Bone age is determined from wrist X-rays which are compared with standardized atlases of bone maturation (such as Greulich and Pyle's *Radiographic Atlas of Skeletal Development of Hand and Wrist* in the USA, and Tanner and Whitehouse's *Assessment of Skeletal Maturity and Prediction of Adult Height (TW2 Method)* in the UK). Female bone age atlas images showing normal carpal bone maturation from 8 months to 9 years.

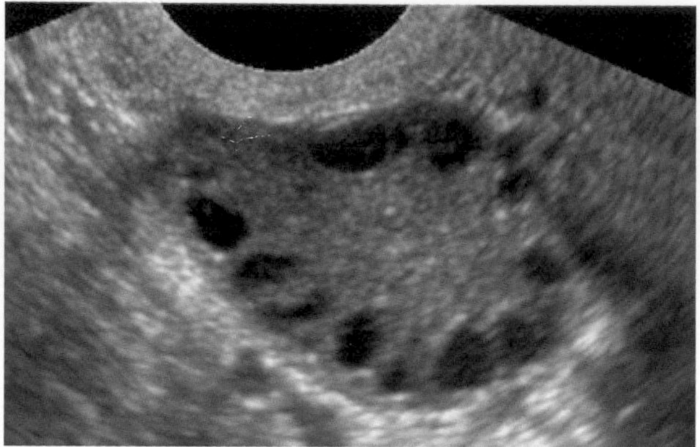

Figure 1.23. Ultrasound scan of the endocrine system: polycystic ovaries.
A pelvic ultrasound scan showing multiple small peripheral cysts diagnostic of polycystic ovaries; these are structural polycystic ovaries but are not necessarily the result of PCOS.

scans give far better pictures and are less influenced by obesity. Other uses of ultrasonography in endocrine diagnosis and management include use of endoscopic ultrasound in the localization of gastroenteropancreatic neuroendocrine tumors (*Chapter 8*), assessment of testicular presence/morphology, presence of hepatic metastatic disease in endocrine oncology, and adrenal imaging.

Computed tomography

Computed tomography (CT) works by taking a series of X-rays which are then reconstructed into two-dimensional pictures to give cross-sectional images of the body. CT imaging can be used to give detailed images of the adrenal glands, neuroendocrine tumors and pituitary lesions (where MRI is contraindicated). CT can also provide information about the thyroid gland, particularly if there is suspicion of compression of the esophagus and trachea (in conjunction with flow volume loops).

Adrenal glands can also be assessed for masses or hyperplasia (*Figure 1.24*), which can indicate underlying disease. Adrenal lesions (or incidentalomas) are common findings as a result of the increased numbers of scans being performed for other reasons. In a basic non-enhanced CT scan of the adrenal glands, if the adrenal mass is less than 10 Hounsfield Units (HU), a diagnosis of adrenal adenoma can be

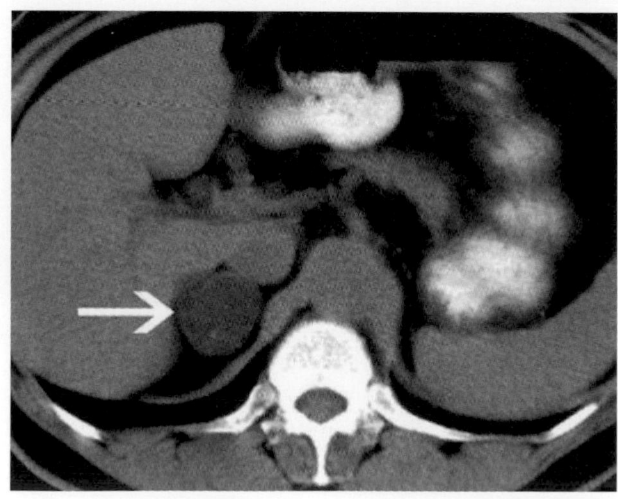

Figure 1.24. Computed tomography image of the endocrine system: adrenal adenoma.
Unenhanced CT image of an adrenal lesion (arrow). The mass is smooth and of low attenuation (less than 10 Hounsfield Units) suggesting a lipid-rich adenoma.

made. If the adrenal mass is more than 10 HU, CT with intravenously administered contrast material should follow, and the washout (washout refers to the difference in attenuation in HU between the initial dynamic scan and a further scan at 15 min) should be calculated; benign lesions typically demonstrate more than 50% washout. CT can also be used to stage endocrine cancers to provide evidence of the extent of tumor involvement and therefore enable appropriate treatment plans to be formulated.

The disadvantage of CT is the radiation exposure involved with each scan. There is evidence that CT, particularly abdominal scans, can increase lifetime risk of malignancy and as a result all scans need to be justified clinically. Often CT scans require intravenous (IV) contrast material which is contraindicated in the presence of significant renal impairment as it is nephrotoxic and may worsen renal failure. CT is also contraindicated in pregnancy due to radiation dose.

Magnetic resonance imaging

MRI involves the use of a strong magnetic field and detects the response of protons within molecules to applied radio waves at the resonant frequency. The images produced are related to the relative water content of the soft tissues. This allows the precise visualization of internal soft tissue structures, such as the pituitary and adrenal glands. Axial, coronal, and sagittal views are possible and because there is no signal from the bone, there is no bone artifact. MRI scans are thus superior to CT scans in the visualization of the posterior fossa and spinal cord structures.

MRI images are often expressed in two sequences: T1- and T2-weighted (T referring to the relaxation time constant). In a T1-weighted image, cerebrospinal fluid (CSF) is dark and fat is white; in a T2-weighted image, CSF appears white. Patients with metallic implants, pacemakers, aneurysm clips, shrapnel or splinters are not suitable candidates for MRI imaging due to the risk of migration given the use of such a strong magnetic field. In addition, the scan is performed in an enclosed space and may pose a problem in claustrophobic patients.

MRI is the imaging modality of choice for the pituitary gland. T1-weighted sequences are obtained prior to and after administration of IV contrast agent (gadolinium). Gadolinium enhances the clarity of soft tissue structures due to its paramagnetic properties. For localization of pituitary adenomas, T1-weighted sequences are more effective. The posterior pituitary (neurohypophysis / pars nervosa) has a bright signal on T1-weighted images due to its high neurophysin content.

Pituitary adenomas can be classified by radiological appearance into microadenomas or macroadenomas according to their diameter: microadenomas are <10 mm in diameter and macroadenomas are >10 mm in diameter. On T1-weighted images pituitary adenomas appear as hypointense (darker) areas compared to the surrounding pituitary tissue. Hemorrhages (seen in cases of pituitary apoplexy) within the gland appear as hyperintense areas (bright signals).

MRI allows visualization of the immediate anatomy of the pituitary gland within the sella turcica (*Figure 1.25*), identifies local invasion of the cavernous sinus, and shows distortion of the optic chiasm by the expanding pituitary mass. This is of great importance in neurosurgical intervention. Although high resolution CT is the initial modality of choice in the imaging of adrenals, MRI can also be used to differentiate cortical from medullary adrenal tumors (*Figure 1.26*).

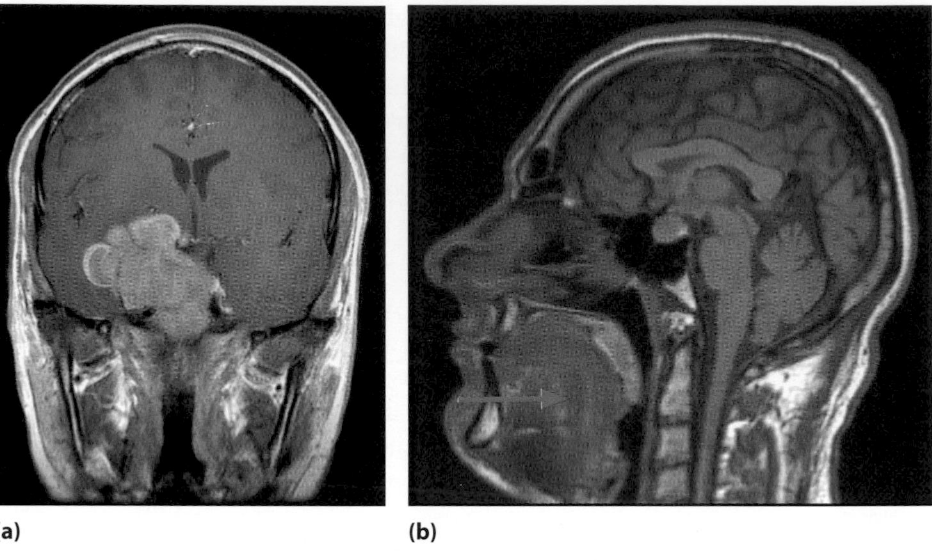

(a) **(b)**

Figure 1.25. Magnetic resonance imaging of the endocrine system: pituitary tumor.
(a) MRI scan showing massive pituitary tumor (arrow) with a large suprasellar extension and invasion of the right cavernous sinus.
(b) MRI scan showing discrete pituitary adenoma (white arrow), enlargement of the sella and significant macroglossia (blue arrow) in a patient with acromegaly.

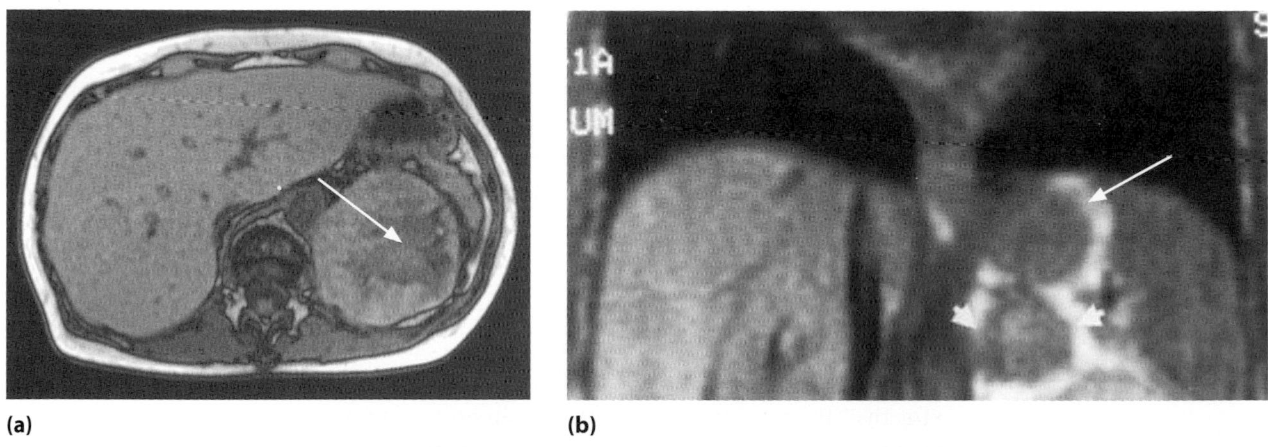

(a) **(b)**

Figure 1.26. Magnetic resonance imaging of the endocrine system: tumors of the adrenal medulla and pancreas.
(a) MRI scan showing a large left-sided pheochromocytoma (arrow).
In the case of carcinoid tumors, the aim of imaging is to identify the sites of primary and metastatic disease. Both MRI and CT are comparable in efficacy. The MRI appearance is isointense on T1-weighted images and hyperintense (bright) on T2-weighted images.
(b) T1-weighted arterial phase gadolinium-enhanced MRI scan showing neuroendocrine tumor in the body of the pancreas.

Scintigraphy

Scintigraphy is a technique whereby two-dimensional images of radioactivity in tissues are generated following the intravenous administration of radiopharmaceutical imaging agents. A scintillation camera is used to capture the energy released by the radioactive isotopes.

Thyroid gland. Radioisotopes, such as ^{123}iodine and ^{99m}technetium pertechnetate, are commonly used in thyroid scans to aid in differentiating causes of thyrotoxicosis (*Chapter 3*). They can be administered either orally (^{123}iodine) or intravenously (^{99m}technetium pertechnetate).

A diffuse, generalized homogenous uptake of the radioisotope would be suggestive of Graves disease. A single area of increased uptake (a 'hot' nodule) compared to the rest of the gland would be indicative of a solitary toxic adenoma, whereas a toxic multinodular goiter would appear as multiple areas of increased uptake of radioisotope ('hot' nodules) on the scintigram. An absent or low radioisotope uptake in the thyroid gland indicates thyroiditis, or an extra-thyroidal source should be considered. Areas of non-radioisotope uptake are termed 'cold' nodules and these can include benign causes (80%) such as cysts, inflammatory lesions, hemorrhages, and colloid nodules. The remaining 20% can be malignant (papillary, follicular, medullary, and anaplastic carcinomas). 'Hot' nodules may be associated with a lower incidence of thyroid cancer, although their presence does not exclude malignancy.

Both ^{123}iodine and ^{99m}technetium pertechnetate have short half-lives and maximum thyroid uptake occurs within 30 minutes of intravenous administration of ^{99m}technetium pertechnetate. Foods (i.e. seaweed, kelp), supplements (i.e. multivitamins, cough syrups), and medications (i.e. amiodarone) containing iodine need to be omitted a few days prior to the thyroid scan and patients must be asked if they have had any radiological studies involving the use of iodine-containing contrast in recent weeks. The iodine in these compounds may block the uptake of the radioisotope by the thyroid tissue and affect the thyroid imaging. Anti-thyroid medications (carbimazole, propylthiouracil) may also need to be withheld for a few days prior to the scan.

In ^{123}iodine thyroid scintigraphy, the patient must fast from the night before and the radioisotope can be given as a capsule or liquid to swallow. After 4–6 hours, the patient is asked to lie on the table and the scanner is positioned over the upper chest and neck. Images are taken and then again after 24 hours to obtain a second set of images. For ^{99m}technetium pertechnetate scintigraphy, images can be taken 15–30 minutes after the tracer is injected with a syringe.

Radioisotope scans are not used in pregnant women and it is important to ensure that women of child-bearing age are not pregnant prior to the scan. ^{99m}Technetium pertechnetate, however, can be used in breast-feeding women, although breast feeding needs to be discontinued for the subsequent 24 hours.

Parathyroid glands. ^{99m}Technetium pertechnetate sestamibi scanning was first used in myocardial perfusion studies and has now found a role in pre-operative imaging for localization of abnormal parathyroid tissue. This imaging modality is used in the investigation of primary hyperparathyroidism as suggested by biochemical tests (*Chapter 4*). Sestamibi is a small protein radiolabeled with ^{99m}technetium pertechnetate. It is administered intravenously and absorbed by the overactive parathyroid gland. Images are taken just after administration of the radioisotope and then again approximately 2 hours later. The parathyroid adenoma shows up as a bright spot on the sestamibi scan (*Figure 1.27a*). Sensitivity and specificity vary among institutions but percentages are typically reported as 91% and 99%, respectively.

In cases of biochemical primary hyperparathyroidism and negative sestamibi scans, most patients have a single parathyroid adenoma. In order to aid the endocrine surgeon in minimally invasive parathyroidectomy, further localization can be investigated by thallium subtraction scans, ultrasound scans (*Figure 1. 27b*) and intra-operative jugular venous sampling. Four-dimensional CT scans may provide additional information for the surgical approach.

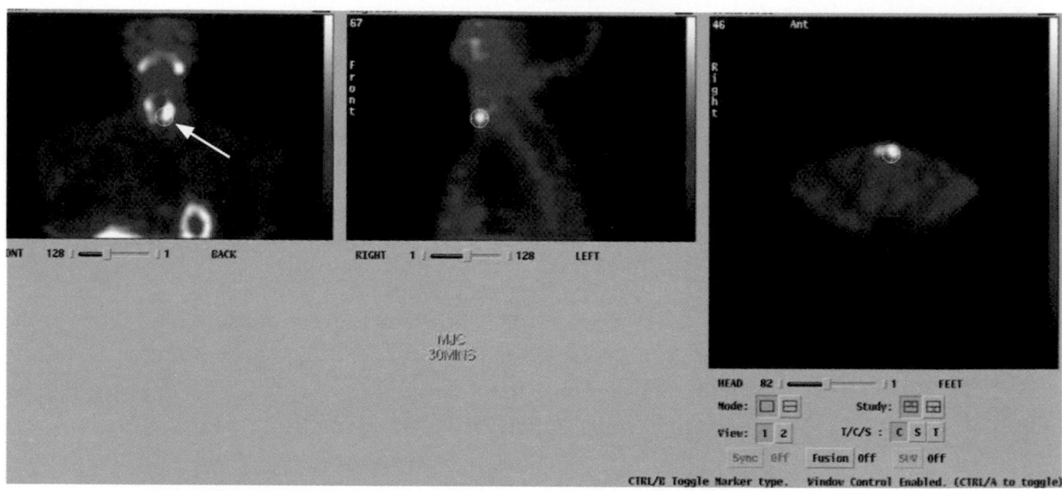

(a)

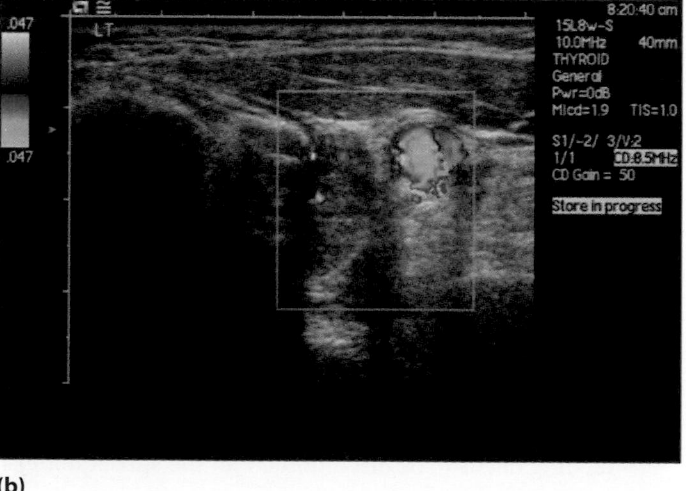

(b)

Figure 1.27. Scintigraphy: sestambi imaging of a parathyroid tumor.
(a) Sestamibi scan demonstrating increased uptake in the region of the lower left pole of the thyroid – this was, in fact, a tumor of a parathyroid gland.
(b) Subsequent ultrasound with color flow Doppler helped to characterize and delineate the lesion.

Adrenal glands. ^{123}Iodine-metaiodobenzylguanidine ([^{123}I]-MIBG) is a guanethidine analog and resembles the neurotransmitter substance nor-epinephrine (nor-adrenaline). It is concentrated in chromaffin cells and is therefore useful in identifying pheochromocytomas, paragangliomas, carcinoid tumors and neuroblastomas. Its sensitivity is 82–88% and specificity is 82–84% in diagnostic assessment of primary and metastatic pheochromocytomas or paragangliomas (*Figure 1.28*). [^{131}I]-MIBG is also a valuable therapeutic adjunct to surgery for malignant pheochromocytomas (see *Chapter 6*).

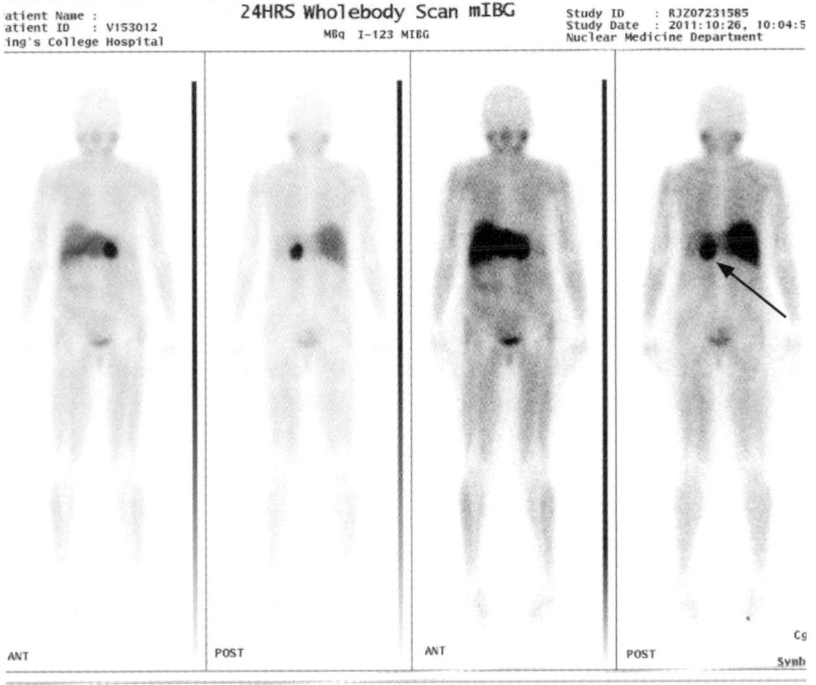

(a)

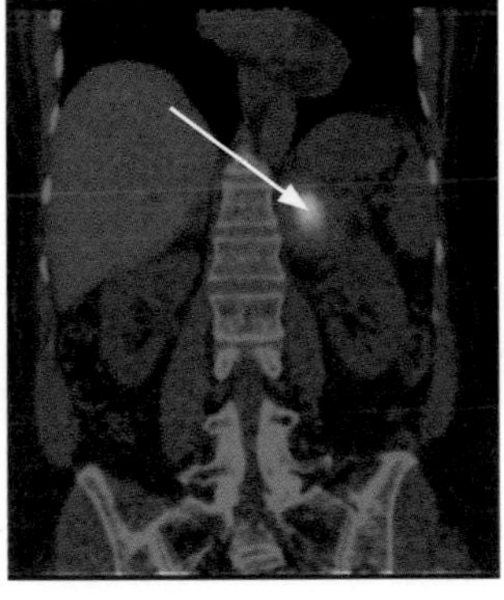

(b)

Figure 1.28. Scintigraphy: [^{123}I]-MIBG scanning of the adrenal gland identifying a pheochromocytoma.
(a) [^{123}I]-MIBG scan demonstrating left-sided pheochromocytoma, best seen on the far right posterior scan (black arrow).
(b) The same patient imaged by whole body [^{123}I]-MIBG with SpeCT and CT co-registered localization (arrow shows pheochromocytoma in left adrenal gland). The other area of uptake represents the physiological uptake of [^{123}I]-MIBG in the liver.

[^{123}I]-MIBG is administered by intravenous injection. The patient is asked to lie on a table under the arm of the scanner. Each scan can take up to 1–2 hours and repeat scans may be required in the subsequent 1–3 days. Before or during the scan, the patient may be given an iodine solution to prevent uptake of the radioisotope by the thyroid gland. Certain medications, including antihypertensive agents, antidepressants, and antipsychotics, need to be stopped for 2–3 weeks prior to the scan as they can affect imaging. Certain foods, including blue-veined cheese and chocolate, should also be avoided on scan days.

^{111}Indium-octreotide scanning and positron emission tomography (PET) with ^{18}fluorodopamine, ^{18}fluorodeoxyglucose, ^{18}fluorodopa or [^{11}C]-hydroxyephedrine are sometimes useful where initial [^{123}I]-MIBG scintigrams have not proved conclusive but clinical suspicion remains, because some studies suggest a marginally higher *sensitivity* (although MIBG is highly *specific*). ^{18}Fluorodeoxyglucose, a PET imaging agent, should not be used for initial diagnostic imaging because it has limited sensitivity and is not specific for pheochromocytomas.

Carcinoid tumors. Studies have shown that most endocrine tumors, especially carcinoid tumors, express a high density of somatostatin receptors. [^{111}In]-pentetreotide or [^{111}In]-DTPA-octreotide (Octreoscan®) are standard somatostatin analogs which bind to normal tissues rich in somatostatin receptors, non-neuroendocrine tumors bearing somatostatin receptors, and primary and metastatic neuroendocrine tumors. Tumors with a high expression of somatostatin receptors include adrenal medullary tumors (*Chapter 6)* and gastroenteropancreatic neuroendocrine tumors: gastrinomas, vasoactive intestinal polypeptide tumors (VIPomas), glucagonomas, insulinomas, and non-functioning tumors (*Chapter 8*). Five human somatostatin receptor subtypes have been cloned so far (SST1–SST5) (*Chapter 8*) and the binding and affinity of ^{111}In-DTPA-octreotide may be dependent on the somatostatin receptor subtypes expressed in different (normal and abnormal) tissues.

[^{111}In]-DTPA-octreotide has been evaluated in several trials, the majority of which have demonstrated high rates of detection of glucagonomas (100%), VIPomas (88%), carcinoids (87%), and non-functioning islet cell tumors (82%). A lower detection rate of 46% was noted for insulinomas and this is thought to be attributed to insulinoma cells containing fewer SST2 somatostatin receptors. There is also reduced sensitivity in poorly differentiated (atypical) carcinoid tumors. Thus somatostatin receptor scintigraphy (SRS) is very useful for the detection, localization, staging and identification of recurrence of neuroendocrine tumors, and is helpful in demonstrating the extent of metastatic disease and extra-hepatic sites which cannot be provided by MRI imaging.

Octreoscan® has a half-life of 3 days and is excreted via the kidneys. This eliminates issues with other radionuclide agents where their normal biliary excretion masks potential hepatic sites of metastatic disease. Hepatic lesions may appear isointense compared to neighboring liver parenchyma. Hence if the SRS appears normal, further single photon emission computed tomography (SPECT) is recommended. The tracer remains within the bloodstream and enables visualization of vascular flow to the metastatic sites. False positives may be seen in patients with respiratory infections, with accumulation of Octreoscan® in pulmonary hilar regions and nasopharynx. It may also occur at recent colostomy or surgical sites and physiological gallbladder activity must not be mistaken for hepatic metastases.

Planar images are usually obtained, using a large-field-of-view gamma camera, 24 hours after intravenous administration of Octreoscan®. Images taken at 4 or 48 hours post-tracer administration is optional. In patients with suspected insulinomas, the risk of hypoglycemia during the SRS is controversial and protocols in institutions should be adhered to.

A multi-modal approach should be adopted in the detection of neuroendocrine tumors which includes CT or MRI imaging, endoscopic ultrasound, SRS, and visceral angiography.

Adrenal vein sampling

In patients with primary aldosteronism, CT imaging of the adrenal glands is performed to identify the presence of an adrenal nodule. However, aldosterone-producing adenomas less than 5 mm in diameter may not be detected by this modality. Patients with biochemical primary aldosteronism and a negative CT scan or bilateral adrenal nodules may only have unilateral adrenal disease.

Adrenal venous sampling is the 'gold standard' test used to help distinguish between unilateral and bilateral adrenal aldosterone hypersecretion. Both adrenal veins and inferior vena cava (IVC) are catheterized in turn via the femoral vein under fluoroscopy guidance. Contrast medium is injected to confirm the site of the catheter tip. Cortisol and aldosterone measurements are obtained from all three sites. The adrenal vein:IVC cortisol concentration ratio should be 3:1 to ensure correct placement. Aldosterone ratios of 4–5 times the opposite side would identify the localized site (left or right adrenal gland) of the aldosterone-producing adenoma. A bolus dose of tetracosactrin (synthetic ACTH; synacthen) may be administered prior to venous sampling to increase cortisol secretion.

Complications of the procedure include groin hematoma, adrenal hemorrhage and adrenal vein dissection. It is an invasive and difficult technique and operator-dependent so correct catheterization may occur in only 75% of patients; however, its diagnostic role is extremely useful in patients suitable for surgery.

PET scans

Positron emission tomography (PET) scans are a type of nuclear medicine scan that gives information about how well the body is functioning rather than its anatomical structure (see *Figure 1.29*). They use an assessment of metabolic processes within the body, for example glucose metabolism or blood flow within tissues. To perform the test radioactive tracer is injected, swallowed, or inhaled depending on the organ being assessed, and then 3D images are constructed to show distribution of this tracer. The radioisotope in the tissue releases gamma rays which are detected by a specialized gamma camera which formulates this information into the 3D images. 'Hot spots' or high uptake areas on images indicate an abnormality.

PET scans are useful for detecting endocrine malignancy, particularly ones which are not obvious on CT or MRI. It is also useful in cancer where the primary

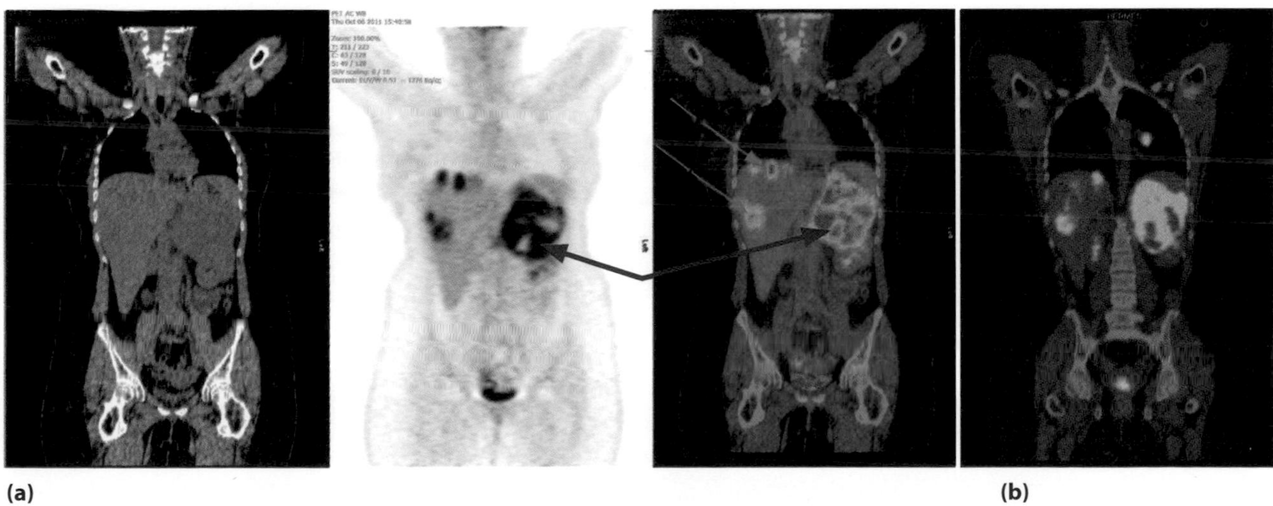

Figure 1.29. Positron emission tomography scans.
Whole body fluorodeoxyglucose PET (a) and CT (b) showing metastatic adrenal carcinoma (red arrows); metastases can be clearly seen in the liver (blue arrows).

CASE 1.1 3 24 31 33 46

- 28 year old woman with increased metabolic rate and a palpable goiter
- Abnormal TFTs
- Check assay
- Check response of pituitary to TRH – no response
- Check suppression of TSH with octreotide – TSH levels reduced
- Suspect pituitary adenoma – confirmation requires imaging
- MRI of pituitary confirms pituitary microadenoma

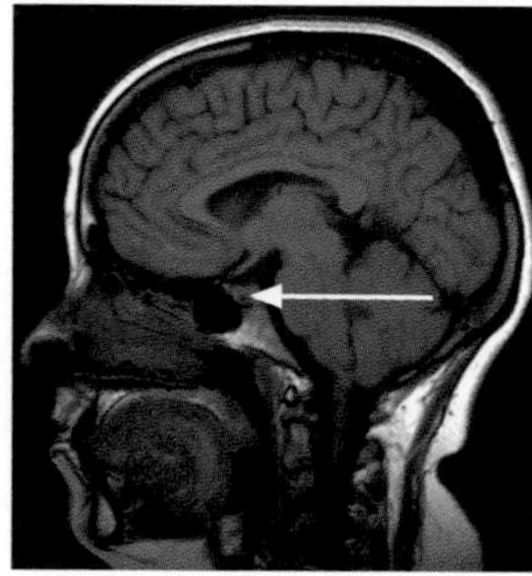

Case figure 1.1. MRI scan of the patient showing a pituitary microadenoma (i.e. an adenoma of <10 mm in maximum diameter) in the anterior pituitary (arrow).

To recap, the patient presented with symptoms of thyrotoxicosis (excess thyroid hormone) and initial tests confirmed this, but with no evidence of a suppressed TSH which would be expected if feedback pathways were intact. Subsequent tests, both basal and dynamic, were strongly suggestive of unregulated TSH excess secretion from the pituitary. The somatostatin analog, octreotide, in a test dose was able to lower TSH secretion. The patient was started on a longer-acting somatostatin analog called lanreotide (*Box 2.3*) which helped control her symptoms while imaging studies were arranged. Because the likely diagnosis of a TSH-secreting pituitary adenoma was highly likely, an MRI scan of the pituitary was carried out first. This confirmed a 9 mm adenoma in the anterior pituitary. As pituitary adenomas are often somatostatin receptor positive (specifically expressing somatostatin receptors 2 and 5, see *Chapter 2*) confirmation was sought with a specific radiolabeled octreotide scan which confirmed high uptake in the pituitary. The patient was discussed at a multidisciplinary pituitary meeting and the decision was made to proceed to surgery (transsphenoidal hypophysectomy). The operation was uncomplicated. Histology confirmed a pituitary adenoma which stained strongly for TSH. Post-operative recovery was uncomplicated and reassessment of basal pituitary hormones revealed no deficit of gonadotropins, growth hormone, ACTH and normal prolactin levels. Posterior pituitary function remained intact with no evidence of loss of arginine vasopressin activity leading to diabetes insipidus (*Chapter 2*). At review 3 months later the patient was asymptomatic, happy and had started a new job and embarked on a new relationship. Off all treatment her thyroid function tests completely normalized, and 18 months later she gave birth to a healthy baby girl.

malignancy is unknown. Fluorodeoxyglucose is used as a radioisotope as well as [^{11}C]-hydroxyephedrine for localization of pheochromocytomas, [^{11}C]-5-hydroxytryptophan, and [^{11}C]-l-dihydroxyphenylalanine for carcinoid tumors and [^{11}C]-metomidate for adrenocortical tumors. Because PET scans give an assessment of function of tissues they can pick up subtle disease before a mass would be seen on CT or MRI. PET is also useful in monitoring for recurrence of disease after treatment. There have been cases where PET scans have been useful in diagnosing ectopic ACTH-releasing carcinoid tumors and for follow-up of thyroid carcinomas after surgery.

1.10 Further reading

Alberts B, Johnson A, Lewis J, Raff M, Roberts K, Walter P (2007) *Molecular Biology of the Cell*, 5th edition. Garland Science. *Chapters 6, 7 and 15 are particularly relevant to endocrinology and the cell signaling (Chapter 15) is well worth a look.*

Herder WW (ed.) (2000) *Functional and Morphological Imaging of the Endocrine System*. Endocrine Updates, Volume 7. Springer-Verlag.

Playfair JHL (2009) *Immunology at a Glance,* 9th edition. Wiley-Blackwell. *This may be useful for understanding the basis for autoimmune diseases of the endocrine system.*

There are two short books on endocrinology which readers might find useful:
Hinson J, Raven P and Chew S (2007) *The Endocrine System,* 2nd edition. Churchill Livingstone.
Porterfield SP and White BA (2007) *Endocrine Physiology,* 3rd edition. Mosby.

Useful websites

You & Your Hormones, a new web-based project by the Society for Endocrinology (UK) that aims to give patients and the general public access to reliable online information on endocrine science: www.youandyourhormones.info

The web site of the Endocrine Society in the USA, useful for Clinical Practice Guidelines: www.endo-society.org

1.11 Self-assessment questions

(1) Which of the following is a steroid hormone?
- (a) Parathyroid hormone
- (b) Vitamin D
- (c) Erythropoietin
- (d) Endothelin
- (e) Thyroxine

(2) What is the half-life of insulin?
- (a) 60 minutes
- (b) Approximately 4 seconds
- (c) 2 hours
- (d) About 4–7 minutes
- (e) Over 3 hours

(3) Which enzyme is responsible for the conversion of pregnenolone to progesterone?
- (a) Aromatase
- (b) 17β-hydroxysteroid dehydrogenase
- (c) 3β-hydroxysteroid dehydrogenase
- (d) Cholesterol side chain cleavage enzyme $P_{450}scc$
- (e) CYP21

(4) Which gland is controlled by hormone secretions of the hypothalamic–pituitary axis?
- (a) Pancreas
- (b) Parathyroid gland
- (c) Thyroid gland
- (d) Adrenal medulla
- (e) Pineal gland

(5) In adaptive immunity, which of the following statements is true?
- (a) Macrophages are activated by pathogens
- (b) Interferon attacks viruses
- (c) Th2 cells differentiate into cytotoxic T cells
- (d) B cells produce antibodies
- (e) Th1 cells are activated by antigen presenting cells

(6) In an enzyme-linked immunosorbent assay (ELISA) the concentration of the hormone in an unknown sample is:
   (a) Directly proportional to the color change
   (b) Measured by binding to a single antibody
   (c) Inversely related to the color change
   (d) Measured by two antibodies that recognize a single epitope
   (e) Measured by the second primary antibody that is labeled with an enzyme

CHAPTER 02 The pituitary gland

After working through this chapter you should be able to:

- Describe the functional anatomy of the hypothalamic–pituitary axis and the hormones produced by the pituitary gland
- Outline the functions of growth hormone and prolactin and the causes, diagnosis, and treatment of an excess or deficiency of their secretions
- Describe the functions of vasopressin and oxytocin and know the pathophysiology and diagnosis of diabetes insipidus
- Outline the etiology, diagnosis, and treatment of hypopituitarism

2.1 Introduction

The pituitary gland is an important endocrine organ, regulating diverse physiological functions including growth, metabolism, reproduction, lactation, and the stress response. The adult pituitary gland consists of the adenohypophysis (anterior and intermediate lobes) and the neurohypophysis (posterior lobe). During development, the anterior and intermediate lobes are distinct structures but in the adult this lobe involutes and the cells become interspersed with cells of the anterior pituitary gland. The anterior lobe (*Figure 2.1*) consists of five different cell types secreting six different hormones:

- thyrotrophs secreting thyroid stimulating hormone (TSH)
- corticotrophs secreting adrenocorticotropic hormone (ACTH)
- gonadotrophs secreting luteinizing hormone (LH) and follicle stimulating hormone (FSH)
- somatotrophs secreting growth hormone (GH)
- lactotrophs secreting prolactin

Cells of the intermediate lobe secrete pro-opiomelanocortin, a precursor to melanocyte stimulating hormone (MSH), MSH, ACTH, and endorphins. The posterior lobe secretes oxytocin and arginine vasopressin (AVP), otherwise known as antidiuretic hormone (ADH).

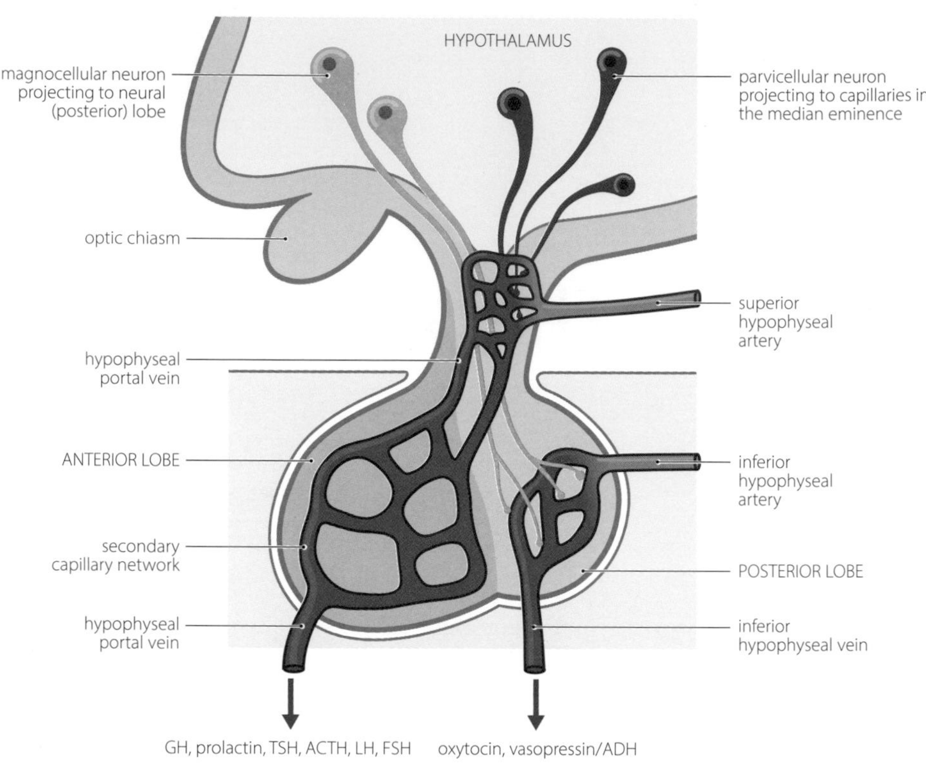

Figure 2.1. Anatomy and functional connections of the hypothalamic–pituitary axis and the hormones secreted by the anterior and posterior lobes of the pituitary gland.
Neurons in the supraoptic and paraventricular nuclei project directly to the posterior lobe. Neurons in other nuclei of the hypothalamus terminate on a capillary network in the median eminence which take up their secretions of stimulatory and inhibitory hormones and transport them to the anterior lobe via the portal veins. Hormone secretions of the anterior lobe are controlled through the secondary capillary bed.

Hormones secreted by the adenohypophysis are controlled by hypothalamic hormones which are released by neurosecretory cells and transported to the anterior lobe by the hypophyseal portal veins (*Table 2.1*). The four trophic hormones, TSH, ACTH, LH, and FSH not only control growth and functional maintenance (hence the term trophic) of the three peripheral target glands, i.e. thyroid, adrenal cortex, and

Table 2.1. **Hypothalamic releasing and inhibitory factors**

Releasing / inhibiting factor	Hypothalamic origin	Function
Corticotropin releasing hormone (CRH)	Paraventricular nucleus	Stimulates ACTH
Dopamine	Arcuate nucleus	Inhibits prolactin/TSH
Growth hormone releasing hormone (GHRH)	Arcuate nucleus	Stimulates GH
Gonadotropin releasing hormone (GnRH)	Preoptic nucleus	Stimulates LH/FSH
Somatostatin release inhibiting factor (SRIF)	Periventricular nucleus	Inhibits GH/TSH
Thyrotropin releasing hormone (TRH)	Paraventricular nucleus	Stimulates TSH / prolactin

gonads, but also control their synthesis and release of hormones. GH and prolactin do not have specific peripheral endocrine gland targets, although some of the actions of GH are mediated by its ability to stimulate the production of insulin-like growth factor-1 (IGF-1) by the liver (see *Figure 2.8*). Similarly hormones secreted by the posterior lobe of the pituitary gland do not target classical endocrine glands.

The four 'trophic' glands are described in detail in *Chapters 3, 6* and *7;* this chapter focuses on the physiology and pathophysiology of GH, prolactin, and the two posterior pituitary hormones, vasopressin and oxytocin.

2.2 Anatomy and embryology

2.2.1 Anatomy

The pituitary gland measures approximately 15 × 10 × 6 mm and weighs about 500–900 mg. The anterior lobe constitutes about two-thirds of the gland's mass. The pituitary sits at the base of the brain in a pocket or fossa of the sphenoid bone, the sella turcica; so named because of its structural likeness to a Turkish horse saddle. Wing-like projections of the sphenoid bone, the anterior and posterior clinoid processes, serve as attachment points of the diaphragma sellae, which is a reflection of the dura mater surrounding the brain. The brain and pituitary gland are surrounded by the dura whilst the arachnoid membrane, which secretes cerebrospinal fluid, is prevented from entering the sella turcica and so the pituitary gland lies outside of the blood–brain barrier (*Figure 2.2*).

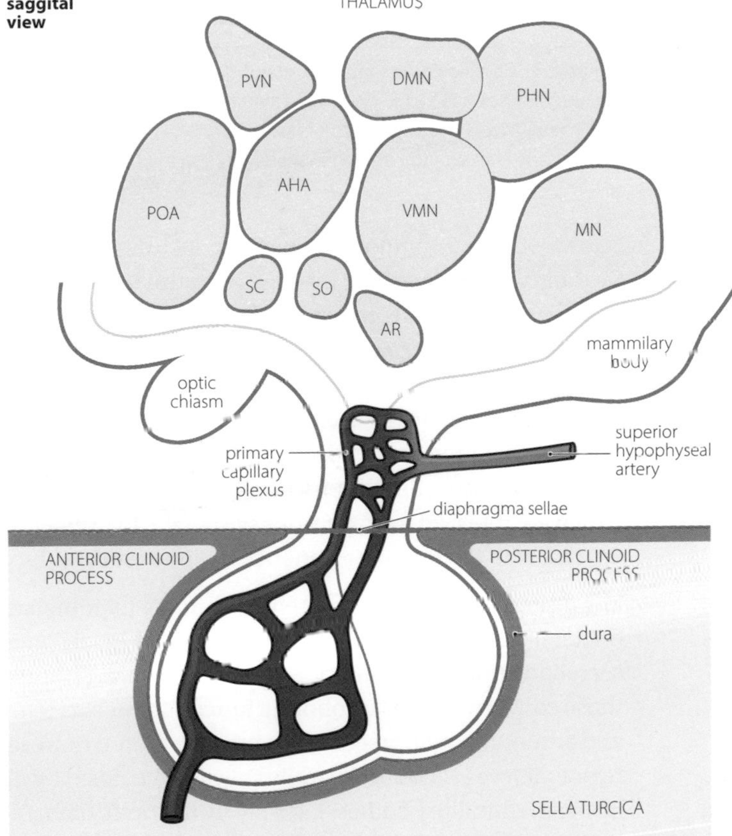

Figure 2.2. Gross anatomy of the hypothalamic–pituitary axis. This diagram shows the major hypothalamic nuclei, the primary capillary plexus in the median eminence and the hypophyseal portal veins which drain into the anterior lobe where they form a secondary capillary plexus. The pituitary gland sits within the sella turcica surrounded by dura mater and is therefore outside the blood–brain barrier. Abbreviations: AHA, anterior hypothalamic area; AR, arcuate nucleus; DMN, dorsomedial nucleus; MB, mammillary body; ME, median eminence; MN, medial nucleus; OC, optic chiasm; PHN, posterior hypothalamic nucleus; POA, preoptic area; PVN, paraventricular nucleus, SC, suprachiasmatic nucleus, SO, supraoptic nucleus; VMN, ventromedial nucleus.

The posterior lobe

The posterior lobe of the pituitary gland is embryologically and anatomically continuous with the hypothalamus: an area of gray matter in the basal part of the forebrain surrounding the third ventricle. Neurons in the supraoptic and paraventricular nuclei of the hypothalamus send axons to the posterior pituitary via the neural stalk and so this lobe of the gland consists of axons and nerve terminals of the hypothalamic neurons. They are surrounded by modified astrocytes known as pituicytes which have an important role in the local control of hormone release.

The anterior lobe

In contrast, the anterior lobe is anatomically distinct and has no direct neural connection with the hypothalamus. It consists of groups of endocrine cells which were initially identified by their ability to take up general histological stains; they were classified as acidophils, basophils, and chromophobes (*Figure 2.3*).

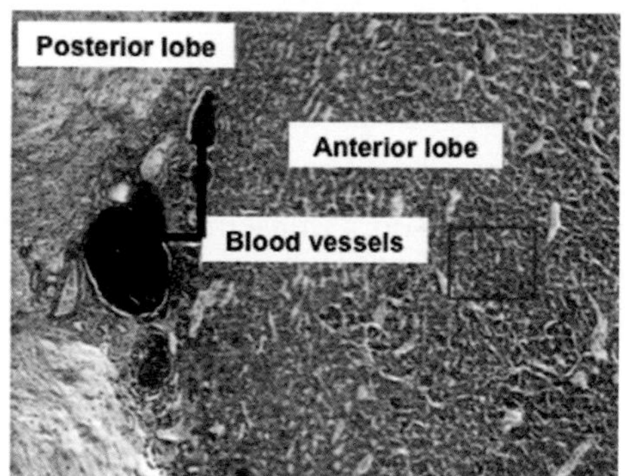

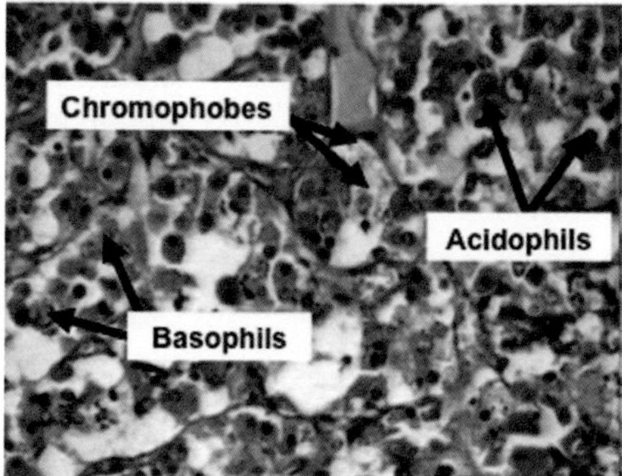

Figure 2.3. Histology of the pituitary gland.
The section has been stained using a modified Azan stain: acidophils stain orange and basophils stain blue/purple; chromophobes take up very little dye. The right-hand section shows a high power microscope image of the area in the red box from the left-hand section.

Subsequently, immunohistochemical techniques allowed classification of cells by their specific secretory products and this showed that there was considerable difference in the percentage of cells secreting GH, prolactin, ACTH, LH, FSH, and TSH (*Table 2.2*). Chromophobes do not secrete identified hormones although these cells contain secretory granules and, like pituicytes, may be important in the local control of hormone release. The functional connection of the anterior lobe with the hypothalamus is via the hypophyseal portal veins. These veins carry distinct stimulatory and/or inhibitory hormones for each pituitary hormone (*Table 2.1*), which are released from neurons of specific hypothalamic nuclei whose axons terminate in the median eminence in apposition to the capillaries (*Figure 2.1*).

The discrete groups of nerve cells within the hypothalamus, the nuclei, are arranged bilaterally around the third ventricle. Those nuclei concerned with hormone secretions from the pituitary gland tend to be distributed more medially, whilst those concerned with autonomic functions such as temperature regulation and adrenomedullary secretions are distributed more laterally. As a whole the hypothalamus is bound rostrally (toward the nose) by the optic chiasm, caudally by the mammillary bodies, laterally by the optic tracts, and dorsolaterally by the thalamus (*Figure 2.2*).

Table 2.2. Major cell types and secretory products of the pituitary gland

Cell type	Secretory products	Cell population (approx. %)
Anterior pituitary		
Somatotroph	Growth hormone	50
Lactotroph	Prolactin	15
Corticotroph	Adrenocorticotropic hormone	15
Thyrotroph	Thyroid stimulating hormone	10
Gonadotroph	Luteinizing hormone / follicle stimulating hormone	10
Posterior pituitary		
Axon terminals of hypothalamic neurons	Vasopressin and oxytocin	

It is important clinically to note that the optic chiasm lies about 5 mm above the diaphragma sellae and that the pituitary gland sits in a restricted pocket of the sphenoid bone. Thus any abnormal growth of the pituitary gland can cause compression of the gland and loss of function as well as upward compression toward the hypothalamus causing visual field defects. Visual defects and structural damage to the hypothalamus only occur with pituitary growths that are large enough to compromise the optic chiasm and extend out of the sella. These large tumors (>10 mm in maximum diameter) are termed macroadenomas, whilst microadenomas (<10 mm) may go undetected unless they are secreting sufficient hormone to result in identifiable clinical features.

The anterior pituitary gland is richly vascularized by the portal veins; these receive their arterial blood from the carotid arteries via the superior hypophyseal arteries which form a primary network of capillaries in the median eminence. These then recombine to form the portal veins carrying blood to the anterior pituitary gland. The pituitary stalk and the posterior pituitary gland receive their blood supply directly from branches of the middle and inferior hypophysial arteries whilst the hypothalamus receives its blood supply from the circle of Willis.

Hormones from the anterior lobe of the pituitary gland reach the systemic circulation via various routes, but veins from the lobe eventually drain into the cavernous sinus, then to the superior and inferior petrosal sinuses and finally to the jugular vein. Blood sampling from the petrosal sinuses can be useful in locating the site of hormone-secreting adenomas of the anterior pituitary gland. Venous drainage of the posterior gland is into the posterior lobe veins and hence into the general circulation, although some capillaries in the neural stalk form 'short' portal veins that drain into the anterior pituitary gland (see *Figure 2.1*).

2.2.2 Embryology

The pituitary gland is formed from neural and oral ectoderm. Between 4 and 6 weeks' gestation there is a thickening of the roof of the oral cavity forming

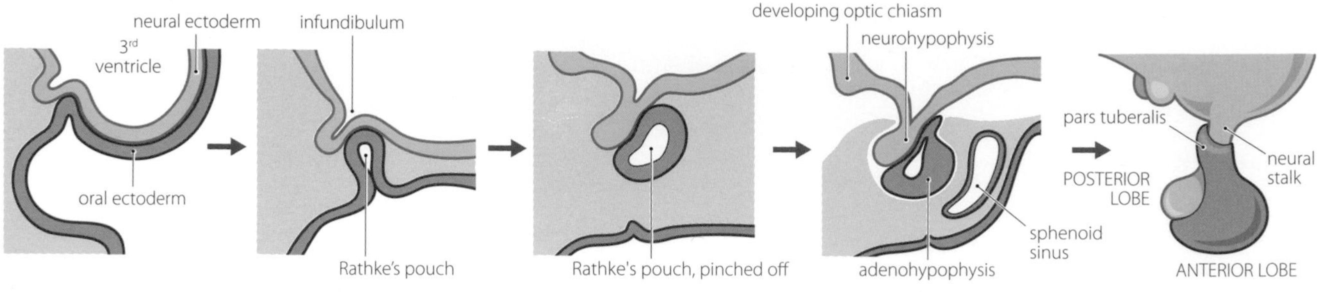

Figure 2.4. Embryology of the pituitary gland.

the pituitary placode. Invagination of this oropharynx (oral ectoderm) forms a rudimentary pouch, Rathke's pouch, which makes contact with an evagination of the floor of the third ventricle of the brain (the neural ectoderm) which forms the neural stalk and the posterior pituitary (*Figure 2.4*). This contact is essential to early development of the pituitary gland and involves activation of transcription factors and expression of signaling molecules which allow communication between the oral and neural ectoderm. Rathke's pouch is eventually pinched off from the oral cavity and becomes separated by the sphenoid bone of the skull. The lumen of the pouch is reduced to a small cavity whilst the upper portion of the pouch surrounds the neural stalk and forms the pars tuberalis. Together with the anterior lobe, the pars tuberalis forms the adenohypophysis. Progenitor cells of Rathke's pouch proliferate and then undergo terminal differentiation. This differentiation is dependent on the timely expression of various transcription factors which determine whether cells will become somatotrophs, lactotrophs, thyrotrophs, gonadotrophs, or corticotrophs. When some cells from Rathke's pouch are left behind they can form tumors known as craniopharyngiomas (see *Section 2.3*).

The lumen of the pouch, formed by the downward evagination of the third ventricle (neural ectoderm) fuses to form the neural stalk, whilst the upper portion of the pouch forms a recess in the floor of the third ventricle, the median eminence. The neural stalk together with the median eminence form the infundibular stem and this, together with the posterior lobe, is collectively called the neurohypophysis.

Transcription factors involved in the development of the pituitary gland include HESX1, PROP1, POU1F1, LHX3, LHX4, PITX1, PITX2, SOX2, and SOX3 and mutations of the genes that code for these transcription factors in humans can lead to congenital hypopituitarism. For example, mutations in *POU1F1* cause GH, TSH, and prolactin deficiencies, and mutations of *PROP1* cause deficiencies of all anterior pituitary hormones. Many other mutations of genes coding for transcription factors involved in the development of the pituitary gland have been identified, giving a variety of abnormalities in hormone secretions and different phenotypes. Thus normal pituitary development is totally dependent on the sequential expression of numerous genes and close signaling interactions between Rathke's pouch and the neural ectoderm (*Figure 2.5*).

Like the development of the pituitary gland, the development of the ventral diencephalon and the neurosecretory cells in the hypothalamus (that control hormone secretions from the anterior pituitary gland) are also under the control

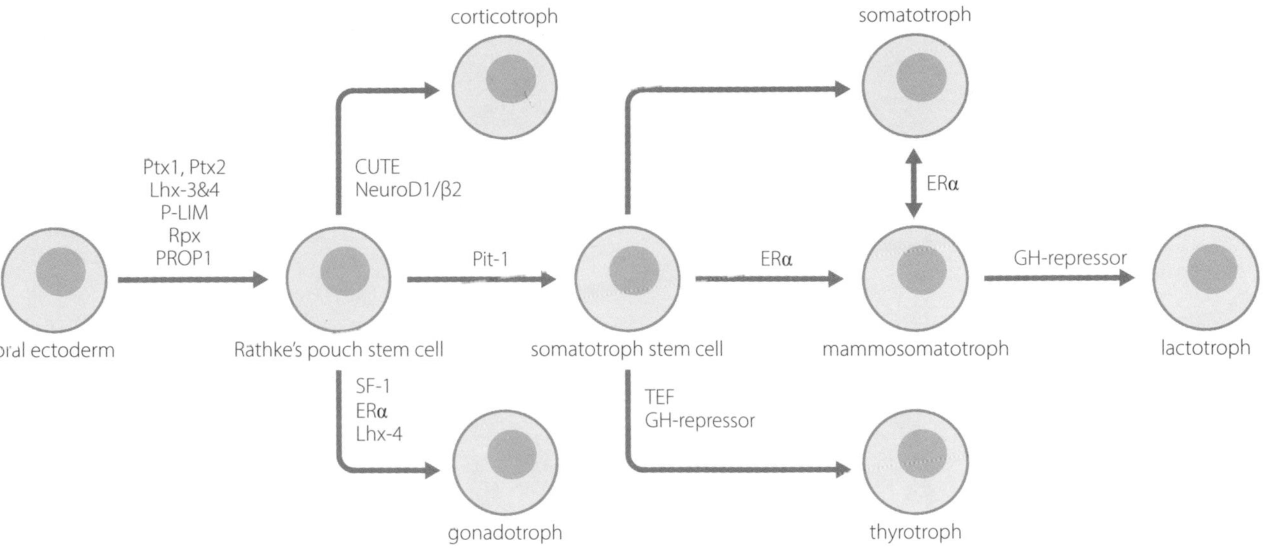

Figure 2.5. Transcription factors involved in the differentiation of different cell types of the anterior lobe of the pituitary gland.

The differentiation of cell types in the anterior lobe of the pituitary gland from the oral ectoderm is controlled by timely expression of a number of genes including those that code for transcription factors. The development of Rathke's pouch involves the expression of early genes as shown. Development of the corticotrophs probably involves the gene *CUTE* (corticotroph upstream transcription binding element) and the CUTE-binding proteins NeuroD1/beta2. This is followed by the development of somatotrophs controlled by Pit-1/POUF-1. Under the influence of estrogen receptor alpha (ERα) and perhaps a GH repressor, somatotroph stem cells can differentiate into lactotrophs. The differentiation of gonadotrophs occurs along a different pathway, with the expression of SF-1 (steroidogenic factor-1) in conjunction with ERα, inducing the development of gonadotrophs from the stem cells of Rathke's pouch.

of a series of transcription factors including Sim1, Otp, Nkx2-1, SF1, and SOX3. Sequential expression of the genes coding for these transcription factors determines the development of different nuclei within the hypothalamus and the fate of neurons that specifically regulate the secretion of prolactin, GH, ACTH, TSH, and the gonadotropins, LH and FSH.

2.2.3 Craniopharyngioma

Craniopharyngiomas are solid or mixed solid/cystic tumors that arise in the region of the sella turcica and are **usually** derived from remnants of Rathke's pouch. They are histologically benign but should probably be regarded as low grade malignancies. They vary in size from small, solid, well-circumscribed masses to huge multilocular cystic lesions that can damage neighboring intracranial structures (*Figure 2.6*). The size of craniopharyngiomas, as evaluated by CT or MRI, has been reported to be larger than 4 cm in 14–20% of cases, 2–4 cm in 58–70% of cases, and smaller than 2 cm in 4–28% of cases. The cysts are filled with cholesterol-containing fluid that is sometimes described as being like engine oil. Malignant transformation is rare but has been reported, particularly in recurrent cases or after incomplete courses of radiotherapy.

The WHO classification of craniopharyngiomas suggests two main categories:

- adamantinomatous craniopharyngiomas (most prevalent in children) and derived from embryonic remnants of Rathke's pouch

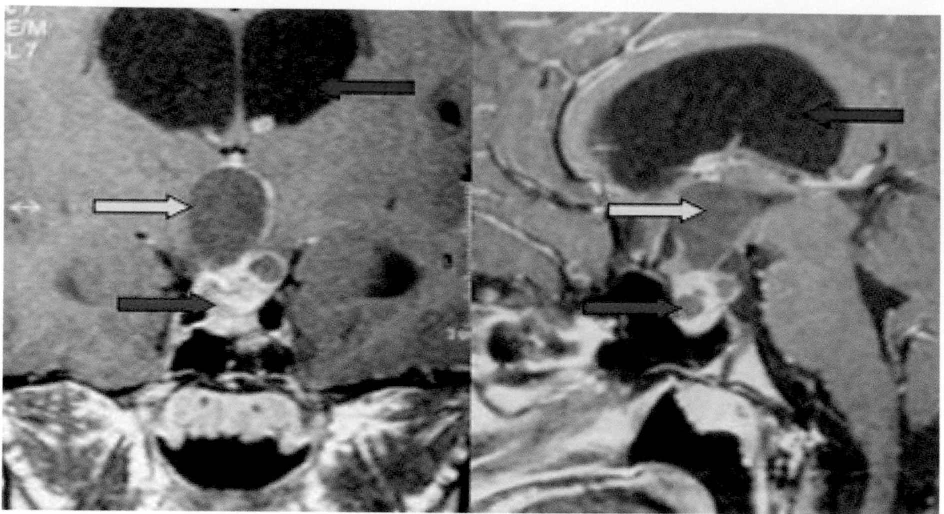

Figure 2.6. MRI scan of a craniopharyngioma.
Yellow arrows point to the cyst; red arrows to the solid part of the tumor; and blue arrows to a dilated lateral ventricle (hydrocephalus).

- papillary craniopharyngiomas (which account for only about 2% of childhood craniopharyngiomas, but up to 50% of adulthood craniopharyngiomas) are derived from metaplastic foci of mature cells of the adenohypophysis.

The histologic subtypes seem to have little difference in terms of survival or tumor progression or, indeed, in response to radiotherapy.

Incidence

Craniopharyngiomas account for about 9% of all intracranial tumors in childhood, and are the most common peripituitary tumor in this age group. In the USA, there are an estimated 350 new cases of craniopharyngioma diagnosed each year (1–3% of all brain tumors). Higher rates have been reported in Japan and Africa. Sex distribution is equal, but there is a bimodal age distribution, with one peak in children between 5 and 14 years, and a second peak in adults between 50 and 75 years. Papillary craniopharyngiomas are more common in adults whereas adamantinomatous craniopharyngiomas are more common in children.

Symptoms and signs

In childhood, craniopharyngiomas may grow relatively rapidly causing more symptoms and being challenging to treat. Symptoms and signs may be due to a rise in intracranial pressure:

- headache – especially early morning (mass effect or hydrocephalus)
- nausea and vomiting (accompanying pressure-related headaches)
- visual field defect (pressure effects on optic chiasm and tracts)

and/or due to destruction of anterior and posterior pituitary tissue with concomitant loss of hormones:

- slow growth during childhood (GH and/or TSH deficiency)
- delayed or arrested puberty, and very occasional precocious puberty

- diabetes insipidus – polyuria and polydipsia (AVP deficiency)
- fatigue (possibly related to cortisol and/or TSH deficiency)
- cold intolerance, constipation, slow pulse, dry skin (TSH/T_4 deficiency)
- sexual dysfunction and amenorrhea in adults (LH/FSH deficiency)

Diagnosis and treatment

A cystic calcified parasellar lesion seen on MRI and CT imaging is very likely to be a craniopharyngioma. It is often useful to compare MRI with CT (which is better at showing calcification) when a suspicious lesion is seen. Around 60% of patients with craniopharyngioma will have calcification in the sellar/suprasellar area and about 75% will show evidence of cysts (*Figure 2.6*). In patients without classical imaging findings, the diagnosis can only be completely confirmed histologically following resection or biopsy. The differential diagnosis includes any of the myriad lesions that may occur in the region of the pituitary (*Box 2.1*).

Box 2.1 | Tumors occurring in the area of the pituitary

- Pituitary macroadenoma
- Craniopharyngioma
- Meningioma
- Optic glioma
- Germinoma
- Teratoma
- Lymphoma
- Metastases
- Non-neoplastic cyst (Rathke's, pars intermedia, and arachnoid)
- Granulomatous lesions, e.g. sarcoidosis and systemic histiocytosis

Treatment is by a combination of relatively aggressive neurosurgery in an attempt to remove the bulk of the tumor followed by radiotherapy. Prior to surgery endocrine dysfunction should be managed by appropriate hormone replacement. Hydrocephalus can be treated with either temporary or permanent shunts. The transphenoidal approach with endoscopic aid can be used for sellar and suprasellar tumors but in some cases a craniotomy is required (*Figure 2.7*).

Advances in radiotherapy have allowed a more targeted approach with less damage to surrounding structures. Techniques such as stereotactic radiotherapy and radiosurgery, intensity modulated radiation therapy (IMRT), and proton beam therapy have increased the cure rate and reduced recurrence rates. Alternatives or adjuncts to conventional external irradiation include intracavity irradiation (with radioisotopes such as phosphorus-32 or yttrium-90) or intracavity chemotherapy (with bleomycin). Cysts can be difficult to deal with and they have a habit of recurring. Aspiration of cyst contents may help alleviate symptoms – an alternative is to place a reservoir to allow intermittent aspiration of persistent cysts.

Following treatment, patients require long-term follow-up (with imaging and endocrine function testing) to look for evidence of recurrence or hypothalamic/pituitary deficit as a result of the condition or its treatment. Panhypopituitarism (see *Section 2.5.1*) is not uncommon and requires adequate hormone replacement. Hypothalamic dysfunction may also result in impaired appetite regulation with

(a)

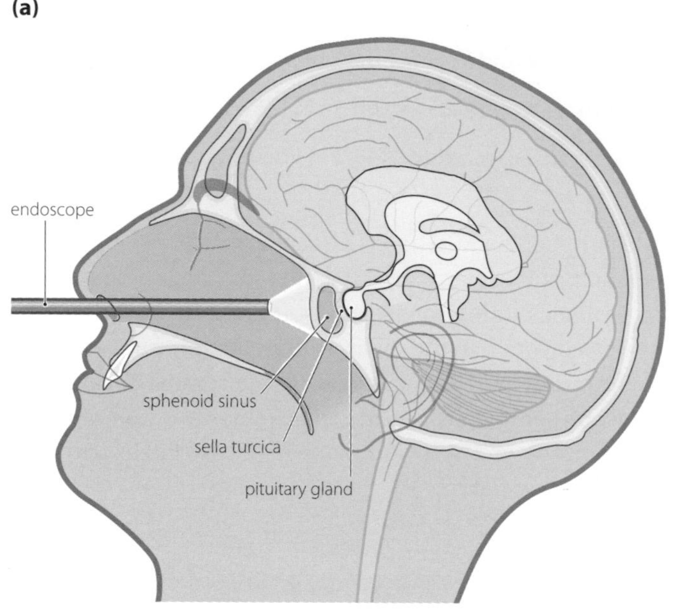

(b)

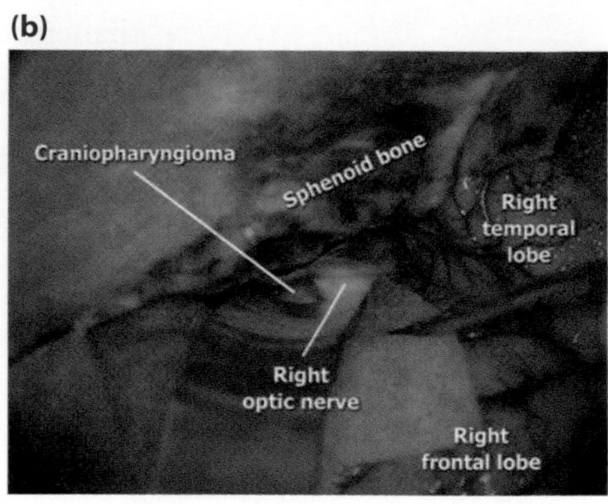

Figure 2.7. (a) Transsphenoidal surgery and (b) an intra-operative photograph during removal of craniopharyngioma using a pterional craniotomy.

development of obesity, disorders of temperature and sleep regulation or diabetes insipidus. Behavioral disorders and impairment of intellectual functioning are frequent in children with craniopharyngiomas. After treatment, visual defects, often present at diagnosis, may worsen or improve and the development of new malignant glial tumors has been reported following radiotherapy treatment of craniopharyngiomas. Recurrent disease is a common problem, either local or distant, possibly as a result of seeding through the cerebrospinal fluid during surgery.

2.3 Basic physiology of growth hormone

CASE 2.1

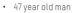

- 47 year old man
- Prognathism, overbite, and wide interdental spacing
- Increasing size of head, hands, and feet
- ? Acromegaly

A 47 year old male motor cycle despatch rider was referred to the endocrinologist by his dentist. He had complained of temporo-mandibular joint pain and the dentist had noted a marked overbite with wide interdental spacing. Over the last few years (particularly when reviewing pictures from his youth) he had noticed marked facial change with prognathism (jaw protrusion), a broadening and enlargement of the nasal bridge and frontal bossing. On direct questioning he admitted that he could no longer wear his wedding ring and his motor cycle boot size had increased. He had tried to return his motor cycle crash helmet to the manufacturers as he claimed it had shrunk in the rain! On examination, all the above facial features were noted. He had a small non-vascular goiter, was hypertensive (blood pressure 155/100) and had soft 'doughy' hands with greasy skin.

Acromegaly was suspected and he underwent confirmatory tests including circulating IGF-1 estimation, an oral glucose tolerance test (*Figure 1.17*) to look for adequate suppression of growth hormone, and measurement of other anterior pituitary hormones.

Case 2.1 illustrates the slow physical changes that occur in acromegaly due to an excess secretion of GH. The disease has an insidious onset and it may be several years before there is sufficient alteration in physical appearance to even suspect acromegaly. The changes that do occur, however, are not surprising knowing the actions of GH.

2.3.1 Actions of growth hormone

The major functions of GH are growth promoting and metabolic, some of which are due to direct actions of GH on target tissues, whilst others are mediated by GH-stimulated production of IGF-1 in the liver. Like GH, circulating IGF-1 is bound to IGF-binding proteins with less than 1% of the total IGF-1 existing in free form. Such binding prolongs the half-life of IGF-1 and regulates the availability of 'free' IGF-1 which can interact with target tissues.

The actions of GH are as follows, with further details given in *Box 2.2.*

- Promotion of somatic growth.
- Growth plate elongation (longitudinal growth) and increased bone mass post-natally and throughout puberty.

Box 2.2 | Actions of growth hormone

GH receptors are highly expressed in liver, skeletal muscle, adipose tissue, cartilage, heart, kidney, intestine, lung and pancreas.

Metabolic actions in liver, skeletal muscle and adipose tissue (see also *Figures 5.3–5.7*)

- Liver – GH stimulates triglyceride uptake by increasing the expression of lipoprotein lipase and/or hepatic lipase and promotes storage of triglycerides. It also antagonizes insulin signaling in the liver and stimulates hepatic glucose production.
- Skeletal muscle – GH stimulates triglyceride uptake by increasing lipoprotein lipase expression. The lipids are either stored as intramyocellular triglycerides or undergo lipolysis or lipid oxidation to produce energy.
- Adipose tissue – GH triggers lipolysis by activation of hormone-sensitive lipase, thereby releasing free fatty acids into the circulation. This effect is predominantly in visceral adipose tissue and, to a lesser extent, in the subcutaneous fat. GH also reduces glucose uptake into adipocytes, an action which may be mediated by its ability to antagonize insulin signaling, and induces the differentiation of pre-adipocytes into mature adipocytes.

Protein metabolism

GH has a net anabolic effect on protein metabolism, stimulating protein synthesis and inhibiting proteolysis. This action is probably mediated by IGF-1.

Insulin resistance

GH induces insulin resistance, but the mechanism causing this effect is not completely understood.

Skeletal growth and bone homeostasis

GH and IGF-1 are important regulators of bone homeostasis and although GH may act directly on bone, most of its actions are mediated by IGF-1. Postnatally and throughout puberty GH and IGF-1 play a critical role in longitudinal growth, stimulating division of chondrocytes and the formation of endochondrial bone; thus children with GH deficiency will have a short stature. GH and IGF-1 stimulate the proliferation and differentiation of osteoblasts (see *Section 2.5*), and they play an important role in bone modeling by depositing matrix at the outer surface of cortical bone, thereby increasing bone width and skeletal strength. This is particularly important in late adolescence and early adulthood, periods which are important in acquiring peak bone mass. Bone remodeling is also stimulated by GH/IGF-1 and GH deficiency in adults causes low bone turnover (leading to osteoporosis) whilst excess GH (acromegaly) is associated with high bone turnover (leading to bone loss).

- Maintenance of bone mass in adults.
- IGF-1 generation in peripheral tissues, primarily the liver.
- Production of a subunit of the ternary complex comprising IGF-1 or -2, IGFBP-3, and the acid labile subunit (ALS). This is a large molecular weight complex which 'holds' IGF in the circulation and markedly extends its half-life.
- Nitrogen retention.
- Amino acid transport into muscle.
- Lipolysis.
- Insulin antagonism and increasing blood glucose levels.
- Sodium and phosphate retention.

2.3.2 Synthesis and secretion of GH

A cluster of genes on chromosome 17 code for different isoforms of GH. Two genes encode variants of GH and are named *GH1* (or *GH-N*) and *GH2* (or *GH-V*) and two other genes, *CS1* and *CS2*, encode chorionic somatomammotropin (CS), otherwise known as placental lactogen. *GH2*, *CS1*, and *CS2* are expressed in the placenta, whilst *GH1* is expressed in the pituitary gland and gives rise to a 191 amino acid 22 kDA protein (22K-GH) with two disulfide bridges. Another isoform derived from the *GH1* gene by alternate splicing of mRNA is a similar protein, but with only 176 amino acids and a molecular weight of 20 kDA (20K-GH). The major isoform secreted by the pituitary gland is the 22K-GH form. GH circulates bound to a GH-binding protein which is a truncated soluble form of the GH receptor and which is mainly synthesized in the liver. Although the function of this binding protein is not completely understood, it may prolong the half-life of GH or reduce its availability to the GH receptor. GH acts on two single chain trans-membrane receptors and binding of GH leads to dimerization of two receptors and subsequent activation of the JAK/STAT pathway (see *Figure 1.8e*).

Control of GH secretion

The synthesis and release of GH is primarily controlled by two hormones secreted by hypothalamic neurosecretory cells and transported to the anterior pituitary gland via the hypophyseal portal veins:

- GH releasing hormone (GHRH) stimulates GH production via a GPCR that activates cAMP and increases intracellular calcium, whilst somatostatin inhibits GH production by inhibiting cAMP generation and therefore reduces intracellular calcium concentrations.
- somatostatin-14 inhibits both GH and TSH secretion (*Figure 2.8*); five G-protein linked somatostatin receptors (SSTRs) have been identified and the major subtypes expressed in the adult anterior pituitary gland are SSTR2 and SSTR5; somatostatin is also widely expressed in other parts of the body (*Box 2.3*).

Ghrelin, a major orexigenic factor produced by the gastrointestinal tract (see *Chapter 8*), is also an endogenous inducer of GH and acts directly on somatotrophs to release GH as well as on the hypothalamus to modulate GHRH secretion. In addition, GH production is under the influence of other hormonal signals, being stimulated by thyroid hormones and sex steroids and inhibited by glucocorticoids. The negative

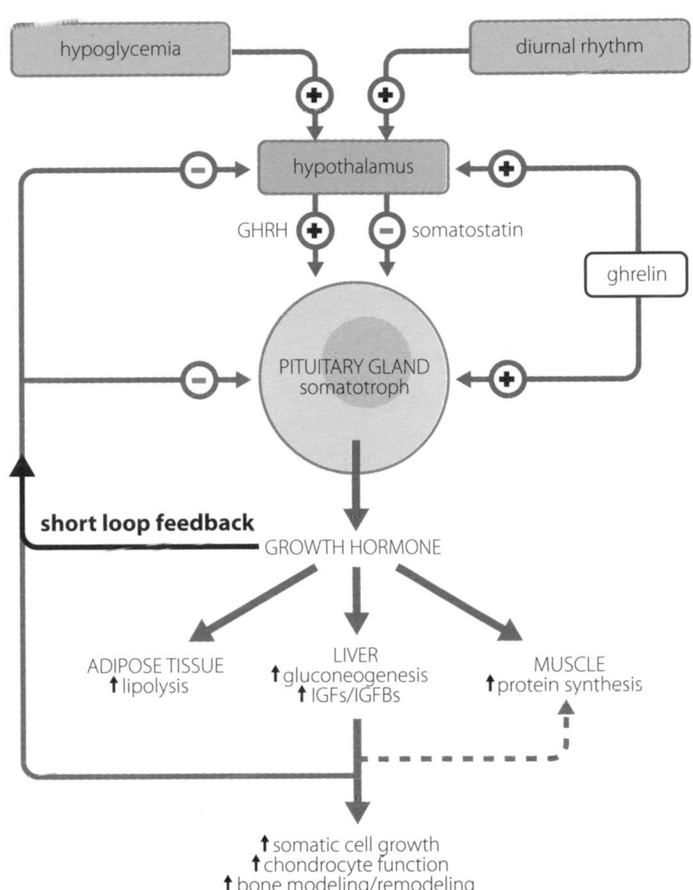

Figure 2.8. Control of growth hormone secretion.

feedback effects on the control of GH secretion are via IGF-1 released by the liver and by a 'short'-loop feedback of GH onto the hypothalamus, although distinguishing between these two feedback loops has been difficult to delineate. Hypoglycemia is a stimulus to GH secretion, whilst hyperglycemia has the opposite effect (*Figure 2.8*).

Under the influence of GHRH and somatostatin, GH is secreted in a pulsatile manner. In the adult human approximately five pulses of GH are secreted during a 24 hour period, with the largest peak occurring at the onset of sleep at night (*Figure 2.9*). Between the peaks, GH concentrations in the circulation are very low. High and sustained levels of GH can result from GH-secreting pituitary adenomas which, if left untreated, can cause gigantism in children and acromegaly in adults.

Serum GH rises after birth with a peak period of secretion during puberty. Levels then decline with age, reaching a nadir by the sixth decade of life such that GH concentrations in older men will have decreased to just 5–20% of that observed in young adults. This decline is more rapid in men than women and the loss of GH and IGF-1 are matched by a progressive loss of muscle mass and strength, an increase in body fat and a decrease in bone mineral density.

2.4 Excess growth hormone – acromegaly

Acromegaly (from the Greek: *akros* – extreme/extremity and *megal* – large) is a rare condition characterized by excess unregulated GH secretion and is nearly always

Box 2.3 | Somatostatin and therapeutic use of analogs

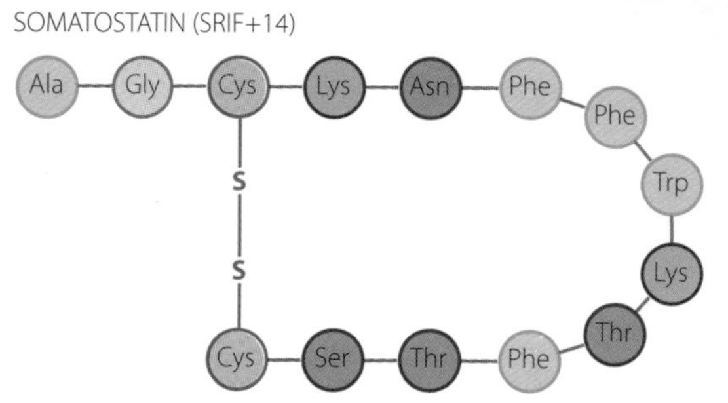

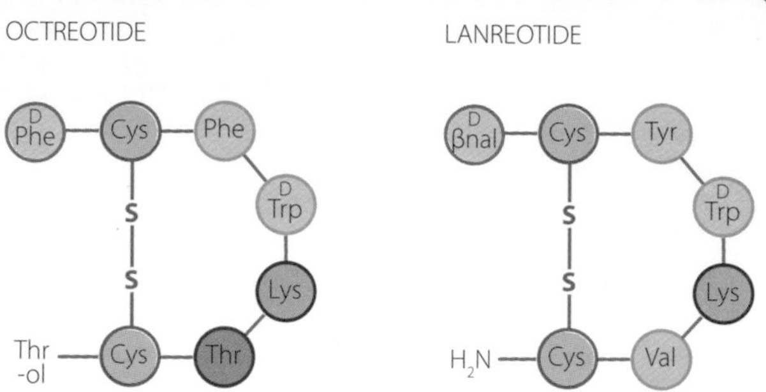

Box figure 2.1. Peptide structure of somatostatin and two long-acting analogs, octreotide and lanreotide.
D-tryptophan (DTrp) is a nonphysiological amino acid which stabilizes the molecule, reduces enzymatic degradation, and prolongs half-life.

Somatostatin (*Box figure 2.1*) or somatotropin release-inhibiting factors (SRIFs) are cleaved from pro-somatostatin to produce either SRIF-14 (14 amino acids) or SRIF-28 which has an additional 14 amino acids at the N-terminus of the molecule. SRIFs are produced in the brain, gastrointestinal tract, liver, pancreas, lungs, immune system, kidneys, adrenal glands, and urogenital tract. Neurosecretory cells in the hypothalamus secrete SRIF-14 into the hypophyseal portal capillaries and this inhibits the release of GH and TSH from the anterior pituitary gland. SRIF from the brain can also inhibit the release of hypothalamic hormones including CRH and TRH. In the gastrointestinal tract SRIFs inhibit the secretion of hormones including insulin, glucagon, gastrin, cholecystokinin, vasoactive intestinal peptide and secretin, as well as exocrine secretions including gastric acid, pepsin and pancreatic enzymes. There are five SRIF receptor subtypes (SSTR1–5), which are typical GPCRs and ubiquitously expressed; in the adult anterior pituitary gland the major subtypes expressed are SSTR2 and 5.

Released SRIF is rapidly inactivated by tissue and blood peptidases and its half-life is about 2 minutes. This limits its therapeutic use. However, long-acting, stable analogs of somatostatin have been developed and are used to treat acromegaly and symptoms arising from gastroenteropancreatic (GEP) tumors (see *Chapter 8*). Octreotide and lanreotide (*Box figure 2.1*) are long-acting analogs of somatostatin that have been clinically approved; they have a high affinity for SSTR2 and a lower affinity for SSTR5. Other analogs such as pasireotide are currently undergoing clinical trials and further analogs are being developed with the aim of obtaining receptor-specific stable analogs of SRIF (for further details see *Section 2.4.2*).

In acromegaly, somatostatin analogs inhibit the excess GH secretion in about 80% of cases and may also reduce the size of the pituitary adenoma. In the different types of gut neuroendocrine tumors such as insulinomas, glucagonomas, gastrinomas, and VIPomas (see *Chapter 8*), treatment with somatostatin analogs inhibits the excess hormone secretions and helps to relieve symptoms associated with such tumors.

(about 99%) due to a benign pituitary adenoma. Very rarely acromegaly may occur as a result of unregulated GHRH secretion, or ectopic GH from non-endocrine sources. Around 5% of cases are familial occurring as part of multiple endocrine neoplasia (MEN-1; see *Section 8.5*), familial acromegaly, Carney's complex, or McCune–Albright syndrome. Figures suggest an incidence of acromegaly in the USA and UK of around 4 cases per million and a prevalence of between 50 and 60 per million. There is an equal sex distribution and most cases are diagnosed between the ages of 45 and 55 years. Mortality is significantly increased compared with the normal population, historically as a result of complications of heart disease, diabetes (secondary to GH-induced insulin resistance) and respiratory disorders. Long-term exposure to

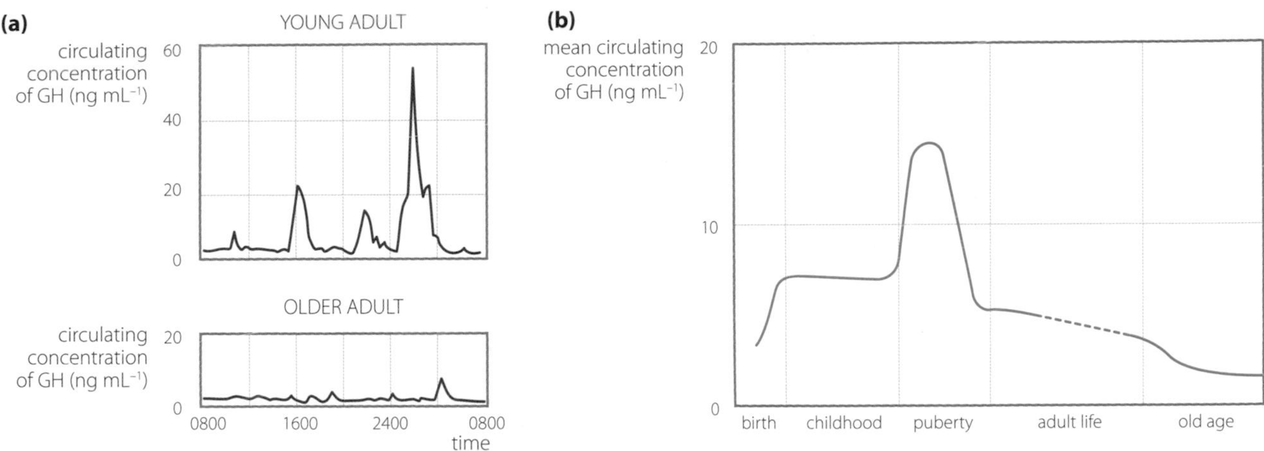

Figure 2.9. (a) Diurnal fluctuations of growth hormone and (b) changes in the mean concentration of growth throughout life.
(a) Growth hormone is secreted in a pulsatile manner during the day, with larger peaks occurring with the onset of sleep. (b) Mean GH levels decline with age and this is the result of smaller pulses of GH secretion.

uncontrolled levels of GH and IGF-1 (a potent mitogenic, anti-apoptotic hormone) results in an increase in the relative risk of cancer (particularly of the colon).

The majority of adenomas (around 70%) resulting in GH excess are macroadenomas (>10 mm in maximum diameter). Acromegaly is an insidious condition and has usually been present for several years prior to presentation. It is often informative to look through previous photographs of patients where changes due to acromegaly may be seen developing over the years (*Box 2.5*). The diagnosis is often suggested by healthcare professionals other than endocrinologists who recognize the classical facies and body habitus.

2.4.1 Symptoms and signs of acromegaly

Headache is a common presenting feature of acromegaly and is often unrelated to the size of the adenoma. Visual field defects occur in up to 20% of patients at presentation and hypogonadism resulting in amenorrhea or loss of libido may be another presenting feature. The hypogonadism can occur as a result of a deficiency of gonadotropins due to mass effects of the adenoma, i.e. as it grows the tumor inhibits normal anterior pituitary function resulting in a loss of gonadotropin activity (gonadotropins are amongst the first of the anterior pituitary hormones to be lost as a result of tumor expansion). Hypogonadism may also occur as a result of co-secretion of prolactin (which occurs in up to 25% of GH-secreting adenomas; prolactin excess results in gonadotropin insufficiency), or of stalk compression resulting in elevated levels of prolactin due to inability of dopamine (prolactin-inhibiting-factor) to exert its effects in the anterior pituitary. Many of the other symptoms and signs of acromegaly (*Box 2.4*) are related to elevated levels of GH, either directly or through generation of IGF-1.

Facial changes lead to a coarsening of the general appearance with widening of the nose, thicker lips and macroglossia, and development of frontal bossing (increase in

Box 2.4 | Symptoms and signs of acromegaly

Symptoms and signs (see also *Box figure 2.2*) are shown in descending order of frequency

- Facial change, enlargement of the extremities (e.g. hands/ feet), soft tissue swelling
- Sweating
- Carpal tunnel syndrome and other neuropathies
- Fatigue
- Sexual dysfunction – subfertility, amenorrhea, loss of libido
- Joint pains
- Impaired glucose tolerance or frank diabetes
- Goiter
- Dental problems
- Heart failure, arrhythmias and/ or hypertension
- Visual field defects

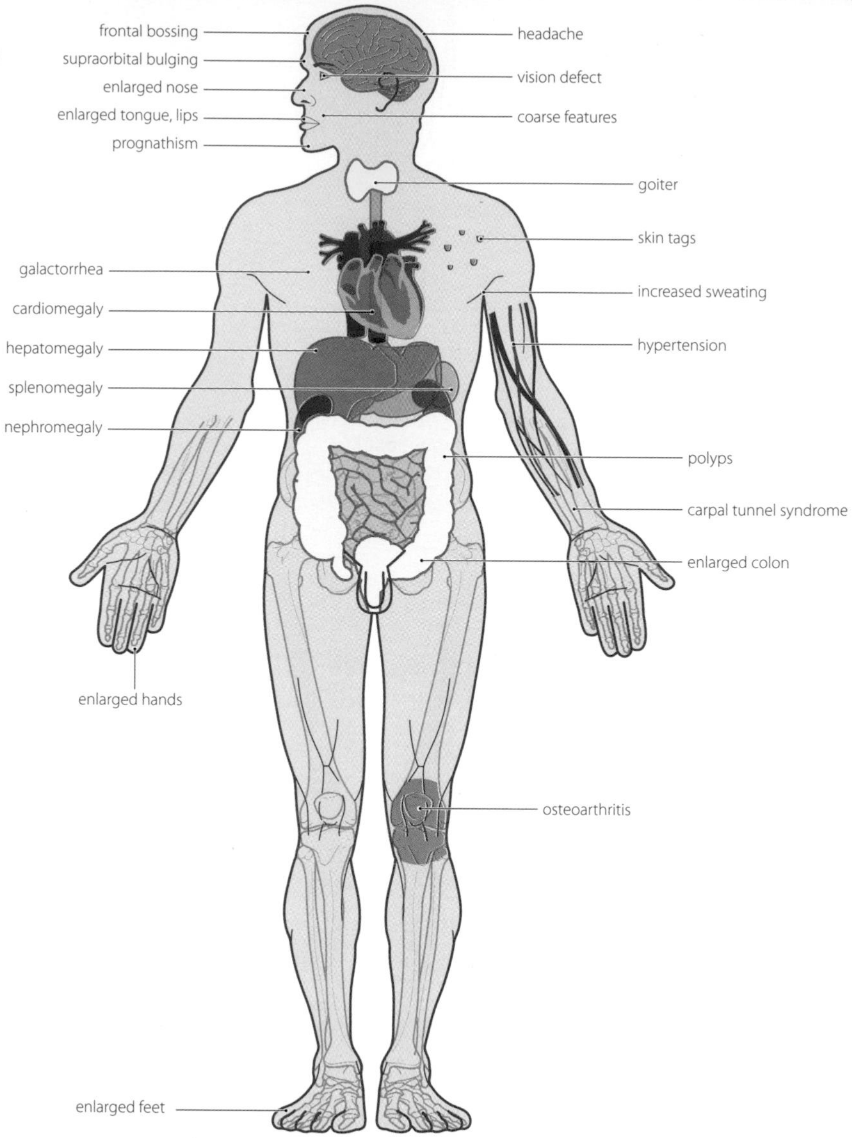

Box figure 2.2. Signs and symptoms in acromegaly.

size of the supraorbital ridge). Enlargement of the jaw results in prognathism, which affects bite (often resulting in temporo-mandibular joint pain), and wider spacing of the teeth. Hands and feet grow, leading to a difficulty in wearing rings and an increase in shoe size. Indeed, ring size (which can easily be measured using a set of jeweler's rings) is a useful objective marker of response to treatment. Skin changes include excess sweating and greasiness of the skin along with skin tags (which have been shown to be a marker of increased likelihood of gastrointestinal polyps). Joint pain is common and mainly affects the load-bearing joints, and kyphoscoliosis can result from differential overgrowth of the thoraco-lumbar vertebral cartilages.

GH is a relatively potent glucoregulatory hormone and impairs the action of insulin resulting in impaired glucose tolerance or even frank diabetes. Control of diabetes often improves with treatment of the acromegaly, if GH levels can be normalized. Insulin resistance may also result in an adverse lipid profile (especially hypertriglyceridemia), potentially contributing to cardiovascular risk. Despite the concerns over an increased risk of cancer as mentioned above, the commonest cause of premature death in acromegaly remains cardiovascular disease due to hypertension, heart failure (secondary to left ventricular hypertrophy) and disturbance of cardiac rhythm.

Multiple adenomas are not uncommon in acromegaly and these occur more frequently in the right colon in contrast with the majority of lesions in the non-acromegalic population where about 65% will occur in the left colon, and it is worth noting that right-sided polyps have a greater risk of malignancy than those in the left colon. Because there is an increased risk of colonic cancer in association with acromegaly (it is generally agreed that the risk is at least threefold; some studies have suggested a relative risk of tenfold or more), it is recommended that all patients are screened with colonoscopy on a regular basis. Other cancers may also be more common in acromegaly, although epidemiological evidence is sometimes contradictory. However, several large population studies indicate that normal individuals with an IGF-1 level in the upper quartile have a significantly higher risk of developing prostate and breast cancer and it is tempting to apply this finding to patients with acromegaly.

Sleep apnea is common, as a result of multiple problems, including macroglossia, hypertrophy (overgrowth) of laryngeal structures and narrowing of large and small airways. This may complicate anesthesia, and many centers will carry out formal sleep studies to assess this risk pre-operatively.

Quality of life is significantly impaired in acromegaly. The combination of significant changes in appearance associated with increased cardio-metabolic risk and numerous other features of the condition make this somewhat unsurprising.

2.4.2 Investigation and management of acromegaly

Investigations

The diagnosis is strongly suggested by the combination of appearance and other classical signs and symptoms (*Box 2.5*), but biochemical confirmation (see *Box 2.6* for details of appropriate tests) is necessary prior to tumor delineation and treatment planning.

In common with all other situations where a hormonal excess is suspected, a suppression test is employed. In this case it is an oral glucose tolerance test (OGTT) because hyperglycemia typically inhibits GH secretion. In response to a 75 g oral glucose load, GH will be suppressed to undetectable levels in most normal individuals, whereas in acromegaly there will be a lack of suppression (in about 35% of cases there is actually a paradoxical rise in GH).

A useful feature of this test is that it also gives an illustration of the degree of insulin resistance – a 2 h post-load glucose of >11 mmol/L being indicative of diabetes mellitus and an intermediate level of 8–11 mmol/L suggesting impaired glucose tolerance (see *Chapter 5*). Measurements of IGF-1 are useful because levels are more stable than GH, but there remains a small crossover between normality and acromegalic ranges.

Box 2.5 | Clinical features of acromegaly

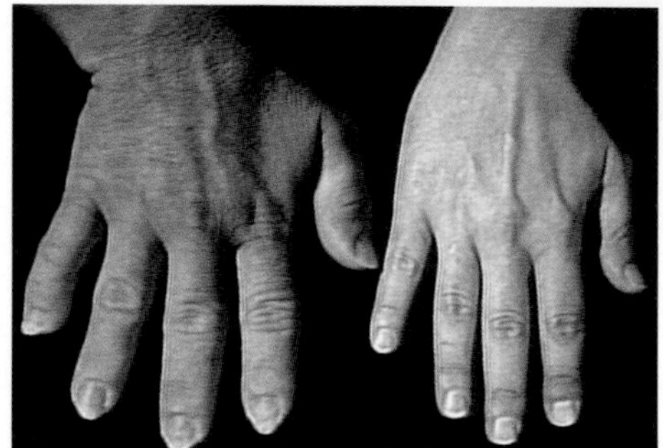

(a)

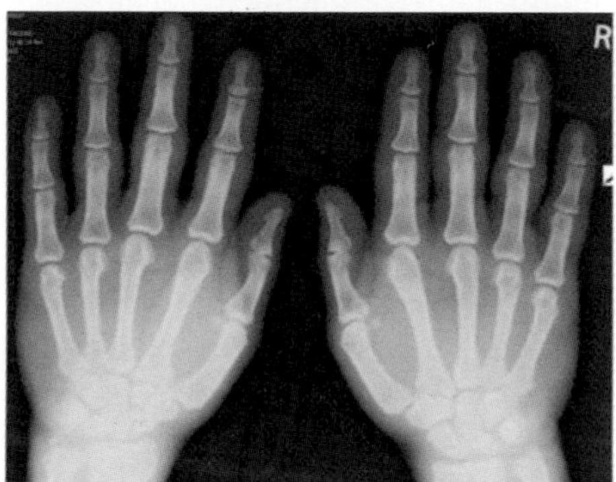

(b)

Box figure 2.3. The hands of a patient with acromegaly.
(a) 'Spade-like' hands (compared with normal-sized hand on the right). (b) X-ray of the hands shows tufting of the terminal phalanges, widening of the bases of distal phalanges, metacarpal osteophytes on radial aspect (metacarpal hooks) and soft tissue hypertrophy.

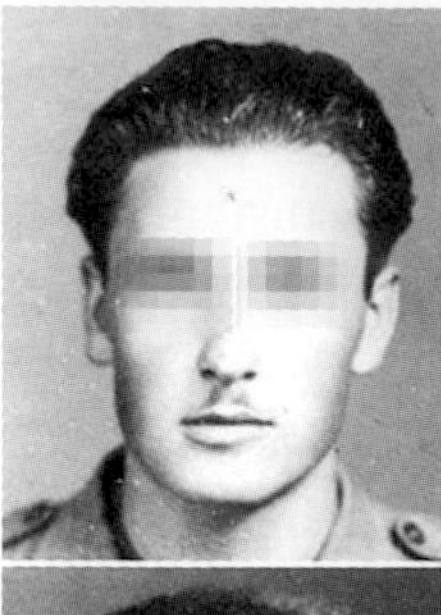

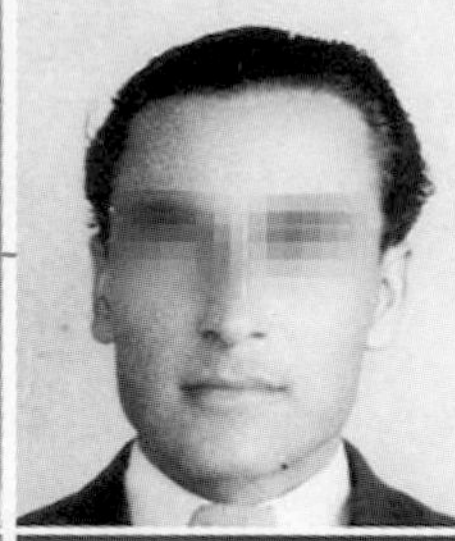

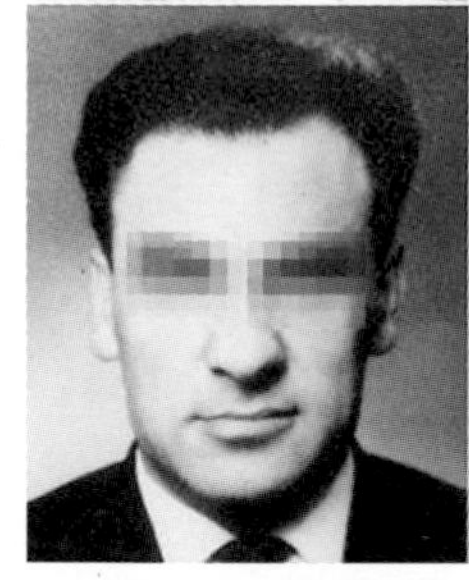

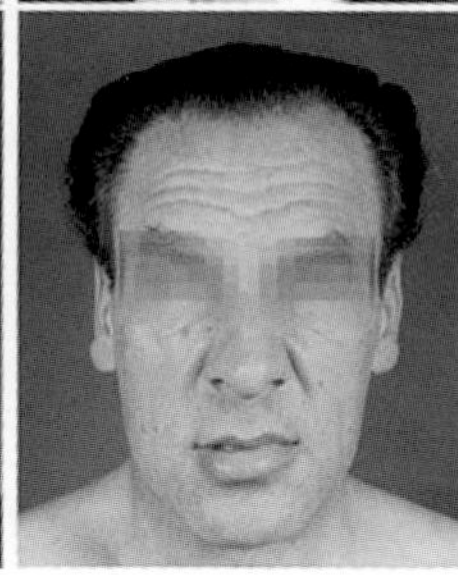

Box figure 2.4. A series of facial photos showing the slow progression of the development of acromegaly.
The classic acromegalic facies eventually result in the prominent supraorbital ridges, thickened lips, prognathism and hypertelorism seen on the bottom right photograph.

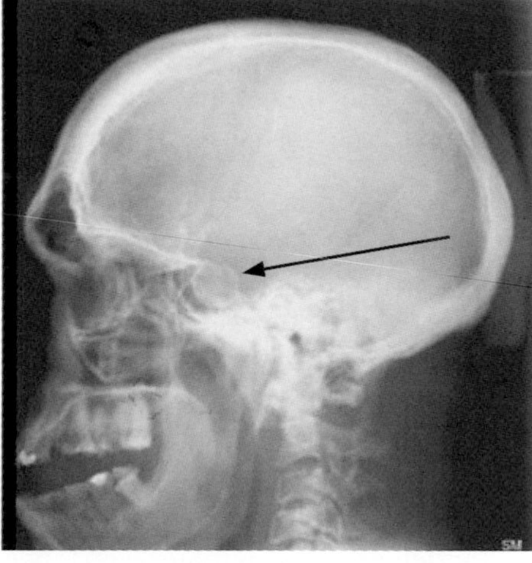

Box figure 2.5. Lateral skull X-ray demonstrating changes seen in acromegaly.
Changes include enlarged frontal air sinuses, frontal bossing, prognathism with interdental separation and enlargement of the sella turcica (arrow).

A GH 'day curve' can also help. This involves taking resting (unstimulated) measurements of GH 4–5 times over a 12 h period, taking blood through an indwelling cannula (to reduce stress as much as possible). In normal subjects, GH will usually be undetectable due to the pulsatile nature of GH secretion (*Figure 2.9*), but in patients with acromegaly GH will be detectable in every sample, and usually at roughly the same value indicating autonomous and unregulated GH output from the pituitary.

The TRH test can also be used with 200 μg of recombinant TRH being given through a cannula and GH measured at 20 minute intervals for 1 hour. Normal individuals do not show any increase in GH secretion, whilst acromegalic patients generally have a paradoxical GH elevation.

Box 2.6 | Tests of growth hormone excess and deficiency

The basic premise of clinical endocrinology is to try and suppress a hormone if hormone excess is suspected, and to stimulate it if there is thought to be a deficiency of hormone secretion.

Acromegaly

The glucose tolerance test (GTT)

The patient fasts overnight. After a basal sample for GH, glucose and IGF-1 is taken, 75 g of glucose in 250–300 mL water is drunk. Blood samples (for GH and glucose) are taken through a cannula at 30, 60, 90, and 120 minutes.

A normal response is suppression of glucose to undetectable limits. Suppression of GH to less than 0.5 ng/mL probably excludes acromegaly. IGF-1 should be in the normal age/sex-matched range. The test has the added benefit of diagnosing abnormalities of glucose homeostasis simultaneously: a glucose level at 2 h of <7 mmol/L is normal and >11 mmol/L is indicative of diabetes (see *Box 5.3*).

The GTT can also be used after treatment (surgery, radiotherapy or medical) to assess response. The same criteria apply.

GH day curve

An alternative to the GTT which may be of use in assessing response to treatment is the GH day curve. There are various protocols but a relatively simple approach is to take five GH samples over a 12 hour period. The majority of values should be undetectable – consistently high levels indicate poor control.

Acceptable levels suggesting adequate treatment of acromegaly are a nadir GH of 0.5 ng/mL on a GTT and a mean GH during a day curve of about 1.5 ng/mL although results from the two tests may be discordant.

TRH test

If the above tests fail to give a clear diagnosis, a TRH test can be used; 200 μg of thyrotropin releasing hormone (TRH) are given intravenously with serum measurements of TSH and GH at 0, 20, and 60 minutes. In normal subjects TRH inhibits growth hormone secretion with a fall in serum concentration, whilst approximately 60% of patients with acromegaly demonstrate a paradoxical rise in growth hormone levels. The measurements of TSH in this instance merely confirm that the TSH has been adequately administered.

GH deficiency

There are several tests employed to confirm GH deficiency.

Insulin stress test

This is the 'gold standard'. For this, 0.15 units of insulin/kg weight are given in the fasted state and serial measurements of GH and glucose taken for 2–3 h. A nadir laboratory glucose of <2 mmol/L indicates a successful test, i.e. adequate hypoglycemia resulting in sufficient stimulus to GH release, a peak response of GH <3 ng/mL indicates severe GHD. In children a peak value of <5 ng/mL is usually taken as indicating GHD. The test is contraindicated in coronary artery disease and epilepsy, or following transcranial neurosurgery.

Glucagon test

In this test,1 mg of glucagon is given intramuscularly (1.5 mg if the patient weighs more than 90 kg). Samples for GH are taken at baseline and then at 90,120,150, and 180 minutes. As in the insulin stress test, a peak response of <3 ng/mL indicates severe GHD and a maximum response of between 3 and 5 ng/mL indicates probable GHD.

Arginine stimulation test

This test is infrequently used in adults. It employs 0.5 mg/kg of L-arginine monohydrochloride infused in normal saline (10% solution) over 30 minutes. Samples for GH are taken at 30, 60, 90, 120, and 150 minutes after the start of the infusion. The interpretation is identical to that of the glucagon test.

Other tests include the arginine–GHRH test (carried out as above but with the inclusion of a bolus dose of 1 μg/kg GHRH given intravenously at the start of the test) or the arginine L-dopa test (where 500 mg L-dopa is given at the start of the arginine infusion).

It is important to assess other anterior pituitary hormone levels: basal levels of LH, FSH (and target hormones estrogen and testosterone), prolactin, cortisol, and thyroid function are generally sufficient. If an early morning cortisol is considered insufficient (i.e. probably less than 450 nmol/L) an insulin stress test may be necessary (see *Section 6.6*).

Once the diagnosis has been confirmed biochemically, imaging is essential. A skull X-ray is often recommended and this can demonstrate an enlargement of the bony floor of the sella turcica, frontal bossing, prognathism, increased interdental spacing, and increased size of frontal air sinuses (see *Figure 1.19*). Nowadays, it is unlikely that a patient with biochemically proven acromegaly would leave the clinic without an MRI scan request in their rather spade-like hands. MRI scans are used to demonstrate the presence and extent of the adenoma and its relationship with surrounding structures (specifically the optic chiasm and the cavernous sinuses). MRI images will show a lower signal intensity of an adenoma compared with surrounding tissue and reduced enhancement after injection of gadolinium contrast (see *Section 1.9.3*).

Assessment of vision is important. Visual field defects are not uncommon and can be tested at the bedside with the aid of a red pin, and more formally by established perimetry studies (e.g. Goldmann or Humphrey automated visual field test as shown in *Box 2.7*).

Box 2.7 | Visual field testing in pituitary adenomas

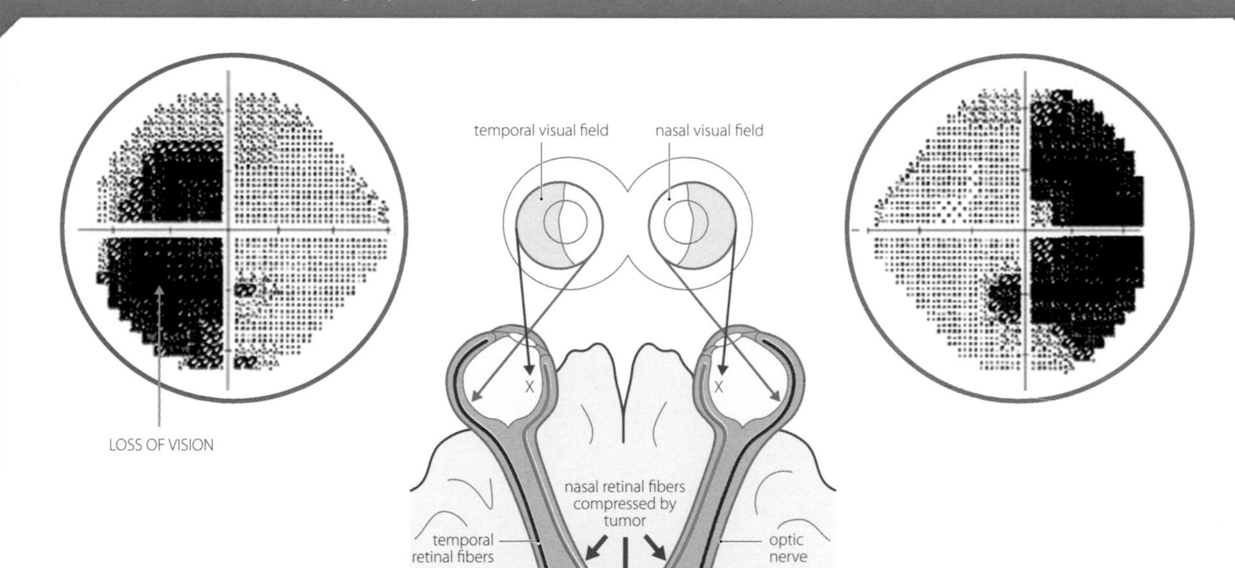

Box figure 2.6. Effect of macroadenomas of the pituitary on vision.

The tumor compresses the nasal retinal fibers which convey peripheral vision. Example of the Humphrey eye test, with the black squares highlighting the loss of peripheral vision.

Macroadenomas of the pituitary gland can cause compression of the optic chiasm when the growth on the pituitary gland (enclosed in the sella turcica) presses up into the hypothalamic region. This region is in close proximity to the optic chiasm which conveys nasal retinal fibers (receiving peripheral light/images) to the opposite retinal cortex. As a result there is a loss of peripheral vision associated with macroadenomas.

Loss of peripheral vision is tested by the Humphrey or Goldmann eye tests. Patients tend to prefer Goldmann perimetry, whereas technicians prefer the fully automated Humphrey technique, even though the latter may take 30% longer to complete. Sensitivity and specificity for visual field defects is claimed to be slightly better with Humphrey testing.

Management

Acromegaly requires treatment for resolution of established symptoms, including mass effects of the pituitary adenoma, normalization of GH/IGF-1 secretion, and prevention of future potential complications. Treatment is planned following biochemical diagnosis and tumor localization and characterization. In common with most pituitary pathology, treatment is by one or more of surgical, medical or radiotherapeutic approaches (and not uncommonly all three). At the moment, surgery is still the first-line treatment, and transsphenoidal approaches have an excellent success rate with minimal complications. The success of surgery depends on the skill of the operator, the size of the tumor, and pre-operative GH/IGF-1 levels. In experienced hands success rates should be in the order of 80–90% for microadenomas and 40–50% for macroadenomas. Medical treatment (with somatostatin analogs) is often employed prior to surgery in order to reduce the size of the tumor (by up to 50%).

Although surgical treatment remains the mainstay of treatment, three main medical therapies are of value:

- somatostatin analogs (somatostatin inhibits pituitary GH secretion)
- dopamine agonists (particularly useful in tumors that co-secrete prolactin and GH)
- GH receptor antagonists (that do not prevent GH excess but ameliorate its actions by blocking the GH receptor)

Dopamine agonists provided the first effective medical treatment for acromegaly and have been used since the early 1970s. They are not universally effective and probably need to be given in higher doses than those used for true mono-secreting prolactin adenomas (see *Section 2.6.2*). They do have a place in the treatment of tumors that co-secrete GH and prolactin (somatomammotroph adenomas diagnosed either biochemically with concomitant hyperprolactinemia or post-operatively with histological evidence of GH and prolactin antibody positivity) and may improve the efficacy of somatostatin analogs. The most frequently used dopamine agonist is probably cabergoline which is usually given twice a week in doses up to a total of 3 mg a week.

Somatostatin analogs reduce GH secretion from adenomas (*Box 2.3*). The vast majority of adenomas resulting in GH excess express the somatostatin receptor subtypes SSTR2 and, to a lesser extent, SSTR5. Native somatostatin has a half-life of a few minutes, whereas octreotide (an 8 amino acid analog) has a half-life of about 2–3 hours and can be given three times a day. Although now made largely redundant by longer-acting analogs, it can be usefully employed as a test dose to assess potential benefit of long-term therapy. The longer-acting somatostatin analogs (Sandostatin LAR and Somatuline autogel) are given as a depot injection every 3–4 weeks (sometimes with longer dose intervals depending on response). About 75% of patients will show a favorable response as assessed by normalization of IGF-1 levels and suppression of mean GH levels to less than 2 ng/mL (6 mIU/L).

Newer somatostatin-based treatments are being made available.

- SOM 230 (Pasireotide) is a hexapeptide analog which can bind to multiple somatostatin receptors (SSTR1,2,3, and 5) and can therefore mimic endogenous somatostatin more effectively. It is promising not only in the treatment of acromegaly, but also of Cushing disease and neuroendocrine tumors.

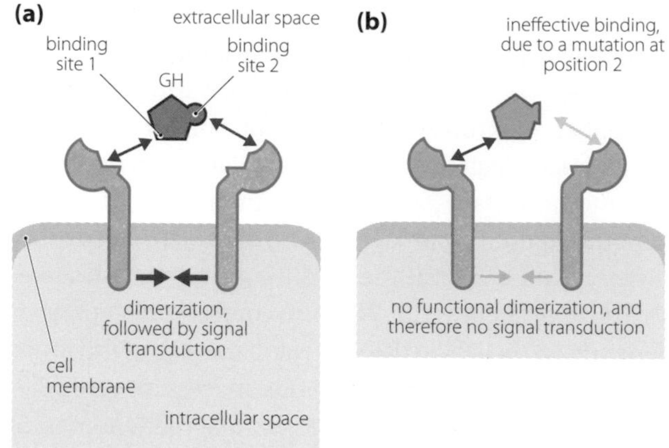

Figure 2.10. The mechanism of action of the growth hormone antagonist pegvisomant. (a) Growth hormone (GH) binds to the receptor dimer at binding sites 1 and 2 and activates signal transduction pathways, leading to the production of IGF-1. (b) Pegvisomant binds to binding site 1, and so competitively inhibits the binding of native endogenous GH, but does not bind to the second receptor. Dimerization of the receptor is prevented and signal transduction is inhibited.

- Chimeric compounds (somatostain analogs plus dopaminergic moieties) are being developed. These can preferentially bind to SSTR2 and 5 and also to the dopamine D2 receptor, which would theoretically increase efficacy.

Side-effects of somatostatin analogs generally relate to the widespread inhibitory effects of somatostatin. Gallstones may occur due to reduced gall bladder contractility and alteration in bile composition. There is a direct inhibitory effect of somatostatin on insulin secretion, but this is usually offset by reducing the insulin-antagonistic effects of excess GH. Flatulence, diarrhea, abdominal pain and nausea are often encountered, although these side-effects usually resolve with time.

A different approach to targeted blockade of the dopamine and somatostatin receptors (with somatostatin analogs and dopaminergic drugs) is to block the actions of GH directly. A relatively new compound, pegvisomant, achieves this by affecting receptor dimerization. GH binds to one half receptor at site 1 and

CASE 2.1

58 70

- 47 year old man
- Prognathism, overbite, and wide interdental spacing
- Increasing size of head, hands, and feet
- ? Acromegaly

The patient underwent baseline biochemical screening. His IGF-1 level was 355 μg/L, which is elevated when compared against an age/sex-matched reference range of 80–250 μg/L. After an OGTT his baseline GH (17 ng/mL) rose at 2 h to 33 ng/mL. A 4-point GH day curve gave a mean GH level of 19 ng/mL with no undetectable values. All other anterior pituitary hormone levels were normal including a prolactin level of 222 mIU/L. An MRI scan revealed a 20 mm macroadenoma.

He initially refused surgery and was treated with a long-acting somatostatin analog (Sandostatin LAR) at a dose of 30 mg every 4 weeks. His IGF-1 normalized and mean GH reduced to 4 ng/mL. At this point he agreed to surgery. The tumor had reduced in size to 11 mm in maximum diameter and surgery was uncomplicated. Post-operatively his mean GH reduced further (after stopping somatostatin analogs) to 1.5 ng/mL and his IGF-1 was measured in the normal range at 155 μg/L. He subsequently refused radiotherapy and further somatostatin treatment, but he has attended regularly for review and his acromegaly remains in remission to date.

then binds to a second receptor at site 2, resulting in receptor dimerization and signaling. Pegvisomant has a mutated site 1 binding domain with *increased* affinity and a mutated site 2 binding domain with markedly *reduced* binding affinity, thus preventing receptor dimerization and GH signaling (*Figure 2.10*). Pegvisomant is well tolerated, effective, and to date there have been few reports of tumor growth on treatment. In the UK it is currently used as a fourth-line treatment when surgery, radiotherapy and somatostatin analogs have been ineffective at achieving adequate control of acromegaly. Its use in Europe is more widespread. The drawbacks are the need for once daily injection and the cost, which is about 20 times more expensive per annum than effective doses of somatostatin analogs.

2.5 Growth hormone deficiency

Growth hormone (acting both directly and through generation of IGF-1) has important growth-promoting effects on the epiphyseal growth plates of long bones. GH deficiency (GHD) in childhood leading to postnatal growth failure has therefore been recognized for decades. Only more recently has the syndrome of adult GHD and its significance on several metabolic parameters and quality of life been understood.

2.5.1 Childhood growth hormone deficiency

The causes of short stature are numerous and GHD accounts for a very small percentage of these (*Box 2.8*). Indeed, the largest of the population-based growth studies (the Utah study) suggests that only about 5% of the short stature cohort had any form of endocrine disease. The most common causes are as follows:

- Familial short stature – this refers to small children of small parents; they will usually have normal bone maturation (bone age in keeping with chronological age), normal growth velocity, and normal progression of puberty.
- Constitutional growth delay – this is a term used for those children who are somewhat behind their peers in terms of growth; this often runs in families, and children will have a delayed bone age and may enter puberty somewhat later than the average, with final adult height perhaps not being reached until the age of 18–19 years.

Box 2.8 | Causes of childhood growth hormone deficiency

- Genetic
- Idiopathic
- Congenital – structural defects
  - Septo-optic dysplasia
  - Arachnoid cyst
  - Corpus callosum agenesis
  - Associated with midline facial defects
- Acquired
  - Peri- or postnatal trauma
  - CNS infections
- Cranial irradiation
- Tumors of the hypothalamus or pituitary regions
  - Craniopharyngiomas
  - Glioma/astrocytoma
  - Germinoma
  - Lymphoma
- Histiocytosis

- Chronic disease including malnutrition – probably the commonest cause of weight loss and growth failure worldwide.
- Chromosomal abnormalities including Turner syndrome (45XO, see *Chapter 7*) and Down syndrome (trisomy 21) are usually associated with short stature, as are numerous other genetic diseases.
- Endocrine causes include hypothyroidism, panhypopituitarism with GHD, and isolated GHD.

The prevalence of GHD in children is around 1:3000–3500 in the USA and UK. Incidence figures are unclear, but the incidence is probably rising as a result of higher indices of suspicion, improved diagnosis, and a larger cohort of patients surviving treatment (including radiotherapy) for cancers acquired in childhood.

The majority of cases have long been thought to be idiopathic, although there is now a better understanding of the genetic basis of pituitary growth and development, and of the transcription factors involved in embryonic development of specific pituitary cell subtypes. Abnormalities of genes encoding transcription factors such as *Pit-1, HESX1, Lhx3* and *4*, and *PROP1*, have been implicated in abnormalities of pituitary development (*Figure 2.5*) and in multiple hormone deficiencies (TSH, GH, and prolactin). In addition, there are at least four described gene defects in the *GH1* gene giving rise to various clinical pictures of GHD of varying severity. Recent reports have also suggested that biologically inert GH may be produced as a result of subtle point mutations on the *GH1* gene; this results in measurably high levels of GH but very low IGF-1 – a situation analogous to that seen in abnormalities of the GH receptor (Laron syndrome). Defects in the GHRH receptor have also been described (most notably in small and often consanguineous families from Brazil and India), leading to a lack of GHRH-mediated pituitary GH release.

Congenital structural defects of the pituitary and/or hypothalamus may occur; the best known of these is probably septo-optic dysplasia which leads to hypopituitarism associated with optic nerve defects and agenesis of the septum pelucidum. In familial cases this is usually due to an inactivating mutation in the homeobox gene *HESX1*.

Acquired causes of GHD also occur. Congenital infections (for example with rubella, toxoplasmosis and cytomegalovirus (CMV) or perinatal trauma (complicated instrumental deliveries) may result in GHD. The most common tumor causing hypopituitarism in childhood is craniopharyngioma (*Section 2.2*) and GHD is the most common endocrine abnormality associated with this tumor in children (found in 70–75% of cases). The treatment of craniopharyngioma (with surgery and radiotherapy) will also almost certainly render the child GH deficient, and so careful endocrine follow-up is essential. Other tumors that cause childhood GHD include optic gliomas and germinomas.

Finally, it should be remembered that many children will have received radiotherapy for cancers, either as prophylactic irradiation for leukemias, or as treatment for solid tumors in the region of the pituitary of the hypothalamus (including tumors that did not in themselves cause GHD). Approximately 85% of children who have received more than 30 Gy of radiation will develop GHD within 5 years, which highlights the importance of surveillance clinics for childhood cancer survivors.

2.5.2 Investigation and management of childhood GHD

Investigations

A basic tenet of adult endocrinology is that if you think a hormone is low then stimulate it, and if you think it is high then suppress it. The range of stimulatory tests available for GH is vast and their popularity varies from country to country. Whereas the insulin stress test (*Box 2.6* and *Figure 1.17*) is the 'gold standard' test in adults, fear of side-effects and complications means it is used less often by pediatricians. The most commonly used tests in children are the glucagon or clonidine stimulation tests. In both these tests (as well as the insulin stress test) a peak level of less than 5 ng/mL is considered diagnostic of GHD. Measurements of the GH-dependent peptides IGF-1, IGFBP-3 and the ALS (which binds with IGF-1 and IGFBP-3 to form a high molecular weight stable ternary complex) are of use in confirming the diagnosis, although there is a wide range of 'normal' values and these may cross-over with pathologically low values.

Imaging studies will usually include a pituitary MRI scan along with X-rays of the wrist to determine bone age (see *Figure 1.22*). In the case of early onset multiple pituitary hormone deficiencies or familial GHD it is worth considering molecular investigation of the *GH1*, homeobox, or *GHRH* genes.

Management

The treatment of GHD is obviously GH replacement therapy; recombinant GH is used and administered as a daily single subcutaneous injection. A variety of formulations exist, with different injecting devices. In cases of multiple hormone deficiency other hormones will also need to be replaced. The aim of treatment is to normalize adult height and this will usually require something in the region of 0.2–0.3 IU/kg/day (0.07–0.1 mg/kg/day). With appropriate dosing and medical supervision, significant side-effects are rare, but may include problems at the injection site (erythema and swelling), temporary mild elevations of blood glucose, headache, hematuria and worsening of thyroid function.

2.5.3 Adult growth hormone deficiency

Historically, GH treatment in childhood was stopped at the point where either final adult height or peak bone mass was reached, and for many years it was thought that GHD in adulthood was irrelevant because linear growth had been completed. Although the metabolic effects of GH had been understood for some time, the impact of deficiency in adulthood was not fully appreciated. Over the last two decades our understanding has increased and early work in the 1990s led to the description of the syndrome of adult GHD. The work stemmed from the realization that patients with hypopituitarism, although adequately replaced with 'standard' hormones, including cortisol, thyroid hormone, and sex steroids, continued to demonstrate a measurable decrease in both quantity and quality of life.

The etiology of GHD in adulthood is essentially that of hypopituitarism (*Box 2.9*) and, in reality, about 90% of cases of adult GHD are due to the effects of, or consequences of, treatment of a pituitary adenoma. There is a hierarchy of hormone loss in pituitary disease as a result of treatment or mass effects: somatotroph and gonadotroph cells are the first affected, with ACTH, TSH, and prolactin loss following in order. Consequently, patients with structural pituitary/hypothalamic disease that has resulted in ACTH deficiency will almost always have GHD.

Box 2.9 | Causes of hypopituitarism

Pituitary diseases

- Mass lesions – pituitary adenomas, cysts, other benign lesions
- Pituitary surgery or irradiation
- Infiltrative disease – lymphocytic hypophysitis, hemochromatosis
- Apoplexy
- Genetic disease – *Pit1* mutation

Hypothalamic disease

- Mass lesions – craniopharyngiomas and malignant tumors
- Radiation for CNS or nasopharyngeal malignancies

Sarcoidosis, histiocytosis, tuberculosis

Box 2.10 | Symptoms and signs of adult growth hormone deficiency

- Decreased quality of life including:
  - low mood
  - anxiety
  - decreased energy levels
  - social isolation
  - lack of positive well-being
- Alteration in body composition including:
  - increased body fat
  - decreased muscle mass
- Metabolic abnormalities including:
  - decreased insulin sensitivity and increased prevalence of impaired glucose tolerance
  - increased LDL cholesterol and apolipoprotein B and decreased HDL cholesterol
  - increased concentration of plasma fibrinogen and plasminogen activator inhibitor type I
- Other cardiovascular effects including:
  - decreased cardiac muscle mass
  - reduced stroke volume
  - atherosclerosis
  - decreased total and extracellular fluid volume
- Decreased bone density and (possibly) an increased fracture risk

The prevalence of GHD is unknown, but approximately 35 000 adult patients in the USA are on GH with a further 5-6000 starting treatment annually. The symptoms and signs are somewhat variable and are outlined in *Box 2.10*. The majority of these parameters improve with GH replacement treatment, both in placebo-controlled crossover studies and in the real clinical world. The diagnosis of adult GHD is essentially the same as in childhood, although the insulin stress test (IST) is used much more widely in adulthood (particularly in the UK). In those with contraindication to IST (e.g. patients with coronary artery disease or epilepsy), the glucagon test is used most frequently. Other tests include provocation with arginine, GHRH, dopamine, or clonidine, or combinations of these secretagogues (see *Box 2.6*). Basal measurements of IGF-1 and the GH-dependent peptide IGFBP-3 can help in the confirmation of diagnosis, and they are also used to assess effectiveness of GH replacement therapy. As a primary diagnostic tool, however, these measurements are of limited use because of the wide range of normal values and the crossover between low 'normal' values and pathologically low values.

Treatment of adult GHD is with recombinant GH. This is given (as in childhood GHD) by once daily subcutaneous doses, but much lower doses are usually required; the majority of patients can be commenced on 0.3 mg GH once daily and the dose titrated at 4 weekly intervals (based on clinical response and IGF-1 levels). The aim is to titrate the dose up to that resulting in an IGF-1 in the top tertile of the age/sex-matched normal range. The average dose for men is around 0.4 mg a day, and is a little higher in women (especially those on estrogen replacement).

Side-effects occur mainly as a result of fluid retention (in itself a result of the correction of salt/water deficit present in patients with GHD). Consequently edema, arthralgia, myalgia and carpal tunnel syndrome are often encountered (particularly in male patients). These adverse effects usually disappear on dose reduction. Benign intracranial hypertension is far less common than in children, but persistent severe headache warrants investigation (i.e. brain MRI scan) to exclude raised intracranial pressure. There is always a theoretical risk of increasing cancer risk by elevating IGF-1 levels (as IGF-1 is a potent mitogenic peptide, and prevents apoptosis). Long-term studies, however, have failed to show any compelling evidence of an excess risk of either *de novo* tumor formation or re-growth of sellar/parasellar tumors.

There are two main groups of patients with adult GHD: those who were diagnosed in childhood and in whom GH is continued and those where the condition occurs and is diagnosed in adulthood. It is important that patients diagnosed in childhood attend a dedicated transitional clinic to allow further treatment and follow-up in the adult service; many will need re-testing in late teenage years prior to continuation of treatment.

GH treatment in adulthood, however, is not universally accepted, even by endocrinologists. Costs are high and some studies have tended to show little sustained benefit. Nevertheless, objective evidence probably does support a significant and cost-effective improvement in quality and quantity of life. In the UK it is the reduced quality of life that allows GH replacement to be commenced in adulthood: before GH replacement is prescribed, NICE guidelines require the demonstration of both:

- GHD, using a provocative stimulation test, and
- a reduced quality of life, that improves with GH replacement using disease-specific validated questionnaires – the AGHDA score.

In the USA, the Endocrine Society recommends treatment for all patients with proven GHD, particularly those with more severe biochemical and clinical abnormalities.

2.6 Basic physiology of prolactin

Case 2.2 illustrates the effects of excess prolactin, which can stimulate milk production in a non-lactating woman with associated irregular menstruation and suppression of hormone secretions. Prolactin is a homologous hormone to GH and human placental lactogen, with a similar structure and comprising 198 amino acids compared with the 191 amino acids in GH. It was originally identified by its ability to stimulate mammary gland development and lactation but now more than 300 different actions of prolactin have been reported in various vertebrate species, including on growth and development, metabolism, brain and behavior, salt and water balance, reproduction and immune modulation. In humans, however, the only clearly defined physiological role of prolactin is stimulation of lactation during pregnancy when prolactin levels are raised. Post-partum prolactin levels normalize within about 6 months in nursing mothers and within weeks in non-nursing mothers.

CASE 2.2 76 84

- 27 year old woman
- History of oligomenorrhea (4y) and problems conceiving
- Low FSH and high prolactin

A 27 year old woman was referred from the subfertility clinic with a 4 year history of oligomenorrhea (she was having approximately four menstrual periods per annum) and difficulty getting pregnant. Her partner had a normal semen analysis. Apart from the menstrual disturbance she had no other symptoms and was on no medication (either prescribed or 'over the counter'). Initial examination revealed normal visual fields, normal BMI (25 kg/m^2) and bilateral galactorrhea (which she had been unaware of until it was demonstrated to her in the clinic). Investigations revealed the following results:

- LH: 1.9 IU/L
  (NR luteal phase: 0.8–10.4)
- FSH: 2.1 IU/L
  (NR luteal phase: 2.6–9.5)
- Prolactin: 3200 mIU/L
  (NR: 100–550)
- Estradiol: 90 pmol/L
  (NR: 70–1100)

Further biochemical analysis revealed the prolactin to be entirely monomeric (i.e. biologically active) with no evidence of macroprolactin. Macroprolactin is a biologically inert form of the hormone which is bound to IgG and interferes with many assays for prolactin, giving a falsely high value; it is important to reassess samples either in assays not subject to interference, or after removal of macroprolactin complexes using polyethyleneglycol.

A pituitary MRI scan with gadolinium enhancement (see *Section 1.9.3* for details of the use of gadolinium) was arranged for the patient.

2.6.1 Synthesis, action, and control of prolactin secretion

Prolactin is primarily synthesized by the lactotrophs in the anterior pituitary gland, although extra-pituitary sites of prolactin synthesis have been identified including immune, mammary, epithelial and fat cells.

In humans there are seven recognized isoforms of the prolactin receptor (PRLR) resulting from alternate splicing of RNA. These single-pass transmembrane receptors are identical in their extracellular domain but differ in the lengths and sequences of their intracellular domains. They are generally classified as the 'long' forms or 'short' forms of the receptor. The long PRLRs are widely distributed in the body, not only in the mammary gland but also the ovary, adrenal gland, kidney, small intestine, and pancreas, whilst the short forms are expressed in organs such as the liver. Prolactin signaling is initiated by one prolactin molecule binding to two cell surface receptors leading to their dimerization and subsequent activation. The long PRLR isoforms activate the JAK2/STAT signaling pathway (see *Figure 1.8e*); the short PRLRs cannot activate STAT although, like the long isoforms, they can activate PI3K/Akt and MEK as downstream targets. The action of prolactin on the mammary gland is largely the result of activity of the long isoforms via JAK2/STAT, although the function and signaling mechanisms of the short isoforms have not been defined; they may act by inhibiting the function of the long PRLRs or as positive regulators in the mammary gland.

Like GH, prolactin is controlled by two hypothalamic neurohormones released into the hypophyseal portal capillaries. The predominant hypothalamic control is via

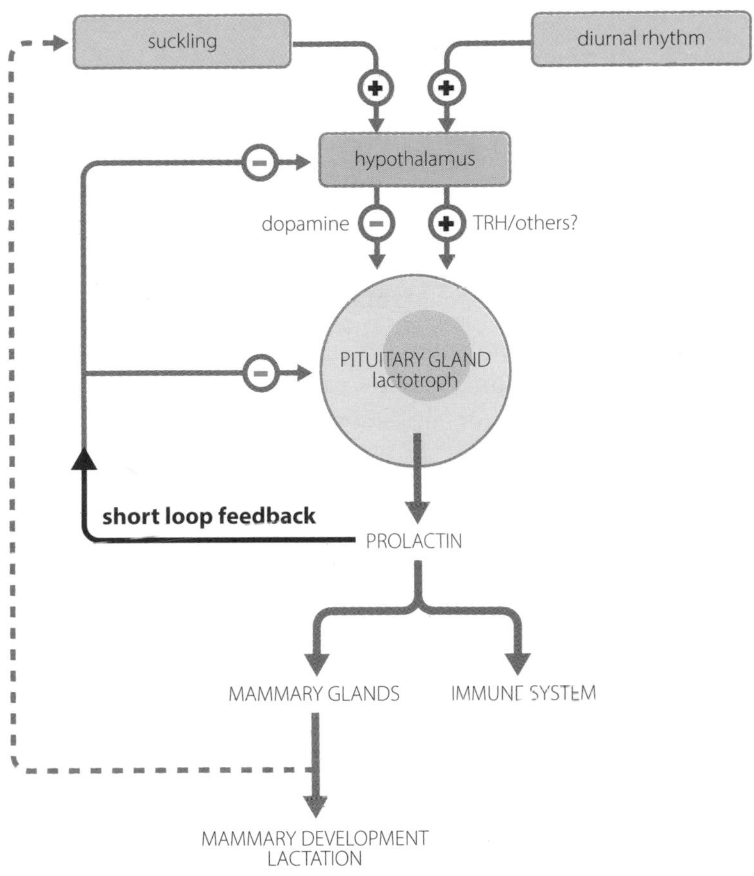

Figure 2.11. Control of prolactin secretion.

dopaminergic neurosecretory cells which inhibit prolactin release, whilst several hypothalamic factors can stimulate prolactin release including TRH (*Figure 2.11*). Chronic increases in 17β-estradiol also stimulate prolactin secretion through actions on the pituitary gland and through hypothalamic mechanisms. Drugs which block dopaminergic receptors, e.g. antipsychotic drugs, will induce elevated prolactin concentrations and the reverse occurs with dopamine agonists which are used for the medical treatment of prolactinomas (see *Section 2.7.1*). Prolactin secretion is controlled by a short loop feedback and its synthesis and secretion are stimulated by suckling. Like GH it shows a diurnal rhythm in its secretory pattern.

2.7 Hyperprolactinemia

Case 2.2 demonstrates the relative paucity of symptoms associated with high levels of prolactin in humans. The majority of women with hyperprolactinemia present with irregular menstruation (or amenorrhea) with or without galactorrhea. Men usually present later (due to the absence of these obvious signs) and may complain of loss of libido, erectile dysfunction or gynecomastia. A female patient presenting with amenorrhea and/or galactorrhea and male patients presenting with loss of libido, signs suggestive of acquired hypogonadism or (rarely) gynecomastia, should be screened for hyperprolactinemia.

It should be remembered that prolactin differs from other hormones of the anterior pituitary in that its secretion is mainly under inhibitory control (predominantly by dopamine) rather than stimulation by a hypothalamic-releasing hormone. Nevertheless, there are a number of stimuli to prolactin release which can be a cause of hyperprolactinemia. The causes of 'true' hyperprolactinemia are many and varied and are summarized in *Box 2.11*, but it can be seen that most causes are the result of unregulated production of prolactin by the pituitary gland (e.g. prolactin-secreting adenomas) or inefficient dopaminergic inhibition of prolactin secretion. The loss of dopamine inhibition may be due to:

- a true dopamine deficiency at the level of the hypothalamus (e.g. tumors or inflammatory processes resulting in diminished or defective dopamine synthesis or release) or drugs that may deplete dopamine stores (e.g. methyldopa)
- a defect in transport of dopamine from the hypothalamus to the pituitary lactotroph, e.g. a pituitary or stalk tumor or indeed section of the pituitary stalk, for example, during surgery
- antagonism of the action of dopamine by certain drugs, most commonly antipsychotic medications (e.g. sulpiride, haloperidol) and antiemetics (metoclopramide and domperidone)
- unregulated stimulation of lactotrophs, e.g. by excess TRH in hypothyroidism (TRH acts as a prolactin-releasing factor), or by chest wall injury which results in a 'suckling' reflex similar to that seen in lactating women.

Box 2.11 | Causes of hyperprolactinemia

- Stress
- Pregnancy and breast-feeding
- Hypothyroidism
- Drugs:
  - estrogen (e.g. oral contraceptive pill)
  - antiemetics (e.g. metoclopramide)
  - antipsychotic medications
  - major tranquilizers
- Impairment of metabolism/excretion, e.g. liver disease and renal failure
- Chest wall trauma
- Hypothalamic disease
  - trauma
  - radiotherapy
  - infiltration (sarcoidosis, histiocytosis)
  - metastatic disease
  - craniopharyngioma
  - glioma, meningioma, astrocytoma
- Pituitary disease
  - microprolactinoma
  - macroprolactinoma
  - mixed lactotroph/mammotroph adenoma
  - stalk compression (from any pituitary/sellar pathology associated with a macroadenoma)
- Spurious results including interference by macroprolactin

In women, levels of less than 550 mIU/L are considered normal. It should be remembered that prolactin is a stress hormone and levels below 1000 mIU/L should be checked in a stress-free manner, ideally by measuring prolactin in a sample withdrawn from a cannula where the cannula has been inserted at least 1 hour before the sample is taken. Levels of between about 600 and 3500 mIU/L may be associated with pituitary secreting microadenomas (tumors <10 mm in diameter), in response to dopamine antagonistic drugs, or in association with stalk compression. Levels above 5000 mIU/L are usually associated with macroadenomas (tumors >10 mm). It is imperative to exclude pregnancy in women with high prolactin to avoid costly, unnecessary and potentially dangerous investigations.

2.7.1 Prolactinomas

Prolactinomas (pituitary adenomas secreting prolactin) are the most common functioning (i.e. hormone-secreting) pituitary tumors. They account for up to 70–75% of all pituitary adenomas in women under the age of 60 years and have an incidence of around 40 per 100 000 population in the UK. They are much more common in women; men tend to present much later with an increased frequency of macroadenomas being encountered, perhaps as high as 60% macroadenomas in males compared with around 10% in females. In common with all pituitary tumors, the consequences of a prolactinoma can be considered in terms of the biological effects of the hormone excess and the mass effects of the tumor. The clinical features of prolactinomas are shown in *Box 2.12*.

Box 2.12 | Clinical features of prolactinomas

Related to hormone excess

- Menstrual disturbance (usually oligo- or amenorrhea)
- Anovulatory subfertility
- Galactorrhea (spontaneous or expressive)
- Hypoestrogenism (vaginal dryness, osteoporosis, dyspareunia)
- Delayed menarche if it occurs pre-pubertally
- Male hypogonadism (erectile dysfunction, libido loss, subfertility)
- Gynecoid (female body) habitus if it occurs pre-pubertally (along with small testicles)

Related to mass effects

- Headache
- Visual problems – field defects (most commonly bitemporal hemianopia but occasionally blindness or ophthalmoplegia due to involvement of the IIIrd, IVth, and VIth cranial nerves)
- Loss of other anterior pituitary hormones

Diagnosis

The diagnosis of prolactinomas is based on appropriate imaging (*Figure 2.12*) secondary to the demonstration of an elevated prolactin level and exclusion of other causes of hyperprolactinemia (*Box 2.11*). Difficulties can sometimes arise in patients on long-term dopamine antagonistic therapy (e.g. antipsychotic medications) who have a level of prolactin that causes concern. Some of these will already have had a pituitary MRI scan which may show a pituitary lesion. The problem here is that a significant percentage of individuals undergoing scans for unrelated reasons will have a pituitary lesion – this is termed a pituitary incidentaloma (*Box 2.13*). Pituitary incidentalomas are common and it is sometimes impossible to determine the significance of a small microadenoma unless medication can be stopped or changed to something with no dopamine antagonism.

Biochemical testing includes prolactin estimation (repeated on a stress-free sample from a cannula if necessary), measurement of TSH (hypothyroidism can be associated with hyperprolactinemia), measurement of testosterone and gonadotropins (LH and FSH) in hypogonadal males, and measurement of other

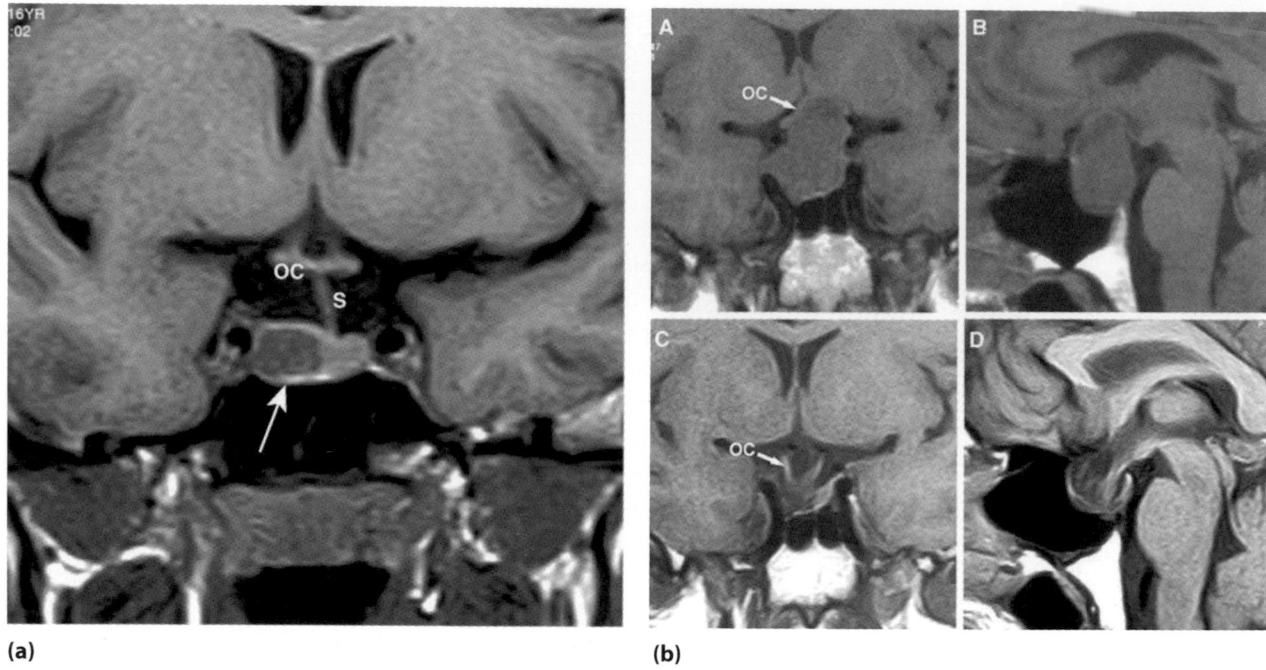

(a) (b)

Figure 2.12. MRI scans of (a) a microprolactinoma and (b) a macroprolactinoma.
(a) A microprolactinoma measuring 9 mm in its widest diameter. The lesion remains within the sella turcica and is not compromising the optic chiasm.
(b) Coronal (left) and sagittal (right) MRI images of the pituitary. Panels A and B demonstrate a large pituitary adenoma with suprasellar extension abutting and stretching the optic chiasm. After 6 months of cabergoline treatment (500 μg twice a week, panels C and D) the tumor has shrunk dramatically, decompressing the optic chiasm which has prolapsed into the fossa.
Abbreviations: OC, optic chiasm; S, pituitary stalk.

anterior pituitary hormones if clinically or radiographically indicated. Chronic renal failure and liver cirrhosis may be associated with hyperprolactinemias and it is important to assess hepatic and renal function if clinically indicated.

Once hyperprolactinemia has been confirmed (and other causes ruled out), imaging with MRI is usually indicated, although hyperprolactinemia due to microadenoma in women is very common and some might suggest that imaging in every case of presumed microprolactinoma is not necessary and definitely not cost-effective. However, the problem with that approach is that occasionally patients may present with a relatively modest elevation of prolactin (e.g. <3000 mIU/L) and no other obvious symptoms or signs of mass effect, but may still have a non-functioning macroadenoma causing 'bystander' hyperprolactinemia by stalk compression. MRI scanning with gadolinium enhancement will detect all significant prolactinomas.

Treatment

Unlike for the majority of pituitary adenomas, the treatment of prolactinomas is primarily medical with surgery and/or radiotherapy reserved for cases where medical treatment fails or is not tolerated. Medical treatment is with dopamine agonists which inhibit the synthesis and secretion of prolactin and which also reduce the rate of mammotroph cellular division and the growth of individual mammotrophs. Note, however, that hyperprolactinemia secondary to stalk

Box 2.13 | Pituitary incidentalomas

By definition a pituitary incidentaloma is a lesion in the pituitary which has been discovered serendipitously, i.e. it was not suspected before imaging was carried out for something (probably) entirely unrelated (such as headache, trauma, or head and neck neurological complaints rather than visual field defects or a clinical suspicion of hormonal excess or deficiency). In keeping with all pituitary tumors, incidentalomas are either microincidentalomas (less than 10 mm in maximum diameter) or macroincidentalomas (>10 mm). They may be solid (usually adenomas), cystic (usually Rathke's cleft cysts or craniopharyngiomas), or mixed.

Most incidentalomas will not require surgical intervention so final histological diagnosis remains unclear. Nevertheless, evidence suggests that the majority of apparently non-functioning incidentalomas will either be 'null-cell', i.e. no staining for pituitary hormones, or gonadotroph-positive on immunocytochemical histological analysis.

It is difficult to get accurate data on the incidence of incidentalomas, but studies suggest that about 0.2% of patients undergoing CT or MRI for unrelated neurological symptoms will have an incidentaloma. In contrast, autopsy data put the overall incidence of pituitary adenomas at about 10%.

Evaluation

It is reasonable to assess all incidentalomas both clinically and biochemically for evidence of either excess or deficiency of hormone secretion.

Excess hormone secretion

Prolactin secretion is highly variable, with some studies suggesting that up to 10% of incidentalomas secrete excess prolactin. This secretion should be treated with dopamine agonists if clinically warranted. Because prolactin secretion may be secondary to other factors such as stalk compression, it is sensible to follow up the incidentaloma with further biochemical assessment and imaging because it may continue to grow.

Screening for 'silent' somatotroph secretion is warranted because the treatment for this is generally surgical. In the light of any clinical features or an elevated IGF-1, formal testing for GH excess should be carried out (*Box 2.6*). Incidentalomas that are positive for GH staining or associated with abnormal GH regulation are relatively commonly reported: autopsy studies suggest a prevalence of about 2% GH positivity in all incidentalomas.

Adrenal incidentalomas are frequently associated with abnormal cortisol regulation with a retrospective realization that the patients exhibit hypertension and glucose intolerance. It is not unreasonable to approach pituitary incidentalomas with the same thought process, and a dexamethasone suppression test is often justified.

If there is any suggestion of familial disease, the possibility of MEN should be considered with appropriate further investigation (see *Chapter 8*).

Hormone deficiency

Screening for hypopituitarism is equally important. Baseline tests for IGF-1, TSH, free T_4, cortisol, LH, FSH and testosterone are often sufficient.

A low gonadotropin level in a post-menopausal woman will suggest hypogonadotropic hypogonadism. A low testosterone level in a man also suggests loss of LH and FSH (secondary) rather than primary gonadal failure. An IGF-1 level may be useful in assessment of possible GH deficiency, but due to the large cross-over between 'low–normal' and pathologically low values, further tests for GH deficiency may be indicated if there is a strong clinical suspicion. It is reasonable to assess for GH deficiency only if there is a clear view that GH treatment will be possible or effective.

If the incidentaloma compromises the optic chiasm, formal visual field assessment (*Box 2.7*) should be carried out with automated perimetry.

If the incidentaloma was initially identified by CT it is worth further delineating the anatomy with contrast pituitary-dedicated MRI scanning.

Follow-up

If there is no indication for surgery and no hormonal excess or compromise, follow-up can be limited to recurrent scanning to assess change in size. It is probably reasonable to re-scan a macroincidentaloma after 6 months and then yearly, reducing in frequency if stable. A microincidentaloma should be re-scanned after 1 year and then every 2–3 years, again reducing in frequency if stable.

If there is growth of a macroincidentaloma, re-testing of endocrine function is warranted, particularly if there is any clinical suggestion of abnormality. Microincidentalomas with no change in MRI appearance and no change clinically do not need re-testing.

Indications for treatment

Recent guidelines from the Endocrine Society suggest the following indications for surgery for incidentalomas:

Box 2.13 | continued

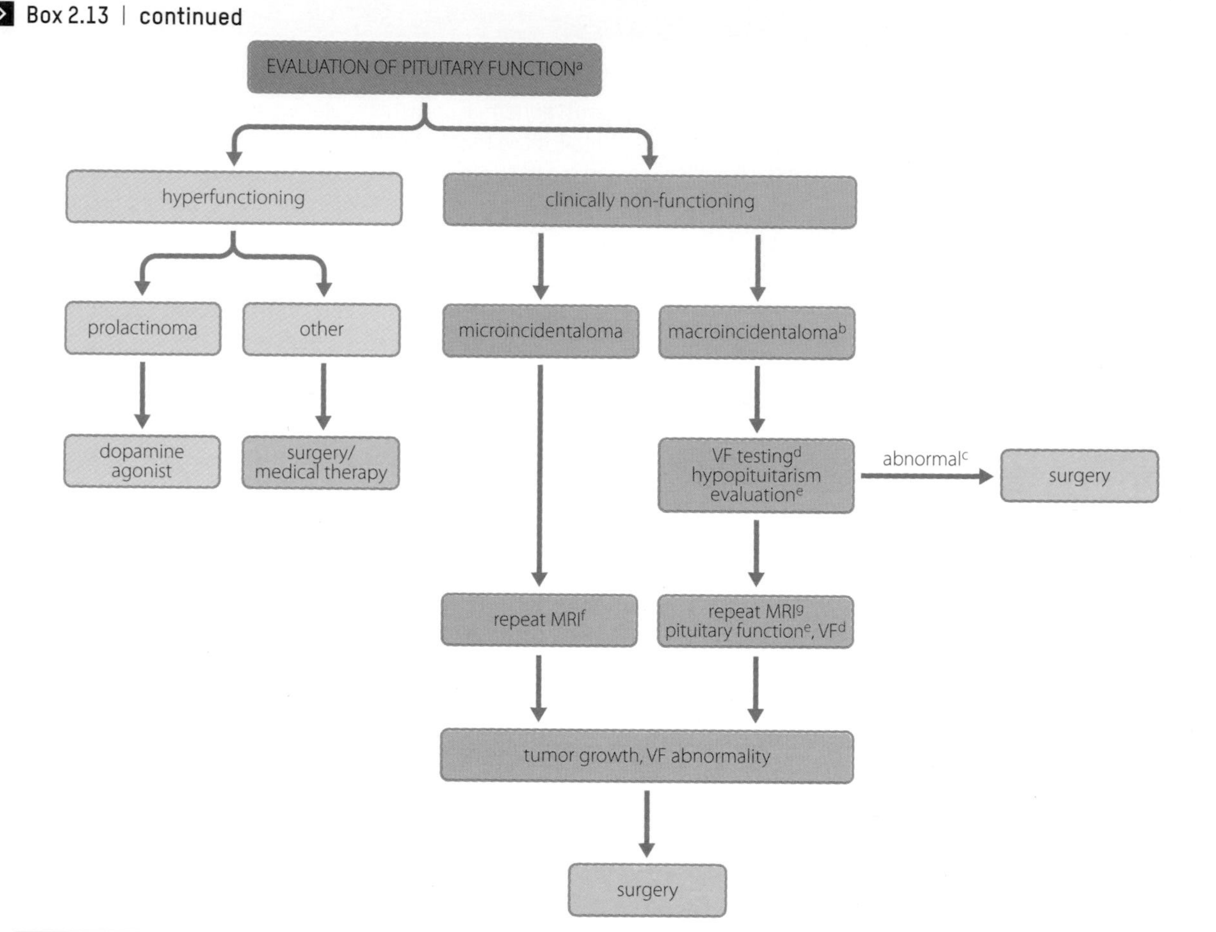

Box figure 2.7. Flow diagram for the evaluation and treatment of pituitary incidentalomas.
[a]Baseline evaluation in all patients should include a history and physical examination evaluating for signs and symptoms of hyperfunction and hypopituitarism and a laboratory evaluation for hypersecretion.
[b]This group may also include large microlesions.
[c]The recommendation for surgery includes the presence of abnormalities of visual fields (VF) or vision and signs of tumor compression.
[d]VF testing is recommended for patients with lesions abutting or compressing the optic nerves or chiasm at the initial evaluation and during follow-up.
[e]Evaluation for hypopituitarism is recommended for the baseline evaluation and during follow-up evaluations. This is most strongly recommended for macrolesions and larger microlesions.
[f]Repeat MRI in 1 year, yearly for 3 years, and then less frequently thereafter if no change in lesion size.
[g]Repeat the MRI in 6 months, yearly for 3 years, and then less frequently if no change in lesion size.
Reproduced from *J. Clin. Endocrinol. Metab.* (2011; **96**: 894–904) with permission from the Endocrine Society.

- Visual field defects
- Ophthalmoplegia
- Lesion touching the chiasm or compressing the optic nerves
- Pituitary apoplexy
- Biologically active lesions (with the exception of prolactinomas)
- Clinical significant growth of the lesion
- Loss of endocrine function
- A lesion close to the chiasm in a fertile woman planning a family
- Unremitting headache

Dopamine agonist therapy for an incidentaloma that is discovered to be prolactin secreting is reasonable. There is no evidence, however, for medical treatment of other incidentalomas with, for example, dopamine agonists, somatostatin analogs, or combination therapy.

compression by a non-prolactin secreting macroadenoma will usually require surgical intervention.

Two dopamine agonists are in common use:

- Bromocriptine – has been used for nearly 4 decades and is clinically effective in doses starting at 1.25 mg a day and building up to 2.5 mg three times a day; side-effects (including nausea, postural hypotension, dizziness) are not uncommon.
- Cabergoline – this is a newer longer-acting dopamine agonist. Cabergoline has higher affinity for the D2 dopamine receptor and probably has greater efficacy and fewer side-effects than bromocriptine and so has become the first-line treatment. It is given in doses starting at 250 μg twice a week increasing (rarely) to up to 3 mg a week in divided doses in resistant cases.

Dopamine agonists will usually restore normoprolactinemia and can result in impressive and rapid reductions in tumor size, even in large macroadenomas (*Figure 2.12b*).

Although well tolerated, recent evidence suggests that cabergoline may be associated with fibrotic adverse reactions, including cardiac valvular fibrosis, pleuropulmonary and retroperitoneal fibrosis. Some of this evidence is somewhat contradictory (particularly in the low doses used in hyperprolactinemia, compared with the much higher doses used in Parkinson's disease) and we await the outcome of long-term prospective studies. However, it is reasonable to reconsider the duration of treatment. Dopamine agonists cause tumor shrinkage and some microadenomas will effectively disappear after a period of treatment. Given the potential risk of protracted dopamine agonist therapy, it is reasonable to reassess the situation after about 2 years with cessation of treatment and follow-up clinically (maintained restoration of menses and absence of galactorrhea) and biochemically with prolactin measurements (which are an effective tumor marker).

Microadenomas are extraordinarily slow growing and in some cases (e.g. post-menopausal women) could probably be left untreated and simply monitored using serial prolactin measurements and imaging. In younger women, however, it is important to treat the associated hyperprolactinemia in order to restore menstruation, estrogen levels and fertility, and to treat the sometimes unacceptable symptom of galactorrhea. Macroprolactinomas will always require treatment to obviate mass effects.

The incidence of prolactinomas is highest in women of reproductive age and it is these women who are most likely to present with amenorrhea or subfertility. It is reasonable to continue therapy whilst trying for a baby with the aim of stopping it after a positive pregnancy test. There is a theoretical risk with cabergoline of miscarriage or fetal malformation, although evidence of numerous conceptions on cabergoline treatment does not support this.

The pituitary doubles in size during pregnancy. This is not a problem with microadenomas, but a macroadenoma may grow sufficiently to compromise the chiasm. Monitoring during pregnancy is clinical, supported by serial measurements of visual fields in patients with macroadenomas; there is no point in trying to use prolactin as a tumor marker in this situation. Many endocrinologists will continue dopamine agonist treatment throughout pregnancy in patients with large macroadenomas to minimize the risk of significant optic chiasm involvement.

Some tumors will remain resistant to medical treatment and some patients may be intolerant of dopamine agonists. In some patients, hitherto undiagnosed or *de novo* psychotic symptoms may develop. In these cases it is necessary to resort to surgical and/or radiotherapeutic approaches (although radiotherapy alone is rarely effective). Transsphenoidal hypophysectomy is associated with low mortality and morbidity. Complications (common to surgical resections of all pituitary adenomas) include hemorrhage, CSF rhinorrhea, diabetes insipidus (*Section 2.10*) and hypopituitarism (*Table 2.4*). Initial cure rates in tertiary centers with experienced and dedicated pituitary surgeons approach 90% with a recurrence rate of 15–20%. In some resistant cases, for example those with extensive tumor growth into areas not amenable for surgical excision, cytotoxic chemotherapy may be considered. Early results with temezolamide, an alkylating agent, are highly encouraging.

CASE 2.2 76 

- 27 year old woman
- History of oligomenorrhea (4y) and problems conceiving
- Low FSH and high prolactin
- Successful treatment with cabergoline

The patient underwent MRI scanning which revealed an enhancing 9 mm adenoma in the left side of the anterior pituitary with minimal stalk deviation and no optic chiasm involvement. She was treated with cabergoline (250 µg twice a week) and her periods resumed within a month. After 5 months of treatment she became pregnant and after two positive pregnancy tests the cabergoline was stopped. The pregnancy progressed without incident and she delivered a baby boy at term. Clinical and imaging reassessment are planned for when she has finished breast-feeding.

2.8 Trophic hormones of the anterior pituitary gland – ACTH and the glycoprotein hormones

ACTH is a hormone synthesized from the pro-opiomelanocortin gene, *POMC*, and produced by the action of peptidases which split up the prohormone into different products via post-translational processing: ACTH, MSH, and endorphins are therefore produced from the same RNA translation. ACTH, a 39 amino acid peptide, is the major hormone produced from the POMC prohormone in the anterior pituitary gland and its synthesis and secretion are controlled by CRH and vasopressin secreted by hypothalamic neurosecretory cells. ACTH acts on the adrenal cortex to stimulate the synthesis and secretion of cortisol and androgens, but not aldosterone under normal physiological conditions. The actions of ACTH and the control of its secretion are described in more detail in *Chapter 6*.

There are three homologous glycosylated hormones produced by the anterior pituitary gland: TSH and the two gonadotropins, FSH and LH. Each is made up of two subunits, α and β, joined by disulfide bridges attached to cysteine residues on the subunits. There is a common gene, structurally identical in all three hormones, that codes for the α unit. The β units are coded on separate genes and they confer biological specificity to the hormones. TSH is synthesized in thyrotrophs, whilst both FSH and LH are co-produced in the gonadotrophs. The synthesis and secretion of TSH is stimulated by TRH secreted from the hypothalamus and inhibited by somatostatin. FSH and LH are controlled by a single hypothalamic neurohormone, GnRH; their differential release is dependent on the feedback effects of gonadal steroids on the pituitary gland and the amplitude and frequency of GnRH pulses reaching the pituitary gland, which is also under feedback control by gonadal steroids.

The actions of these adenohypophyseal hormones (TSH on the thyroid gland and FSH and LH on the gonads) and the control of their secretions are described in detail in *Chapters 3* and *7*.

2.9 Basic physiology of oxytocin and vasopressin

2.9.1 Oxytocin

Oxytocin is synthesized from a single gene which neighbors the vasopressin gene. The prohormone protein transcript consists of oxytocin and neurophysin I (Np1) interspaced with a tripeptide linker. The prohormone is cleaved to give oxytocin and NP1, both of which are released upon secretion. Oxytocin is a 9 amino acid peptide which is homologous to vasopressin and differs by only 2 amino acids. In the hypothalamus oxytocin, like vasopressin, is expressed in neurons of the supraoptic and paraventricular nuclei although peripheral *OXY* gene expression and oxytocin synthesis have been identified in the uterus, ovary, testis, epididymis, prostate, heart, and adrenal glands. In hormone-dependent tissues, expression of the *OXY* gene is dependent on gonadal steroids and this is particularly marked in the uterus during pregnancy as a result of the rising levels of estrogen.

The most well-defined physiological functions of oxytocin are in labor and lactation (*Figure 2.13*). Although it is not understood exactly what initiates labor in humans, it

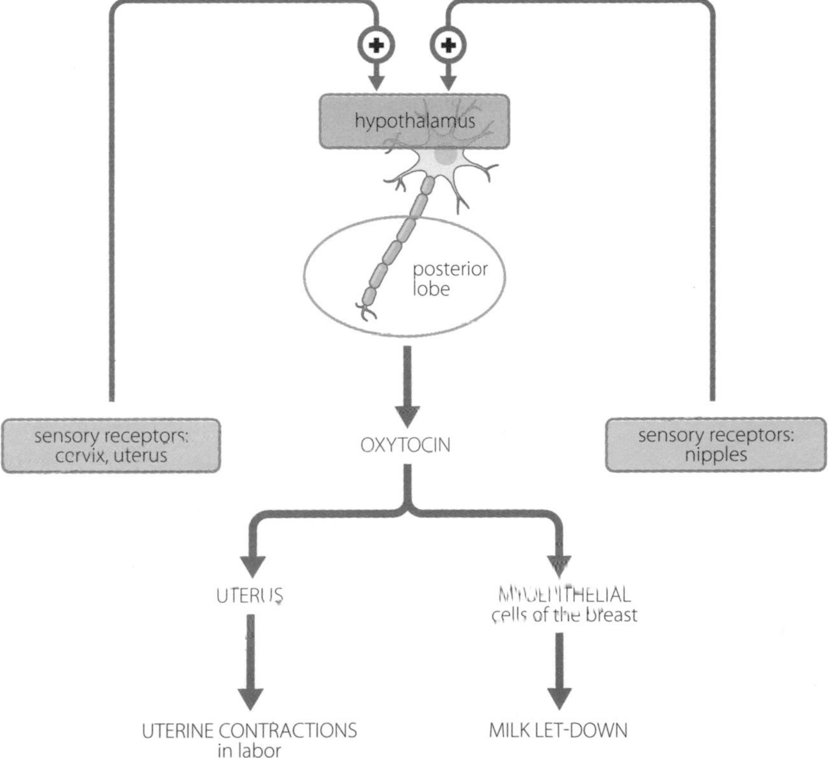

Figure 2.13. Control of oxytocin secretion.

is recognized that many hormones are involved, including oxytocin. This hormone, secreted from the pituitary gland in response to cervical sensory inputs, stimulates uterine smooth muscle contractions and is clearly important in the progression of labor. Clinically, synthetic oxytocin is widely used to induce cervical ripening and labor (an alternative to the use of prostaglandins) and in the treatment of post-partum hemorrhage. In lactation, oxytocin stimulates the milk let-down reflex. In response to suckling, the oxytocinergic neurons in the hypothalamus receive sensory information from the nipples, oxytocin is then secreted from the posterior pituitary gland and this causes contraction of the myoepithelial cells of the ducts in the mammary gland.

Animal studies have shown that oxytocinergic neurons project to higher brain centers and there is evidence from human studies suggesting that central oxytocin can modulate maternal, sexual, social, and stress-related behavior. More recently defects in the oxytocinergic system have been associated with autism, anxiety, and depression. Peripheral actions of oxytocin, derived through local production or from the neurohypophysis, are commonly associated with smooth muscle contraction, particularly in the male and female reproductive tracts.

2.9.2 Vasopressin

Vasopressin (VP), alternatively known as antidiuretic hormone (ADH), is the second neurohypophyseal hormone and like oxytocin is a 9 amino acid peptide which includes two cysteine residues bridged by a disulfide bond. It is synthesized from a single gene on chromosome 2 which is transcribed into a large prohormone consisting of VP, a short linker sequence and a carrier protein, neurophysin II (Np2). The prohormone is synthesized in magnocellular neurosecretory cells in the paraventricular and supraoptic nuclei of the hypothalamus and, once packaged into secretory granules, they are transported down the axons and then stored in the nerve terminals of the posterior pituitary gland. During this transit the prohormone is cleaved to produce VP and Np2 which are co-secreted following activation of the hypothalamic neurons.

In the circulation the half-life of VP is between 20 and 30 minutes and it is metabolized in the liver. Plasma VP concentrations vary between individuals but are usually around 1–5 pg/mL, although night-time levels of VP are double those during the day.

VP receptors (VPR) are widely distributed in the body and three distinct receptor subtypes have been identified.

- V1 receptors (also referred to as V1aR) are found primarily on vascular smooth muscle cells especially in the mesentery, skin, and skeletal tissues. Their activation causes vasoconstriction. They are also present on platelets (where they promote platelet aggregation), the adrenal gland (where they promote aldosterone and cortisol release), and on other organs including the liver, GI tract, kidney, and the brain.
- V2 receptors (V2R) predominate in the kidney and are concentrated on cells of the distal convoluted tubule and collecting duct. Their activation increases gene transcription and insertion of water channels (aquaporins) into the luminal membrane of tubular cells. Aquaporins increase water retention by the kidney. V2 receptors are also located on the vascular endothelium and release the blood clotting factors, von Willebrand, factor VIII, and plasminogen-activating factor.

- V3 receptors (also referred as V1bR) are predominantly found in the anterior pituitary gland and their activation stimulates ACTH release by potentiating CRH (see *Chapter 6*). Brain V3 receptors are likely to mediate the effects of VP on social behaviors (e.g. aggression) and social communication, for which there is some evidence for the role of VP in humans.

All receptors are linked GPCRs. V1R (V1aR) and V3R (V1bR) act via the phosphatidyl-inositol pathway, stimulating the production of inositol triphosphate (IP3) and diacylglycerol which in turn stimulate an increase in intracellular Ca^{2+} concentration and activation of protein kinase C, respectively. V2 receptors activate the adenyl cyclase/cAMP pathway (see *Figure 1.8*). VP can also regulate its own receptors by uncoupling the G proteins and internalization of its receptors.

Control of vasopressin secretion

The major control of VP secretion is plasma osmolality which is precisely regulated between 285 and 295 mOsmol/kg H_2O (osmolarity, mOsmol/L H_2O). Changes in osmolality are sensed by central osmoreceptors surrounding the third ventricle and by peripheral receptors near the hepatic portal vein, and there is a linear relationship between increasing plasma osmolality and the secretion of VP. Thus increases in osmolality stimulate VP secretion, increase water retention in the kidney and thereby dilute osmotically active constituents in plasma (*Figure 2.14*).

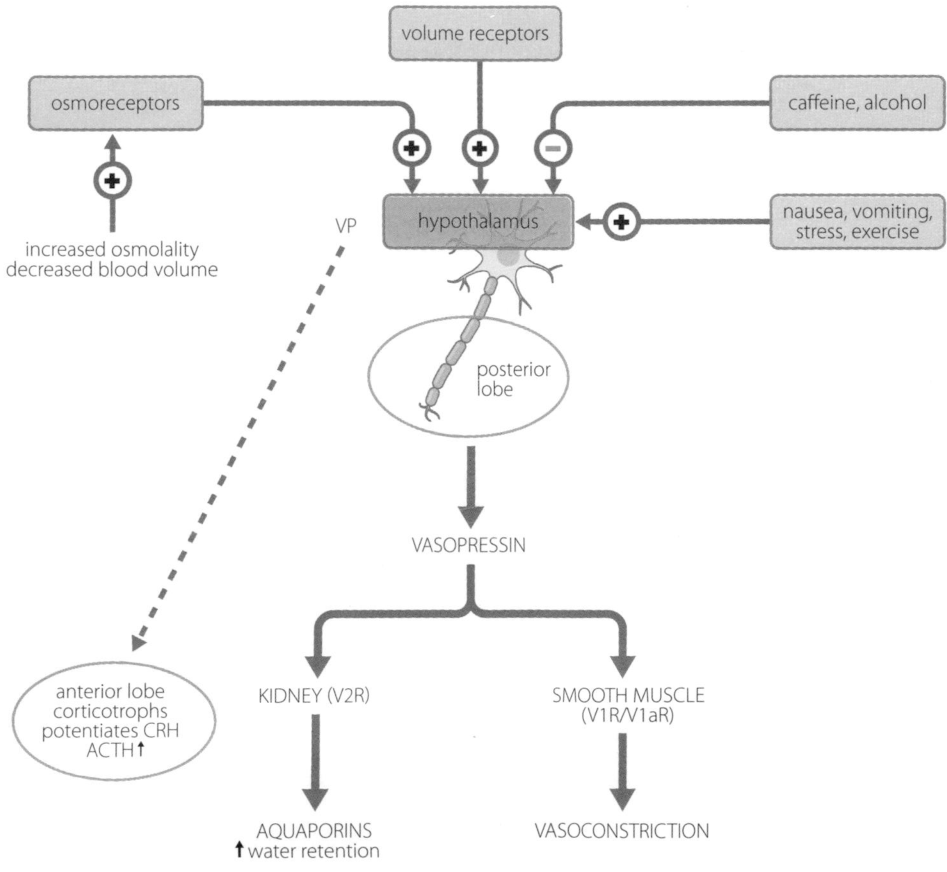

Figure 2.14. Control of vasopressin secretion.

VP secretion is also stimulated by a reduction in blood pressure/blood volume which is sensed by baroreceptors in the left heart, aortic arch and carotid sinuses. This effect is only observed when blood pressure drops by at least 10%, contrasting the stimulation of VP secretion when osmolality increases by 1%. It is therefore considered that VP has a limited role in blood pressure regulation under normal physiological conditions. Several other non-specific factors are known to stimulate VP secretion and these include pain, nausea and hypoglycemia, whilst caffeine and alcohol are known to inhibit VP secretion, leading to diuresis (*Figure 2.14*).

2.10 Disorders related to vasopressin secretion and action

Vasopressin is essential for maintaining the homeostatic mechanisms regulating sodium concentrations and fluid balance. Consequently, impaired production or inhibition of the action of VP results in an inability to concentrate urine, leading to polyuria (dilute urine, >3 L/24 h). The polyuria leads to plasma hyperosmolality and an intense thirst with a very high fluid intake (polydipsia). This is known as diabetes insipidus. In contrast, VP can be secreted inappropriately and this can lead to hyponatremia – this is known as the syndrome of inappropriate ADH secretion.

There are no recorded clinical consequences of oxytocin deficiency.

2.10.1 Diabetes insipidus

A deficiency of VP secretion is known as cranial or central diabetes insipidus (DI) whilst a resistance to the action of VP at the kidney is known as nephrogenic DI.

Polyuria may also occur as a result of compulsive water drinking, a condition known as dipsogenic DI or psychogenic polydipsia. The causes of psychogenic polydipsia are often psychiatric – most commonly schizophrenia. Patients will often demonstrate an inability to suppress thirst at low levels of plasma osmolality and they have an exaggerated thirst response to osmotic challenge. These causes of excessive thirst contrast with the polyuria seen in diabetes mellitus which is caused by glucose in the glomerular filtrate preventing water reabsorption in the kidney due to the osmotic effects of the glucose (see *Chapter 5*).

The causes of cranial DI, resulting from a loss of VP secretion in response to increasing plasma osmolality, are varied (*Box 2.14*). Although there are congenital forms of cranial DI, most are acquired and result from a brain or pituitary tumor, hypothalamic–pituitary damage, from infection, or after pituitary surgery. Resistance to the action of VP at the kidney results in loss of its antidiuretic effect. The usual cause of nephrogenic DI (*Box 2.15*) is drugs or acquired metabolic disease, but familial forms occur due to mutations in either the V2 receptor gene or the aquaporin-2 gene (*AQP-2*). Drugs or metabolic derangement lead to milder nephrogenic DI than familial forms.

Diagnosis

Patients will usually present with polyuria and polydipsia and it is important to exclude other causes of these symptoms such as hyperglycemia or hypercalcemia. Measurement of VP is difficult and the water deprivation test is usually used to confirm DI and to differentiate cranial from nephrogenic (or dipsogenic) DI. For this test (*Figure 2.15*) the patient is allowed to drink freely up until the start of the test (usually at about 0800h). At this point the patient is weighed and access to fluid prevented. The test continues for 8 h but is stopped if the patient loses >4% of their

Box 2.14 | Causes of cranial diabetes insipidus (DI)

Congenital

- Genetic:
  - DIDMOAD
  - rare autosomal dominant or recessive syndromes
- Developmental:
  - septo-optic dysplasia
- Idiopathic

Acquired

- Trauma:
  - head injury
  - surgery
- Tumor:
  - craniopharyngioma
  - germ cell tumors
  - metastatic disease
- Vascular:
  - aneurysm
  - Sheehan syndrome
  - infarction
- Inflammation
  - hypophysitis
  - neurosarcoid
  - histiocytosis
  - other granulomatous disease
  - infection
- Pregnancy

Trauma (including surgery) can lead to posterior pituitary, hypothalamic or stalk damage. Up to 22% of patients presenting with acute traumatic brain injury (TBI) may have DI and this is persistent in around 7%.

Hypothalamic tumors and pituitary metastases may present with DI, but it is uncommon for a primary pituitary tumor to be associated with DI.

Congenital or familial forms of DI are rare. DIDMOAD syndrome (DI, DM, optic atrophy, and deafness) is also known as Wolfram syndrome and is due to a mutation in the *WFSI* gene which encodes a protein called Wolframin. Autosomal dominant DI usually presents in childhood. It is due to inactivating mutations in exon 1 and 2 of the *VP* gene. Symptoms may be relatively slow to appear, and presentation in later life is common and depends on the speed of loss of *VP* functionality.

Box 2.15 | Causes of nephrogenic diabetes insipidus (DI)

- Familial
  - V2 receptor mutations
  - AQP2 mutations
- Idiopathic
- Chronic kidney disease
  - polycystic kidneys
  - renal outflow obstruction
- Metabolic
  - high calcium, low potassium
- Drugs
  - lithium
  - demeclocycline
- Pregnancy

Loss of function mutations of the *V2-R* gene are inherited in an X-linked recessive manner and are rare: they probably account for <1% of nephrogenic DI. Autosomal recessive and dominant families with nephrogenic DI have been described with mutations in the *AQP2* gene. Far more commonly, the defect results from drugs or metabolic derangement.

starting weight. Plasma and urine osmolality are measured at 2-hourly intervals. After 8 h, 1 μg of intramuscular DDAVP (a long-acting analog of AVP) is injected and the patient allowed to eat and drink (it is recommended that the fluid intake is no more than 1.5 times the volume of urine passed in the first 8 h); urine and plasma osmolality are then measured hourly for 4 h and then again the following morning at 0900h.

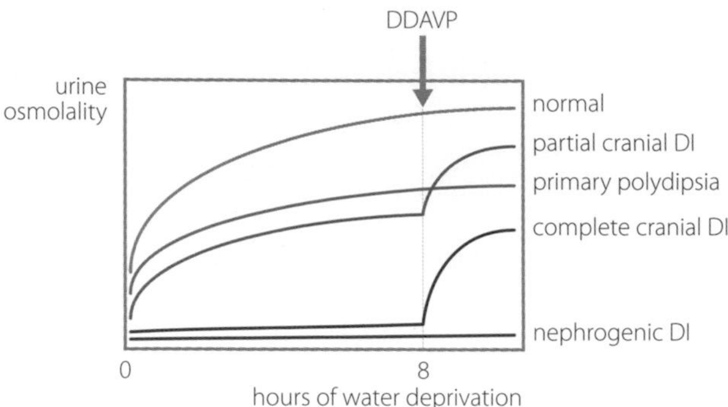

Figure 2.15. The water deprivation test.
During an 8 hour water deprivation test, urine osmolality in normal subjects increases due to an increase in vasopressin secretion in response to an increased plasma osmolality. In complete cranial diabetes insipidus there is no response to the water deprivation, so whilst plasma osmolality increases there is no increase in urine osmolality due to lack of vasopressin. However, these patients will respond to the long-acting vasopressin analog, DDAVP, added at 8 hours. Patients with nephrogenic DI are unable to respond to vasopressin and so their urine osmolality does not increase, even with the addition of DDAVP. In primary polydipsia the ability to concentrate urine is impaired due to deleterious effects of compulsive water drinking on the kidney.

- In cranial DI the plasma osmolality will typically rise to >290 mOsm/kg and urine osmolality will remain dilute (<300 mOsm/kg). After the DDAVP injection, urine osmolality rises (to >700 mOsm/kg).
- In nephrogenic DI the initial pattern will be the same (i.e. concentrated plasma, dilute urine) but there will be no rise in urine osmolality after DDAVP administration.
- In psychogenic polydipsia (primary polydipsia) the urine will gradually concentrate during the initial (dehydration) phase of the test.

Often the water deprivation test may give results that are difficult to interpret: 'partial' cranial DI may produce a 'normal' set of results, and prolonged polyuria from any cause may result in mild nephrogenic DI. In such cases there are two options:

1. *Hyperosmolar stress with measurements of VP in serum.* Hypertonic sodium chloride is infused in order to increase plasma osmolality. Normal individuals will demonstrate a rise in VP as plasma osmolality increases, as will those with psychogenic polydipsia. Patients with cranial DI will have a markedly *reduced* secretion of VP and those with nephrogenic DI will show a brisk and exaggerated response of VP because the kidneys are insensitive to the action of VP, but cranial secretion in response to increased osmolality is still possible.
2. *A trial of DDAVP.* In borderline symptomatic cases where the water deprivation test has not absolutely confirmed or refuted a diagnosis it is reasonable to undertake a trial of DDAVP (administered intranasally in a dose of 10–20 μg per day) with close monitoring of sodium and symptoms. Those with true cranial DI will show an improvement in polydipsia and polyuria, and sodium levels will fall. Patients with psychogenic polydipsia will gradually reduce plasma

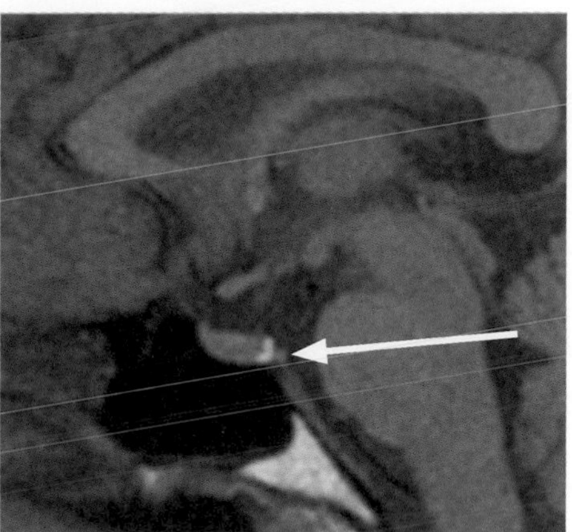

Figure 2.16. Sagittal MRI demonstrating a normal posterior pituitary 'bright spot'.

sodium levels as they dilute their serum. Those with nephrogenic DI will have no benefit.

Once the diagnosis of cranial DI is confirmed, imaging of the pituitary/hypothalamus is necessary to demonstrate the presence/absence of mass lesions in the area. Additionally, MRI may demonstrate an absence of the posterior pituitary 'bright spot' in familial or idiopathic cases (*Figure 2.16*). In T1 weighted MRI the brightness of the posterior pituitary correlates well with VP levels.

Treatment

The mainstay of treatment for cranial DI is a long-acting analog of vasopressin, desmopressin (1-deamino-8-D-arginine vasopressin, DDAVP). This is the only clinically available VP agonist with V2 receptor specificity. DDAVP can be given intranasally (10–80 μg per day), orally (100–800 μg/day), or by parenteral injection (0.1–2 μg/day).

Treatment of nephrogenic DI can be challenging. The offending drug needs to be stopped if the DI is drug-induced and any metabolic abnormalities corrected. In cases of partial nephrogenic DI high doses of DDAVP may be effective. Thiazide diuretics and non-steroidal anti-inflammatory drugs have some benefit in selected cases. In all cases it is important to stress the need for maintenance of adequate hydration.

In psychogenic DI, DDAVP administration could have devastating effects because increased intake without the ability to excrete free water would result in significant electrolyte disturbance, mainly hyponatremia. DDAVP must therefore be avoided and fluid limitation is the only viable treatment.

2.10.2 Hyponatremia and the syndrome of inappropriate antidiuretic hormone secretion

Hyponatremia (a plasma sodium <130 mmol/L) is common in hospitalized patients and unquestionably leads to increased length of stay and increases in mortality and morbidity. There are several causes, but a reduction in plasma sodium must, basically, be due to defects in the normal homeostatic regulatory mechanisms including thirst, action of VP, and renal salt handling. To assess the etiology of hyponatremia it is useful to think in terms of the broad categories that each underlying diagnosis may fall into in terms of changes in total body water, extracellular fluid volume, and total body sodium (*Table 2.3*).

Table 2.3. **Classification of hyponatremia**

Type of hyponatremia	Total body water	Extracellular fluid volume	Na^+	Edema
Hypovolemic	↓	↓	↓↓	-ve
Euvolemic	↑	Minimal ↑	No change	-ve
Hypervolemic	↑↑	↑↑↑	↑	+ve
Redistributive*	No change	↑	No change	
Pseudo**	No change		No change	

*Redistributive hyponatremia occurs where other moieties are contributing to excess osmolality and a fall in sodium is an understandable physiological response to hyperosmolality (e.g. in hyperglycemia or after excessive contrast medium usage). In this situation measured osmolality would be high.

**Pseudohyponatremia is essentially an artifact where, historically, measurements of sodium were affected by high levels of triglycerides or globulins; newer methodologies using ion-specific electrodes have removed this problem.

- *Hypovolemic hyponatremia* occurs where sodium loss exceeds water loss – this may be through renal loss (diuretics, aldosterone deficiency, nephritis, some cases of renal tubular acidosis, cerebral salt wasting) or extra-renal loss (vomiting, diarrhea, burns, extreme sweating, pancreatitis). Renal or extra-renal causes can be differentiated by measurement of renal sodium excretion – levels of 25–30 mmol/L or more suggest renal sodium loss. Renal loss can be treated by stopping any offending diuretic medication and restoring circulating volume with normal (0.9%) saline (in extreme cases higher concentrations of NaCl may be used, e.g. 1.8% or 3%). Fluid restriction is clearly contraindicated in this situation.
- *Hypervolemic hyponatremia* occurs when total body water has increased to a greater extent than total sodium, for example in liver, heart, and renal failure. Treatment is directed at the underlying cause with fluid and salt restriction and use of loop diuretics.
- *Euvolemic hyponatremia* may occur in psychogenic polydipsia and here the urinary sodium loss will be <25–30 mmol/L. Where urinary sodium loss is >30 mmol/L the differential includes hypothyroidism and glucocorticoid deficiency (normal thyroid hormone and cortisol levels are necessary for adequate free water excretion), drugs, stress, and the syndrome of inappropriate ADH secretion (SIADH).

Syndrome of inappropriate ADH secretion

SIADH is a condition in which patients have euvolemic hyponatremia and urine osmolality greater than plasma osmolality. This is caused by unregulated, non-osmotic secretion of VP and dilution of the total body sodium content. Patients with SIADH continue to drink normal amounts of fluids despite low plasma osmolalities, due to a downward resetting of their osmotic threshold for thirst.

It is important to realize that secretion of VP is not always 'inappropriate'. Sometimes it is difficult clinically to identify mild hypovolemia, and the secretion of VP may be as a result of baroreceptors detecting hypovolemia rather than osmoreceptors detecting high osmolality, i.e. the physiological response to perceived hypovolemia may worsen the hyponatremia by conserving free water and further diluting the plasma sodium.

Like other types of hyponatremia, SIADH is commonly diagnosed in hospitalized patients and frequently observed in post-operative patients when pain may contribute to the excess VP secretion. There are numerous causes of SIADH (*Box 2.16* shows the major causes) including drugs, brain damage or infections, ectopic production of VP, and a number of malignancies that lead to excess pituitary VP secretion through poorly understood mechanisms.

Box 2.16 | Causes of SIADH

- Drugs (numerous) – some of the more commonly encountered are:
  - diuretics (loop and thiazide)
  - opiates
  - dopamine agonists
  - ecstasy
  - antidepressants (tricyclic, MAOI, and SSRI)*
  - anticonvulsants
- Cancer
  - bladder, bronchus, prostate, pancreas
  - carcinoid
  - lymphoma, leukemia
  - thymoma
  - mesothelioma
- Neurological
  - trauma (neurosurgery and TBI)
  - brain tumor or abscess
  - meningitis, encephalitis
  - seizures
  - alcohol withdrawal
  - intracranial bleeds
  - hydrocephalus
- Chest
  - TB
  - pneumonia
  - empyema
  - cystic fibrosis
- Other
  - psychosis
  - idiopathic
  - porphyria

*MAOI, monoamine oxidase inhibitors; SSRI, selective serotonin reuptake inhibitors.

The diagnosis of SIADH requires the combination of euvolemia, absence of significant hypotension, inappropriately elevated urine osmolality, urinary sodium loss in excess of 30 mmol/L, and reduced plasma osmolality. Normal cardiac, renal, liver, thyroid, and adrenal function should be confirmed. Most cases of SIADH are temporary and may be managed by fluid restriction, e.g. 1–1.5 L/day.

Clinical features, management, and treatment of hyponatremia

Symptoms of hyponatremia are uncommon until the plasma osmolality falls below 268 mOsmol/kg H_2O, but the symptoms are generally neurological with a hierarchy depending on the sodium level (*Box 2.17*). Thus patients may initially experience headaches and nausea but, as the water intoxication becomes more severe, cerebral edema develops causing drowsiness, lethargy, and mental confusion with fits and coma being the most profound features. Normally the fall in serum sodium is slow but rapid falls are potentially fatal.

The management of hyponatremia is somewhat challenging. It is imperative that correction of sodium should not be attempted too quickly. Any increase in excess of about 12 mmol/day carries a serious risk of central pontine myelinolysis

Box 2.17 | Symptoms and signs of hyponatremia*

- Headache
- Nausea
- Muscle aches and pains
- Lethargy
- Vomiting
- Confusion
- Seizure
- Coma
- Death

* Symptoms/signs occur in this hierarchy dependent upon the degree of hyponatremia

(demyelination as a result of rapid osmotic shifts across the blood–brain barrier leading to rapid changes in brain volume) and this can have devastating consequences such as quadriplegia, coma, and death.

In relatively mild cases of hyponatremia, fluid restriction (to about 1 liter/day) is often sufficient, although this is sometimes surprisingly difficult to achieve. Regular measurements of sodium are necessary and it is important, for the reasons mentioned above, to restore sodium levels slowly and certainly by no more than 12 mmol/day. If the hyponatremia is severe and symptomatic it may be necessary to use hypertonic (3%) NaCl, but again avoiding any increase in sodium >1–2 mmol/h; as a rule of thumb, around 1 mL/kg/h of 3% saline should increase sodium by this amount. Hypertonic saline infusion should be stopped when the clinical situation improves and certainly once a sodium level of 125 mmol/L has been attained.

It is obviously important to stop any offending drugs (if possible) and to seek an underlying cause, which may or may not be treatable. Despite these measures, hyponatremia often recurs and long-term tight fluid restriction is not always possible or acceptable to the patient. In these cases options include the use of the tetracycline, demeclocycline, which antagonizes the action of VP and thus causes nephrogenic DI, or the use of specific vasopressin receptor antagonists generally called 'vaptans'. These non-peptide VP antagonists have either V1a/V2 selectivity, V2 selectivity, or V1a/b selectivity. All V2 antagonists increase urine output and raise serum sodium concentrations. Vaptans are not yet proven in long-term clinical use, but studies to date are encouraging. It is worth noting that they can promote an effective diuresis in heart failure, with rapid and important clinical improvement, and without the reno-toxic effects of some other drug-based therapies for heart failure. In SIADH they are effective, although sodium levels tend to drift back to starting values on cessation of treatment. Long-term treatment is currently lacking data and would be immensely expensive given the current cost of about $1000 (£625) per day.

2.10.3 Adipsia

Adipsic patients have reduced or absent thirst because the osmotic stimulation for thirst is impaired. Due to the co-location of regulatory centers for thirst appreciation and VP release, this may occur in conjunction with cranial DI, causing a potentially life-threatening situation that can result in significant hypernatremia. There are many causes of adipsia/hypodipsia and these are shown in *Box 2.18*.

Treatment is difficult and tailored to the individual. The aim is to ensure adequate fluid intake despite the absence of thirst mechanism and, in some cases, VP control

Box 2.18 | Causes of adipsia/hypodipsia

- Neoplastic lesions in the region of the anterior hypothalamus
  - craniopharyngiomas
  - pinealomas
  - germinomas
  - histiocytomas
  - gliomas
- Granulomatous disease
  - sarcoidosis
  - histiocytosis
- Congenital lesions associated with adipsia include:
  - microcephaly
  - ectrodactyly-ectodermal dysplasia-cleft lip/palate (EEC) syndrome
  - empty sella syndrome
  - malformation of the septum pellucidum
- The following can also produce adipsia:
  - meningoencephalitis
  - subarachnoid hemorrhage
  - hydrocephalus
  - pseudotumor cerebri
  - psychogenic abnormalities

of antidiuresis. DDAVP can be used to control urinary loss (plus insensible loss) to around 2 liters/day and this can be matched by intake with regular monitoring of sodium. Fine tuning may require adjustments for daily weight, based on an ideal weight where sodium and osmolality is known to be normal, i.e. intake is 2 liters plus/minus the difference between daily weight and ideal weight.

2.11 Hypopituitarism

CASE 2.3 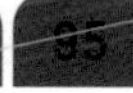 101

- 65 year old man
- Intense headache and loss of vision (over 24h)
- 3rd and 4th cranial nerve involvement
- MRI scan shows pituitary macroadenoma
- Test revealed low IGF-1, undetectable LH and FSH, low testosterone, and low free T_4
- Treatment initially with hydrocortisone, then thyroxine, followed by testosterone and GH

A 65 year old man presented to the emergency department complaining of a 24 hour history of intense headache which had occurred suddenly. This was associated with loss of vision in the right eye. Over the last 24 hours he had felt extremely fatigued, was confused, had recurrent vomiting and a mild pyrexia of 37.6 degrees. Examination revealed a palsy of the right 3rd cranial nerve (dilated pupil, inability to move the affected eye inwards or upward) with ptosis (drooping of the affected eyelid), and a probable 4th cranial nerve palsy (inability to move the affected eye downward). Visual field examination revealed severe visual impairment in the right eye (light perception only), and a left temporal visual field loss.

An emergency CT scan without contrast revealed a hyperdense mass in the area of the pituitary gland and optic chiasm. MRI scanning confirmed the existence of a pituitary macroadenoma with acute hemorrhage.

Because of the patient's acute visual loss, neurosurgeons performed an emergency transsphenoidal resection.

Hypopituitarism simply means a deficiency of secretion of hormones from the pituitary, usually either as a result of pituitary disease or its treatment, or hypothalamic abnormalities associated with reduced stimuli to hormonal secretion. Best estimates suggest about 75% are caused by pituitary lesions, with the other 25%

comprising extra-pituitary tumors, granulomatous disease, pituitary infarction or hemorrhage, rare genetic syndromes, or idiopathic etiology (see *Box 2.9*).

Clinical manifestations are variable depending on the chronicity of the underlying lesion and the hormones affected. For example, many patients may merely present with fatigue, but pituitary apoplexy (infarction or hemorrhage usually in the presence of an adenoma) can occur suddenly with devastating consequences due to sudden loss of ACTH and therefore cortisol deficiency. In contrast, radiation therapy may take several years to cause hypopituitarism.

Severity is variable and partial ACTH deficiency may only manifest in the light of severe stress, unrelated illnesses, surgery, trauma, etc. Hypopituitarism may be complete (affecting all anterior and posterior pituitary hormones) or partial, and there is a general hierarchy of pituitary hormone loss with secretion of gonadotropins and GH being affected more readily than that of ACTH and TSH. However, there are certain situations when pituitary hormone loss does not follow this pattern, for example, isolated ACTH deficiency, which is not uncommon in association with lymphocytic hypophysitis (see *Box 2.19*). Symptoms and signs vary from subtle to profound and are summarized in *Table 2.4*.

- *ACTH deficiency* presents essentially as cortisol deficiency (see *Chapter 5*). This is the most serious aspect of hypopituitarism because vascular collapse may occur in the absence of cortisol, which is important in peripheral vascular

Table 2.4. **Symptoms associated with hypopituitarism due to deficiency of specific pituitary hormone**

Growth hormone (GH)	**Gonadotropins (LH / FSH)**
Weight gain (abdominal adiposity) Decreased muscle strength Decreased exercise capacity Increased cardiovascular risk Impaired psychological well-being Growth retardation (children)	Amenorrhea/oligomenorrhea Infertility Dyspareunia Breast atrophy Loss of secondary sexual hair Decreased libido Impotence Small, soft testes Decreased muscle mass and strength Decreased erythropoiesis Osteoporosis
Thyroid stimulating hormone (TSH)	**Adrenocorticotropin (ACTH)**
Sensitivity to cold Dry skin Constipation Decreased energy	Weight loss Fatigue Pallor Hypoglycemia Nausea / vomiting Circulatory collapse
Prolactin	**Vasopressin (ADH)**
Poor or absent lactation	Urinary frequency Thirst

tone. In milder forms, postural hypotension may be seen, often in association with fatigue, anorexia, weight loss, and hypoglycemia. Clinical presentation of ACTH deficiency is different from primary adrenal failure in two important ways: it does not cause excessive hypovolemia and hyperkalemia because there is no associated aldosterone loss; and there is no pigmentation because ACTH is deficient rather than in excess. Hyponatremia secondary to SIADH may also occur.

- *TSH deficiency* essentially presents as T_4 deficiency, i.e. hypothyroidism (see *Chapter 3*). Classic symptoms of cold intolerance, lethargy, poor appetite, dry skin, constipation and bradycardia may all be present. Often the symptoms are insidious.
- *Gonadotropin deficiency* in women causes ovarian failure with anovulation (subfertility) and associated estrogen deficiency resulting in oligo- or amenorrhea, hot flushes, vaginal dryness and breast atrophy. Androgen secretion can be severely impaired (especially if there is concomitant ACTH deficiency) resulting in loss of libido and reduced bone density. In men, subfertility and testosterone deficiency (decreased energy, well-being, muscle and bone strength, decreased frequency of shaving and loss of libido) may be seen.
- *GH deficiency* is described in detail in *Section 2.5.*
- *Prolactin deficiency* appears to have very few effects apart from the inability for women to lactate post-partum.
- *Vasopressin deficiency* causes diabetes insipidus (see *Section 2.10.1*).

Best estimates as to the incidence/prevalence of hypopituitarism suggest an incidence of around 4 per 100 000 per annum, with a prevalence of about 50 per 100 000 in the UK and USA.

2.11.1 Causes of hypopituitarism

Pituitary lesions

Any lesion in the sella (adenomas, cysts, metastases, hypophysitis) can cause hypopituitarism by pressure effects on normal pituitary cells. Surgery may reverse this situation by allowing normal pituitary cells to restore function once pressure effects are removed, but may also cause hypopituitarism by destroying normal pituitary tissue where differentiation from pathological tissue cannot be made visually or where, during excision, damage to normal pituitary tissue is unavoidable.

Irradiation of the pituitary (following surgery, as primary treatment of inoperable pituitary lesions or where the pituitary is included in a wide field for unrelated radiation treatment) may result in loss of pituitary function over a variable time frame, hence the need for long-term follow-up of any patient after radiotherapy treatment.

Infiltrative disease (hemochromatosis, lymphocytic hypophysitis) can cause pituitary failure. Hereditary hemochromatosis, or iron deposition acquired following multiple transfusions tends to affect gonadotrophs leading to hypogonadotropic hypogonadism. Lymphocytic hypophysitis (*Box 2.19*) occurs most frequently in late pregnancy or the post-partum period and is probably autoimmune in origin.

Box 2.19 | Miscellaneous lesions of the hypothalamus/pituitary gland

Lymphocytic hypophysitis

This is the most common form of primary hypophysitis (i.e. inflammation of the hypophysis). It is most common in women, especially in pregnancy or the early post-partum period. It is likely that a number of cases originally ascribed to Sheehan syndrome (necrosis of the pituitary secondary to blood loss and hypovolemia following complicated delivery) were in fact due to lymphocytic hypophysitis.

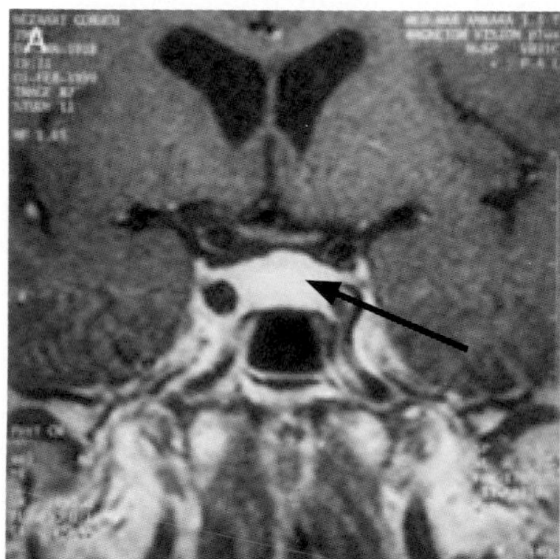

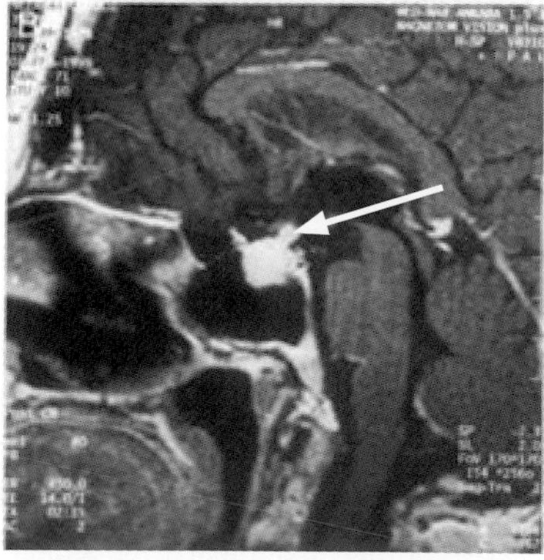

Box figure 2.8. MRI scan from a patient with lymphocytic hypophysitis.
The coronal image (top) illustrates homogenous uptake of gadolinium and the sagittal scan (bottom) shows thickening of the stalk. The arrows point to the pituitary showing uniform uptake of gadolinium (top) and the thickened pituitary stalk (bottom).

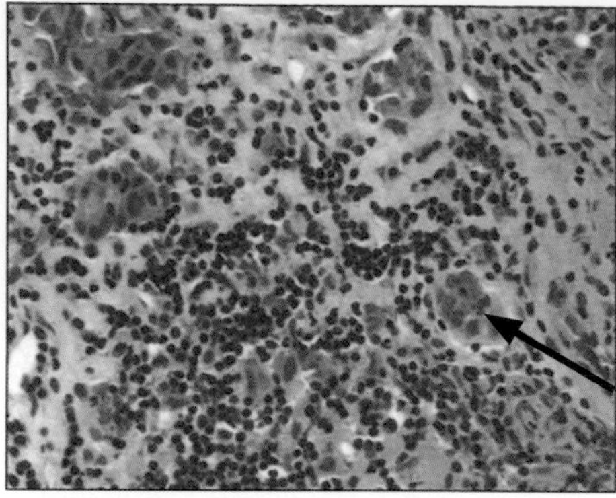

Box figure 2.9. Histology of lymphocytic hypophysitis showing a diffuse inflammatory infiltrate composed mainly of lymphocytes and plasma cells forming occasional lymphoid follicles (arrow).

Interestingly, the normal hierarchy of anterior pituitary hormone loss is not followed on lymphocytic hypophysitis. ACTH loss is the most common pathology, followed by TSH loss causing secondary hypothyroidism. GH and gonadotropin deficiency is rare. Diabetes insipidus is not uncommon. The histological features (diffuse infiltration of the pituitary with lymphocytes that form lymphoid follicles) resemble other autoimmune endocrine disease, and an autoimmune pathology is likely.

Many patients will undergo surgical resection, either as a result of diagnostic uncertainty or because of potential visual compromise, and this may result in post-operative hypopituitarism. The condition itself may cause hypopituitarism secondary to continued destruction of pituicytes by the inflammatory process. Sometimes, if the diagnosis is made without recourse to surgery, and the patient is closely followed-up, resolution may occur. Improvement in pituitary function and cessation of the inflammatory process is also sometimes seen with high-dose glucocorticoid treatment.

Lesions in the region of the hypothalamus

Numerous lesions arise in the region of the hypothalamus, many of which can extend into the pituitary fossa leading to visual defects and hormone abnormalities. In contrast to primary pituitary lesions, hypothalamic tumors are frequently associated with posterior pituitary pathology, i.e. diabetes insipidus. Full blown and devastating hypothalamic syndromes may ultimately arise from hypothalamic lesions, with hydrocephalus secondary to blockage of the foramen of Monro (ultimately leading to coma), temperature and appetite dysregulation leading to massive obesity, and loss of thirst mechanisms.

Box 2.19 | continued

Structural lesions in the region of the hypothalamus are numerous and include:

- Developmental abnormalities
  - craniopharyngioma (*Section 2.3*)
  - germinoma
  - hamartoma
  - chordoma
  - epidermoid and dermoid cysts
- CNS tumors
  - ependymoma
  - optic glioma
  - meningioma
- Malignant CNS disease
  - Hodgkin and non-Hodgkin lymphoma
  - leukemia
  - histiocytosis X (Langerhans cell histiocytosis)
  - eosinophilic granuloma
- Vascular tumors
  - hemangioblastoma
  - hemangiopericytoma
  - cavernous hemangioma
- Granulomatous disease
  - sarcoidosis
  - Wegener's granulomatosis
  - TB

Chordomas are rare tumors, thought to arise from notochord remnants. If they arise close to the clivus (i.e. in the sellar area) they can cause endocrine dysfunction. Treatment is by surgery and radiotherapy and the overall prognosis remains rather poor.

Hypothalamic hamartomas are rare, occurring exclusively in childhood where they may lead to precocious puberty (due to secretion of GnRH) or gigantism (if secreting GHRH).

Malignant CNS disease (Hodgkin and non-Hodgkin lymphoma, histiocytosis X, and eosinophilic granuloma) can occur in the suprasellar area and give rise to anterior pituitary dysfunction associated with diabetes insipidus and visual disturbance. Treatment is of the primary disease, although hormone replacement may occasionally be required.

Granulomatous CNS disease due to neurosarcoid can give rise to diabetes insipidus, high prolactin and anterior pituitary hormone loss. More extreme hypothalamic syndromes include somnolence, appetite and temperature dysregulation, and obesity. The diagnosis is made on MRI. CSF protein estimations may help with the diagnosis although serum ACE (used in the diagnosis of systemic sarcoid) is not usually helpful. The diagnosis may only be made after a pituitary biopsy. Steroid treatment using prednisolone, both as an immunosuppressive and to combat ACTH deficiency, may put the condition into remission.

This is an unusual form of hypopituitarism in that ACTH (and less frequently TSH) deficiency often occurs with preservation of GH and gonadotropin function.

Pituitary infarction (Sheehan syndrome) after post-partum hemorrhage has long been recognized as a cause of hypopituitarism, but advances in obstetric practice have made this a less common cause in developed countries. Nevertheless, in any case of hypopituitarism it is important to take an obstetric history because in mild cases the diagnosis can be delayed for years. The classic presentation is of failure to lactate after a difficult delivery associated with blood loss sufficient to require transfusion. Menstruation may not return after delivery, and there may be associated symptoms of loss of sexual characteristics, lethargy and weight loss. Diabetes insipidus is rare. Imaging will usually show a normal sized sella (no pre-existing pituitary pathology) with an atrophic pituitary or empty sella.

Pituitary apoplexy is a sudden hemorrhage into the pituitary gland usually in association with an underlying adenoma. This can present abruptly with a sudden onset excruciating ('thunderclap') headache associated with diplopia and hypopituitarism, usually manifesting as circulatory collapse due to sudden cortisol deficiency (secondary to ACTH loss). Apoplexy should be considered a neurosurgical emergency because decompressive surgery may lead to rapid improvement of visual dysfunction and, occasionally, reversal of hypopituitarism. Less severe cases can be managed conservatively with hormonal replacement as necessary; resorption of blood may lead to reduction in compressive symptoms.

Pituitary abscess is a rare cause of hypopituitarism usually presenting with headache, variable hypopituitarism and diabetes insipidus.

Genetic diseases

Defects in genes encoding transcription factors that are essential for the differentiation of anterior pituitary cells (*Figure 2.5*) can result in congenital deficiency of pituitary hormones.

- Mutations in *HEXS1*, *LHX3*, and *LHX4* cause combined pituitary hormone deficiency (GH, FSH, LH, TSH, prolactin all reduced).
- Mutations in the *PROP1* gene are the commonest cause of congenital combined pituitary hormone deficiency. Older patients with defects in the *PROP1* gene may present with ACTH deficiency. Otherwise the age of onset and progression of pituitary hormone loss is variable. Most patients will have short stature due to GHD.
- Dominant and recessive mutations of the gene that encodes PIT-1 (*POU-1F1*) lead to congenital deficiencies of GH, prolactin and, sometimes, TSH. The secretion of ACTH, FSH, and LH is preserved.
- The *TPIT* gene is necessary for differentiation of pituitary corticotrophs and mutations can cause isolated ACTH deficiency which may have devastating neonatal consequences if not detected quickly.

Hypothalamic diseases

Hypothalamic diseases with concomitant reduction in the secretion of hormones controlling anterior pituitary function can result in hypopituitarism. However, DI due to loss of vasopressin secretion occurs much more frequently than loss of anterior pituitary hormone secretions. The causes of hypothalamic dysfunction include:

- Any mass lesion (e.g. craniopharyngiomas, secondary deposits from breast or lung tumors).
- Irradiation of the hypothalamus (e.g. in treatment of nasopharyngeal tumors or brain tumors). Survivors of childhood irradiation require close follow-up for development of anterior pituitary hormone loss in later life.
- Sarcoidosis and Langerhans cell histiocytosis can cause deficiencies of anterior pituitary hormones and DI, and the loss of anterior pituitary function may often post-date the onset of DI by several years.

Traumatic brain injury

Severe skull base injury can cause hypothalamic damage, but recent studies suggest that other forms of traumatic brain injury may also have immediate and longer-term effects on anterior pituitary function. Some studies suggest that up to 75% of patients with severe traumatic brain injury may have acute loss of one or more pituitary hormones which persist in about 10%. GHD is probably the most studied and prevalent longer-term effect of severe brain injury. DI is not uncommon in acute brain injury and occasionally persists after recovery. SIADH is very commonly associated with brain trauma, but again is rarely persistent.

Ischemic stroke and subarachnoid hemorrhage may occasionally be associated with hypopituitarism and again the commonest manifestation is impaired GH response to stimulatory tests (*Box 2.6*), although hypogonadism and even hypoadrenalism have been reported.

2.11.2 Treatment of hypopituitarism

Treatment of hypopituitarism is based on replacement of missing target hormones.

ACTH deficiency is treated with hydrocortisone (or occasionally another glucocorticoid hormone such as prednisolone or dexamethasone). With hydrocortisone therapy the aim is to try to mimic normal secretion of cortisol, so it is usually given in divided doses (two or three times a day) with the majority given in the morning and the last dose given no later than early afternoon.

TSH deficiency requires thyroxine replacement. It is important (in pan-hypopituitarism) to restore normal cortisol levels before starting thyroxine. Also, TSH cannot be used to monitor thyroxine requirements – the aim is to get the fT_4 into the upper quartile of the normal range.

Gonadotropin deficiency is treated by replacing the target hormone, i.e. testosterone in men and estrogen (with or without progesterone depending on the presence of a uterus) in women. It is important to remember that young women with hypopituitarism require estrogen/progestogen replacement therapy not solely for symptomatic relief (as in post-menopausal women); the aim is to ensure that the benefits of long-term estrogen replacement (until the age of the natural menopause) are achieved. Unopposed estrogen (without progestogen) is contraindicated due to the risk of endometrial hyperplasia and possible cancerous change (see *Chapter 7*), so the normal method is to give a combined sequential oral form (which

CASE 2.3

95 

- 65 year old man
- Intense headache and loss of vision (over 24h)
- 3rd and 4th cranial nerve involvement
- MRI scan shows pituitary macroadenoma
- Test revealed low IGF-1, undetectable LH and FSH, low testosterone, and low free T_4
- Treatment initially with hydrocortisone, then thyroxine, followed by testosterone and GH

The patient was reviewed following surgery by the endocrine team. Histology from the surgical specimens confirmed a pituitary adenoma with positive staining for LH, FSH and alpha subunit.

Close questioning revealed a gradual loss of sexual function over several years prior to presentation, with decreased frequency of shaving, decreased libido and impaired erectile function. Clinically the patient was pale and hypogonadal. Post-operative assessment revealed:

- pan-hypopituitarism with undetectable cortisol
- low IGF-1 (GHD was confirmed later with a glucagon test)
- undetectable LH and FSH
- testosterone: 4.6 nmol/L (NR 14–28)
- TSH: 0.4 mIU/L (NR 0.4–4.2)
- fT_4: 7 pmol/L (NR 10–20)
- prolactin was normal

The patient initially received hydrocortisone given in divided doses (15 mg in the early morning, 5 mg at lunchtime and 5 mg in the early afternoon) and after a week thyroxine was introduced at a dose of 100 μg daily. He was also started on testosterone replacement and then GH replacement. At review 2 months later he was well and happy with the outcome.

contains estrogen throughout the pack and progestogens from day 16 to day 28), or continuous estradiol by transdermal patch with progestogen taken orally from day 1 to day 10 of each calendar month. If fertility is required, gonadotropins or pulsed gonadotropin-releasing hormone (if the defect is hypothalamic and the pituitary is intact) can be used.

2.12 Non-functioning pituitary adenomas

Non-functioning pituitary adenomas (NFPAs) describe those tumors that have no demonstrable clinical features of hormone excess, i.e. there is no evidence of Cushing disease, acromegaly, significant hyperprolactinemia, TSH or gonadotropin excess. Although there may be no clinical evidence of hormone excess, up to 80% of NFPAs will show histological evidence of positive staining for glycoprotein hormones, most commonly LH and FSH. These are often called 'silent gonadotropinomas'. Approximately 20% of NFPAs show absolutely no hormone staining (and indeed no evidence of hormonal mRNA generation or hormone secretion into the media on cell culture) and are called 'null-cell tumors'.

NFPAs are usually monoclonal in origin, i.e. arising from a single abnormal cell line. It is likely that both hypothalamic stimulatory factors and locally produced growth factors promote tumorigenesis. There are numerous oncogenes involved in tumor progression in a variety of sites, and attention has understandably been focused on defining the influence of oncogenes on NFPAs. To date there is no evidence that mutations in the *MENIN* gene are important in NFPAs and, in contrast to somatotropinomas, Gs-alpha mutations are rare (<10%). Two 'new' genes, which may be relevant, have been described: *PTTG* (pituitary tumor transformation gene) and *PTAG* (pituitary tumor apoptosis gene). The latter is poorly expressed in NFPAs and may contribute to the lack of apoptosis in NFPAs.

2.12.1 Clinical signs and symptoms

The absence of hormone excess means that symptoms are usually only apparent once the tumor has grown to sufficient size to cause headache or visual symptoms: hemianopia if the optic chiasm is compromised or ophthalmoplegia if the 3rd, 4th, and 6th cranial nerves are compromised within the cavernous sinus. Stalk compression by large pituitary adenomas can result in hyperprolactinemia, which can contribute to the genesis of hypogonadism. Hypogonadism is the most common presenting feature of NFPA, although it is mainly due to loss of gonadotropins resulting in amenorrhea, loss of libido or secondary sexual function/characteristics. The somatotrophs are the most sensitive cells in terms of loss of function secondary to NFPA growth, but the symptoms of GHD in adulthood are subtle, and may only be recognized once GH has been replaced. ACTH deficiency is less common but may occur acutely if pituitary apoplexy occurs (e.g. in situations of surgery, extreme stress, infection, or hemorrhage). TSH deficiency resulting in secondary hypothyroidism is rarer still.

2.12.2 Treatment

Surgery is the mainstay of treatment. Hypogonadism caused (at least in part) by hyperprolactinemia secondary to stalk compression may improve post-operatively. Other hormone deficiencies (caused by pituitary compression) are less likely to improve. Visual field defects (*Box 2.7*) will usually improve rapidly after surgery.

If resection is incomplete (e.g. if there is tumor in the cavernous sinuses which is not easily accessible or if there is a significant residual and further operative intervention is deemed unsafe) post-operative radiotherapy may be necessary. There is some concern that radiotherapy may result in more frequent cerebrovascular mortality/morbidity, but it is clear that it has a place in preventing tumor recurrence. There is no compelling evidence that radiotherapy worsens vision or leads to an increase in the incidence of *de novo* intracranial tumors. It is likely that highly focused radiotherapy (i.e. gamma knife) will cause fewer problems than conventional radiotherapy.

Some evidence suggests that post-operative (and post-radiotherapy) treatment of NFPA with selective dopamine agonists will lengthen the time to recurrence. Tumors may also express receptors for Type 2 and Type 5 somatostatin receptors, suggesting that treatment with the combined D2 agonist/SSR agonist dopastatin may be effective.

2.13 Further reading

Ben-Schlomo A and Melmed S (2010) Pituitary somatostatin receptor signalling. *Trends Endocrinol. Metabol.* **21:** 123–33.

Binart N, Bachelot A, and Bouilly J (2010) Impact of prolactin receptor isoforms on reproduction. *Trends Endocrinol. Metabol.* **21:** 362–8.

Daly AF, Tichomirowa MA, and Beckers A (2009) The epidemiology and genetics of pituitary adenomas. *Best Pract. Res. Clin. Endocrinol. Metabol.* **23:** 543–54.

Debono M and Newell-Price J (2010) New formulations and approaches in the medical treatment of acromegaly. *Current Op. Endocrinol. Diab. Obesity,* **17:** 350–5.

Giustina A , Mazziotti G, and Canalis E (2008) Growth hormone, insulin-like growth factors, and the skeleton. *Endocrine Reviews,* **29:** 535–59.

Gueorguiev M and Grossman AB (2011) Pituitary tumors in 2010: a new therapeutic era for pituitary tumors. *Nature Rev. Endocrinol.* **7:** 71–3.

Holt NF and Haspel KL (2010) Vasopressin: a review of therapeutic applications. *J. Cardioth. Vasc. Anaes.* **24:** 330–47.

Klibanski A (2010) Prolactinomas. *New Engl. J. Med.* **362:** 1219–26.

Melmed S (2008) Update in pituitary disease. *J Clin. Endocrinol. Metabol.* **93:** 331–8.

Melmed S (2009) Acromegaly pathogenesis and treatment. *J Clin. Invest.* **119:** 3189–202.

Richmond E and Rogol AD (2010) Current indications for growth hormone for children and adolescents. *Endocrine Devel.* **18:** 92–108.

Tom N and Assinder SJ (2009) Oxytocin in health and disease. *Int. J. Biochem. Cell Biol.* **42:** 202–5.

Vijayakumar A, Novosyadlyy R, Wu Y, Yakar S, and LeRoith D (2010) Biological effects of growth hormone on carbohydrate and lipid metabolism. *Growth Hormone IGF Res.* **20:** 1–7.

2.14 Self-assessment questions

(1) Which is the predominant hormone secreting cell type of the adenohypophysis?
   - (a) Lactotrophs
   - (b) Somatotrophs
   - (c) Thyrotrophs
   - (d) Gonadotrophs
   - (e) Corticotrophs

(2) Which one of the following adenohypophyseal hormones is predominantly controlled by a hypothalamic inhibitory neurohormone?
(a) Prolactin
(b) Thyroid stimulating hormone
(c) Growth hormone
(d) Luteinizing hormone
(e) Adrenocorticotropin

(3) Growth hormone secretion is inhibited by which one of the following?
(a) Octreotide
(b) Cabergoline
(c) Ghrelin
(d) Hypoglycemia
(e) Arginine

(4) Which is the most specific diagnostic test for acromegaly?
(a) A pituitary MRI scan
(b) Measurement of IGF-1 levels
(c) A visual field test
(d) Measurement of GH levels during a 2h glucose tolerance test
(e) An insulin stress test

(5) The following treatments are commonly used in the treatment of craniopharyngiomas with the exception of which one?
(a) Surgery
(b) Radiotherapy
(c) Octreotide
(d) Hormone replacement therapy
(e) Insertion of cerebral shunts

(6) In acromegaly, pegvisomant works by which one of the following mechanisms?
(a) Inhibiting GH release by activating the somatostatin receptor
(b) Inhibiting GHRH release from the hypothalamus
(c) Competitively inhibiting GH binding to and activation of the GH receptor
(d) Blocking the peripheral action of IGF-1
(e) Shrinking the pituitary adenoma

(7) A 45 year old bank clerk presented with polyuria and polydipsia. Her fasting blood glucose was 4.4 mmol/L (NR 3.5–6.1) and ionized serum calcium was 1.2 mmol/L (NR 1.15–1.27) and diabetes insipidus (DI) was suspected. Which one of the following results from an 8 hour water deprivation test would indicate that she had central DI as opposed to nephrogenic DI?
(a) A rise in serum osmolality after 4 hours of water deprivation
(b) A decrease in urine osmolality after 8 hours of water deprivation
(c) A rise in urine osmolality after DDAVP administration
(d) No change in urine osmolality after 8 hours water deprivation
(e) An increase in serum osmolality after DDAVP administration

(8) A 12 year old girl complains of frequent headaches, nausea and vomiting, and loss of peripheral vision. She is sent for CT and MRI imaging which reveals a cystic calcified parasellar lesion. What is the most likely diagnosis?
(a) Non-functioning pituitary tumor
(b) Macroadenoma
(c) Lymphocytic hypophysitis
(d) Craniopharyngioma
(e) Pituitary apoplexy

(9) A 61 year old man has noted a gradual loss of peripheral vision and complains of frequent headaches, feeling tired and a diminished capacity for exercise over the past year or so. An MRI scan reveals a 4 cm pituitary mass extending superiorly.
(a) What is the most likely diagnosis?
(b) What is the cause of the loss of peripheral vision?
(c) How would his loss of pituitary function be assessed?
(d) What are the treatment options?

(10) A 19 year old girl presents with a milky discharge from her breasts and has noted that her periods stopped about 7 months ago although she had a normal menarche at the age of 13. Otherwise she is fit and healthy and takes no medication. Her prolactin level was 6000 mIU/L (NR 100–550).
(a) What is the most likely cause of her hyperprolactinemia?
(b) What is the cause of the loss of menstruation?
(c) What are the hypothalamic hormones that regulate the secretion of prolactin?
(d) What is the most likely treatment option for a prolactinoma?

CHAPTER 03 The thyroid gland

After working through this chapter you should be able to:

- Describe the physiological roles of thyroxine and triiodothyronine and consequently the signs and symptoms of excessive and insufficient thyroid hormone secretion
- Describe the synthesis of thyroid hormones, their transport and metabolism, and the control of thyroid growth and hormone secretion
- Outline the importance of iodine in thyroid metabolism and the consequences of iodine deficiency
- Know the causes and clinical effects of hyper- and hypothyroidism
- Outline the investigation and treatment of thyroid disease

3.1 Introduction

The thyroid gland secretes two hormones, thyroxine (T_4) and triiodothyronine (T_3); T_3 is the biologically active form of these two hormones, with T_4 being converted to T_3 after its secretion from the gland. Thyroid hormones act on virtually every cell of the body to stimulate the resting metabolic rate. They also have important effects on the cardiovascular system and in development.

Disorders of thyroid physiology affect about 5% of women and 0.5% of men and thus they are amongst the most common disorders in endocrinology. Whatever the etiology, symptoms of thyroid disorders are manifest as those relating to:

- an excess of thyroid hormones (hyperthyroidism or thyrotoxicosis) – the clinical features are typically tachycardia, heat intolerance, warm moist skin, goiter, increased appetite and weight loss, anxiety and tremor (see *Cases 3.1* and *3.2*)
- a deficiency of thyroid hormones (hypothyroidism) – the clinical features are typically bradycardia, cold intolerance, dry thin hair and skin, goiter, fatigue and depression (see *Case 3.6*)

To understand the clinical features of thyroid diseases and their treatment it is important to know about basic thyroid anatomy, embryology and physiology.

3.2 Anatomy and embryology

3.2.1 Anatomy

The thyroid gland is one of the largest classical endocrine organs in the body and weighs approximately 25 g (it is slightly larger in women than men). It has variously been described as 'U' or 'H'-shaped, with two lobes lying on either side of the ventral aspect of the trachea connected by a band of connective tissue called the isthmus (*Figure 3.1*). The four parathyroid glands (in two pairs - superior and inferior) usually lie in close association with the thyroid. The lateral parts of the thyroid are covered by the sternothyroid muscles and, anteriorly, the sternohyoid and omohyoid muscles can be found. The gland is supplied with blood from the superior thyroid arteries (arising from the external carotids) and the inferior thyroid arteries (arising from the subclavian arteries) and, because it has to trap iodine avidly for thyroid hormone synthesis, it takes more blood per unit weight than the kidneys. In fact, when there is excessive growth of the gland - termed a goiter (see *Box 3.2* in *Section 3.4.5*) - the blood flow to the gland may be heard with a stethoscope and the sound is termed a bruit.

The superior laryngeal nerve follows the course of the superior thyroid artery and the recurrent laryngeal nerve is closely associated with the inferior thyroid artery (although there is a great deal of individual variability). These nerves are easy to damage during thyroid surgery. The thyroid itself has parasympathetic innervation

(a)

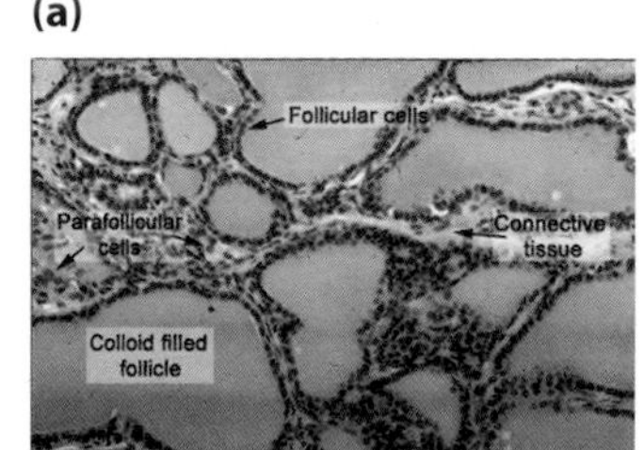

(b)

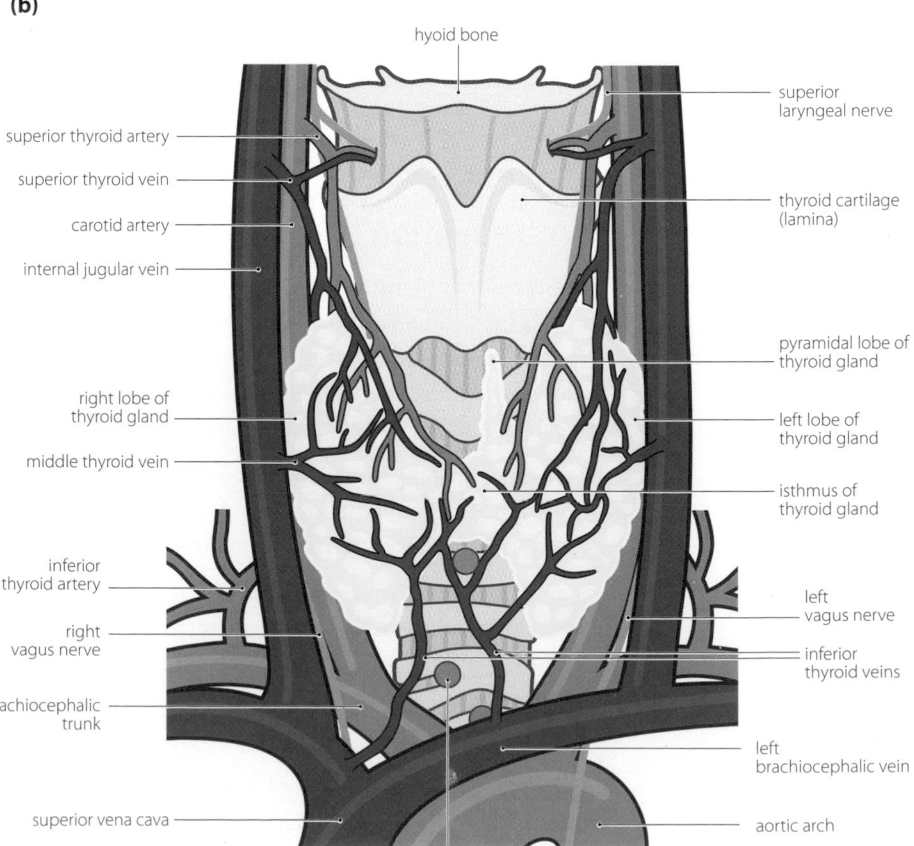

Figure 3.1. (a) Histology and (b) anatomy of the thyroid gland.

from the vagus and sympathetic innervation from the superior, middle, and inferior ganglia of the sympathetic trunk.

3.2.2 Embryology

The thyroid gland is one of the first endocrine organs to develop, beginning at around 24 days of gestation. Like the pituitary gland (see *Chapter 2*), it develops from proliferation of endodermal cells on the pharyngeal floor (1st and 2nd pharyngeal arches) and, as the embryo grows, the thyroid gland descends into the neck. For a short time the gland is connected to the developing tongue by a narrow tube, the thyroglossal duct. The gland has assumed its definitive shape by around 7 weeks and has also reached its final destination in the neck. By this time the thyroglossal duct has normally disappeared, although its remnants persist as a small pit, the foramen cecum (*Figure 3.2*).

The parathyroid glands that are closely associated with the thyroid gland also develop from the pharyngeal endoderm, in this case the 3rd and 4th pharyngeal

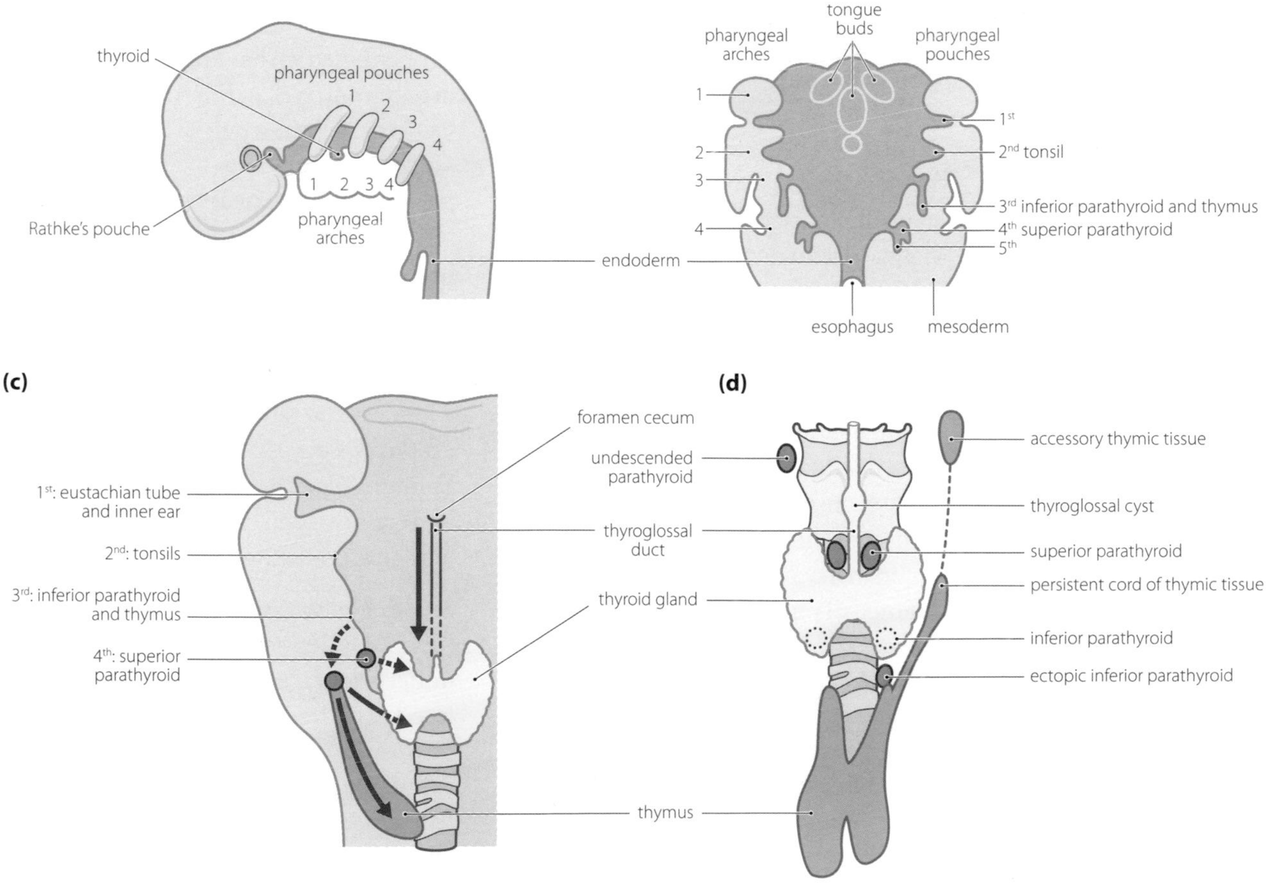

Figure 3.2. Embryology of the thyroid and parathyroid glands.
(a) Sagittal and (b) transverse views of the pharyngeal regions of a human embryo during the fifth week of gestation, showing the endodermal pharyngeal pouches and mesodermal pharyngeal arches; the embryonic origin of the thyroid gland and parathyroid glands is shown.
(c) Migration of the thyroid gland and parathyroid glands (anterior view). (d) Illustrates various abnormalities which can occur during embryonic development. Diagrams are not drawn to relative scale.

pouches (*Figure 3.2*). The inferior parathyroid glands (sitting at the lower poles of the two lobes of the thyroid gland) migrate along with the thymus gland, and the superior parathyroids from the 4th pharyngeal pouch migrate laterally.

The embryology of these glands results in important clinical sequelae. If the thyroglossal duct does not disappear completely this may result in mid-line thyroglossal cysts, and the persistent connection with the tongue means that such cysts move upwards when the tongue is protruded. The descent of the thyroid and parathyroid glands can also result in ectopic thyroid and parathyroid tissue in a number of positions from the tongue to the chest. Finally, it should be noted that thyroid surgery can result in the removal of parathyroid tissue, subsequently leading to hypoparathyroidism (see *Chapter 4*).

3.3 Hyperthyroidism

CASE 3.1 110 127 128

- Caucasian female of 26 years with 4 months of weight loss and lack of menstrual period
- Symptoms and examination suggested Graves disease: bilateral tremor, heat intolerance, tachycardia, non-tender vascular swelling in neck, thyroid bruit, and lid lag
- TFTs ordered

A 26 year old Caucasian woman presented to her family doctor having not had a menstrual period for 4 months; pregnancy was excluded. She had also lost 5 kg over 4 months despite an increased appetite. The persistent bilateral tremor in her hands was causing her significant problems in her work as a dentist. Both she and her friends and family had noticed that she had been lethargic and irritable over the last 4–5 months as well as noting a slight change in her facial appearance. Despite being winter, she found that she only needed to wear a light jacket to go outside instead of her usual winter coat, and she claimed to feel uncomfortable when in a warm room. Finally, she complained of palpitations and increased shortness of breath when she exerted herself, causing problems when she trained in the gym. She had no other significant medical problems and was not on any form of regular medication. Her mother has insulin-independent diabetes mellitus and her maternal grandmother was said to have had a large goiter.

On examination, her fingers were warm to touch and well perfused. A regular tachycardia (pulse rate 96 b.p.m.) was noted. There was a small amount of palmar erythema bilaterally. Neck examination revealed a small symmetrical non-tender vascular swelling in the neck which moved upwards on swallowing. On auscultation, a thyroid bruit was clearly audible. She had lid lag of approximately 2 mm with lid retraction and bilateral proptosis. Graves disease (primary autoimmune hyperthyroidism) was suspected and confirmation was sought by arranging specific investigations.

Blood tests to assess thyroid function (thyroid function tests or 'TFTs') were undertaken, including measurement of free T_3 and free T_4 levels, thyroid peroxidase (TPO) and TSH receptor antibody status, and a nuclear medicine scan using radiolabeled technetium 99m was considered (see *Section 3.4.3*).

CASE 3.2 111 129

- Afro-Caribbean female of 35 years with 2 day history of neck pain
- Symptoms and examination suggested thyroiditis: bilateral tremor, muscle weakness, tachycardia

A 35 year old Afro-Caribbean woman presented to her family doctor complaining of a 2 day history of neck pain around the thyroid region which appeared suddenly and radiated up to her jaw. She described the pain as constant and throbbing in nature, causing her significant distress. As well as feeling feverish, she was experiencing subtle signs of thyroid hormone excess including bilateral tremor and muscle weakness. She had just recently recovered from a suspected viral illness during which she suffered from a sore throat, myalgia, malaise, and lethargy. Apart from endometriosis, she had no other significant past medical or family history and took no form of regular medication. On examination her neck was extremely tender and warm to touch. She was found to be tachycardic with warm and well perfused peripheries. Neurological examination demonstrated significant proximal muscle weakness.

The combination of acute thyrotoxic symptoms following a viral illness and associated with exquisite tenderness in the neck suggested a diagnosis of thyroiditis. This was investigated by testing her blood for thyroid hormone levels and by undertaking a nuclear medicine scan.

3.4 Basic physiology

The two cases above illustrate some of the symptoms of hyperthyroidism, such as tachycardia, heat intolerance, goiter and tremor. They also illustrate differences in the etiology of hyperthyroidism, with *Case 3.1* being an example of a chronic autoimmune disease and *Case 3.2* an example of acute hyperthyroidism.

This section covers:

- the actions of thyroid hormones to explain the symptoms of hyper- and hypothyroidism
- thyroid hormone receptors to show how thyroid hormones exert their effects and to demonstrate the consequences of thyroid hormone receptor resistance
- the synthesis of thyroid hormones and the importance of iodine trapping in relation to diagnosis and treatment of thyroid disorders, the action of drugs to treat hyperthyroidism and the consequences of iodine deficiency
- the metabolism of thyroid hormones and the regulation of T_4 and T_3 concentrations in target tissues
- the control of thyroid hormone synthesis and secretion to understand biochemical diagnosis of thyroid disorders.

3.4.1 Thyroid hormones and their actions

The thyroid gland secretes three iodinated hormones (see *Figure 3.3* for their structures):

- thyroxine – typically referred to as T_4 (tetraiodothyronine) because it contains four iodine atoms

- triiodothyronine – typically referred to as T_3 because it contains three iodine atoms
- reverse T_3 – a biologically inactive isomer of T_3

T_3 is by far the most potent hormone and binds to thyroid hormone receptors with a 10-fold higher affinity than T_4. However, ten times more T_4 is secreted by the gland daily.

T_4 is converted to active T_3 in peripheral tissues and in the brain and pituitary gland. T_3 acts on virtually every cell in the body and its main actions are:

- regulation of the resting metabolic rate
- inotropic and chronotropic effects on the heart
- a role in fetal development, particularly development of the brain
- a role in skeletal development during childhood
- regulation of bone turnover and mineralization

Knowing these actions of thyroid hormones the clinical features of hyper- and hypo-thyroidism can be predicted (see *Box 3.1* for more details).

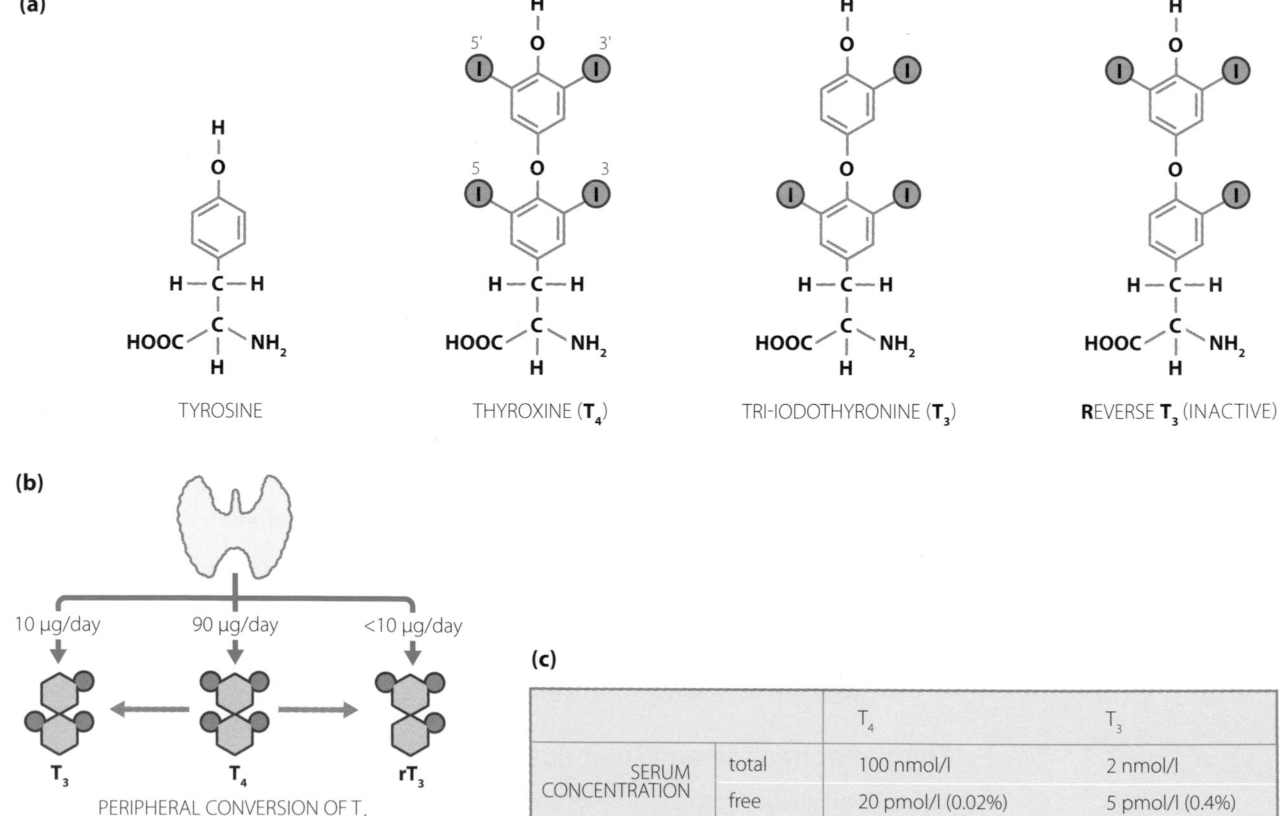

		T_4	T_3
SERUM CONCENTRATION	total	100 nmol/l	2 nmol/l
	free	20 pmol/l (0.02%)	5 pmol/l (0.4%)

Figure 3.3. (a) Structure of thyroid hormones, (b) their approximate daily secretion rates and (c) comparison of the transport of T_4 and T_3.

Box 3.1 | Actions of thyroid hormone

In most tissues (exceptions include the brain, spleen, and testis) thyroid hormones stimulate the metabolic rate by increasing the number and size of mitochondria, stimulating the synthesis of enzymes in the respiratory chain, and increasing the cell membrane Na^+ and K^+-ATPase concentration (pumping Na^+ out in exchange for K^+) to maintain the electrochemical gradient between the interior of the cell and the extracellular fluid. Thus the resting metabolic rate may increase by 100% in hyperthyroidism or decrease by as much as 50% in hypothyroidism, causing heat or cold intolerance, respectively (see *Cases 3.1* and *3.6*).

Thyroid hormones also stimulate heart rate and force of contraction and these chronotropic and inotropic effects are mediated through both nuclear receptors and cell surface receptors. T_3 increases the expression of Ca^{2+} channels in the sarcoplasmic reticulum in addition to other membrane ion transporters and voltage-gated K^+ channels. The increased number of Ca^{2+} channels increases the amount of calcium released from the sarcoplasmic reticulum during systole and probably accounts for the increased contractile activity observed in hyperthyroidism (see *Cases 3.1–3.5*). Thyroid hormones may also increase the speed of contraction by increasing the expression of α-myosin. Non-genomic effects of thyroid hormones include increased activity of the Ca^{2+}-ATPase and Na^+/K^+-ATPase pumps. Thyroid hormones also lower arterial resistance by up to 50% in hyperthyroidism. This, in turn, lowers diastolic pressure so that in hyperthyroidism there are only minor effects on mean arterial pressure, despite an increase in systolic pressure caused by the inotropic effects of thyroid hormones. Conversely, hypothyroidism leads to reduced heart rate and stroke volume but increased diastolic pressure.

Thyroid hormones (T_3) play a key role in fetal mammalian brain development and the developing brain is sensitive to thyroid hormone deficiency. In the absence of thyroid hormone, brain development is retarded leading to deficiencies in motor skills and reduced intellectual development; these are attributed to maldevelopment of specific cell types and regions of the brain, including the cerebral cortex and cerebellum. In early gestation the fetus is dependent on maternal T_4 which can cross the placenta via specific transporter proteins (see *Figure 3.4*) and be converted to T_3 by the fetal brain. Even mild to moderate maternal hypothyroidism can lead to sub-optimal neurodevelopment. Thyroid hormones are also important in placental tissues where they modify their metabolism, differentiation and development.

During childhood, T_3 is required for skeletal development (see *Case 3.6*), and in adults it regulates bone turnover and mineralization. The primary T_3 targets in bone are the growth plate chondrocytes and osteoblasts (cells that build up bone), where thyroid hormone receptors are expressed. Bone turnover also involves osteoclasts which are responsible for bone resorption, but it is thought that thyroid hormones stimulate osteoclastic activity by inducing paracrine signals from the osteoblasts. Thyrotoxicosis is an established risk factor for osteoporosis.

3.4.2 How do thyroid hormones exert their cellular effects?

Many of the actions of thyroid hormones are mediated by their binding to nuclear receptors that have a preferential affinity for T_3. T_3 receptors are, like all the steroid hormone receptors, members of a family of nuclear transcription factors that regulate gene expression in target cells (*Figure 3.5*). The genes *THRA* and *THRB* code for two different thyroid hormone receptors – TRα and TRβ; there are two major isoforms for each receptor generated by alternate splicing of the mRNA (*Figure 3.5*). *THRA* is expressed fairly ubiquitously but *THRB* is restricted more to the liver, the pituitary, the retina, and areas of the brain.

Thyroid hormones can also have rapid actions that do not involve gene transcription. Such non-genomic effects include stimulation of sugar and amino acid transport, increased Ca^{2+}-ATPase activity and increased Na^+ transport. Ten per cent of THRs are in the cytoplasm and their activation has been shown to stimulate the PI3 kinase/Akt signaling pathway (see *Figure 1.8d*) which has numerous downstream targets. An integrin molecule, αVβ3 has also been identified as a thyroid hormone binding site in the plasma membrane and can activate signaling pathways, facilitating membrane transport functions and MAPK-mediated transcriptional activity. Thus it can be seen that there are many ways in which thyroid hormones may regulate cellular activity which involve both genomic and non-genomic effects.

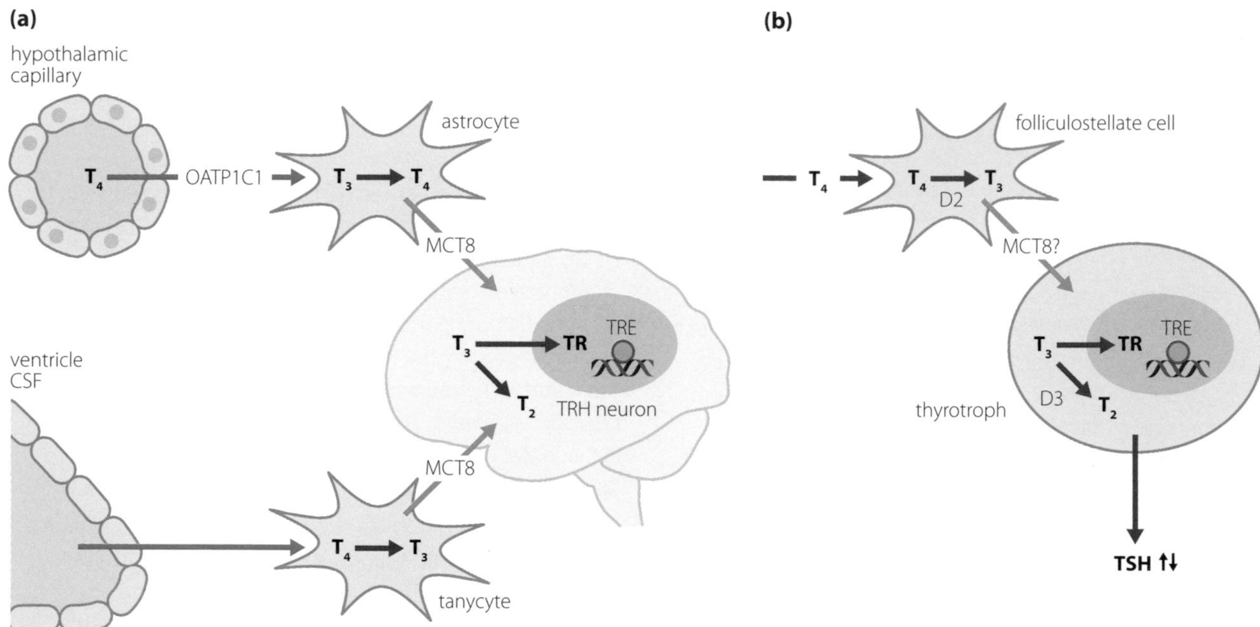

Figure 3.4. Thyroid hormone transporters in (a) the brain and (b) the pituitary gland.

The illustrations show the role of OATP1C1 and MCT8 in controlling the feedback effects of thyroid hormones on the hypothalamus and pituitary gland.

It was originally thought that thyroid hormones passively diffused through the lipid bilayer of the plasma membrane, but more recently it has been shown that thyroid hormones are actively transported into cells by high affinity, low capacity transporters. There are different transporters for T_4, T_3, and rT_3 except in the pituitary gland where the thyroid hormones share the same receptors. These transmembrane receptors include members of the Na^+/taurocholate co-transporting polypeptide (NTPC), the (Na^+ independent) organic anion transporting polypeptide (OATP), L-type amino acid transporter (LAT1 and 2), and the monocarboxylate transporter (MCT) families. Amongst these families of transporters, OATP1C1and MCT8 have been identified as specific thyroid hormone transporters. OATP1C1 is widely expressed in capillaries throughout the brain and also in the testis. It has a high affinity and specificity for T_4 and is thought to be important in regulating T_4 uptake into the hypothalamic-pituitary axis (notably astrocytes and folliculostellate cells, respectively) and thus regulating feedback effects. MCT8 is a very active and highly specific thyroid hormone transporter and shows a preference for T_3. It is highly expressed in liver and brain but is also widely distributed in other tissues. The *MCT8* gene is located on the X chromosome and recently mutations of this gene in humans have been associated with severe X-linked psychomotor retardation and elevated serum T_3 concentrations. The explanation for raised serum concentrations is that if T_3 is unable to enter cells expressing D3 there will be a decreased T_3 metabolism. Both transporters are also expressed in the placenta and they are thought to be important in transporting maternal thyroid hormones.

Key: D2, D3, deiodinase type 2 and type 3; TR, thyroid hormone receptor; TRE, thyroid hormone response element on the DNA.

(a)

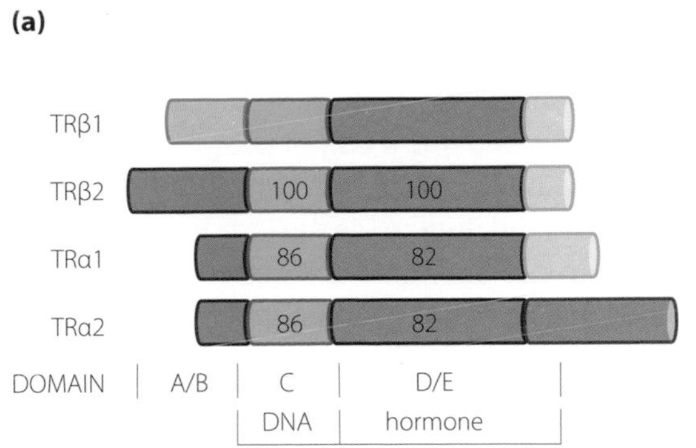

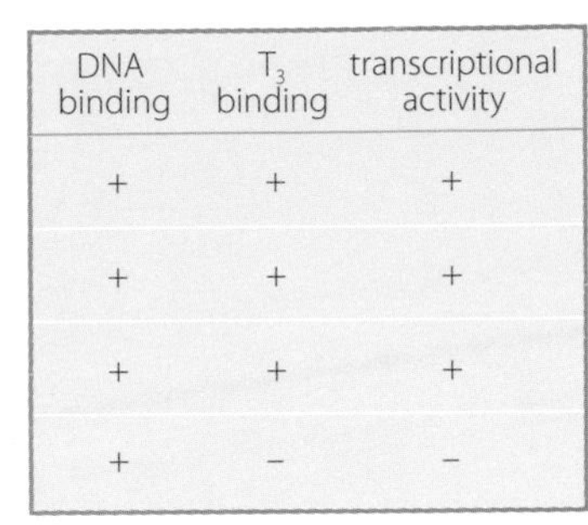

DNA binding	T_3 binding	transcriptional activity
+	+	+
+	+	+
+	+	+
+	–	–

(b)

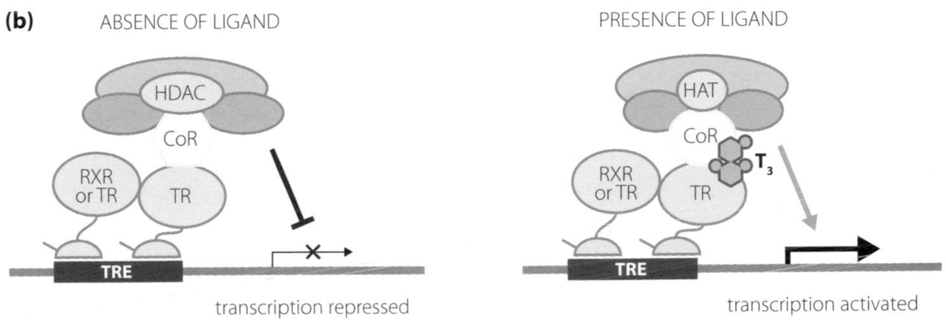

Figure 3.5. Thyroid hormone receptors.

(a) *THRA* and *THRB* are the two genes which code for TRα and TRβ receptors respectively, and each gene encodes for two major proteins generated by alternate splicing of the mRNA. TRs show high sequence homology in the DNA binding domain and the T_3 binding domain (the percentage sequence similarity is shown), but the N-terminal A/B domains are variable (different colors represent totally dissimilar sequences). TRβ1, TRβ2, and TRα1 are T_3 binding proteins and have transcriptional activity whilst TRα2 (the oncogene is *c-erbAα-2*) does not bind T_3 or have transcriptional activity, though it may act as a dominant negative regulator of thyroid hormone action by binding to thyroid hormone response elements (TREs). TR isoforms have differential expression in different tissues but it is not known whether specific TR isoforms have gene-specific effects on transcription.

(b) Thyroid hormone receptors form homodimers or heterodimers with the retinoic acid receptor (RXR). In the absence of thyroid hormones, TRs can bind to TREs and repress basal transcriptional activity by recruiting co-repressor molecules (CoR). These in turn recruit other complexes that harbor histone deacetylase (HDAC) activity which holds the chromatin structure in a closed conformation limiting access of basal transcriptional machinery. Ligand-dependent transcriptional activity involves the binding of co-activators (CoA) to the dimerized receptors as well as other complexes with histone acetylation activity (HAT). Histone acetylation causes a conformational change in the nucleosome (DNA coiled round a histone complex), increasing accessibility of chromatin to transcriptional factors and increased promoter activity. Thyroid hormones also exert non-genomic actions (see text for details).

3.4.3 Synthesis and release of thyroid hormones and mechanisms of control

Thyroid hormones, like epinephrine and nor-epinephrine, are synthesized from tyrosine molecules, but their synthesis also requires iodine (a rare element ranking 61st in the list of most common elements). The thyroid gland not only traps this element effectively from dietary sources but also maintains a large store of the iodinated tyrosines to allow the secretion of thyroid hormones during periods of relative iodine deficiency. In 1994, nearly 30% of the world's population was at risk of iodine deficiency, but a policy of iodine supplementation of salt reduced the population at risk to less than 15% by 1997. However, a review by the World Health Organization in 2005 indicated that 2 billion people still have insufficient iodine intake. The normal dietary intake of iodine is about 150 μg per day of which 125 μg is taken up by the thyroid gland. Iodine (as the iodide I^-) is plentiful in seafood, and fruit and vegetables also contain significant concentrations of iodine, although these levels are reduced in fruit and vegetables grown at high altitude and with increasing distance from the sea.

Synthesis of thyroid hormones takes place in thyroid follicles which are the functional units of the gland. Each follicle comprises a single layer of cells surrounding a protein-rich colloid material, and synthesis and storage of thyroid hormones occurs between the follicular cells and the colloid (see *Figures 3.1* and *3.6*). The follicular cells are orientated with their bases near the capillary blood supply and the apices abutting the colloid; less active follicles contain cells with a more cuboidal appearance, whilst the active follicles contain columnar cells.

The thyroid gland traps iodine by a Na^+/K^+-ATPase-dependent Na^+/I^- symporter on the basal surface of the follicular cells, and this active transport system allows iodide to be taken up from capillary blood into follicular cells against both a concentration and an electrical gradient (*Figure 3.6*). This system means that the thyroid gland can concentrate iodide to 30–50 times that of the circulating concentration. This activity also allows radioactive isotopes of iodine to be used to image the thyroid in patients with thyroid disorders (see *Figure 3.13*) and, at high doses, to treat both benign and malignant thyroid disease by destroying thyroid tissue (see *Section 3.5.5*). Other ions such as bromide, chlorate, or pertechnetate (though not fluoride) may also compete with iodide for this uptake process and an isotope of pertechnetate (which has a shorter half-life than radioactive iodine and which is not incorporated into thyroid hormone synthesis) is frequently used to image overall and regional activity in the thyroid gland rather than iodine (see *Figure 3.13*).

Once inside the follicular cells the iodide moves from the basolateral surface to the apical surface where it is transported across the apical membrane to the follicular lumen by a transporter known as pendrin (other unknown systems are also involved). This process is known as iodide efflux. The synthesis of thyroid hormones is complex (*Figure 3.6*) and involves:

- activation (oxidation) of thyroid peroxidase (TPO) by hydrogen peroxide
- formation of iodinating intermediates from the trapped iodide by the oxidized heme group on TPO
- iodination of tyrosine residues in the thyroglobulin molecule
- coupling reaction between pairs of iodinated tyrosine residues

The thyroglobulin molecule contains about 140 tyrosine residues of which about 25% can be iodinated. The coupling of two tyrosine residues, each iodinated at two positions (di-iodotyrosine, DIT), produces tetraiodothyronine or thyroxine (T_4), whilst the combination of DIT with mono-iodotyrosine (MIT) produces triiodothyronine (T_3). Antithyroid drugs, known as thionamides (still the cornerstone in the management of hyperthyroidism (see *Case 3.1*) inhibit thyroid synthesis by interfering with TPO-mediated iodination of tyrosine residues (*Figure 3.6*).

Thyroid hormones are stored in this coupled state and they are secreted when droplets of colloid are taken back into the cell and T_4 and T_3 are released by thyroglobulin by the action of lysosomal enzymes (*Figure 3.7*).

The synthesis and release of thyroid hormones is controlled by thyroid stimulating hormone (TSH) and this pituitary hormone stimulates many stages in the synthesis and release of thyroid hormones (see below). Another factor that controls thyroid hormone synthesis is iodine itself and this process is known as autoregulation. Excess iodine given to a person with normal thyroid gland activity leads to an initial reduction in the incorporation of iodine into the thyroglobulin molecule, and thus reduced hormone synthesis and secretion; this is known as the Wolff–Chaikoff effect (see also *Section 3.5.3*). 'Escape' from this inhibition generally occurs after several days. The exact mechanism(s) of such autoregulation is unknown but the Wolff–

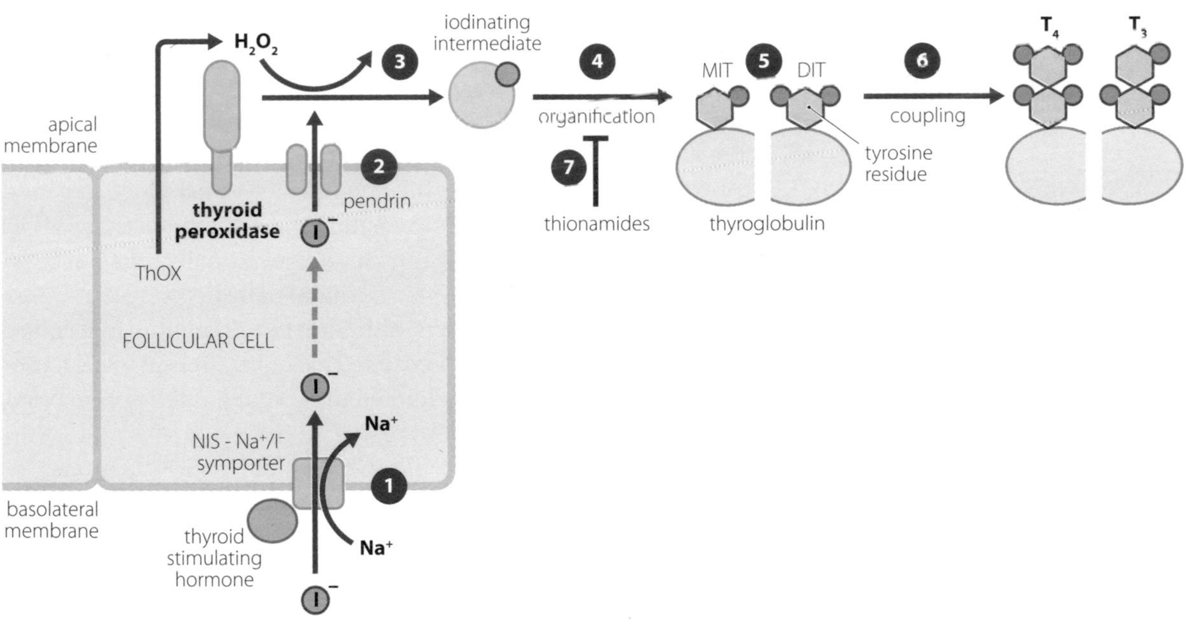

Figure 3.6. Synthesis of thyroid hormones.

(1) Active uptake of iodide (I^-) by the Na^+/I^- symporter (NIS) from the circulation against an electrical and concentration gradient. Action stimulated by TSH.

(2) **Iodide** is transported across the apical membrane by a transporter, pendrin, and other unknown mechanisms (iodide efflux).

(3) **Hydrogen peroxide** (H_2O_2) generated by the NADPH oxidase system, ThOX, oxidizes the heme group on the thyroid peroxidase (TPO) enzyme that is anchored in the apical membrane. This oxidized heme group reacts with the trapped iodide to form iodinating intermediates.

(4) **The iodinating** intermediates then iodinate tyrosine residues on the thyroglobulin (TG) molecules – a process known as organification.

(5) **The tyrosine** residues may be iodinated at one or two positions forming mono- and di-iodotyrosines (MIT and DIT) respectively.

(6) **Coupling of** the iodinated tyrosine molecules to produce T_4 (coupling of two DITs) and T_3 (coupling of MIT and DIT). These are stored within the colloid until they are secreted.

(7) **Thionamides inhibit** thyroid synthesis by interfering with TPO-mediated iodination of tyrosine residues.

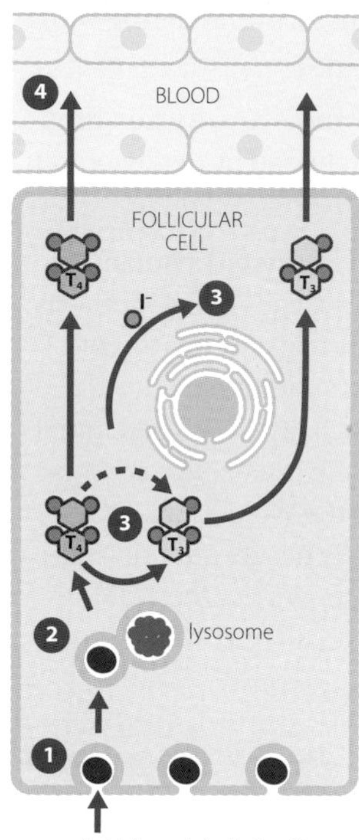

Figure 3.7. Secretion of thyroid hormones.
Under the influence of TSH, colloid droplets consisting of thyroid hormones within the thyroglobulin molecules are taken back up into the follicular cells by pinocytosis.
Fusion of colloid droplets with lysosomes causes hydrolysis of thyroglobulin and release of T_3 and T_4.
About 10% of T_4 undergoes mono-deiodination to T_3 before it is secreted. The released iodide is re-utilized. Several-fold more iodide is reused than is taken from the blood each day, but in states of iodide excess there is loss from the thyroid.
On average approximately 100 μg T_4 and about 10 μg T_3 are secreted per day.

Chaikoff effect is useful clinically because pharmacological doses of iodine may be used in an acute situation to reduce the activity of the thyroid gland. When dietary intake of iodine is insufficient, overactivity of the thyroid gland is a more common initial response to excess iodine.

3.4.4 Transport, peripheral metabolism, and excretion of thyroid hormones

The iodothyronines are virtually insoluble in water and, once released from thyroglobulin, they are rapidly bound to the plasma proteins, thyroxine-binding globulin (TBG), transthyretin (previously called thyroxine-binding prealbumin), and albumin (*Figure 3.3*). These plasma proteins vary in their capacity and affinity for T_3 and T_4. About 70% of circulating thyroid hormones are bound to TBG and only a tiny fraction (<0.5%) of released thyroid hormones exist in a free form in the circulation; this is in equilibrium with the bound forms of thyroid hormones (see *Box 1.1*).

It is the free fraction which determines overall thyroid hormone activity in the body and the assessment of hyper- or hypothyroidism typically involves measuring 'free' rather than the total concentration of circulating thyroid hormones.

Approximately 100 μg of thyroid hormones are secreted from the gland each day, mostly in the form of T_4 with about 10% as T_3 and smaller amounts as rT_3 (*Figure 3.3*). T_4, however, is a precursor molecule and must be deiodinated to generate the biologically active T_3. This deiodinase pathway in peripheral tissues is a major determinant of plasma T_3 because all T_3 generated eventually exits the cells, unless it is further metabolized. In fact, the extrathyroidal pathway contributes about 80% of T_3 produced daily in healthy subjects, although the circulating free concentrations of T_3 and T_4 are roughly similar because T_4 is tightly bound to carrier proteins in the circulation. T_4 can also be deiodinated to rT_3 that has little or no biological activity (*Figure 3.3*).

Deiodination of thyroid hormones (*Figure 3.8*) involves the iodothyronine deiodinase enzymes type I, II, and III (D1, D2, and D3). 3,5,3′5′-tetraiodothyronine (T_4/thyroxine) and 3,5,3′ triiodothyronine (T_3) enter cells through specific transporters and, once in the cell, T_4 can be converted to T_3 by D2 or D1. It is thought that the D2 pathway, rather than the D1 pathway, is the major source of extrathyroid T_3 production in healthy subjects. D1 is a kinetically inefficient enzyme because it can deiodinate both outer (5′) and inner (5) rings of the thyroxine molecule with equal efficiency and thus can activate (T_3 production) or deactivate (rT_3 production) T_4 on an equimolar basis. Alternatively, local T_3 concentrations may be reduced by D3 to convert T_3 to T_2 or T_4 to rT_3. This particular enzyme is highly stimulated during development and may protect against thyroid hormone signaling in developing structures by lowering serum T_3 concentrations.

The actions and expression of deiodinases are integrated to maintain cellular and serum T_3 concentrations and the expression of these enzymes changes according to thyroid hormone status.

Further metabolism of thyroid hormones involves deiodinations at both the 3rd and 5th carbon atoms of both tyrosine rings, producing increasingly inactive diiodo- and monoiodothyronines, whilst conserving iodine. Iodothyronines may be excreted in the urine although some thyroid hormones are conjugated with glucuronide and excreted via bile in the feces. Some T_4 is metabolized by other pathways (e.g. sulfation, decarboxylation, deamination), whilst T_3 may be sulfated or converted to the acetic acid derivative, triiodoacetate (TRIAC), the latter being more potent than T_3.

3.4.5 TSH and the control of thyroid hormone synthesis and secretion

Like the adrenal cortex and the gonads, the thyroid gland is controlled by hormone secretions from the hypothalamic–pituitary axis. The synthesis and secretion of TSH from the thyrotrophs is stimulated by the tripeptide, thyrotrophin-releasing hormone (TRH). This small peptide, cleaved from a larger prohormone, is released

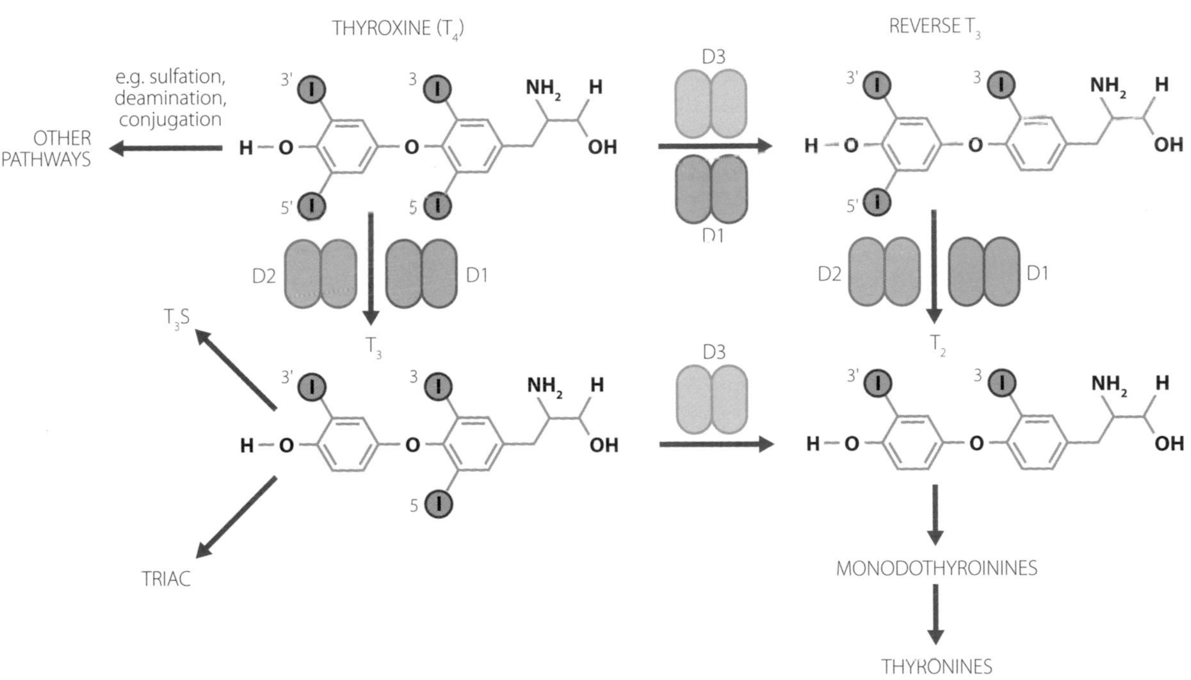

Figure 3.8. Metabolism of thyroid hormones.
Thyroid hormones are metabolized by a series of deiodinations which involve three types of deiodinases (D1, D2, and D3).

- **Type 1:** deiodinates at both 5′ and 5 carbon atoms, converting T_4 to T_3 or rT_3. It is found in the liver, kidney, thyroid, pituitary gland, and central nervous system. With a high K_m for T_4, it is the only iso-enzyme inhibited by PTU. Its activity is increased in hyperthyroidism and reduced in hypothyroidism.
- **Type 2:** deiodinates only at the 5′ position, converting T_4 to T_3. It is found in brain, brown fat, placenta, and pituitary gland. With a lower K_m than Type 1, it is considered to maintain intracellular concentrations of T_3. This is important in the negative feedback actions of T_4 on the pituitary gland. Its activity is decreased in hyperthyroidism and increased in hypothyroidism.
- **Type 3:** deiodinates only at the 5 position and found only in brain and placenta. As it is incapable of converting T_4 to the active T_3, it may protect the brain and fetus from excess active T_3.

Some T_4 is metabolized by being sulfated, decarboxylated, deaminated, or conjugated with glucuronide (other pathways).
Some T_3 may be sulfated (T_3S) or converted to the acetic acid derivative triiodoacetic acid (TRIAC) that is more potent than its parent T_3.
Serum half-lives: T_4 – 7 days, T_3 – 1 day, rT_3 – 4 hours.

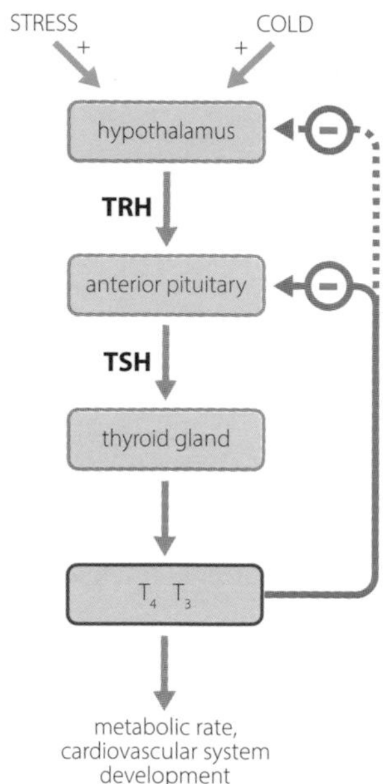

Figure 3.9. Negative feedback control of thyroid hormone synthesis and secretion. Circulating concentrations of thyroid hormones are sensed by the hypothalamus and pituitary gland, though the pituitary gland appears to be the major site for feedback effects. High levels of circulating thyroid hormones suppress TRH/TSH and thus reduce the hormonal stimulus for the synthesis, storage, and release of thyroid hormones. The reverse occurs when thyroid hormone levels fall. This negative feedback loop can also be over-ridden by external factors such as stress and cold.

from neurosecretory cells in the hypothalamus into the hypothalamo-hypophyseal portal capillaries, from where it is transported to the pituitary thyrotrophs (*Figures 2.1* and *3.9*). TSH secretion is inhibited by other hormones, including somatostatin and dopamine (released from neurosecretory cells in the hypothalamus), and also cytokines, particularly IL-1β, IL-6, and TNF-α.

TSH is a complex glycoprotein hormone, containing approximately 16% carbohydrate. It contains 211 amino acids in two subunits. The α unit is identical to that of two other glycoprotein hormones secreted by the human anterior pituitary gland, namely luteinizing hormone (LH) and follicle stimulating hormone (FSH) (see *Section 2.8*). The β unit is unique to TSH and confers biological specificity. The attached sugar moieties are heterogeneous and this affects both its bioactivity and clearance. TSH has a half-life in the circulation of about 1 hour.

The cell surface receptor for TSH is a typical G-protein linked receptor (see *Figure 1.7*) and there are approximately 1000 TSH receptors on the basal surface of each follicular cell. The binding of TSH to its receptor activates the classical G-protein coupled effectors, adenylate cyclase (AC) and phospholipase C (PLC) which regulate different processes in thyroid hormone synthesis (*Figures 1.8* and *3.10*).

Inactivating mutations of this receptor have been described and these lead to hypothyroidism. In contrast, activating mutations have been identified in the transmembrane domain of the receptor and these have been most frequently associated with autonomous 'hot' nodules (areas of increased growth and activity) of the gland. If such activating mutations are heritable (which is extremely rare), they cause familial hyperthyroidism. Mutations of Gs (termed gsp) that result in constitutive activation of the G protein have also been described in 'hot' nodules.

The concentration of thyroid hormones in the circulation is regulated by a homeostatic negative feedback loop involving the hypothalamic-pituitary axis (*Figure 3.9*). This involves the brain and pituitary gland monitoring circulating levels of thyroid hormones and is primarily dependent on specific transporters of T_4 into brain and pituitary cells (the major secretion of the thyroid gland) and their conversion into T_3 (see *Figure 3.4*). T_3 then regulates receptors on TRH neurons and thyrotrophs. In addition, both the brain and pituitary gland can inactivate T_4 and thus may help to modulate thyroid hormone feedback on the hypothalamic-pituitary axis.

A fall in the concentration of circulating thyroid hormones is detected by the hypothalamus and pituitary gland resulting in an increased synthesis and release of TRH and TSH, and an increase in the number of TRH receptors in the pituitary gland resulting in an increased TSH response to TRH. The reverse is true in the presence of high circulating concentrations of thyroid hormones. Whilst the TSH response to a bolus injection of TRH can be used to diagnose causes of hypo- or hyperthyroidism, measurement of free thyroid hormones and TSH, using sensitive modern assays (see *Section 9.1*), is usually sufficient for diagnosis of the most common form of hyperthyroidism, Graves disease (see *Case 3.1*). It should be noted that TSH stimulates growth of the thyroid gland, so any thyroid disorder which causes a rise in TSH secretion, such as primary hypothyroidism (*see Case 3.7*) or autoantibodies stimulating TSH receptors (see *Case 3.1*), will induce a goiter (*Box 3.2*).

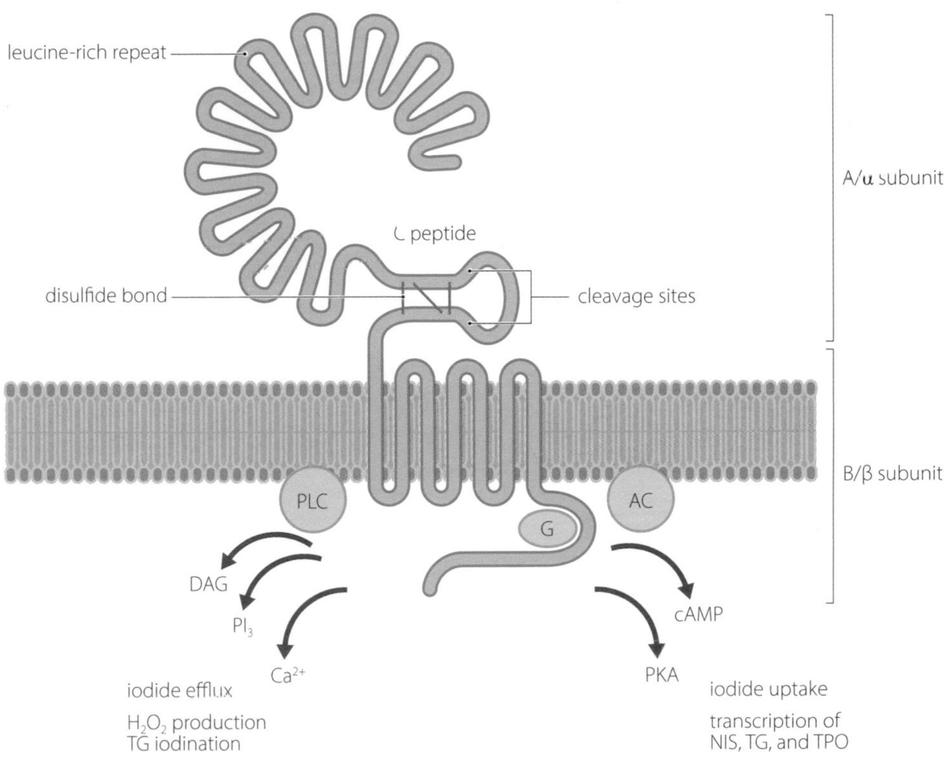

Figure 3.10. Highly simplified diagram of the TSH receptor and its actions.
The TSH receptor (TSHR) is a typical G-protein coupled receptor (G). It has a large highly glycosylated N-terminal ectodomain (the A or α subunit) with a series of leucine-rich repeats. The 7-transmembrane domain with a short cytoplasmic tail forms the B or β subunit. The TSH receptor can undergo intramolecular cleavage which involves the step-wise removal of a looped segment, the C peptide region, between the A and B subunits. Whilst the two subunits may be joined by disulfide bonds there is evidence that the A subunit can subsequently be completely shed from the B subunit. TSH binds with equal affinity to the complete polypeptide and the cleaved form of the receptor (the B subunit only). There is some evidence that the shed A subunit of the receptor is the crucial autoantigen in the generation of thyroid stimulating autoantibodies, i.e. in Graves disease.
Activation of the TSH receptor activates both G_s and G_q proteins which activate adenyl cyclase (AC) and phospholipase C (PLC) respectively. Adenyl cyclase stimulates cAMP formation and activation of protein kinase A, whilst phospholipase C stimulates the conversion of phosphatidyl inositol 4,5-diphosphate (PIP_2) to inositol triphosphate (IP_3) and diacyl glycerol (DAG). Adenyl cyclase and cAMP regulate iodide uptake and transcription of the sodium-iodide symporter (NIS), thyroglobulin (TG), and thyroid peroxidase (TPO). PLC and Ca^{2+} regulate iodide efflux from follicular cells, H_2O_2 production, and thyroglobulin iodination.

This regulatory loop is also affected by internal and external factors that alter the rate at which TSH is secreted. TSH is secreted in a pulsatile fashion with a diurnal variation, peaking around midnight. Environmental temperature may stimulate or inhibit the release of TSH by adjusting TRH secretion, such that after 24 hours of exposure to a cold environment, the plasma concentrations of thyroid hormones increase with a consequent rise in basal metabolic rate. Pharmacologic doses of glucocorticoids, as prescribed in anti-inflammatory therapy or seen in Cushing syndrome (see *Section 6.4*), inhibit thyroid hormone secretions by reducing the TSH secretory response to TRH. In contrast, estrogens have the opposite effect, increasing TSH secretion and, hence, increasing the activity of the thyroid gland.

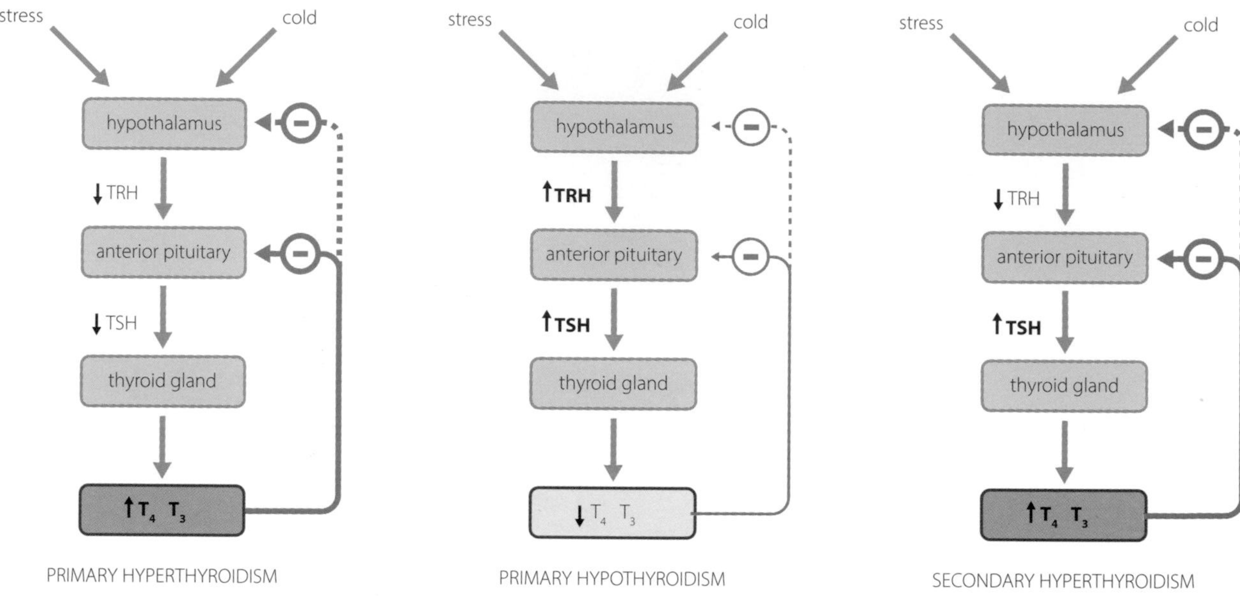

Figure 3.11. Negative feedback effects of thyroid hormones in primary and secondary thyroid disorders – assessing thyroid hormone status.
In primary hyperthyroidism circulating thyroid hormones are raised and these have negative feedback effects on the hypothalamic–pituitary axis suppressing TRH and TSH secretion.
In primary hypothyroidism thyroid hormones are low and the loss of negative feedback effects increases TRH and TSH secretions.
In secondary hyperthyroidism there is an excessive secretion of TSH which drives the thyroid gland to secrete high levels of thyroid hormones. These do not appropriately suppress TSH.
Thus assays of free thyroid hormones and/or TSH provide a sensitive measurement of thyroid hormone status and causes of thyroid hormone disorders.

3.5 Hyperthyroidism

Hyperthyroidism or thyrotoxicosis refers to excess circulating thyroid hormone. This may be due to excess *de novo* thyroid hormone synthesis (e.g. by stimulating antibodies), or by unregulated functional autonomous tissue, or excess release of pre-formed thyroid hormone (e.g. by inflammation of the thyroid gland secondary to a thyroiditis). It is often useful to differentiate causes of thyroid overactivity on the basis of radionucleotide uptake: high uptake occurs where there is new synthesis of thyroid hormone, but uptake is low when there is excessive release of pre-formed thyroid hormone (see *Section 3.4.3* and *Figure 3.13*).

Hyperthyroidism can also be considered as being primary (where the problem is in the thyroid gland itself) or secondary (where, very rarely, there is unregulated TSH stimulation of the thyroid due to a TSH-secreting pituitary adenoma). The causes of thyroid overactivity are summarized in *Box 3.3* and the alteration in thyroid hormone levels, and those of TSH in primary and secondary hyperthyroidism, are shown in *Figure 3.11*.

The most common cause of hyperthyroidism is Graves disease (some studies suggest an incidence of up to 4.6 per 1000 in women of childbearing age). In simple terms, hyperthyroidism is more common in women than men – young women tend to have

Graves disease whereas older patients often present with toxic adenomas or toxic multinodular goiters.

3.5.1 Graves disease

The signs and symptoms of Graves disease are illustrated in *Figure 3.12*. The most common symptoms are irritability, palpitations, tremor, and sweating seen in 90% of hyperthyroid patients. Tiredness, muscle weakness, and weight loss are also common (about 70% prevalence). Common signs are tachycardia, goiter, heat intolerance and warm moist palms which are seen in 95–100% of patients.

Graves disease accounts for approximately 80% of hyperthyroid cases, compared to just 15% of cases with toxic nodular goiters. Other causes are much less common (autonomous nodules, for example, probably account for no more than 3% of cases) or, indeed, rare (for example thyroid follicular carcinoma is found in <0.01% of cases). Graves disease affects women nine times more commonly than men. It is an autoimmune disease which results in the production of autoantibodies that stimulate the TSH receptor. This highly unusual action of an antibody (most block receptor activation) not only stimulates thyroid hormone synthesis and secretion, but also thyroid growth. Graves disease is associated with other autoimmune diseases such as myasthenia gravis, type 1 diabetes mellitus, Addison disease (*Section 6.6*) and vitiligo. A family history indicates a genetic predisposition to autoimmune disease, although a concordance rate of only 30–50% in monozygotic

Box 3.2 | Goiter

A goiter is simply an enlargement of the thyroid gland. The goiter may be a diffuse goiter which means that the entire gland is larger than normal, or it may be a nodular goiter with either a single nodule or it may be multi-nodular.

The causes for a **diffuse goiter** include:

- autoimmune Graves disease and Hashimoto disease
- thyroiditis (inflammation of the thyroid) due to various causes such as a viral infection
- iodine deficiency
- hereditary factors
- problems with making T_4 or T_3

Causes of **nodular goiters** include:

- a cyst
- adenoma (solid benign tumor)
- cancerous tumor (rare)
- iodine deficiency

Patients can develop hyper- or hypothyroidism without evidence of a goiter and some patients may develop a goiter whilst remaining euthyroid.

It is important to remember that activation of TSH receptors by TSH or TSH-stimulating antibodies (Graves disease) stimulates growth of the thyroid follicles. Thus goiters are consequences of both hyper- and hypothyroidism. In Hashimoto disease when thyroid tissue is destroyed by an autoimmune response, thyroid hormone secretions are reduced and, due to loss of negative feedback, TSH secretions increase; this, together with an infiltration of the gland by white blood cells, enlarges the thyroid gland. With iodine deficiency, circulating concentrations of T_4 and T_3 are low and hence TSH is high, again stimulating growth of the thyroid gland.

Blood tests will initially be undertaken to measure circulating concentrations of 'free' thyroxine (T_4), triiodothyronine (T_3), and TSH which may help to find out the cause of some goiters. For example, patients with a diffuse goiter due to Graves disease will have high levels of T_4 and low levels of endogenous TSH. Patients with Hashimoto disease will have high TSH levels and low T_4 concentrations. Further tests may include:

- an ultrasound scan of the thyroid
- a radioactive iodine or pertechnetate scan of the thyroid gland
- biopsy (fine needle aspiration) of a nodular goiter

twins indicates that environmental factors may also trigger the development of this disease.

Graves disease may be differentiated from other causes of hyperthyroidism because it is often associated with eye disorders known variously as Graves eye disease, dysthyroid eye disease, or thyroid-associated ophthalmopathy (*Box 3.4*), and abnormalities of skin and integument (e.g. onycholysis, thyroid acropachy, pre-tibial myxedema).

Box 3.3 | Causes of thyroid overactivity

Excessive synthesis of thyroid hormone

Autoimmune thyroid disease

- Graves disease
- Hashitoxicosis

Autonomous thyroid tissue

- Toxic nodule (adenoma)
- Multinodular goiter

Unregulated TSH excess

- TSH producing pituitary adenoma

HCG-mediated hyperthyroidism

- Hyperemesis gravidarum
- Molar pregnancy

Excessive release or ingestion of thyroid hormone

Thyroiditis

- Subacute granulomatous (de Quervain's thyroiditis)
- Painless (subacute lymphocytic) thyroiditis and post-partum thyroiditis
- Amiodarone-induced thyroiditis
- Radiation and palpation-induced thyroiditis

Exogenous thyroid hormone

- Excessive thyroid hormone replacement (intentional or accidental)
- Factitious hyperthyroidism (e.g. using thyroid hormone to promote weight loss)

Ectopic hyperthyroidism

- Struma ovarii or metastatic thyroid cancer

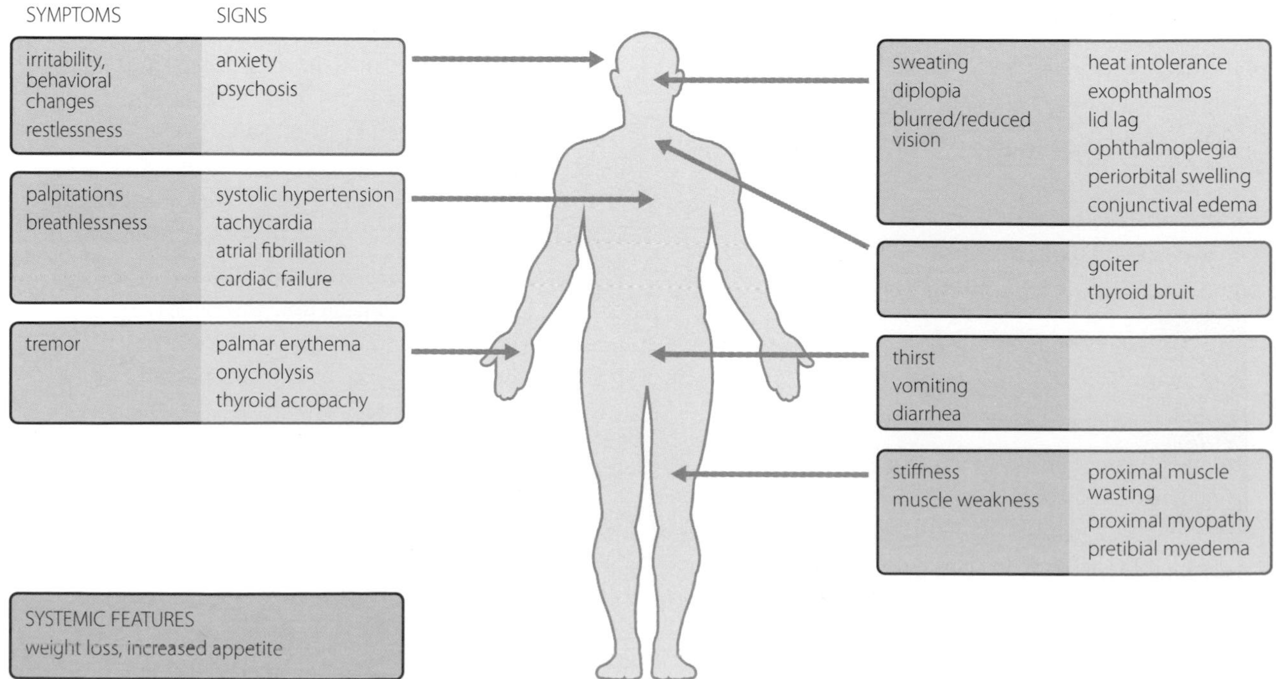

Figure 3.12. Signs and symptoms of Graves disease.

3.5.2 Diagnosis of hyperthyroidism – biochemical measurements of thyroid hormone status

Assays of circulating thyroid hormone concentrations are usually referred to as 'thyroid function tests', often abbreviated to 'TFTs'. It is clear that they do not measure thyroid 'function' because this implies a measure of the effectiveness of thyroid hormone on peripheral tissues, but they are used as surrogate measures. Whilst total (bound plus free) thyroid hormones can be measured this may not reflect the physiological state since changes in the concentration of binding proteins alter the total hormone concentration (*Box 1.1*). It must be remembered that, in the presence of an intact feedback loop, serum TSH concentration reflects the effects of thyroid hormones on the pituitary gland. For this reason serum TSH concentration has been recommended as the first-line assay of thyroid 'function'.

Diagnosis of primary hyperthyroidism is usually straightforward and most patients have raised serum concentrations of free T_4 and T_3 (i.e. above the normal range of 10.0–22.0 pmol/L for T_4 and 2.5–6.2 pmol/L for T_3) and reduced concentrations of TSH (below the normal range of 0.5–5.2 mU/L). In the extremely rare cases of secondary hyperthyroidism due to a TSH-secreting adenoma of the pituitary gland, both TSH and free T_4 and T_3 will be raised. In contrast, in the case of primary

Box 3.4 | Thyroid eye disease

Abnormalities of the eye associated with Graves disease (see *Box figure 3.1*) is variously referred to as thyroid eye disease (TED), Graves eye disease, or thyroid-associated ophthalmopathy (TAO). TED has a prevalence of between 1 and 2% in the UK and affects up to 30% of people with Graves disease. Clinical features include pain, photophobia, diplopia, chemosis (conjunctival swelling), and exophthalmos. The eyes may feel dry and gritty.

The symptoms and signs occur as a result of deposition of glycosaminoglycans (from orbital fibroblasts) in the orbit with concomitant hypertrophy of adipose tissue.

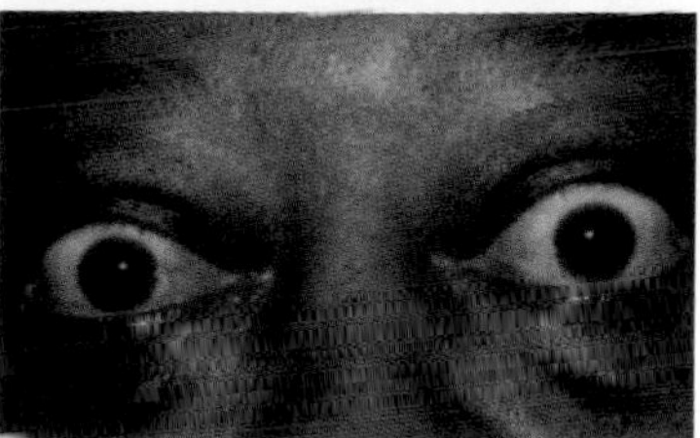

Box figure 3.1. Thyroid eye disease.
The extra-ocular muscles are involved in an order which can be remembered by the mnemonic I'M SLOW (inferior, medial, superior, lateral, obliques).

Fibroblasts are stimulated by a number of cytokines which have been identified in affected orbital tissue; these include IL-1β, TNF-α, IL-8, IL-10, and interferon-γ. Orbital fibroblasts can also differentiate into adipose cells given the appropriate stimuli. Thyroid eye disease is an autoimmune phenomenon and the process of T-cell activation is almost certainly induced by TSH receptor antigen.

Risk factors for development of TED include smoking (by far the most clinically important and potentially reversible risk factor) and radioiodine treatment (there is good evidence that radioiodine treatment of Graves disease can cause a flare-up of pre-existing TED). There is, as yet, no good evidence for a genetic basis for the risk of developing TED, although genetic factors are implicated in the genesis of Graves disease. Also, unlike Graves disease itself (where women are affected about nine times more frequently than men), there is no gender preponderance in TED – if anything older men tend to develop rather more severe eye disease.

Management of TED

There are various classifications of severity of TED and disease activity scores. The ATA (American Thyroid

Box 3.4 | continued

Association) has recommended use of the 'NO-SPECS' classification:

- Class 0 – **N**o symptoms, no signs
- Class 1 – **O**nly signs (lid retraction, lid lag), no symptoms
- Class 2 – **S**oft tissue involvement
- Class 3 – **P**roptosis
- Class 4 – **E**xtra-ocular muscle involvement (see *Box figure 3.2*)
- Class 5 – **C**orneal involvement
- Class 6 – **S**ight loss (due to involvement of the optic nerve)

Alternatively, one point can be given for each of the following signs, which sometimes helps in follow-up of progression or resolution:

- spontaneous retrobulbar pain
- pain on eye movement
- eyelid erythema
- conjunctival injection
- chemosis
- swelling of the carbuncle
- eyelid edema

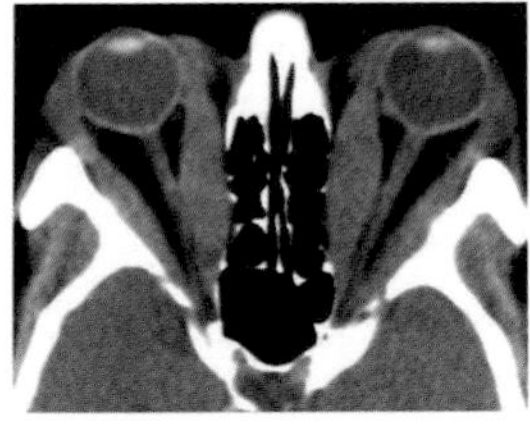
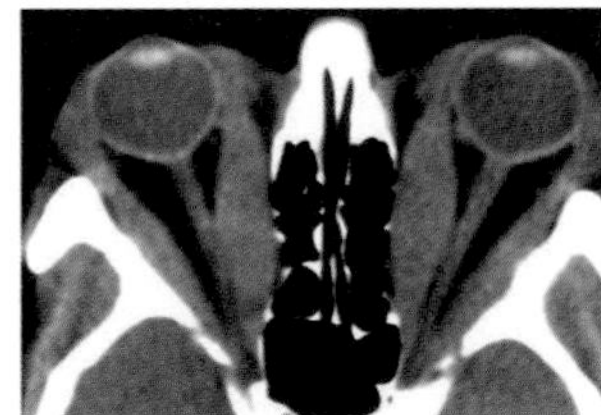

Box figure 3.2.
Axial and coronal CT scans of the orbits showing marked enlargement of the extra-ocular muscles with sparing of the tendons consistent with the diagnosis of TED.

Obviously, hyperthyroidism associated with Graves disease (or hypothyroidism in definitively treated Graves disease) needs to be controlled, but even exquisite control of thyroid function may have little effect on either the severity or progression of the associated TED. Total thyroidectomy clearly treats Graves hyperthyroidism and possibly improves TED, secondary to removing a great deal of the antigenic load.

Specific management of TED is based on the severity of the presentation:

Mild cases (ocular discomfort, mild proptosis)

- Eye lubrication with topical tears
- NSAIDs

Moderate cases (ocular discomfort, eyelid retraction)

- NSAIDs
- Low dose steroid, e.g. prednisolone for 4 weeks
- Marked disease (active diplopiachemosis, ocular motility disorders)
- Oral prednisolone for 4 weeks reducing over 8 weeks
- Longer-term steroid sparing agents (azathioprine, cyclosporine) if persistent diplopia

Severe cases (optic nerve dysfunction, color vision loss, decreased visual acuity)

- intravenous methylprednisolone followed by oral steroid +/- steroid sparing agents
- 10 sessions of orbital radiotherapy
- surgical orbital decompression

Surgery is the last line of treatment and decompression of the eye (where a hole is made in the medial and inferior walls of the orbit allowing the orbital contents to prolapse down into the maxillary sinus) is used only when TED is sight-threatening and other treatment have failed. However, there is a real place for cosmetic surgery in TED in order to improve upper lid retraction or to correct significant peri-orbital edema (see *Box figure 3.3*).

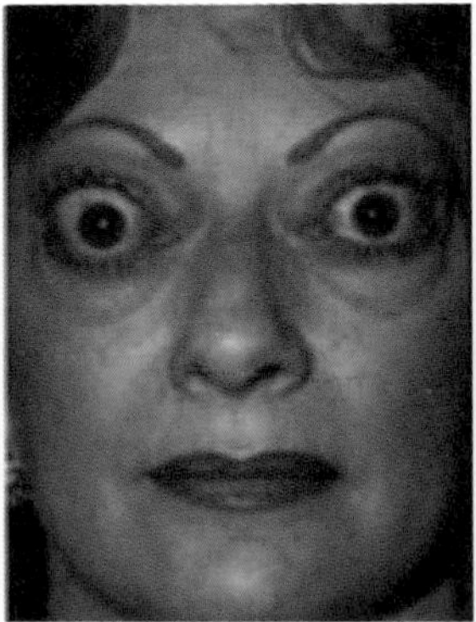
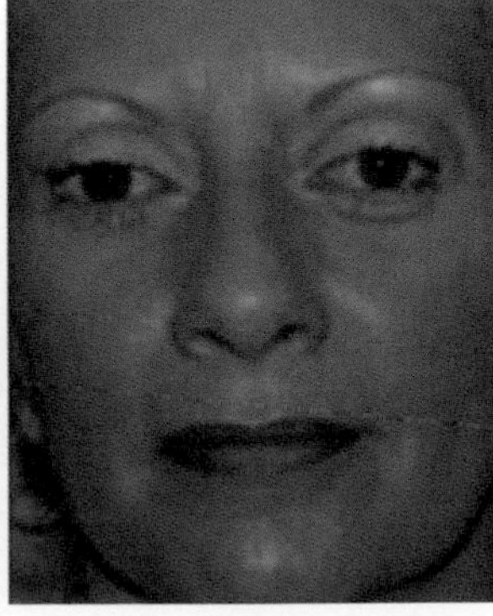

Box figure 3.3. Surgery can be highly effective and produce excellent cosmetic results.

CASE 3.1 110 127 128

- Caucasian female of 26 years with 4 months of weight loss and lack of menstrual period
- Symptoms and examination suggested Graves disease: bilateral tremor, heat intolerance, tachycardia, non-tender vascular swelling in neck, thyroid bruit, and lid lag
- TFTs ordered
- Family history suggests possible genetic susceptibility

The patient showed some of the classic features of hyperthyroidism: bilateral tremor, irritability, heat intolerance, and palpitations.

A quick check on her family history established that her mother had type 1 diabetes mellitus and her grandmother had a large goiter indicating probable thyroid disease, and suggesting a genetic susceptibility. The exact nature of this genetic susceptibility remains uncertain but experimental studies have suggested linkage with a number of genes. The earliest recognized was a relatively weak linkage with certain histocompatibility complex genes on chromosome 6. Evidence suggests that the alleles HLA-DRB1*08 and DRB3*0202 were associated with the disease and that the DRB1*07 allele is protective. More recent studies have shown linkage with specific alleles of the *CTLA-4* gene (cytotoxic T-cell antigen-4) and a B cell co-stimulatory molecule CD40.

In order to investigate the patient further it was first necessary to confirm overproduction of thyroid hormone and then delineate the underlying cause. The initial investigations ordered were therefore blood tests for thyroid hormones and thyroid autoantibodies.

hypothyroidism, levels of T_4 and T_3 will be low whilst TSH levels will be raised due to loss of negative feedback. In rare cases of secondary hypothyroidism due to loss of pituitary function both TSH and thyroid hormones will be low.

Whilst TFTs can provide information about abnormal thyroid function, they do not identify the cause. Measurement of thyroid autoantibodies can be helpful in this regard:

- antibodies directed against the TSH receptor (TSHR-Ab) are specific for Graves disease, but are not always routinely available
- antibodies to thyroglobulin or TPO are often positive in Graves disease but are less specific

3.5.3 Other causes of primary hyperthyroidism

Thyroiditis

Thyroiditis refers to a group of self-limiting conditions characterized by inflammation of the thyroid (see *Box 3.5*). In simple terms, thyroiditis can occur in association with a generalized systemic illness when it is often painful (examples include infectious thyroiditis and de Quervain's thyroiditis), or in situations where there is no obvious inflammation (for example, subacute lymphocytic thyroiditis and postpartum thyroiditis). The nomenclature is complicated and sometimes opaque and so it is probably best to separate the etiologies into painful, painless or drug-induced (e.g. by lithium or amiodarone).

Unlike Graves disease, there is no increase in synthesis of thyroid hormones in thyroiditis, but instead there is a breakdown of stored thyroglobulin and destruction of thyroid follicular cells. This leads to release of thyroid hormone. Because hormone synthesis is not increased (it is in fact inhibited) there is little uptake on nuclear medicine scanning, and the stores of thyroid hormones are soon exhausted – hence the classic pattern of transient thyrotoxicosis followed by a hypothyroid phase. This hypothyroid phase is sustained only rarely (in around 5–10% of cases) and normally there is an eventual return (after 6 weeks or so) to euthyroidism.

CASE 3.1

110 127 

- Caucasian female of 26 years with 4 months of weight loss and lack of menstrual period
- Symptoms and examination suggested Graves disease: bilateral tremor, heat intolerance, tachycardia, non-tender vascular swelling in neck, thyroid bruit, and lid lag
- TFTs ordered
- Family history suggests possible genetic susceptibility
- High T_4 and T_3 with low TSH
- Treat with carbimazole

The results of blood tests for free thyroid hormones on this patient showed that her free T_4 and T_3 levels were 35.7 pmol/L (NR: 10.0–20.0) and 12.2 pmol/L (NR: 2.5–6.2) respectively, and her TSH levels were <0.01 mU/L (NR: 0.4–4.2). Anti-TSH receptor autoantibodies were also detected in her serum.

Additional confirmation that it was Graves disease came from her clinical presentation: a female in her reproductive years with a family history of thyroid disease, a large vascular goiter, eye signs and dermopathy (palmar erythema). In this case no further investigations were necessary to confirm the cause of her hyperthyroidism.

However, in some cases it is useful to carry out nuclear medicine scanning (see *Figure 3.13*) with ^{123}I or technetium 99-m (^{99m}Tc). This patient underwent scanning with ^{99m}Tc which revealed a 12% increased homogenous uptake of tracer (NR: 0.5–4%), confirming increased synthesis of thyroid hormones.

The patient was started on carbimazole and by 5 weeks had become biochemically euthyroid with significant symptomatic improvement. At this point a decision was made to add in thyroxine and continue treatment with 'block and replace' for a further 6 months (see *Section 6.5.3*).

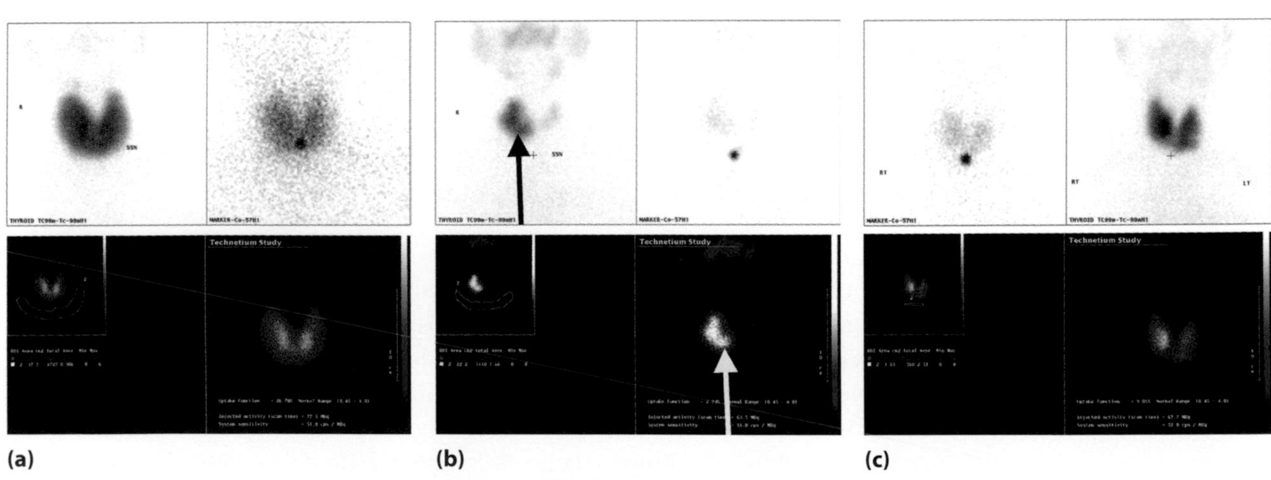

Figure 3.13. Nuclear medicine scans of the thyroid in thyrotoxicosis.
(a) Graves disease with increased homogenous uptake of tracer (total uptake is 27%; (NR 0.4–4%). (b) A toxic nodule (arrowed). The overall uptake is normal (2.73%; NR 0.4–4%) but there is a large 'hot' nodule in the right lobe which is completely suppressing activity within the rest of the gland. The patient had elevated levels of fT_3 and fT_4 with a suppressed TSH, and was successfully treated with radioiodine. (c) A toxic multinodular goiter. The overall uptake is increased (9%, NR 0.4–4%) and there is an irregular outline to the thyroid with heterogenous uptake of tracer (compared with (a)). The patient had elevated levels of fT_3 and fT_4 with a suppressed TSH and was successfully treated with radioiodine.

Painful thyroiditis

Painful thyroiditis can be caused by infectious thyroiditis which is suppurative and usually caused by bacterial infection (staphylococcus or streptococcus). It is more common in immunocompromised patients and is characterized by acute neck pain associated with systemic symptoms of fever or rigors. Unlike de Quervain's thyroiditis (*Box 3.5*), there is no prodrome of a flu-like illness. Treatment is with appropriate antibiotics and (if necessary) drainage of abscesses percutaneously or surgically.

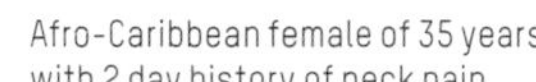
CASE 3.2

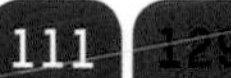
111 129

- Afro-Caribbean female of 35 years with 2 day history of neck pain
- Symptoms and examination suggested thyroiditis: bilateral tremor, muscle weakness, tachycardia
- High T_4 and T_3, low TSH and high ESR
- Nuclear medicine scan showed no tracer uptake
- de Quervain's thyroiditis diagnosed – treat with aspirin and reassurance

This patient presented with the typical symptoms and signs of thyroiditis. She had a throbbing pain around her neck which had appeared suddenly, she was feeling feverish and showing subtle signs of thyrotoxicosis with tremor, tachycardia, warm skin, and muscle weakness. She had recently recovered from a suspected viral illness during which she suffered a sore throat and typical viral prodromal symptoms of malaise, fever, and lethargy.

Blood tests demonstrated elevated levels of free T_4 (41.3 pmol/L) and free T_3 (13.8 pmol/L), and with a TSH level of <0.01 mU/L. Her erythrocyte sedimentation rate (ESR) was 98 mm/h (NR: 2–15). A nuclear medicine scan revealed almost no uptake of tracer (0.1%).

She was diagnosed with de Quervain's thyroiditis (synonyms: subacute thyroiditis and subacute non-suppurative thyroiditis; see *Box 3.5*) and treated with aspirin and reassurance. In severely symptomatic cases, patients can be treated with a short course of a steroidal anti-inflammatory drug such as prednisolone. If the thyroid hormone excess is highly symptomatic, it is reasonable to dampen some of the symptoms with a non-selective β-blocker such as propranolol.

Other causes of painful thyroiditis include radiation thyroiditis (typically, though rarely, occurring a few days after ablative radioiodine treatment for thyroid overactivity or thyroid cancer) or 'palpation'/traumatic thyroiditis occurring after neck surgery, thyroid biopsy or direct neck trauma (e.g. from a car seat belt).

Painless thyroiditis

This form of thyroiditis accounts for up to 10% of cases of hyperthyroidism and is considered part of the spectrum of autoimmune (antibody-mediated) thyroid disease. Painless thyroiditis includes:

- 'silent' thyroiditis (often known as lymphocytic thyroiditis)
- post-partum thyroiditis (essentially just painless thyroiditis that occurs within one year of parturition)
- fibrous thyroiditis (also known as Riedel thyroiditis)
- drug-induced (caused by interferons, lithium, and amiodarone, for example; see below)

As ever, the nomenclature appears designed to make things more complicated than they are. Painless thyroiditis is really hyperthyroidism in someone who has not recently been pregnant, has nothing much in the way of a goiter, and who has none of the other clinical features of Graves disease (e.g. dermopathy or orbitopathy).

Box 3.5 | Subacute thyroiditis

Subacute thyroiditis, first described by Swiss surgeon Fritz de Quervain, is a self-limiting inflammatory thyroid disorder. It is most prevalent among people aged 30–50 years and is more common in females than in males. The disease has a tendency to follow upper respiratory tract infections and clusters of the disease appear alongside outbreaks with Coxsackievirus, mumps, measles, adenovirus, and other viral infections.

Two-thirds of patients with the disease have HLA-B35 suggesting that the susceptibility to subacute thyroiditis is genetically influenced. HLA-B35 is associated with familial occurrence of subacute thyroiditis and increased recurrence of the disease compared to the normal population.

The vast majority of people recover completely and only less than 1% become permanently hypothyroid.

CASE 3.3

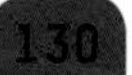

- Male of 55 years with HOCM on long-term warfarin and amiodarone
- No family history of thyroid disease

A 55 year old man was admitted to coronary care with intractable tachycardia associated with breathlessness. For a few weeks prior to admission his family had commented that he had been restless and rather short-tempered. He had a known diagnosis of hypertrophic obstructive cardiomyopathy (HOCM) with intermittent arrhythmias, for which he was on long-term warfarin therapy and treatment with amiodarone. His eldest son also had a diagnosis of HOCM, but there was no family history of thyroid disease, autoimmune disease, or other endocrinopathy. He had no other significant personal history, including no history of thyroid disease. On admission he had atrial fibrillation with a ventricular rate of 140 b.p.m. There was an easily audible 3rd heart sound, bilateral crepitations suggestive of pulmonary edema, and mild ankle swelling (non-pittable edema). There was some bruising to his lower limbs. There was nothing untoward to feel in the neck; certainly no evidence of a goiter or any nodularity in the thyroid gland.

Post-partum thyroiditis, by definition, occurs within one year of giving birth, but it is otherwise identical; the problem here is that recurrence, exacerbation, or *de novo* diagnosis of Graves disease are also much more common in post-partum women. However, there are some clues as to the differential, as shown in *Table 3.1*.

Table 3.1. **Differential diagnosis of thyroiditis and Graves disease in post-partum women**

	Graves disease after delivery	Post-partum thyroiditis
Nuclear medicine scanning	High uptake	Low uptake
Antibodies	TPO and Tg often positive	TSHR-Ab specific
Doppler flow ultrasound	Vascular+++	Decreased vascularity
Clinical signs	Maybe dermopathy, ophthalmopathy	No associated signs
Symptoms	More symptomatic	Less symptomatic
Goiter	Usually large and vascular	Less impressive
Clinical course	Worse if not treated for 2–4 weeks	Most will have improved after 2–4 weeks

Drug-induced thyrotoxicosis

The next significant cause of painless thyroiditis is associated with certain drugs, classically amiodarone and lithium, and less frequently interferon (used in the treatment of hepatitis C) or interleukin-2 (used in the treatment of some metastatic cancers and leukemia).

Amiodarone is an excellent cardiovascular drug, but it can cause real problems in relation to the thyroid. It has an extremely high iodine content; each molecule contains two iodine atoms and a standard dose is equivalent to about 20 times the recommended daily intake of iodine. Because of effects directly related to its iodine content and those due to its intrinsic destructive potential, amiodarone is implicated in both hypo- and hyperthyroid complications (see *Boxes 3.6* and *3.7*).

3.5.4 Thyrotoxicosis associated with structural (nodular) thyroid disease

Thyrotoxicosis can be caused by excess synthesis of thyroid hormone (e.g. in Graves disease) or excess release of thyroid hormone due to a destructive process (e.g. in thyroiditis). In addition, autonomous overproduction of thyroid hormone may occur independently of TSH regulation such as in the case of toxic adenomas and toxic multinodular goiters (*Box 3.2*).

Solitary functioning nodules (variously known as toxic nodules, 'hot' nodules, or toxic adenomas) are autonomously functioning thyroid nodules that produce enough thyroid hormone to suppress TSH. Solitary toxic nodules account for no more than about 2% of hyperthyroid cases; their frequency increases with age and they are more common in women than men. Their autonomous function has been linked to activating mutations of the TSH receptor, or further down in the $G_s\alpha$ protein linked to adenylate cyclase. Diagnosis requires the presence of a unilateral thyroid mass, plus TFTs and nuclear medicine scanning (*Figure 3.13*). When activating mutations in the TSH receptor occur in the germline, the

Box 3.6 | Wolff-Chaikoff and Jod-Basedow effects

It can be difficult to understand how excess iodine can sometimes cause hypothyroidism and sometimes cause hyperthyroidism. In the most simple terms this is due to two independent and eponymous effects: Wolff-Chaikoff and Jod-Basedow (Jod is not actually eponymous but is German for iodine). Underlying established or potential thyroid abnormalities also promote the variable effects of amiodarone.

The Wolff-Chaikoff effect is a protective mechanism whereby sudden exposure to excess iodine is prevented from resulting in thyrotoxicosis by limiting iodine transport and thyroid hormone synthesis. This mechanism ensures that patients do not suddenly become hyperthyroid when, for example, they have an X-ray following ingestion of lots of iodine-based contrast medium, or eat too much sushi. Normal individuals 'escape' from the Wolff-Chaikoff effects when iodine levels normalize; however, those with underlying thyroid disease may fail to escape and so thyroid activity remains closed down, resulting in hypothyroidism.

The Jod-Basedow effect occurs in patients with underlying uncontrolled autonomous thyroid function (e.g. autonomous nodules or multinodular goiters) who may lose the ability to autoregulate iodine, resulting in increased thyroid hormone production in response to an increased iodine load.

To further complicate the situation, amiodarone also has direct intrinsic effects:

- inhibition of 5′ deiodination of T_4 resulting in less T_3 and more rT_3
- blockade of T_3 nuclear receptor binding and therefore reduced activity of T_3
- toxic effects on thyroid follicular cells resulting in a destructive thyroiditis

Box 3.7 | Amiodarone-induced thyroiditis

Because thyroiditis is complicated and because the nomenclature appears to be rather esoteric, it can be helpful to classify hyperthyroidism caused by amiodarone into two types:

- type I AIT (amiodarone-induced thyroiditis), where there is pre-existing thyroid disease (multinodular goiter or latent Graves disease) – the excess iodine substrate leads to increased thyroid hormone synthesis
- type II AIT, where there is no obvious underlying thyroid disorder – the destructive capability of amiodarone results in a thyroiditis with excess release of thyroid hormone

In an ideal world we would be able to distinguish the two types of AIT and tailor treatment accordingly but in practice this is difficult. Nuclear tracer uptake should perhaps be higher in those with underlying disease but in reality the excess of iodine in amiodarone usually mean that tracer uptake is low in both types. TSHR-Ab response may be positive in those with a predisposition to Graves disease and there may be a palpable goiter (smooth or multinodular) but this is not always the case. Often it is impossible to distinguish the two types of AIT and treatments are directed towards the use of thionamides to prevent thyroid hormone synthesis (see *Figure 3.6*) or using immunosuppressive doses of steroids to reduce the effects of amiodarone on thyroid epithelial follicular cells. Amiodarone has a half-life of about 100 days so stopping it does not really help in an acute situation. Eventually many patients will need definitive treatment (usually with surgery because radioiodine is unlikely to be effective in a situation where there is low radioiodine uptake).

CASE 3.4 132

- Caucasian female of 60 years with a 3 week history of difficulty breathing and increasing lump in her throat
- Examination showed tachycardia, warm to touch, with large non-tender mass in neck with many surface nodules
- Thyroid ultrasound scan requested along with TFTs
- Slightly high T_4, normal T_3 and low TSH
- Scan demonstrated typical features of multinodular goiter

A 60 year old Caucasian woman presented to her family doctor with a 3 week history of increasing difficulty in breathing at rest. Furthermore, she felt that a long-standing lump in her throat, which previously caused her no problems, had been starting to get progressively larger for the last few weeks. She described getting significantly short of breath when lying flat on her bed and this was causing her much distress when trying to sleep. She had been experiencing a degree of heat intolerance and was getting occasional palpitations on exertion. She was otherwise well and had no significant past or family history.

On examination, the patient was well perfused with rather warm moist palms and a resting regular tachycardia of 90 b.p.m. She had a relatively large non-tender mass in her neck. On palpation of the thyroid gland, there were many surface nodules of varying size but no obviously dominant nodule. The lower border of the goiter could not be palpated suggesting retrosternal extension. Further investigations of the mass were requested, including a thyroid ultrasound scan (see *Figure 3.14*)

This patient had dyspnea and many surface nodules over the surface of her thyroid gland. Additionally she had some symptoms and signs of thyroid hormone overactivity. Her blood tests revealed a minor elevation of free T_4 (27 pmol/l), a normal level of free T_3 and a low TSH (0.15 mU/l). Thyroid antibodies were negative.

An ultrasound scan of the thyroid in this case demonstrated typical features of a multinodular goiter, with a degree of retrosternal extension (see *Figure 3.14*).

result is familial hyperthyroidism, often inherited as an autosomal dominant trait. The exact frequency of activating mutations is difficult to ascertain as it depends on sampling of tissue and techniques used to screen for mutations.

The diagnosis is usually relatively straightforward. A patient will present with thyrotoxicosis (confirmed biochemically by elevated thyroid hormone levels and suppressed TSH) in association with a palpable nodule. On thyroid scintigraphy there will be increased uptake in the area of the nodule, with suppression of the surrounding normal thyroid tissue. In addition, thyroid autoantibodies (specifically TSHR-Ab) are usually negative. A multinodular goiter is a thyroid gland that has at least two nodules. When at least one nodule is autonomously functioning (i.e. 'hot'), it also produces the signs and symptoms of hyperthyroidism, although most cases reveal normal TSH levels. The exact cause of this disorder is unknown but may be related to mutations in individual cells leading to clonal expansion of cells with autonomous thyroid function. Studies have indicated that multinodular thyroid occurs in around 5% of the population, with a female preponderance of 10:1, and the incidence increases markedly in people over 50 years of age.

Ultrasound of multinodular goiters is useful to:

- determine whether there is an obvious dominant nodule
- determine whether lesions that appear 'cold' (i.e. show no uptake on nuclear scanning) are in fact cystic
- determine whether features suspicious of malignancy are present (e.g. hypoechogenicity, microcalcification, increased vascular flow, irregular borders; see *Section 3.8.3*)
- guide fine needle aspiration/biopsy of suspicious nodules (*Figure 3.14*)

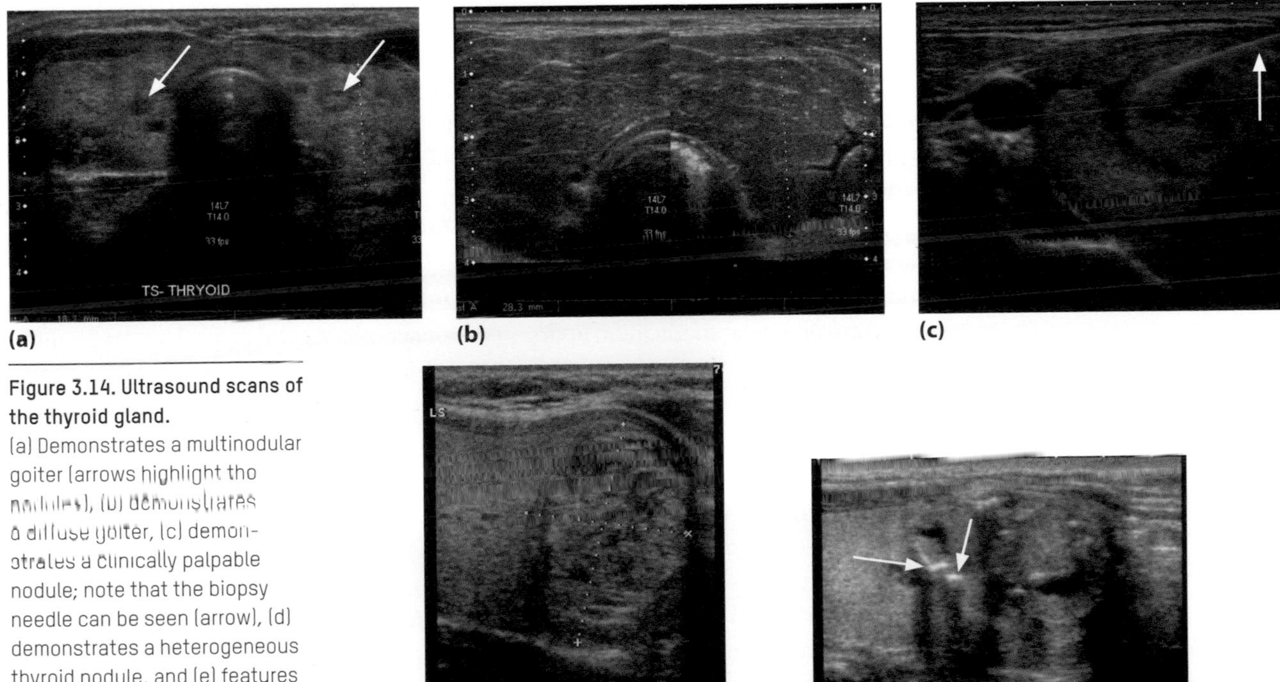

Figure 3.14. Ultrasound scans of the thyroid gland.
(a) Demonstrates a multinodular goiter (arrows highlight the nodules), (b) demonstrates a diffuse goiter, (c) demonstrates a clinically palpable nodule; note that the biopsy needle can be seen (arrow), (d) demonstrates a heterogeneous thyroid nodule, and (e) features of papillary cancer (hypoechogenicity microcalcification).

Thyroid scanning (with ^{125}iodine or ^{99m}Tc) of multinodular goiters (see *Figure 3.13*) shows a heterogeneous pattern of radioactive accumulation with many areas of hyper- and hypoactivity.

The majority of multinodular goiters occur in the presence of euthyroidism. However, up to 25% of patients may have overt or subclinical hyperthyroidism (where TSH is suppressed, although the levels of free T_4 and free T_3 are normal).

Many patients with multinodular goiters are entirely asymptomatic (particularly when the goiter is relatively small and thyroid function is not disturbed). However, as the thyroid grows, and particularly if it is retrosternal, other symptoms may develop due to obstruction of, or pressure on, other structures within the neck/thoracic cavity. Pressure on the trachea can cause stridor/wheezing, if the compression is severe, and cough, and pressure on the recurrent laryngeal nerves can cause hoarseness of the voice and dysphagia. It can sometimes be helpful to group these symptoms together under the umbrella term 'aerophagic'. Typical signs are a slow growing 'lumpy' goiter, tracheal deviation and occasionally dilated neck veins.

3.5.5 Hyperthyroidism in pregnancy

CASE 3.5 134 135

- Caucasian female of 28 years, pregnant, with 2 week history of profound nausea and vomiting
- Symptoms and examination showed sweating and tachycardia, bilateral tremor and muscle weakness, no goiter
- ? Transient hCG-mediated hyperthyroidism – resolved by week 15

A 28 year old Caucasian woman in the 12th week of her first pregnancy, presented to her family doctor following a 2 week history of profound early morning nausea and vomiting. Over this period she had lost 4 kg in weight, she was constantly thirsty and was passing small volumes of very concentrated urine. Further questioning revealed that over the last few weeks she had felt her heart racing on a number of occasions and was sweating despite minimal exertion. She claimed she was also having to open her bowels more than usual. She denied any changes in her vision or facial appearance. She had no significant past medical history and was on no form of regular medication apart from folic acid for the pregnancy.

On examination the patient appeared flushed and anxious. She was tachycardic with a strong bounding pulse. Her hands were warm and a fine bilateral tremor was noted. Neurological examination demonstrated mild proximal muscle wasting and weakness. No lid lag, lid retraction, or exophthalmos was noted. Neck examination excluded the presence of a goiter. Transient hCG-mediated hyperthyroidism was suspected. The patient was reassured and asked to return in a few weeks for a check-up. In her 15th week of pregnancy, the patient was reviewed and her nausea and vomiting had resolved along with her symptoms and signs. Her pregnancy was found to be progressing well.

Pregnancy alters thyroid physiology and, overall, increases circulating concentrations of free thyroid hormones and reduces TSH. The first trimester increase in human chorionic gonadotropin (hCG) has been implicated in this effect because hCG is structurally similar to TSH and its high concentrations may interact with the TSH receptor. Pregnancy is associated with an amelioration of symptoms associated with autoimmune diseases (i.e. immunosuppression) but the causes of this are not understood. The immunological changes that occur post-partum induce a recrudescence of (or, indeed, a first appearance of) autoimmune hyperthyroidism or hypothyroidism. It is estimated that 2–15% women become thyrotoxic (often transiently) post-partum and those that do develop post-partum thyroiditis (as opposed to Graves disease) frequently have antithyroid antibodies in the circulation.

Graves disease accounts for 80–85% cases of hyperthyroidism in pregnancy and 1–5% of neonates born to women with this disease have hyperthyroidism due to transplacental transfer of TSH receptor-stimulating antibodies. Treatment of Graves disease with antithyroid drugs should be carefully monitored by TFTs, particularly in the 3rd trimester of pregnancy when antibody titers may be low, and the lowest possible dose of antithyroid treatment should be used in order to minimize the risk of fetal hypothyroidism. In contrast, untreated Graves disease can have an adverse effect on fetal pituitary development resulting in central congenital hypothyroidism due to high levels of maternal thyroid hormones suppressing fetal TSH secretion. Thus the goal of antithyroid drug treatment for Graves disease during pregnancy should be to maintain free T_4 in the upper normal range using the lowest possible dosage. Although the issue of screening remains controversial, women with a history of thyroid disease or other autoimmune disease should be carefully monitored every 4–6 weeks of pregnancy.

CASE 3.5 134 135

- Caucasian female of 28 years, pregnant, with 2 week history of profound nausea and vomiting
- Symptoms and examination showed sweating and tachycardia, bilateral tremor and muscle weakness, no goiter
- ? Transient hCG-mediated hyperthyroidism – resolved by week 15

The pregnant woman showed typical signs and symptoms of hyperthyroidism: tachycardia, anxiety, proximal muscle wasting, weight loss, sweating, and loose bowels, although there was no indication of Graves ophthalmopathy. Her blood tests showed a free T_4 value of 32.0 pmol/L and a serum TSH value of <0.01 mU/L. No further tests were carried out and her transient hyperthyroidism resolved by the 2nd trimester. Fetal blood sampling for TFTs is only indicated in women with Graves disease if the mother has high maternal TSH receptor-stimulating antibodies, fetal signs suggestive of thyroid disease, and a history of a prior baby with hyperthyroidism. Radionuclide imaging is contraindicated in pregnant women. Occasionally there can be some difficulty in differentiating pregnancy-associated thyrotoxicosis (which is generally transient and requires no active treatment) from Graves disease (which of course may require treatment during pregnancy). A prior or family history of autoimmune thyroid disease, presence of TSHR-Ab, dermopathy or orbitopathy, and lack of improvement with time all suggest Graves disease (*Table 3.1* illustrates some of the differences between thyroiditis in pregnancy and Graves disease in pregnancy).

Whilst changes in thyroid hormone status in relation to pregnancy are now well recognized, maternal thyroid hormones have not been thought to play a major role in the development of the fetal CNS. However, appreciable thyroid hormones are only detectable in the human fetal circulation from 14 to 16 weeks of gestation and recent epidemiological evidence suggests that even relatively mild sub-clinical maternal hypothyroidism (elevated TSH with normal or low normal levels of free T_3 and free T_4), particularly in early pregnancy, may adversely affect neurological development in the offspring. The prevalence of subclinical hypothyroidism in early pregnancy is about 2–4%, although the leading cause of maternal hypothyroidism worldwide is iodine deficiency.

3.5.6 Treatment of hyperthyroidism

The treatment of thyrotoxicosis aims to alleviate the symptoms as quickly as possible and then to try and achieve remission (or ideally cure). Symptomatic relief of symptoms associated with sympathetic nervous system hyperactivity, such as tremor, palpitations, and heat intolerance, can usually be achieved with a non-selective β-blocker (e.g. propranolol or atenolol). Then a treatment strategy designed to result in remission or cure is initiated – this treatment may be medical (drug therapy) or definitive and destructive (surgery or radioactive iodine). The treatment of hyperthyroidism in pregnancy is given in *Box 3.8*.

Antithyroid drugs

There are three types of drugs used to inhibit thyroid hormone synthesis and release: thionamides, iodine and iodinated contrast agents, and radioiodine.

Thionamides

The thionamides are the most widely used antithyroid drugs, having been noted to inhibit thyroid hormone synthesis as long ago as the early 1940s. Thionamides are actively transported into the thyroid gland where they inhibit formation of thyroid hormone by blocking the iodination of tyrosine residues within thyroglobulin and then inhibiting the coupling reaction between iodotyrosines (*Figure 3.6*).

The synthetic thionamides now used are:

- methimazole (in the USA)
- carbimazole (in the UK and Europe) – this is completely metabolized to methimazole but approximately 40% more carbimazole is require to yield an equivalent dose of methimazole
- propylthiouracil (PTU)

Carbimazole and methimazole are more widely used because they only need to be taken once daily whereas PTU needs to be taken more often as it has a very short half-life (1–2 hours). Also, despite the potential benefit of PTU in terms of its ability to block deiodination of T_4 to T_3, the intrathyroidal concentration of the active drug achieved with methimazole/carbimazole is higher and their efficacy in terms of inhibiting iodine organification is greater. However, PTU tends to be prescribed to pregnant and lactating women because:

- it binds to plasma proteins and less crosses the placenta or enters the breast milk
- there are potential teratogenic risks with carbimazole/methimazole
- it also has the added advantage of reducing the hepatic conversion of the less active T_4 to T_3

The aim of treatment with thionamides is to reduce circulating thyroid hormone levels to normal and to maintain euthyroidism for a period of 6–18 months prior to stopping therapy and ascertaining whether the patient has achieved remission. The starting dose is usually relatively high (e.g. 40 mg carbimazole). Two treatment methods are utilized:

- titration – where the dose is gradually reduced on the basis of symptoms and TFTs to the lowest possible maintenance dose

- 'block and replace' – where the higher dose is continued and the thyroxine that is being blocked is replaced by oral levothyroxine treatment, in addition to the thionamide

There are no clear benefits of one treatment strategy over the other, although 'block and replace' is usually used for a shorter period of time (6–8 months) and gives a steadier state of thyroid hormones. It cannot, however, be used in pregnancy as the higher doses used can cross the placenta more effectively than the thyroxine and this puts the fetus at risk of acquired hypothyroidism. It is also not sensible to use 'block and replace' in patients that are highly likely to go on to radioiodine treatment as the exogenous thyroxine may inhibit uptake of the radioactive iodine.

The ultimate remission rate of thionamide therapy is a little disappointing at no more than 30%. This means that many patients will eventually require definitive treatment. The identification of patients likely to relapse is difficult (clues may be male sex, presence of significant ophthalmopathy, titer of TSHR-Ab at cessation of treatment, HLA haplotype). It is also difficult to give patients detailed information on when they may relapse, although most will relapse within the first year or two after stopping treatment.

Thionamides are generally useful in the management of autoimmune thyroid disease but are not without side-effects, including rash, urticaria, arthralgia, nausea, and (the most serious) agranulocytosis (0.5%). Patients must be warned about agranulocytosis and instructed to stop thionamide treatment and seek medical help (i.e. a full blood count) if they develop any significant infection during treatment. There is also evidence of potential (but perhaps questionable) teratogenicity with carbimazole/methimazole: aplasia cutis (a rare fetal scalp defect), tracheo-esophageal fistulas, and choanal atresia have been reported. However, it is extremely important to fully inform pregnant women that the risk to the fetus of untreated maternal Graves disease clearly outweighs the small risk of problems associated with thionamide therapy in pregnancy.

As thionamides block synthesis of thyroid hormones they are only really of value in the treatment of thyrotoxicosis associated with excess thyroid hormone synthesis (*Case 3.1*). In the case of hyperthyroidism caused by toxic 'hot' nodules or toxic multinodular goiters, radioactive iodine (or occasionally surgery) is used for definitive treatment rather than antithyroid drugs because, unlike Graves disease, remission does not occur in these patients.

Iodine and iodinated contrast agents

The fastest acting antithyroid agents are iodinated radio-contrast agents which can block synthesis and release of thyroid hormones, and also block conversion of T_4 to T_3 (they are potent inhibitors of 5′-mono-deiodinase). This form of treatment is no longer widely used but is particularly useful in the short term in hyperthyroid 'storm' where the degree of thyrotoxicosis becomes life-threatening. Iodinated contrast agents used in radiology (e.g. ipodate and iopanoic acid) are used in the UK and Europe, but these are not available in the USA where options include use of supersaturated solutions of potassium iodide, 'Lugol's solution' which contains potassium iodide and iodine, or (rarely and if oral medication is contraindicated) sodium iodide intravenous solution. Iodine itself is more commonly used in the preparation of patients for thyroid surgery where a decrease in vascularity of the gland is a welcome effect. In this case an iodine elixir (e.g. 10 drops or so of a saturated solution of potassium iodide) is used.

Box 3.8 | Treatment of thyroid dysfunction during pregnancy

Hyperthyroidism

The diagnosis of hyperthyroidism in pregnant women should be based on a serum TSH value of < 0.01 mU/L and also a high serum free T_4 value. A favorable maternal and fetal outcome requires the mother's hyperthyroidism to be well controlled. The goal of treatment is to maintain normal thyroid function. To achieve this, serum free T_4 should be assessed regularly with appropriate adjustment of medication.

- Beta blockers may be given to ameliorate the symptoms of moderate to severe hyperthyroidism in pregnant women. However, due to occasional reports of fetal growth restriction, hypoglycemia, respiratory depression, and bradycardia after maternal administration, the dose should be weaned down when possible.
- Anti-thyroid medications are recommended for treatment of moderate to severe hyperthyroidism complicating pregnancy. Treatment should aim to maintain the mother's serum-free T_4 and TSH concentrations in the normal range using the lowest drug dose to ensure that fetal thyroid function is minimally affected. Maternal anti-thyroid drug treatment may result in fetal goiter and hypothyroidism. These cases may be managed by decreasing the maternal anti-thyroid dose if safe to do so, or by intra-amniotic injections of thyroid hormone. When serious adverse reactions such as allergy or agranulocytosis occur with anti-thyroid medication, or persistently high doses of drugs are required to control maternal hyperthyroidism, subtotal thyroidectomy should be considered.
- Radioiodine is absolutely contraindicated because fetal thyroid tissue which is present by 10 to 12 weeks of gestation could be ablated.
- Surgery during pregnancy is associated with an increased risk of spontaneous abortion or premature delivery. The operation should take place in the second trimester to minimize these risks. Prior transient therapy with potassium iodide solution for 10–14 days before surgery is recommended to reduce vascularity of the thyroid gland and is believed safe during this period of exposure.

hCG-mediated hyperthyroidism

Serum chorionic gonadotropin (hCG) concentrations rise soon after fertilization and peak at 10–12 weeks of gestation in normal women, after which they decline. hCG causes an increase in serum thyroxine-binding globulin (TBG) concentrations and stimulation of the thyrotropin (TSH) receptor and thus acts as a weak thyroid stimulator. High serum concentration of hCG during pregnancy can therefore cause subclinical hyperthyroidism characterized by a slight increase in serum-free T_4 concentrations and low serum TSH concentrations. This phenomenon is called gestational transient thyrotoxicosis.

Hyperemesis gravidarum is a syndrome characterized by severe vomiting in early pregnancy, causing more than 5% weight loss, dehydration, and ketonuria. This condition is associated with higher serum hCG than in normal pregnant women and so many of these women have either subclinical or mild overt hyperthyroidism. Thyroid function should be measured in all patients with hyperemesis gravidarum. Gestational transient thyrotoxicosis in women with hyperemesis gravidarum rarely requires treatment because it is mild and subsides as hCG production falls.

On the other hand, a few women do need anti-thyroid medication when there are clearly elevated thyroid hormone levels with clinical evidence of hyperthyroidism. Treatment with anti-thyroid medication is required for as long as clinically necessary. If overt hyperthyroidism persists for more than several weeks or beyond the first trimester, it is unlikely to be hCG-mediated and another cause should be explored.

Thyroid cancer and nodules

The diagnostic evaluation of a thyroid nodule discovered during pregnancy should be similar to that of non-pregnant patients (see *Section 3.8.2*). Ultrasound-guided fine needle aspiration biopsy should be performed for thyroid nodules >1 cm discovered during pregnancy. Subsequent management varies according to the biopsy results. Thyroid radionuclide scanning is contraindicated during pregnancy.

The majority of thyroid nodules are cytologically benign lesions that do not require surgery and should instead be regularly followed up / reviewed. When nodules exhibiting rapid growth, or found to be malignant on cytopathologic analysis are discovered in the first or early second trimester, total thyroidectomy should be offered. The safest time for any type of surgery during pregnancy for both the patient and the fetus is the second trimester before fetal viability. During the first trimester, there is concern over the possible teratogenic effects on the fetus, and surgery of any type is associated with increased early fetal loss. Surgery in the third trimester

>

Box 3.8 | continued

is associated with a higher incidence of pre-term labor. Ideally, however, surgical procedures should be post-poned until after delivery to minimize maternal and fetal complications.

Given the typically indolent nature of most well-differentiated thyroid cancers, thyroidectomy is usually delayed until the post-partum period. In particular, when cytology studies indicate papillary cancer or follicular neoplasm without evidence of advanced disease, it is preferable to wait until the post-partum period for definitive surgery. This approach does not appear to have a negative impact on prognosis and in fact surgical complication rates are lower. Several other considerations must be taken into account when deciding the most appropriate treatment option, including the gestational age, the apparent tumor stage, and the personal inclination of the patient.

If a nodule is discovered during the third trimester, even if highly suspicious of cancer, it is generally accepted that treatment can be delayed until after delivery. The exceptions include a rapidly growing lesion, an anaplastic tumor (which are fortunately very rare in this age group), or if waiting until after delivery causes immense psychological stress to the mother.

Hypothyroidism

It is unusual to find overt hypothyroidism complicating pregnancy for two main contributory factors: some women with hypothyroidism are anovulatory and thus unlikely to become pregnant and, secondly, hypothyroidism is also associated with a high rate of first trimester spontaneous miscarriage. In those women with hypothyroidism and a continuing pregnancy, there is an increased risk of several complications including pre-eclampsia, ante-partum hemorrhage, pre-term delivery, and low birth weight.

A number of studies have shown a significant increased risk of impairment in neuropsychological developmental, IQ scores, and school learning abilities in the offspring of hypothyroid mothers. This suggests that thyroid hormone is extremely important for normal fetal brain development and so it is clearly very important to correct maternal hypothyroidism.

Women need more thyroid hormone during pregnancy and, unlike normal women, those with hypothyroidism are unable to increase serum free T_4 and T_3 secretion. Those with pre-existing hypothyroidism usually require an increase in their daily thyroxine dosage by, on average, 30–50% above preconception dosage. Ideally, thyroxine treatment should be titrated to reach a serum TSH value less than 2.5 mU/L.

Once normalized by treatment, thyroid function tests should be monitored every 6–8 weeks with thyroxine dosage adjusted accordingly. After delivery, most hypothyroid women need to decrease the thyroxine dosage they received during pregnancy over a period of approximately 4 weeks post-partum. Serum TSH should be measured 4–6 weeks later to confirm that the reduction was appropriate.

Radioactive iodine

As described above, patients with autoimmune thyroid disease have a habit of relapsing following thionamide treatment. In addition, thionamides are not appropriate in the long term for patients with hyperthyroidism due to autonomous overproduction of thyroid hormone (e.g. in toxic nodules or toxic multinodular goiters). In the USA, some 70% of patients are offered definitive treatment with radioiodine from the outset, but only 20% of patients are in the UK and Europe.

Radioiodine is simple to administer; it is given in the form of a capsule containing ^{131}I. The iodine is rapidly incorporated into the thyroid where β-emissions cause local destruction of thyroid tissue. It is absolutely contra-indicated in pregnancy and used with caution in putative and pre-existing thyroid eye disease as this may worsen after administration of radioiodine – this effect can be completely ameliorated by co-administration of steroids (see *Box 3.4*). In other situations it is perfectly safe with a very low incidence of significant morbidity or mortality (although it will generally render the patient hypothyroid – see *Section 3.6*). One side-effect is radiation thyroiditis (see

Section 3.5.3) where there may be acute tenderness in the neck associated with a recurrence or exacerbation of hyperthyroid symptoms for 2–3 weeks after treatment. This is a rare complication (<1%) and most patients respond well to steroid treatment. Precautions after radioiodine include avoiding close contact (<1 meter radius) with pregnant women and children for up to 3 weeks following the treatment, and avoidance of sharing cooking and eating utensils with family members.

There is disagreement as to whether it is useful (or indeed possible) to estimate the dose that can cure the thyroid overactivity without rendering the patient hypothyroid. Some centers advocate measuring thyroid volume and isotope uptake and trying to calculate an individualized dose, whereas others give a fixed dose (e.g. 550 MBq or 15 mCi). In patients with an autonomous nodule, the uptake in surrounding 'normal' thyroid tissue is endogenously suppressed and the uptake in the autonomous nodule is increased – this is one of the few situations where euthyroidism is the norm after radioiodine treatment.

Temporal responses are variable, but an effect is usually seen in 6–18 weeks. It is important to monitor the patient for evidence of hypothyroidism (which will require introduction of thyroid hormone replacement with thyroxine) or evidence of treatment failure (which may require a further dose of radioiodine).

There are several myths associated with radioiodine treatment and so many patients will ask 'will I get cancer?' and/or 'will I be subfertile?'. The answer to both these questions is 'No'.

Thyroid surgery

Thyroid surgery for hyperthyroidism is very much a third-line treatment and generally reserved for:

- those patients who cannot tolerate medical treatment (if it is appropriate)
- patients in whom radioiodine would be impractical (e.g. pregnant women intolerant to thionamides, women with small children where alternative care arrangements cannot be made, or patients with severe thyroid eye disease which may be worsened by radioiodine (see *Box 3.4*)
- those with very large goiters causing aerophagic symptoms (or in some cases cosmetic distress)

There is no absolute agreement on the extent of surgery in the management of Graves disease. Many advocate a total thyroidectomy whereas some surgeons take a more conservative approach. Clearly the rate of hypothyroidism is proportional to the amount of thyroid tissue removed. The corollary is that the less tissue removed, the higher the incidence of recurrence of hyperthyroidism or persistence of subclinical hyperthyroidism (persistently suppressed TSH levels in association with normal free T_4 and free T_3 levels). Subclinical hyperthyroidism is at least a theoretical risk factor for the development of cardiac rhythm abnormalities and reduced bone mineral density.

Complications of thyroid surgery can be divided into those common to any operative procedure (risks of anesthetic, hemorrhage, and infection) and those peculiar to operating in this area of the neck (transient or persistent damage to the recurrent laryngeal nerves (1–3%) and damage to the parathyroids resulting in hypocalcemia).

Overall, the incidence of significant complications is less than 1%, but prolonged hypocalcemia may occur in up to 6% and can occasionally be challenging to treat effectively.

Prior to surgery the patient should be rendered euthyroid, either with pre-operative thionamide stabilization or, where this is problematic or contraindicated, treatment for 7–10 days with Lugol's iodine and β-blockade.

3.6 Hypothyroidism

Hypothyroidism is a common condition which can be caused by a defect anywhere in the hypothalamic–pituitary–thyroid pathway (*Figure 3.15*). By far the most common cause is disease of the thyroid itself, known as primary hypothyroidism (*Case 3.6*). Secondary hypothyroidism is much more rare and is due to decreased secretion of TSH from the pituitary or, vanishingly rarely, to hypothalamic disorders resulting in reduced TRH secretion. The etiology of hypothyroidism can be divided up into congenital and acquired causes and this is particularly pertinent to pediatric endocrinology (*Box 3.9*).

Box 3.9 | Causes of hypothyroidism

In adults:

- chronic autoimmune hypothyroidism
- following thyroid surgery
- following radioiodine treatment
- iodine deficiency or excess
- drugs (thionamides, lithium, amiodarone, perchlorate, interleukin-2, interferon-α)
- following thyroiditis (lymphocytic, granulomatous, post-partum) – this may be transient (see text)
- TSH deficiency
- TRH deficiency (vanishingly rare)
- resistance to thyroid hormone

In children and adolescents:

- chronic autoimmune hypothyroidism
- iodine deficiency or excess
- damage to or infiltration of the thyroid gland (e.g. surgery, radioiodine, external radiation therapy, histiocytosis-X, cystinosis)
- thyroid dysgenesis
- hemangiomas of the liver
- TRH/TSH deficiency
- resistance to thyroid hormone

In neonates:

- thyroid dysgenesis, aplasia or hypoplasia
- inborn errors of thyroid hormone synthesis ('dyshormonogenesis')
- maternal antibodies crossing placenta during gestation
- pituitary (central) hypothyroidism
- thyroxine binding globulin deficiency (causes low T_4 but **not** true hypothyroidism)
- iodine deficiency or excess

Congenital causes include developmental abnormalities of the thyroid gland (agenesis, hypoplasia, ectopy, for example), disorders of thyroid hormone synthesis or transport, congenital central (hypothalamic–pituitary) hypothyroidism, and some transient forms. Acquired hypothyroidism can be overt, where there is a reduction in levels of free T_4 and free T_3 with a concomitant increase in TSH as a result of feedback, or subclinical (sometimes called compensated) with low levels of free T_4 and free T_3 but normal TSH levels (*Box 3.9*). The symptoms and signs of hypothyroidism are summarized in *Figure 3.15*.

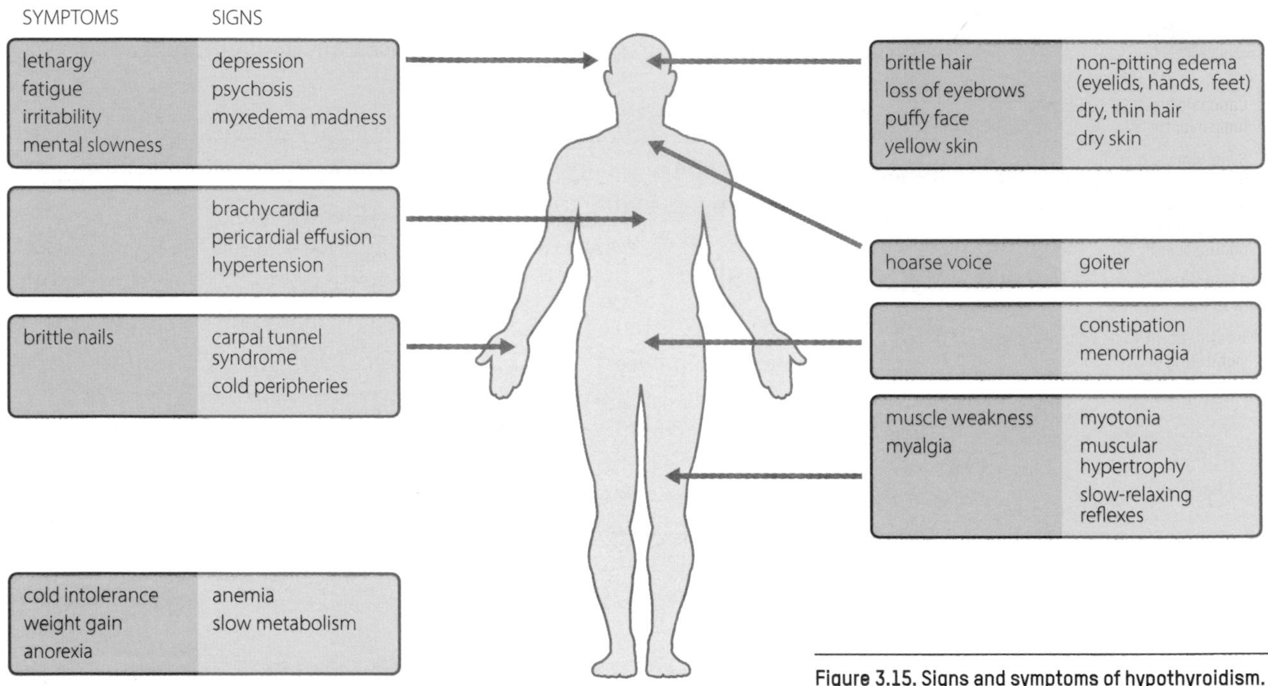

Figure 3.15. Signs and symptoms of hypothyroidism.

CASE 3.6

142 147

- Male child of 14 years with excessive tiredness
- Symptoms and examination: intolerance to cold, increasing weight, lethargy, puffiness around eyes, dry and thin hair
- ? Primary hypothyroidism – TFTs ordered

A previously well 14 year old boy presented with his mother to the family doctor with excessive tiredness. He found it increasingly difficult to keep up in class and complained that his memory had also been deteriorating. Previously a keen sportsman, he had been missing training sessions at school, partly due to his constant lethargy and also his increasing intolerance to the cold outdoors.

His mother commented that he had been putting on weight, despite not having any change in appetite. However, he attributed this to his reduced physical activity. Having previously been one of the tallest in the class, his peers had now overtaken him in linear height and he felt that he was being bullied about his short stature.

On inspection, the doctor noticed some puffiness around his eyes and dry, thin hair, which the patient said he had noticed but not paid much attention to. There was no visible goiter. Other than an uncle who has type 1 diabetes mellitus, he had no significant family history.

Throughout the session, the boy appeared easily distracted and replied to questions slowly, albeit appropriately. When asked about his mood and general well-being, the boy said he felt 'depressed all the time' and was losing interest in school and becoming more withdrawn from his friends.

The doctor suspected primary hypothyroidism and this was checked by blood tests.

3.6.1 Autoimmune hypothyroidism

In areas of adequate iodine intake, by far the most common cause of an underactive thyroid is chronic autoimmune thyroiditis. In common with thyroiditis nomenclature, the aim appears to be to make the nomenclature as opaque as possible so this condition can be found described as chronic autoimmune

CASE 3.7

143 145 148

- Caucasian male of 16 years with lump over thyroid
- Symptoms and examination: hyperactive, frequent bowel opening, warm, ear infections, tachycardia, small non-tender nodule over thyroid
- ? Thyroid hormone resistance –TFTs ordered
- Treatment with thyroxine and close monitoring of SHBG and ferritin

A 16 year old Caucasian man with learning difficulties presented with his mother to the family doctor after his parents noted a lump overlying the thyroid region. The mother claimed that over the last few weeks he had been quite boisterous and hyperactive and had been difficult to manage both at home and at his special learning needs school. She also noted that he had been opening his bowels more frequently and complaining of being warm a lot of the time. He had had a number of ear infections over the last few months.

On general inspection, the patient appeared flushed and was very fidgety. Examination found warm and well-perfused peripheries and tachycardia was noted. Neck examination revealed a small, warm, non-tender nodule over the thyroid region.
Ear examination showed that the left tympanic membrane was red, bulging and was exuding purulent fluid consistent with an ear infection. Thyroid hormone resistance (see *Box 3.10*) was suspected. Thyroid function tests were ordered.

---

thyroiditis, Hashimoto disease, autoimmune hypothyroidism, primary autoimmune thyroid failure, and primary atrophic hypothyroidism. Autoimmune hypothyroidism is as good a descriptive term as any other and is now used most commonly. Autoimmune hypothyroidism has a female:male ratio of 5–8:1 and a prevalence of about 0.1–2 per 100 which increases with increasing age.

Autoimmune hypothyroidism is caused by cell or humoral-mediated destruction of functional thyroid tissue, with lymphocytic infiltration and follicular destruction. The majority of patients will have measurable antibodies to TPO, to thyroglobulin or to the thyroid Na^+/I^+ transporter. Whether antibodies to thyroglobulin and to TPO have a role in causation, or whether they are secondary to thyroid damage caused by T cells, is debatable. Some patients will also have TSHR-Ab which are inhibitory, as opposed to the TSHR-stimulating antibodies seen in Graves disease (see *Section 3.5.1*). The role of these TSHR-blocking antibodies is not entirely clear, as they are common in the normal population, whereas TSHR-stimulating antibodies are specific for Graves disease.

The condition is often, but by no means invariably, associated with goiter formation. The end result is usually hypothyroidism (except in the rarer transient forms of painless and post-partum thyroiditis described in *Section 3.5.3*) but occasionally the destructive process may lead to an initial and transient period of hyperthyroidism (known as 'Hashitoxicosis').

The risk factors for development of autoimmune hypothyroidism are not entirely clear. It is most common in older women, but there is no proven link to estrogen deficiency. It is also more common in patients with Turner syndrome (45 XO – see *Section 7.4*) and Down syndrome (trisomy 21). A family history of autoimmunity is common, but this is not necessarily or exclusively of autoimmune thyroid disease (a family history of insulin-dependent diabetes or adrenal failure may also be recorded). There is a weak association with certain HLA haplotypes (e.g. DR3). Environmental factors such as iodine intake, stress, radiation exposure, infections, and pregnancy may have an impact but these are by no means proven or universally accepted.

In summary, autoimmune hypothyroidism is secondary to immune-mediated destruction of the thyroid with thyroid epithelial cell apoptosis. Thyroid failure is gradual and may or may not be associated with goiter formation. Most patients will have measurable antibodies directed against one or more thyroid-associated antigens. Genetic predisposition probably interacts with environmental stimuli to result in lymphocytic infiltration of the thyroid and follicular destruction.

3.6.2 Other causes of primary hypothyroidism

The causes of hypothyroidism are summarized in *Box 3.9.* Iatrogenic hypothyroidism is relatively common and results from treatment of hyperthyroidism with either surgery or radioiodine (see *Section 3.5.6*). External beam radiotherapy to the neck for other reasons (e.g. in the treatment of Hodgkin lymphoma, or head and neck cancers) may also cause hypothyroidism; the timing of onset is variable and the effects are probably dependent on the dose of radiation used.

Both iodine deficiency and excess can cause hypothyroidism, but these states are relatively rare in the USA and Western Europe. Iodine deficiency is not rare in mountainous areas of South America and Africa and the effects here can be exacerbated by concomitant ingestion of certain foodstuffs rich in cyanoglucosides such as cassava root. Iodine excess causes hypothyroidism secondary to failure to escape from the protective Wolff–Chaikoff effect (see *Box 3.6*). This usually occurs in individuals with underlying thyroid pathology, for example, those with chronic thyroiditis, previous partial thyroidectomy, or a history of painless thyroiditis. Sources of excess iodine include certain health foods and diet supplements (e.g. kelp), regular use of topical iodine-containing disinfecting substances, X-ray contrast media and some drugs (e.g. amiodarone, see *Box 3.7*). Drugs may also cause hypothyroidism either intentionally (i.e. overzealous use of thionamides) or as an unwanted side effect (e.g. lithium, amiodarone).

Occasionally, infiltrative diseases (such as sarcoid, tuberculosis, amyloid, hemochromatosis) have been cited as the cause of hypothyroidism. In many of these cases, however, there is presence of thyroid autoantibodies making an autoimmune pathology much more likely.

3.6.3 Central (secondary) hypothyroidism and resistance to thyroid hormone

Thyroid function test results in primary hypothyroidism typically show a high TSH level with low free T_4 and low free T_3. Occasionally a patient may have a low TSH with low thyroid hormone levels and this is usually a result of the pituitary's inability to respond to hypothyroidism (this is an indication of hypothalamic–pituitary dysfunction or secondary hypothyroidism and may be caused by any of the myriad causes of hypo-pituitarism (see *Section 2.11*). Very rarely TSH deficiency may be isolated, but far more commonly it occurs in association with other pituitary hormone deficiencies (indeed TSH is often the last of the pituitary hormones to become deficient in pituitary disease).

Thyroid hormone resistance is rare at about 1:40 000 live births, and is almost exclusively autosomal dominant on transmission and therefore has an equal sex distribution. Approximately 85% of cases will have mutations in the TRβ gene and those that do not probably have mutations in co-factors associated with thyroid hormone receptors (*Box 3.10*). Because of variable resistance to the action of thyroid hormone, a feature of thyroid hormone resistance is the general lack of signs; despite high free T_3 and free T_4 concentrations the symptoms are often few and far between. Overall, goiter is the most common sign, along with a degree of hyperactivity and tachycardia, the latter probably as a result of the fact that the non-mutated TRα receptor is more prevalent in the heart. This can often lead to a diagnosis of hyperthyroidism which is reasonable given the high levels of thyroid hormone. Symptoms of hypothyroidism may be present: classically growth retardation, learning difficulties, mental retardation, deafness, and delay in bone maturation (see *Case 3.7*).

Resistance to thyroid hormone shows another unusual pattern of TFT results. Here the levels of free T_4 and free T_3 may be high, and a lack of suppression of TSH means that the TSH level is inappropriately in the normal range or indeed high. Historically this condition has been divided into either 'generalized resistance', 'pituitary resistance', or 'peripheral tissue resistance', although these divisions are not particularly useful and do not reflect the genetic basis of the condition.

CASE 3.7 143 145 148

- Caucasian male of 16 years with lump over thyroid
- Symptoms and examination: hyperactive, frequent bowel opening, warm, ear infections, tachycardia, small non-tender nodule over thyroid
- ? Thyroid hormone resistance –TFTs ordered
- Treatment with thyroxine and close monitoring of SHBG and ferritin

The child presented with a number of symptoms suggestive of hypothyroidism, but the association with hyperactivity, tachycardia and developmental delay led to a suspicion of something less common. Recurrent ear infections are common in resistance to thyroid hormone, but associated deafness may be a result of TRβ malfunction itself. The diagnosis of resistance to thyroid hormone was suspected following the finding of high free T_4 and free T_3 in association with non-suppressed TSH, and it was confirmed by genetic analysis of the TRβ gene. There is a relatively strong association of resistance to thyroid hormone with ADHD (attention deficit hyperactivity disorder) and other learning difficulties, and it is certainly good practice to check thyroid function in any child presenting with this constellation of symptoms.

The differential diagnosis of high or inappropriately normal TSH levels with high levels of free T_4 and free T_3 includes pituitary tumors secreting TSH, and abnormalities in the assays for thyroid hormones as a result of abnormalities of thyroid hormone binding in serum (e.g. by thyroxine binding globulin excess or by familial dysalbuminemic hyperthyroxinemia). Abnormalities in hormone binding in serum can be excluded by repeating the hormone estimations using an assay that measures free T_4 and free T_3 by equilibrium dialysis. Pituitary tumors secreting TSH should be suspected when there are high levels of the common alpha subunit of glycoprotein hormones (i.e. TSH, LH and FSH – see *Chapter 1* and *Section 3.4.5*) and where there is evidence of excess thyroid hormone action despite non-suppressed TSH (the patient will appear hyperthyroid and there will be high levels of thyroid hormone-dependent proteins such as SHBG and ferritin).

3.6.4 Symptoms and treatment of hypothyroidism

Signs and symptoms

The signs and symptoms of hypothyroidism are shown in *Figure 3.15*. Common symptoms include fatigue, lethargy, mental slowness, and cold intolerance, with a prevalence of between 70 and 90% of all hypothyroid cases. Less common symptoms are muscle weakness, hoarse voice, and brittle hair, with a prevalence of between 40 and 60%. Common signs are depression, puffy eyes, dry skin and dry, thin hair. Less common signs are bradycardia, constipation, and menorrhagia. As described earlier, it typically affects women more than men at a ratio of 5–8:1.

Treatment

Treatment of hypothyroidism involves simply replacing the lack of thyroid hormones. Typically thyroxine (T_4) is given because this is the major hormone secreted by the thyroid gland; the thyroxine should be taken first thing in the morning on an empty stomach. Efficacy of treatment is monitored by measuring TSH levels and adjusting the thyroid hormone replacement dose to keep these within the normal range (0.4–4.2 mU/L). Overtreatment will result in suppression of TSH with a potential risk of development of atrial arrhythmias and reduction in bone mineral density. Undertreatment will result in an increase in TSH levels above the normal range and is associated with a recurrence of symptoms.

Liothyronine (T_3) therapy is usually reserved for those patients with thyroid cancer where post-treatment surveillance scans require a high TSH level - the half-life of liothyronine is shorter than thyroxine and so TSH levels rise much faster after cessation of liothyronine treatment, allowing scans to be carried out with reduced time without treatment.

Some patients continue to have symptoms despite biochemical normalization of TFT results and these patients can be challenging because they insist that they are still suffering from hypothyroidism. It has been suggested that these patients may benefit from a combination of T_4/T_3 treatment, but there is no compelling evidence for this at present and most learned societies (including those in the USA and UK) do not currently recommend combination treatment. Very occasionally some patients may have a defect in processing (deiodination) of T_4, such as a relative deficiency of type 2 deiodinase (see *Section 3.4.4*), and in theory these patients could benefit from combination therapy. Treatment of these patients with desiccated pig thyroid extract (e.g. Armour thyroid) is not recommended because there is no demonstrable benefit over traditional treatment with thyroxine alone, and there is potentially a variation in the active forms of thyroid hormone in different batches and different preparations.

Once euthyroidism has been established it is unusual that thyroid hormone requirements will change in hypothyroid patients, except in pregnancy where maternal requirements often increase by 25–50%, and in unrelated concurrent gastrointestinal disorders where absorption is impaired. Excretion of thyroid hormone is increased in nephritic syndrome and metabolism of thyroid hormone can be increased by drugs such as rifampicin, phenytoin, and carbemazepine.

3.7 Fetal, neonatal, and childhood hypothyroidism

The importance of thyroid hormones in nervous system and skeletal development means that hypothyroidism during developmental stages can have marked effects (see *Case 3.6*). Congenital hypothyroidism occurs in 1:2000–4000 births and although iodine deficiency is the most common cause of neonatal hypothyroidism worldwide, there are other causes including thyroid dysgenesis (a deficiency of thyroid-binding globulin reducing the levels of free thyroid

CASE 3.6

142 147

- Male child of 14 years with excessive tiredness
- Symptoms and examination: intolerance to cold, increasing weight, lethargy, puffiness around eyes, dry and thin hair
- ? Primary hypothyroidism – TFTs ordered
- Normal T_4, high TSH and strongly positive anti-TPO antibodies
- Treatment started with levothyroxine

This case was atypical in that the patient was a young male, but he showed some of the classic symptoms and signs of hypothyroidism: mental slowness, lethargy, cold intolerance, puffy eyes, dry thin hair, and depression. Although his uncle had type 1 diabetes there was no other history of a first degree relative having had any autoimmune disease.

Investigation revealed a free T_4 of 3.0 nmol/L with a highly elevated TSH level of 120 mU/L. Anti-TPO antibodies were strongly positive. He was treated with levothyroxine. Within weeks his energy levels had improved and he became far more attentive in class. At review 6 months later he had grown 7 cm and was advancing into puberty normally.

Box 3.10 | Thyroid hormone resistance

Forty years have elapsed since the first description of resistance to thyroid hormone action but, with the application of molecular biology techniques, several different causes of hormone resistance in this axis have since been described. It should, however, be pointed out that all syndromes related to resistance are extremely rare. A few cases of resistance to TRH action have been identified and young patients present with short stature and low T_4 associated with normal TSH levels. As expected, there is an absent or impaired response to a bolus injection of TRH. Resistance to thyrotropin is characterized by an impaired sensitivity of thyrotrophs to TSH and is classically associated with mutations in the gene encoding the TSH receptor, although mutations in the G protein linked to the TSH receptor have also been described. The biochemical profiles depend on the degree of impairment in the TSH receptor and can range from very high TSH and low free T_4 to mildly elevated TSH and normal T_4, correlated with profound hypoplasia to normal pathology of the thyroid gland, respectively. Resistance to both TRH and TSH is treated with thyroxine (if required), but in the case of TRH resistance (central hypothyroidism), TSH levels cannot be monitored to titrate the correct dose of the thyroxine replacement as is the case with primary hypothyroidism.

Three different types of genetic mutations that result in resistance to thyroid hormone actions have so far been identified. These are:

i. mutations in the thyroid receptor TRβ
ii. mutations in the MCT8 thyroid transporter that transports T_3 into neurons of the brain and thyrotrophs of the anterior pituitary gland *(Figure 3.4)*
iii. mutations in a binding protein (SECISBP2) that allows the incorporation of selenium into deiodinases allowing enzyme activity

Patients with mutations of the TRβ gene are biochemically characterized by high levels of free T_4 and T_3 in the presence of measurable TSH concentrations, although patients present with very variable clinical features. The biochemical profile of patients with mutations in the *MCT8* gene is characterized by high levels of total and free T_3 with unsuppressed TSH levels (loss of negative feedback effects) and low concentrations of total and free T_4. Patients with mutations of *SECISBP2* show low serum total and free T_3 in the presence of high levels of T_4 and rT_3 with high/normal levels of TSH as a result of loss of activity of deiodinase type 2 activity.

hormone), dyshormonogenesis, and maternal transfer of antibodies. Congenital hypothyroidism requires treatment as soon after birth as possible and thus capillary blood that is obtained from a heel puncture is not only screened for phenylketonuria (the Guthrie test) but also for measurement of TSH levels. If the results show high TSH or even borderline results, thyroxine replacement must be started immediately. Unfortunately, the most severely affected infants will be left with permanent learning disabilities (see *Section 3.4.1*). In childhood, acquired

CASE 3.7

143 145 148

- Caucasian male of 16 years with lump over thyroid
- Symptoms and examination: hyperactive, frequent bowel opening, warm, ear infections, tachycardia, small non-tender nodule over thyroid
- ? Thyroid hormone resistance –TFTs ordered
- Treatment with thyroxine and close monitoring of SHBG and ferritin

This case illustrates the combination of symptoms seen in resistance to thyroid hormone, where some are suggestive of hyperthyroidism whereas others are more compatible with hypothyroidism. He was treated with thyroxine which was closely monitored by measurement of thyroid hormone-dependent surrogate markers (SHBG and ferritin) along with measurements of mental development and bone maturation (wrist X-rays for bone age).

hypothyroidism is usually autoimmune and characteristically presents with poor growth, epiphyseal dysplasia or poor school attainment as seen in *Case 3.6*.

3.8 Structural thyroid disease and thyroid cancer

Many patients will present with structural abnormalities of the thyroid gland such as obvious solitary nodules (see *Case 3.8*) or multinodular disease (*Box 3.2*) but they will be euthyroid. The challenge here is to determine which of these patients have suspicious pathology that may require further investigation and treatment, and which patients can be reassured. It is also important to note that thyroid cancer may present with abnormal thyroid function tests as well as abnormalities of structure.

CASE 3.8

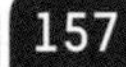

148 157

- Woman of 50 years with 3 week history of increasingly hoarse voice
- Symptoms and examination showed increasing swelling in her neck with single nodule
- ? Thyroid malignancy – TFTs ordered, along with ultrasound scan, FNAC and nuclear medicine scan

A 50 year old woman presented to her family doctor with increasing hoarseness of voice over the past 3 weeks. At first she had attributed this to having the 'flu' as she had felt generally unwell. Her flu-like symptoms had since resolved, although her voice was 'starting to go'. She was clearly distressed as this had been affecting her job as a receptionist answering telephone calls. Also, she complained of a swelling in her neck that she first noticed 6 months ago. It had not caused her any pain or discomfort, and did not bother her too much until she realized it was getting larger. She was worried that the swelling might be causing her change of voice.

On direct questioning, the patient said her grandmother apparently had a thyroid problem, for which she had her thyroid completely removed. Other than that no one else in her family had any significant history of thyroid problems or cancer. As far as she was aware, she had never been exposed to excessive radiation.

On examination, the doctor felt a single nodule on the left anterior aspect of her neck, which had a hard and irregular surface and measured approximately 1.5 cm in diameter. The doctor also palpated her cervical and supraclavicular lymph nodes and noted some enlargement in the anterior chain. The doctor suspected malignancy and requested urgent investigations which included TFTs, an ultrasound scan, an ultrasound-guided fine needle aspiration with biopsy, and a nuclear medicine thyroid scan with ^{125}I.

3.8.1 Thyroid nodules

Thyroid nodules (see *Box 3.11*) are increasingly seen in daily endocrine practice. Patients may present with nodules they have felt themselves, nodules that have been pointed out to them by friends and family (or doctors), or nodules picked up during imaging for other pathologies ('incidentalomas'). They may be solitary or multiple and occur in an otherwise normal gland or a goiter. Multinodular goiters may contain one obviously dominant nodule. Non-malignant nodules are often found in patients with thyroid hyperplasia, and inflammatory or autoimmune thyroid disease.

3.8.2 Investigation of thyroid nodules

Measurement of levels of TSH, along with free T_3 and free T_4, helps to determine the investigation pathway of the nodules and indicates whether to perform thyroid uptake scans (see *Figure 3.13*). These measurements also help to determine the biochemical thyroid status of the patient and the presence of hypo- or hyperthyroidism.

Thyroglobulin measurement has no role in the diagnostic work-up for thyroid cancer (*Box 3.12*). It correlates with the size rather than the nature of the thyroid nodule. Its role in the post-operative period is discussed elsewhere (see *Section 3.8.3*). On the other hand, measurement of calcitonin in patients with thyroid nodules could potentially help with the diagnosis of medullary thyroid cancer (see *Section 8.5.2*), although there is no supporting evidence suggesting that this should be performed routinely. Other causes of elevated calcitonin need to be taken into consideration when interpreting calcitonin levels, such as renal failure, ectopic

Box 3.11 | Thyroid nodules

Thyroid nodules are a common clinical problem, often discovered incidentally on physical examination or an ultrasound scan for an unrelated condition. Their prevalence in the general population is around 4–7%, they are more common in women, and their prevalence increases with age.

Most are not palpable and are asymptomatic. Patients may present with a solitary nodule or multiple nodules which can cause an enlargement of the thyroid gland – a multinodular goiter. Studies of populations (such as Whickham in northern England or Framingham in the USA) have indicated that multinodular thyroids occur in around 5% of the population, with a marked female preponderance (10:1). Autopsy studies have indicated a much higher incidence of nodular thyroid disease (up to 50%), with multinodular disease outnumbering single nodules by about 4:1. The incidence increases markedly in people over 50 years of age. It is much higher in areas of iodine deficiency, indicating the importance of iodine in the etiology of nodularity.

Several types of nodule can develop, with the most common being colloid nodules (benign overgrowths of thyroid tissue), thyroid cysts (fluid-filled areas of thyroid tissue), and inflammatory nodules as a result of chronic inflammation of the thyroid gland (thyroiditis). Benign follicular adenomas account for about 10–15% of thyroid nodules whilst thyroid carcinoma is rare and occurs in only 5% cases of thyroid nodules. Twelve per cent of thyroid nodules are hyperfunctioning autonomous nodules (toxic adenoma, toxic multinodular goiter) and most of these are due to activating mutations of the TSH receptor which leads to stimulation of adenylate cyclase in the absence of TSH and hence hyperthyroidism (thyrotoxicosis).

Controversy exists as to the differential diagnosis and treatment of thyroid nodules, particularly in the case of a solitary or dominant nodule which may be malignant; investigations include measurement of free T_4, T_3 and TSH, scanning and fine needle aspiration (see *Figure 3.14*).

Box 3.12 | Features of thyroid nodules that suggest malignancy

Evaluation of thyroid nodules is with careful history and physical examination. Thyroid ultrasound is an accurate method to assess thyroid nodules for features of malignancy. Features to suggest malignant thyroid nodules are as follows.

- History:
  - of thyroid cancer in one or more first-degree relatives
  - of exposure to ionizing radiation during childhood or adolescence
  - of external beam radiation as a child
  - of rapid growth
  - of discovery of thyroid cancer in a previous hemithyroidectomy sample
- Physical examination:
  - hoarseness
  - hard and irregular consistency
  - ipsilateral cervical lymphadenopathy
  - fixation of the nodule to extrathyroidal tissues
- MEN2/familial medullary cancer-associated *RET* proto-oncogene mutation (*Section 8.5.2*)
- Calcitonin level >100 pg/mL
- Ultrasound:
  - hypoechogenicity
  - microcalcifications
  - absence of peripheral halo
  - irregular borders and infiltrative margins
  - intranodular hypervascularity
  - regional lymphadenopathy
- ^{18}FDG avidity on PET scanning

calcitonin production from non-thyroid neuro-endocrine tumors, hypergastrinemia, Hashimoto thyroiditis and interference from heterophilic antibodies.

After detection, thyroid nodule(s) should be evaluated with ultrasonography. This helps to identify size, position, consistency, the presence of suspicious features, and/or lymph node involvement. When the TSH level is low or undetectable in patients with multinodular goiter, thyroid uptake scans (^{99}Tc, ^{123}I) are useful to determine the functionality of a nodule because they can demonstrate the presence of autonomous functioning nodules. Other imaging modalities (CT, MRI) may also be required in a small number of patients to assess local invasion and/or distant metastases.

During an ultrasound scan an assessment of the need for further investigation by fine needle aspiration cytology (FNAC) can be made. Features of the nodules suggesting that an FNAC is indicated are set out in *Table 3.2.*

FNAC is operator dependent and the best results are usually obtained from an ultrasonographer experienced in the technique working in conjunction with a cytopathologist with significant experience in reporting thyroid cytological specimens (*Figure 3.16*). A series of numerical codes are used to describe the histology:

- Thy1: non-diagnostic – repeat FNAC
- Thy2: non-neoplastic (usually repeat in 3–6 months to be confident)
- Thy3: follicular lesion/suspected follicular neoplasm (discuss at multidisciplinary meeting)
- Thy4: suspicious but not diagnostic of malignancy (papillary, medullary, anaplastic, or lymphoma)
- Thy5: diagnostic of malignancy – surgical intervention required

Table 3.2. Indications for FNAC

Clinical or ultrasound features	Nodule threshold for FNAC
High risk history	
• nodule with suspicious US features	>5 mm
• nodule without suspicious US features	>5 mm
• abnormal cervical lymph nodes	All
• microcalcifications present in nodule	≥1 cm
Solid nodule	
• and hypoechoic	>1 cm
• and iso- or hyperechoic	≥1–1.5 cm
Mixed cystic-solid nodule	
• with any suspicious US features	≥1.5–2 cm
• without suspicious US features	≥2 cm
Spongiform nodule	≥2 cm
Purely cystic nodule	FNAC not indicated

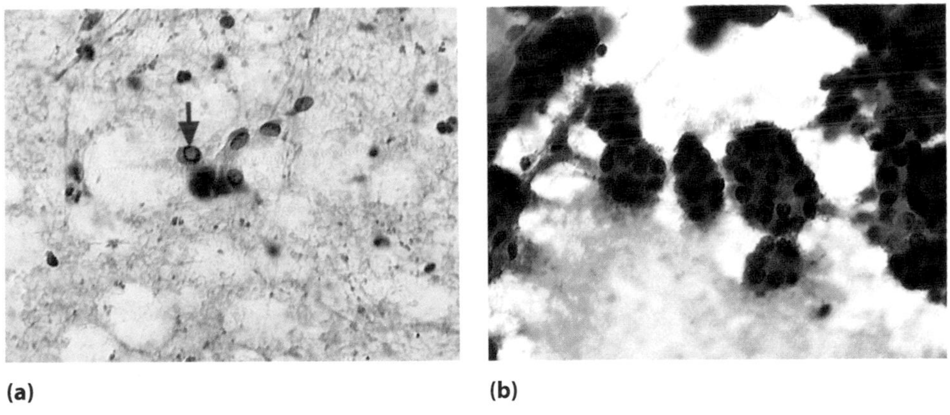

Figure 3.16. FNAC showing (a) papillary thyroid cancer and (b) follicular cancer.
(a) The malignant cells including the one at the tip of the arrow are very loosely arranged. (b) The follicles are composed of small clusters of cells. The colloid cannot be identified easily in this preparation. The nuclei are monotonous without obvious atypia.

3.8.3 Thyroid cancer

Thyroid cancer (see *Box 3.13*) comprises 0.5–1% of all malignancies in adults and accounts for 3% of childhood cancers. It is more common in females compared to males (a ratio of 2.5:1) with a peak incidence in the 4th and 5th decades of life. It is the most common endocrine malignancy and its incidence has shown a steady increase during the last 15–20 years. However, only about six deaths per million people per year can be attributed to thyroid cancer.

The development of thyroid cancer may be as a result of genetic or environmental factors (or a combination of the two). Thyroid cancer occurs more frequently in those with prior exposure to radiation (especially childhood exposure). Survivors of the atomic bombs in Hiroshima and Nagasaki had a higher incidence of thyroid cancer, as did survivors of the nuclear power plant disaster in Chernobyl. There is, however, absolutely no evidence for increased risk of cancer following radioactive ^{131}I therapy. In addition, several oncogenes have recently been identified in the etiology of thyroid cancer. Mutations of the *RET* proto-oncogene, which codes for a membrane-spanning protein with two intracellular protein kinase domains, have been particularly linked to papillary thyroid carcinoma and familial medullary thyroid carcinoma. Other oncogenes have also been identified and these include *TRK, BRAF, Ras, PAX8/PPAR*γ, and β-*Catenin*. In addition, tumor suppressor genes have also been identified and mutations in *p53* in particular have been linked with undifferentiated (anaplastic) tumors of the thyroid gland.

Box 3.13 | Classification of thyroid cancer

1. Thyroid cancers are classified according to their origin (based on the WHO classification):
   a. primary epithelial tumors
   b. benign follicular adenoma
   c. malignant
      i. follicular carcinoma
      ii. papillary carcinoma
      iii. medullary carcinoma (C-cell carcinoma)
      iv. undifferentiated (anaplastic) carcinoma
2. Non-epithelial tumors
3. Malignant lymphomas
4. Miscellaneous tumors
5. Secondary tumors
6. Unclassified tumors

Papillary carcinoma is the most common type, accounting for about 80% of cases followed by follicular carcinoma at 15%. Anaplastic carcinoma comprises about 5–10%.

Box 3.14 | Thyroid cancer

Follicular carcinoma. Follicular cancer (*Box figure 3.4*) is the second most common thyroid neoplasia, accounting for 15% of all thyroid cancers. It originates from the thyroid epithelium and exhibits follicular differentiation. Presentation is usually with a firm and solitary encapsulated nodule. It metastasizes via the hematogenous route. The 10 year survival rate is 75–85%.

Some tumors exhibit features similar to follicular cancer but they show the characteristic nuclei of papillary cancer. These tumors are called the 'follicular variant' of follicular carcinoma and behave like papillary carcinomas.

Papillary carcinoma. Papillary carcinoma accounts for 80% of all thyroid cancers. They are more common in women (with a ratio of 3:1). Their incidence peaks twice (in the 2nd to 3rd decade and again later in life). Histologically (*Box figure 3.5*) they consist of cuboidal cells with intranuclear cytoplasmic inclusions, nuclear grooves, prominent nuclei with marginated chromatin ('Orphan Annie' eyes), and round collections of calcium (psammoma bodies). Papillary carcinoma usually presents as a firm nodule (*Box figure 3.6*). Lesions tend to infiltrate and they rarely have a capsule. The carcinoma may adhere to adjacent structures and has no distinct margins. More than 50% are multifocal within the thyroid gland. Metastasis is via the lymphatic route. The 10 year survival after treatment is over 90%.

Medullary carcinoma. Medullary cancers arise from the parafollicular cells (also called C-cells) of the thyroid and thus are different from papillary or follicular cancers which arise from thyroid hormone producing cells. C-cells produce the hormone calcitonin which is involved in calcium homeostasis (see *Section 4.4.7*). Medullary cancers of the thyroid are the third most common, accounting for about 6–9% of all thyroid cancers. Survival rates are worse than those for follicular or papillary cancer but, if the lesion is confined to the thyroid, 10 year survival of 90% is not uncommon; rates fall to around 65% if there is spread to cervical nodes (which usually occurs early in the disease process), and around 25% if distant spread is present.

Medullary cancers may occur sporadically or in association with other endocrinopathies: pheochromocytomas with hyperparathyroidism (multiple endocrine neoplasia (MEN) type II-a) or with mucosal ganglioneuromas (MEN type II-b). There is also a familial form of isolated medullary thyroid cancer without other

Box 3.14 | continued

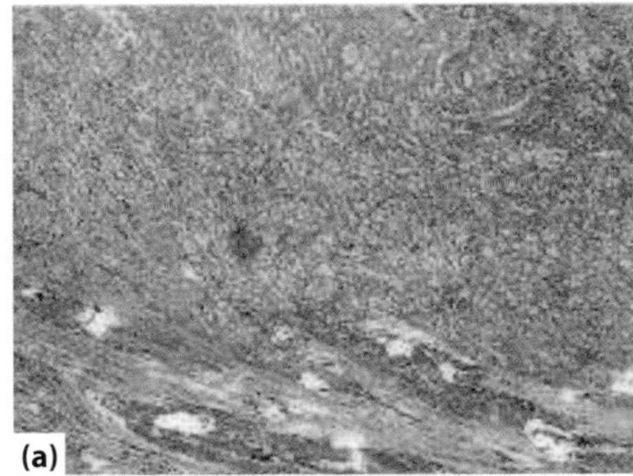

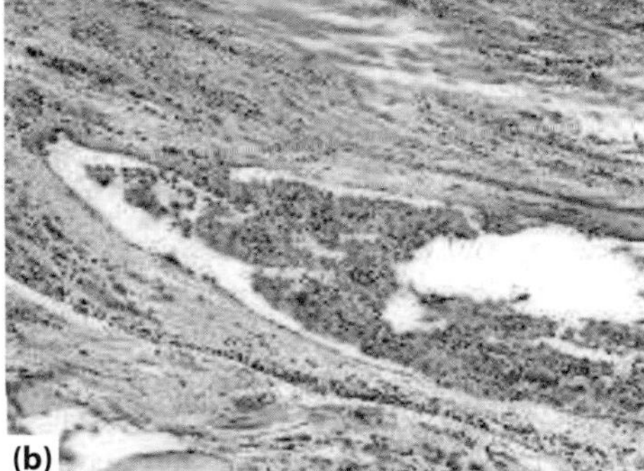

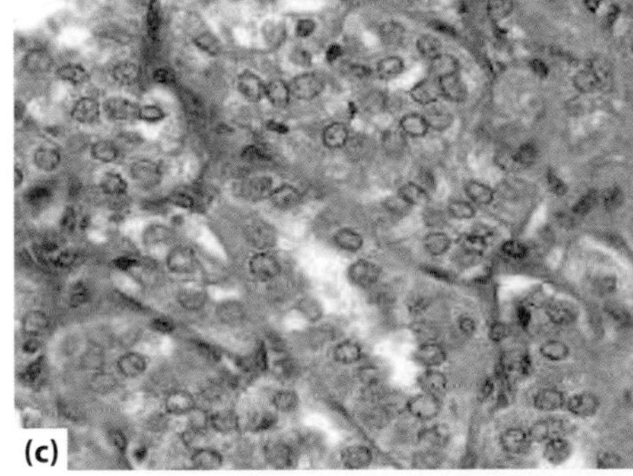

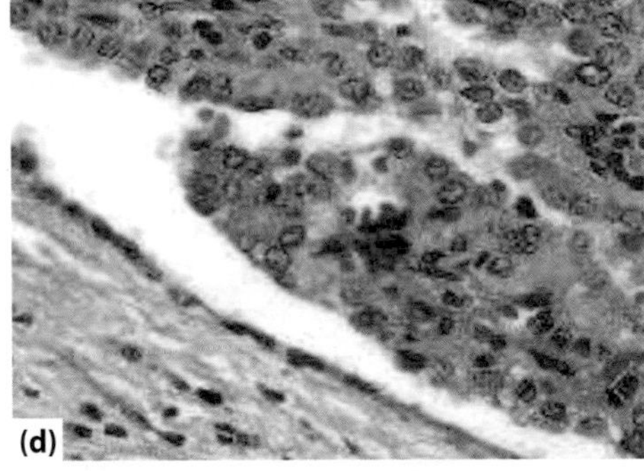

Box figure 3.4. Follicular carcinoma.
Hematoxylin and eosin staining showing characteristic features of follicular carcinoma (a,b). The thyroid nodule shows a thickened capsule and small thyroid follicles can be seen in the other nodule. Notice that the edges of the follicle are irregular and appear to infiltrate into the fibrous capsule. (c) Shows the morphology of the carcinoma with relatively small follicular architecture and somewhat enlarged cells. (d) A higher magnification showing tumor cells within the vascular space confirming a vascular invasion.

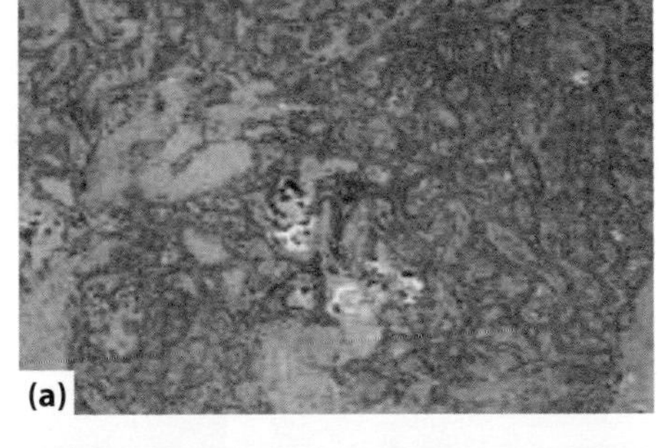

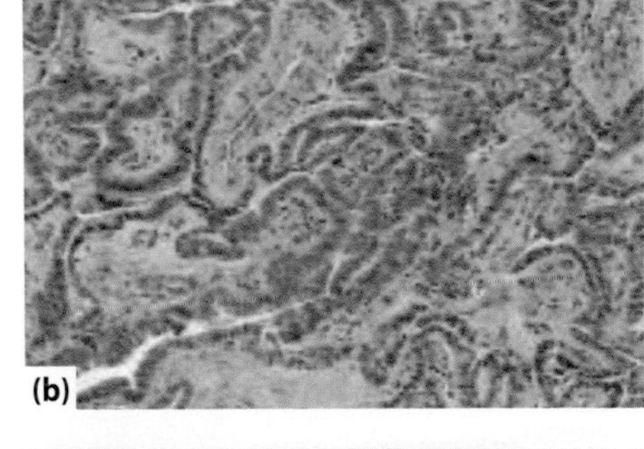

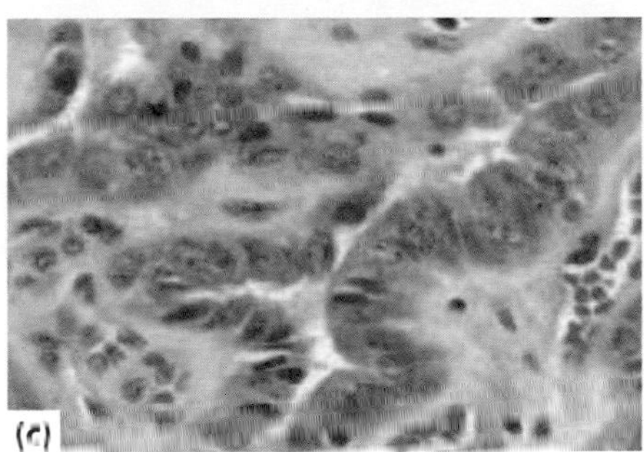

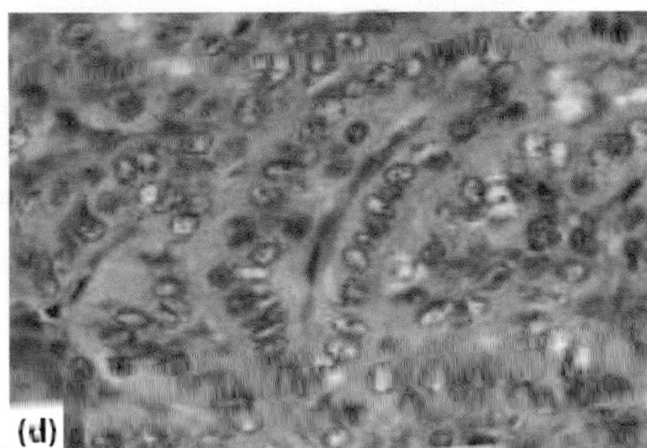

Box figure 3.5. Papillary carcinoma.
This is a classic papillary carcinoma with focal psammona bodies (laminated calcification), papillary structures and cells with nuclear grooving, cellular crowding, cellular enlargement, and nuclear inclusions.

features of MEN-II. Treatment is by surgical excision because the cancer arises from cells that do not have the necessary machinery for iodine organification so there is no place for radioactive iodine ablation.

Anaplastic cancer. Anaplastic cancers are poorly differentiated carcinomas, most commonly presenting in the elderly with a rapidly expanding mass involving the surrounding structures (*Box figure 3.7*). Local and distant metastases are usually present at the time of diagnosis. They account for more than half the mortality of thyroid cancers; the prognosis is poor, with median survival of 2–12 months.

Box 3.14 | continued

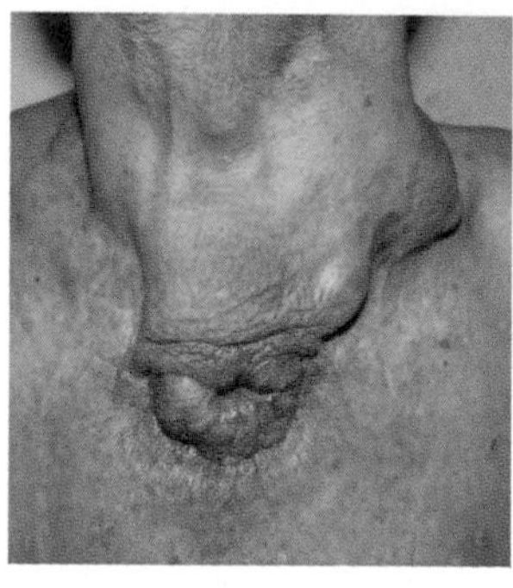

Box figure 3.6. Unusually aggressive papillary cancer. Carcinoma of thyroid with sinus extending downwards and opening in front of the manubrium. The metastatic nodal disease on the left side of the neck can also be appreciated. Reproduced from *J. Med. Case Rep.* (2008) **2**: 64 with permission.

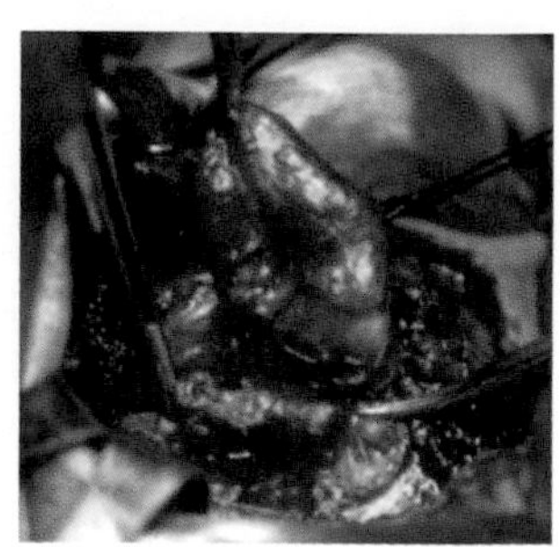

Box figure 3.7. Anaplastic cancer. Intraoperative picture showing mobilization of an aggressive anaplastic thyroid cancer.

Lymphoma. Thyroid lymphoma can arise *in situ* as a result of autoimmune thyroiditis or as part of a more extensive systemic lymphoma. They represent less than 5% of thyroid malignancies. Thyroid lymphomas occur most commonly in women and in patients aged 40 years and above. The majority of thyroid lymphomas are diffuse, large cell lymphomas, diffuse mixed small and large cell lymphomas, or diffuse small cleaved-cell lymphomas. Clinically they present with rapidly expanding neck masses which usually involve the surrounding structures. Patients may notice pain, hoarseness, dysphagia, and dyspnea or stridor. The prognosis of thyroid lymphomas is excellent with appropriate chemotherapy and external beam radiotherapy.

Hurthle cell cancer. According to the WHO and American Thyroid Association, Hurthle cell cancer is classified as a type of follicular carcinoma. It accounts for 5% of thyroid malignancies. It consists of sheets of large eosinophilic granular cells with much cytoplasm (*Box figure 3.8*). Less often it follows the follicular pattern. They are more aggressive than follicular carcinomas and spread via the lymphatic route. They tend to be multicentric. Following treatment, the 10 year survival is approximately 60–70%.

Clinical features and treatment

Typical signs of thyroid cancer include a painless nodule, hoarseness/loss of voice, a persistent cough (not associated with a cold) and difficulty in swallowing and breathing. Symptoms include a progressive increase in nodule size (this is more rapid in patients over 45 years), typically a single nodule which is fixed and solid with an irregular edge, and enlarged cervical lymph nodes.

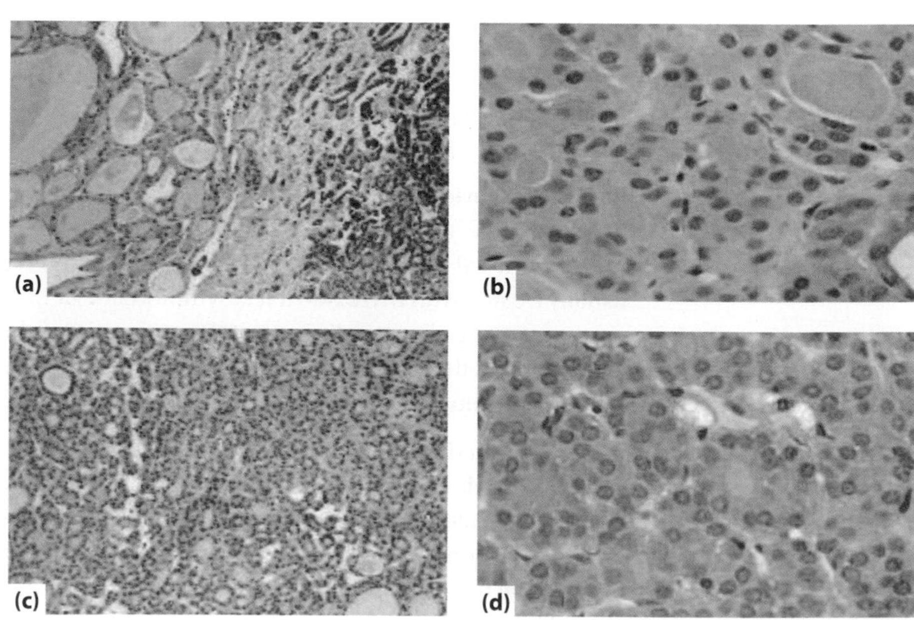

Box figure 3.8. Follicular adenoma with Hurthle cell change.
A follicular adenoma (a) and thyroid tissue with Hurthle cell change (b) in which each of the thyroid cells is enlarged with eosinophilic cytoplasm and variably sized nucleus. Some of these cells may show aneuploidy; however, this is not a definite diagnostic criteria for malignancy. The adenoma is composed of small thyroid follicles (c) with minimal cellular pleomorphism (d).

Box 3.14 | continued

The treatment of thyroid cancer is total thyroidectomy, with neck dissection to examine/remove affected lymph nodes. Surgery is followed by an ablative dose of ^{125}I. Follow-up is with regular clinical examination, measurement of thyroglobulin and whole-body ^{131}I scans. Thyroid hormone replacement is given at a level adequate to suppress TSH. Prior to follow-up scans the TSH needs to be elevated, either by stopping thyroid hormone replacement, or by administering recombinant TSH.

In poorly differentiated disease the basic treatment is the same, although the efficacy of ^{131}I therapy is more debatable. Advanced or inoperable cases have been managed with external beam radiation and chemotherapy. Newer (and somewhat experimental therapies) include:

- kinase inhibitors which affect multiple signaling pathways, such as motesanib diphosphate, vandetanib, sorafenib, axitinib, imatinib, gefitinib, and XL184
- antivascular agents which inhibit angiogenesis or disrupt existing tumor vasculature, such as thalidomide and combretastatin A4 phosphate
- intranuclear targeting for reversal of receptor or epigenetic abnormalities; these can have implications in re-establishing the capacity of tumor cells to take up radioiodine
- gene therapy targeting the suicide-inducing genes

3.9 Abnormal thyroid function test results

Usually, thyroid hormone test results are relatively easy to interpret (see *Table 3.3*):

- in primary hyperthyroidism, thyroid hormone levels are high but TSH levels are low or undetectable (see *Section 3.4.5, Case 3.1, Figure 3.11*)
- in primary hypothyroidism thyroid hormones are low with elevated TSH due to feedback (see *Section 3.6.2, Case 3.6, Figure 3.11*)
- in hyperthyroidism secondary to TSH excess, both thyroid hormone and TSH levels are high (see *Section 3.4.5, Figure 3.11*); this pattern is also seen in resistance to thyroid hormone (see *Section 3.6.4, Box 3.10, Case 3.7*).
- in central hypothyroidism, both thyroid hormone and TSH levels are low (see *Section 3.6.3*)

Rather less obvious situations occur when there is 'compensation.' In compensated (or 'borderline' or 'subclinical') hypothyroidism, thyroid hormone levels remain normal, but TSH levels are high due to increased pituitary hormone drive. This is usually treated with thyroxine if it is symptomatic or if the anti-TPO titer is high; this measurement gives an indication of the propensity to develop overt hypothyroidism with time and there is little point in delaying the almost inevitable need to introduce thyroid hormone replacement.

In compensated or subclinical hyperthyroidism, the TSH level is low and thyroid hormone levels are normal. The significance of this is less well understood than with compensated hypothyroidism. This pattern of TFT results may be seen during treatment of hyperthyroidism with thionamides, or in the few months after radioiodine treatment, but may also arise *de novo*. The latter situation may be caused by a developing autonomous nodule and, if found, this could be treated with targeted low dose radioiodine treatment. Compensated hyperthyroidism in

Table 3.3. **Patterns of thyroid function tests**

Serum TSH	Serum fT_4	Serum fT_3	Diagnosis
Normal	Normal	Normal	Euthyroid
Normal or high	High or (rarely) normal	High or (rarely) normal	Resistance to thyroid hormone TSHoma Anti-iodothyronine antibodies, anti-TSH antibodies Familial dysalbuminemic hyperthyroxinemia* Acute psychiatric disease (really rare)
Normal or low	Low	Low or low-normal	Central hypothyroidism (pituitary failure or rarely TRH deficiency)
High	Low	Low	Primary hypothyroidism
High	Normal	Normal	Compensated hypothyroidism Heterophile antibodies (interfering with hormone assays) Drugs – amiodarone, cholestyramine, iron TSH resistance
Low	High	High	Primary hyperthyroidism
Low	Low or normal	Low or normal	Non-thyroidal illness During treatment of hyperthyroidism or soon after radioiodine Congenital TSH deficiency
Low	Normal	Normal	Compensated hyperthyroidism Rarely: thyroxine treatment or ingestion Non-thyroidal illness Drugs (e.g. steroids/dopamine)

*Familial dysalbuminemic hyperthyroxinemia (FDH) is a genetic disorder, most often occurring in patients of Hispanic background, in whom it occurs in perhaps 0.2% of the population. It is characterized by production of mutant albumin molecules that have a low affinity but high capacity for T_4, but not T_3. Affected patients have high serum total T_4 concentrations but are euthyroid and usually have normal serum TSH concentrations.

the elderly may be treated with thionamide in an attempt to normalize the TSH and, theoretically at least, reduce the risks of osteopenia and atrial dysrhythmia, which are associated with suppressed TSH.

Other more obscure examples of abnormal thyroid function tests may be due to:

- drugs that alter thyroid hormone metabolism or affect the assays used to measure thyroid hormones (see *Table 3.4*)
- endogenous antibodies or abnormalities of thyroid binding proteins which can affect assays
- poor compliance with treatment which can give a unusual picture dependent on whether the treatment is designed to reduce (thionamide) or increase (thyroxine) thyroid hormone levels

CASE 3.8

148 157

- Woman of 50 years with 3 week history of increasingly hoarse voice
- Symptoms and examination showed increasing swelling in her neck with single nodule
- ? Thyroid malignancy – TFTs ordered, along with ultrasound scan, FNAC and nuclear medicine scan
- TFT results normal; ultrasound scan showed single solid lump confirmed as a cold nodule by nuclear medicine scan; FNAC revealed a Thy4 lesion suspicious of papillary cancer
- Treatment included a total thyroidectomy and dissection of lymph nodes, followed by ^{131}I ablation

The patient showed hoarseness and loss of voice and a single hard nodule on the left side of her neck and enlarged lymph nodes. Her blood tests showed normal levels of free thyroid hormones and TSH and the ultrasound scan confirmed a single solid lump in the thyroid gland with a diameter of 1.5 cm. The nuclear medicine scan confirmed a cold nodule, and a biopsy (FNAC) revealed a Thy4 lesion (in this case the histo-cytopathology was highly suspicious of papillary cancer). After discussion in a multidisciplinary meeting (attended by endocrinologists, thyroid surgeons, histopathologists and nuclear medicine physicians) her treatment followed a typical pathway and included total thyroidectomy and dissection of the lymph nodes followed by radioiodine (^{131}I) ablation to eliminate disease remnants.

She was given thyroxine replacement therapy in a dose adequate to suppress the TSH (remaining TSH can stimulate re-growth in any remnant disease) and kept under regular review with clinical examinations, measurements of TFTs and thyroglobulin (a useful post-operative tumor marker) and annual whole body ^{131}I scans.

Table 3.4. **Drugs affecting thyroid hormone tests or thyroid function**

Drugs that cause hyperthyroidism	
Stimulation of TH release or synthesis	Amiodarone, iodine
Effects on immune regulation	Inteferon-α, interleukin-2
Drugs that cause hypothyroidism	
Inhibition of thyroid hormone synthesis or release	Thionamides, lithium, perchlorate, thalidomide Iodine-containing drugs: amiodarone, radiographic agents, potassium iodide, kelp, cough medicines, topical antiseptics
Decreased absorption of T_4	Cholestyramine, omeprazole, calcium carbonate, sucralfate, iron sulfate, raloxifene
Suppression of TSH	Dopamine
Thyroiditis	Suntinib
Decreased conversion of fT_4 to fT_3	Glucocorticoids, propranolol, amiodarone, iodinated radiographic contrast agents
Drugs causing abnormal thyroid function tests (without affecting thyroid function)	
Lowering of TH binding proteins (TBG)	Androgens, danazol, nicotinic acid
Increasing TBG	Estrogen, SERMS (tamoxifen, raloxifene), opiates (heroin, methadone), clofibrate
Increasing clearance of T_4	Phenytoin, rifampicin, phenobarbitone, carbemazepine
Decreasing binding of T_4 to TBG	Salicylates, furosemide, heparin, NSAIDs

Key: TH = thyroid hormones (fT_4 and fT_3).

Thyroid function tests taken in seriously ill patients are very difficult to interpret. This has variously been termed 'sick euthyroid syndrome' or 'non-thyroidal illness' (NTI). Most ill patients will have low thyroid hormone levels and low TSH levels. Outside of severe illness such results may suggest secondary or central (hypothalamic-pituitary) hypothyroidism and it is possible that this is happening, at least transiently, in severe illness. In the light of severe illness with an associated hyper-catabolic state it seems entirely sensible to turn off hormones that promote increases in metabolic rate (i.e. reduce free T_3 levels), and to reduce metabolism of free T_4 to its more biologically active form (free T_3) by reducing 5′-monodeiodinase activity or switching to production of reverse T_3. Also, of course, severely ill patients are often on many drugs which may affect thyroid hormone status (*Table 3.3*). In summary, it is probably best not to measure TFTs in the seriously ill patient unless there is a good chance that thyroid dysfunction (e.g. thyroid storm or severe hypothyroidism) is contributing to the pathology.

3.10 Further reading

Bahn RS (2010) Graves' ophthalmopathy. *N. Engl. J. Med.* **362:** 726–738.

Beck-Peccoz P, Persani L, Calebiro D, Bonomi M, Mannavola D, and Campi I (2006) Syndromes of hormone resistance in the hypothalamic-pituitary-thyroid axis. *Best Pract. Res. Clin. Endocrinol. Metab.* **20:** 529–546.

Bizhanova A and Kopp P (2009) Minireview: The sodium-iodide symporter NIS and pendrin in iodide homeostasis of the thyroid. *Endocrinology,* **150:** 1084–1090.

Brent GA (2008) Graves' disease. *N. Engl. J. Med.* **358:** 2594–2605.

Chiamolera MI and Wondisford FE (2009) Minireview: Thyrotropin-releasing hormone and the thyroid hormone feedback mechanism. *Endocrinology,* **150:** 1091–1096.

Gärtner R (2009) Thyroid disease in pregnancy. *Curr. Opin. Obstet. Gynecol.* **21:** 501–507.

Kharlip J and Cooper DS (2009) Recent developments in hyperthyroidism. *Lancet,* **373:** 1930–1932.

Oetting A (2007) New insights into thyroid hormone action. *Clin. Endocrin. Metab.* **2:** 193–208.

Tonacchera M, Pinchera A, and Vitti P (2009) Assessment of nodular goitre. *Best Pract. Res. Clin. Endocrinol. Metab.* **24:** 51–61.

Warner MH and Beckett GJ (2009) Mechanisms behind the non-thyroidal illness syndrome: an update. *J. Endocrinol.* **205:** 1–13.

Yen PM, Shinichiro A, Feng X, Liu Y, Maruvada P, and Xia X (2006) Thyroid hormone action at the cellular, genomic and target gene levels. *Mol. Cell. Endocrinology,* **246:** 121–127.

3.11 Self-assessment questions

(1) Goiter formation can be stimulated by which one of the following?
- (a) Hypopituitarism
- (b) Methimazole
- (c) Compression of the pituitary stalk
- (d) Hyperparathyroidism
- (e) Primary hypothyroidism

(2) Concerning thyroid hormone synthesis, which one of the following statements is correct?
   (a) Iodide diffuses into the follicular cells
   (b) Thyroid perioxidase (TPO) stimulates the uptake of iodine into the colloid of follicles
   (c) Thionamides stimulate the organification of tyrosine residues of thyroglobulin
   (d) TPO is activated by hydrogen peroxide
   (e) Triiodotyrosine is the predominant hormone stored in the colloid of thyroid follicles

(3) Which one of the following statements concerning Graves disease is true?
   (a) It stimulates TSH secretion
   (b) It causes heat intolerance
   (c) It causes loss of peripheral vision
   (d) It inhibits somatostatin secretion
   (e) It results from autoimmune antibodies stimulating the TRH receptor

(4) In the treatment of Graves disease which one of the following statements is true?
   (a) The relapse rate following a course of medical treatment is less than 10%
   (b) Carbimazole is contraindicated in pregnancy
   (c) Radioiodine is contraindicated in pregnancy
   (d) There is a 50% risk of developing thyroid cancer after radioiodine treatment
   (e) There is less than 5% risk of becoming hypothyroid after radioiodine treatment

(5) Concerning thyroid eye disease (thyroid-associated ophthalmopathy), which one of the following statements is true?
   (a) Women are affected more seriously than men
   (b) Radioiodine relieves many of the symptoms
   (c) High dose steroids may be used in the treatment
   (d) Symptoms may be relieved by keeping the eyes dry
   (e) There is a strong genetic basis

(6) In thyroid carcinoma which one of the following statements is incorrect?
   (a) Thyrotoxicosis is rarely seen
   (b) Different types of cancers tend to affect different age groups
   (c) Anaplastic carcinoma is the commonest type
   (d) Treatment is usually by surgery and radioiodine ablation
   (e) Papillary cancer is always part of a familial syndrome

(7) Which one of the following endocrine disorders is most likely to be associated with increased TSH secretion?
   (a) Hashimoto disease
   (b) Thyroiditis
   (c) Graves disease
   (d) A thyroid 'hot' nodule
   (e) Hypopituitarism

(8) Thyroid function tests were performed on a 53 year old woman and the following results were obtained:
   Serum TSH 6.0 mU/L (NR 0.4–4.2)
   Serum free T_4 45 pmol/L (NR 10–20)
   Serum free T_3 14 pmol/L (NR 2.5–6.2)
   Which one of the following conditions is most likely to be associated with these results?
   (a) Primary hyperthyroidism
   (b) A thyroid hot nodule
   (c) Hashimoto disease
   (d) TSH-secreting adenoma
   (e) Thyroid medullary cell carcinoma

(9) A 32 year old woman arrived at outpatients with her 5 month old baby because she had noted increased irritability, weight loss, and palpitations. On examination she had a moderate diffuse goiter with an audible bruit and a resting tachycardia of 100 bpm. Her eyes were prominent and puffy. Thyroid function tests showed her serum concentration of free T_4 was 56 pmol/L (NR 10–20) and her TSH was 0.1 mU/L (NR 2.5–6.2).

(a) What is the most likely diagnosis of this case? Explain the results of the biochemical investigations.

(b) Why did she have weight loss and tachycardia and what is the cause of her diffuse goiter and audible bruit?

(c) Outline the treatment of thyroid eye disease according to its severity.

(10) A 41 year old woman presented to the endocrine clinic with symptoms of moderate anxiety, tremor, and palpitations. Thyroid function tests carried out in primary care revealed thyrotoxicosis with the following results:

Free T_3 of 9 pmol/L (NR 2.5–6.2)
Free T_4 of 25 pmol/L (NR 10–20)
Suppressed TSH of <0.01 mIU/L (NR 0.4–4.2)

Two weeks previously she had been unwell with flu-like symptoms and a sore throat which had been treated with antibiotics. Her neck had been acutely painful at this time. There was no family history of thyroid or other endocrine disease. TSH-receptor and anti-TPO antibodies were negative. On examinatuion she was tachycardic with a smooth firm goiter, no thyroid bruit, and no eye signs.

(a) What is the most likely diagnosis?

(b) What confirmatory test(s) would be useful?

(c) What is the most appropriate management?

CHAPTER 04 Endocrine control of calcium and phosphate:

the skeleton, parathyroid glands, and vitamin D

After working through this chapter you should be able to:

- Describe the functions and turnover of calcium and phosphate
- Understand the process of bone remodeling and the endocrine control of bone formation and bone resorption
- Identify the hormones secreted from bone, parathyroid glands, and kidney and describe their integrated functions
- Know the major causes of hyper- and hypocalcemia
- Describe the etiology of primary, secondary, and tertiary hyperparathyroidism, their symptoms and their treatment
- Know the causes of vitamin D deficiency and describe the symptoms and its treatment
- Understand the basics of metabolic bone disease including osteomalacia, osteoporosis, and Paget disease of bone

4.1 Introduction

The control of calcium and phosphate are intimately connected, with an inverse relationship between calcium and phosphate levels in the circulation. The calcium ion (Ca^{2+}) has a major function in many physiological processes including:

- bone growth and remodeling (mineralization)
- muscle contraction
- stabilization of membrane potentials
- secretion, e.g. of hormones and neurotransmitters from secretory granules
- as an enzyme co-factor, e.g. in blood coagulation
- as a second messenger in signaling pathways, e.g. activation of calmodulin

Similarly phosphate, which exists as either HPO_4^{2-} or $H_2PO_4^-$ (collectively referred to as P_i) has multiple functions including:

- formation of high energy compounds such as ATP and creatinine phosphate
- formation of active signaling molecules such as cAMP, inositol triphosphate and phosphorylated kinases
- as an important intracellular anion
- as a major component of DNA/RNA and phospholipid membranes
- in bone mineralization (formation of hydroxyapatite crystals)

In the adult human body there is about 1–2 kg of calcium, of which 99% resides in the skeleton and teeth in the form of hydroxyapatite crystals. Most of the intracellular calcium is sequestered in the endoplasmic reticulum, mitochondria, or sarcoplasmic reticulum (skeletal muscle), such that the intracellular concentration of free Ca^{2+} is only approximately 0.1 µmol/L, which is far less than the concentration in extracellular fluid. Extracellular calcium represents 0.99% of the total calcium, of which 45% exists in the free ionized form and 55% bound to plasma proteins and anions (*Figure 4.1*). Ionized calcium is closely regulated and ranges from 1.15 to 1.27 mmol/L and the total calcium, including the bound forms, ranges from 2.2 to 2.58 mmol/L. The levels of free (ionized) calcium are regulated by parathyroid hormone (PTH), which is secreted by the parathyroid glands and vitamin D, the active form of which is released by the kidneys. Hypercalcemia can lead to diffuse precipitation of calcium and phosphate in tissues (e.g. renal stones and bone cysts), gastrointestinal disturbances, depression, lethargy, anorexia, and increased contractility of the heart and shortened ventricle systole. Clinical signs of hypocalcemia include increased neuromuscular excitability causing muscle spasms, tetany, and cardiac dysfunction, which all reflect calcium's ability to stabilize membrane potentials.

Most of the body's phosphate is also in the skeleton (95%), with a considerable proportion of the remaining extraskeletal phosphorus being in combination with proteins, lipids, sugars, nucleic acids, and other organic compounds. Less than 0.03% exists in the circulation, of which approximately 50% is in the free form and 50% bound to plasma proteins (<10%), Ca^{2+}, Na^+, and Mg^{2+} (*Figure 4.2*). The concentration of total serum phosphate ranges from 0.8 to 1.5 mmol/L and the kidneys play an important part in maintaining phosphate homeostasis via type I and type II

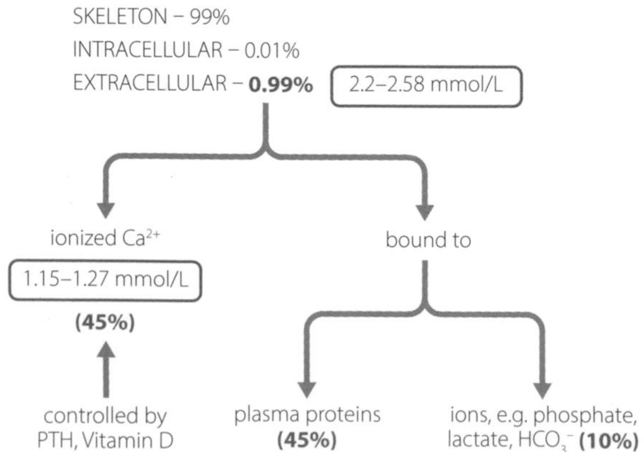

Figure 4.1. Distribution of calcium in the body.

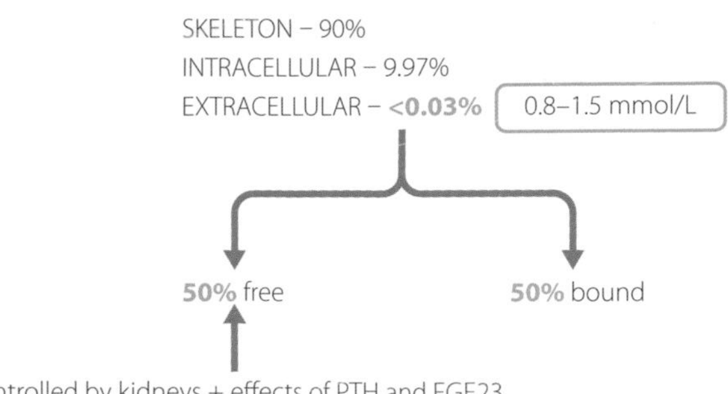

Figure 4.2. Distribution of phosphate in the body.

sodium–phosphate co-transporters. Renal phosphate reabsorption/excretion is tightly controlled by PTH and a newly recognized hormone secreted by the skeleton, fibroblast growth factor 23 (FGF23).

4. 2 Turnover of calcium and phosphate

The recommended daily intake for calcium is 1000 mg although pregnancy, lactation, and growth increase requirements. The average daily intake of P_i is between 800 and 1500 mg which well exceeds homeostatic requirements. The daily turnover of Ca^{2+} and P_i is shown in *Figure 4.3*, the net balance being determined by

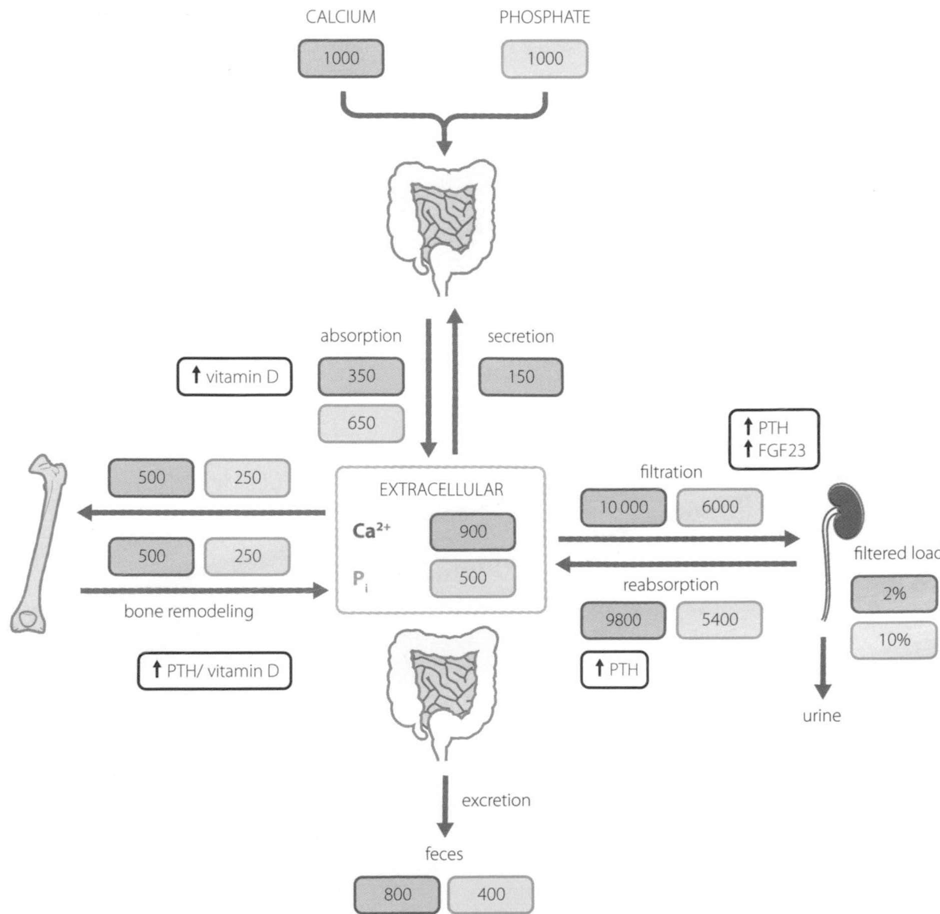

Figure 4.3. Daily turnover of calcium and phosphate. Daily turnover of calcium and phosphate in humans with a dietary intake of 1000 mg/day. All numbers represent mg/day with those for calcium in orange and for phosphate in green. Vitamin D increases the absorption of calcium from the gut, parathyroid hormone (PTH) and vitamin D increase the release of calcium and phosphate from bone, PTH increases calcium <u>re</u>absorption and phosphate <u>ex</u>cretion by the kidneys, whilst fibroblast growth factor (FGF23) increases phosphate excretion.

their absorption in the gut, their retention or excretion by the kidneys, their loss in feces and the rate of bone metabolism. These processes are tightly regulated by PTH, vitamin D, and FGF23 in response to changes in circulating concentrations of ionized Ca^{2+} and P_i. The bound and ionized forms of Ca^{2+} are in equilibrium, so factors that affect Ca^{2+} binding affect ionized Ca^{2+} concentrations.

Normally total serum Ca^{2+} and P_i concentrations are measured in the clinic, although ionized Ca^{2+} can also be measured. Various factors have been used to adjust serum Ca^{2+} measurements when there are changes in serum albumin concentrations or pH because these parameters can change levels of free calcium. For example, when the serum albumin level is low, a higher percentage of total serum calcium will be free and metabolically active. Therefore, even though the total serum calcium may be low the patient may not be metabolically hypocalcemic. Because the ionized serum calcium level is a direct measure of the amount of metabolically active serum calcium, no other calculation is required when it is available. However, if only total serum calcium measurements are available, a correction can be made for the prevailing serum albumin level. pH can also change the ratio of bound to free calcium with acidosis increasing free ionized calcium and alkalosis reducing it.

4.3 Anatomy and embryology of the parathyroid glands

4.3.1 Anatomy of the parathyroid glands

There are usually four parathyroid glands sitting on the posterior aspect of the thyroid gland on the superior and inferior poles of each lobe, though numbers can vary from 2 to 6 *(Figure 4.4)*. Of these supernumerary glands, most are in close

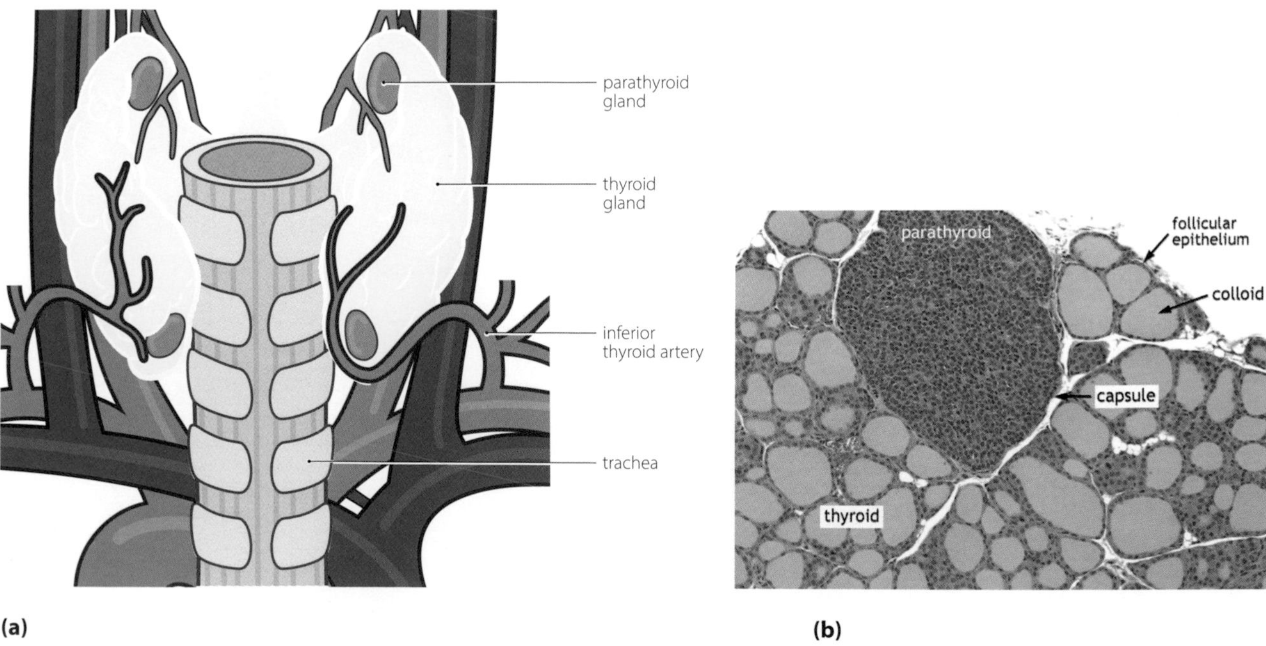

Figure 4.4. Gross anatomy and histology of the parathyroid glands.
(a) Posterior view of the trachea with two small paired parathyroid glands embedded in the connective tissue of the thyroid gland. Blood to all four glands is supplied by the inferior thyroid artery.
(b) Histology of the parathyroid gland showing it in relation to the thyroid gland. Reproduced from the Deltabase Histology Atlas with permission from Deltagen Inc.

relationship with the thyroid gland although about 10% of them, invariably the inferior glands, are aberrant.

The parathyroid glands are yellowish-brown, about the size of a split pea and weigh 30–50 mg. They comprise two types of densely packed cells:

- chief cells which secrete PTH
- oxyphil cells (less numerous) which appear at puberty but have no known physiological function

Both the superior and inferior glands are supplied by the inferior thyroid artery and if a surgeon wants to leave functional parathyroid tissue after thyroidectomy this blood supply must be preserved *(Figure 4.4)*.

4.3.2 Embryology of the parathyroid glands

The superior and inferior parathyroid glands originate from the fourth and third pharyngeal pouches respectively and are vertically transposed during embryogenesis (see *Figure 3.2*). They differentiate between 5 and 6 weeks and lose their connection to the pharynx around gestational week 7. They descend in association with the thyroid gland and thymus.

4.4 Basic physiology

CASE 4.1 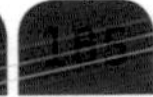 182 190

- Woman of 62 years with 4 month history of polyuria and polydipsia
- Poor appetite and weight loss of 6 kg
- Normal fasting blood sugar, slightly raised creatinine and raised calcium
- ? Hypercalcemia

A 62 year old woman was referred by her family doctor with a 4 month history of polyuria and polydipsia associated with fatigue, mental 'fogginess', and constipation. Her appetite had been poor for several months and this was associated with a weight loss of about 6 kg. On close questioning she admitted to a long history of non-specific symptoms, including general malaise and aches and pains. She had no significant past medical history and denied any family history of note.

Initial investigations had revealed:

- fasting blood sugar: 4.5 mmol/L (NR 3.5–6.1)
- creatinine: 110 μmol/L (NR 53–106)
- total calcium: 3.4 mmol/L (NR 2.2–2.58)

Other blood tests (including albumin, globulins, full blood count, and film) were all normal.

The initial results and symptoms are typical of hypercalcemia.

In this section we will look at:

- the actions of PTH on bone and the kidney
- the synthesis and control of PTH secretion
- PTH-related peptide
- the major actions of vitamin D on the gut and bone
- the synthesis of vitamin D and its control
- the role of fibroblast growth factor in regulating phosphate homeostasis
- the synthesis and actions of calcitonin

4.4.1 Actions of parathyroid hormone

PTH is an 84 amino acid protein hormone that increases calcium reabsorption in the kidney and stimulates calcium and phosphate release from mineralized bone (bone resorption). Its basic action is to raise blood calcium levels and patients with persistently elevated levels of PTH (hyperparathyroidism) will have hypercalcemia, such as in Case 4.1.

There are two GPCRs for PTH, designated PTH-1 receptor (PTHR1) and PTHR2. PTH and its sister hormone PTH-related peptide (see *Section 4.4.7* and *Figure 4.12*) act on PTHR1 but only PTH acts on PTHR2. Stimulation of PTHR1 activates the stimulatory GPCR, Gs, which activates adenylate cyclase (AC)/cAMP pathway as well as another stimulatory GPCR, Gq, which activates phospholipase (PLC) and the inositol signaling pathway, although it has been difficult to attribute these signaling pathways to different functions of PTH.

In the kidney

PTH affects the tubular reabsorption of Ca^{2+}, P_i, and bicarbonate. The bulk of Ca^{2+} and Na^+ is reabsorbed in the proximal tubule, but the fine tuning occurs in the distal tubule where PTH markedly increases the reabsorption of Ca^{2+} (*Figure 4.5*). At the level of the proximal tubules, PTH stimulates internalization of the sodium-phosphate co-transporters which inhibits the reabsorption of P_i (*Figure 4.6*). The result is phosphate wasting and hypophosphatemia. Also in the proximal tubule the action of PTH leads to bicarbonate wasting by inhibiting the Na^+/H^+ exchanger and

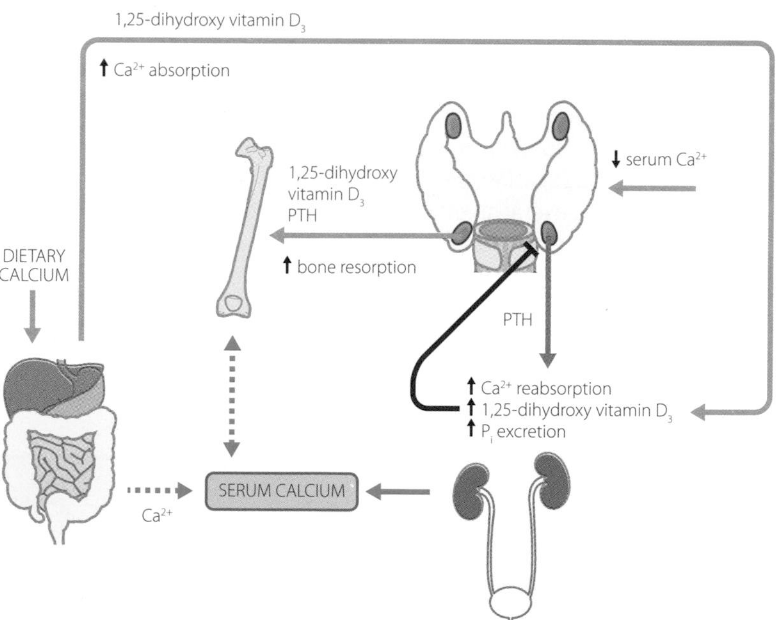

Figure 4.5. Control of serum calcium concentration by vitamin D (1,25-dihydroxyvitamin D) and parathyroid hormone.
1,25-dihydroxyvitamin D increases Ca^{2+} reabsorption from the gut. A drop in serum calcium stimulates PTH secretion which, together with 1,25-dihydroxyvitamin D, increases bone resorption and the release of Ca^{2+} and phosphate (P_i) from bone. PTH also increases Ca^{2+} reabsorption in the kidney, increases phosphate excretion, increases the activity of 1α-hydroxylase which in turn increases the synthesis of active vitamin D by the kidney. The increased production of 1,25-dihydroxyvitamin D can inhibit the synthesis and secretion of PTH.

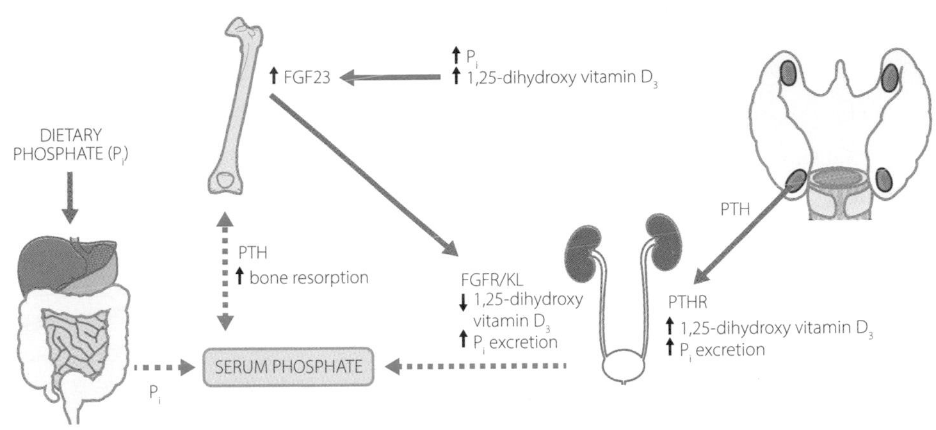

Figure 4.6. Control of serum phosphate concentration by FGF23, PTH, and vitamin D (1,25-dihydroxyvitamin D).

The kidney regulates serum phosphate concentrations via type I and type II sodium–phosphate co-transporters. In addition, serum phosphate levels are controlled by PTH and FGF23. A rise in serum P_i stimulates bone to release FGF23 and, with the synergistic action of PTH, increases P_i excretion in the kidney. 1,25-dihydroxyvitamin D also increases FGF23 secretion and, through a feedback loop, FGF23 inhibits the synthesis of 1,25-dihydroxyvitamin D.

Na^+/K^+-ATPase activity, and it increases Cl^- efflux from the epithelial cells. Overall, prolonged elevations of PTH can lead to mild hyperchloremic metabolic acidosis.

In bone

Continuous exposure to PTH, as occurs in hyperparathyroidism (see Case 4.1), induces bone resorption by increasing the number and activity of osteoclasts. Osteoclasts do not have PTH receptors and activation of bone resorption occurs indirectly through the osteoblasts. PTH stimulates the expression of RANK ligand

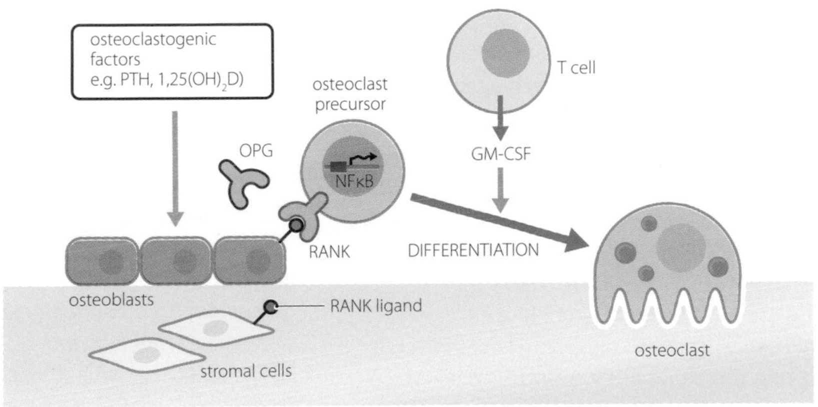

Figure 4.7. Induction of osteoclast differentiation by RANK ligand.

PTH, PTHrP, and 1,25-dihydroxyvitamin D act on marrow stromal cells and osteoblasts to induce RANK ligand. RANK ligand binds to RANK (receptor of activation of nuclear factor kappa B ligand, NFκB) on osteoclast precursors. This, in conjunction with GM-CSF, activates the transcription factor NFκB in osteoclast precursors, which induces their differentiation into mature osteoclasts. A decoy receptor, osteoprotogenin (OPG), can block RANK ligand binding to RANK and inhibit the formation of mature osteocytes.

Box 4.1 | Bone and its remodeling

The four major functions of bone are:

- rigid support of limbs and body cavities
- locomotion
- to act as a large reservoir of ions such as calcium, phosphorus, magnesium, and sodium that are critical to life and can be mobilized when the external environment fails to provide them
- as an endocrine organ (see *Figure 8.8*).

There are two types of bone:

- cortical bone composed of densely packed layers of mineralized collagen; this is the major constituent of long bones
- trabecular or cancellous bone, which has a spongy appearance and constitutes the major portion of the axial skeleton.

Two-thirds of the weight of bone is mainly in the form of hydroxyapatite crystals [$Ca_{10}(PO_4)_6(OH)_2$]. The other third is due to collagen type I and other non-collagenous proteins such as proteoglycans, glycosylated proteins, and alkaline phosphatase – generally referred to as osteoid or bone matrix. Bone is also a source of growth factors and hormones.

Bone is a dynamic tissue and continually undergoes remodeling which underpins the development and maintenance of the skeletal system. The tightly coordinated events of remodeling require the integrated activity of different bone cells to ensure that bone resorption (removal) and formation occur sequentially.

Cells involved in bone remodeling

Osteoclasts: these comprise 1–2% of bone cells. They are multinucleated cells derived from the monocyte–macrophage lineage and are responsible for resorbing bone. They express acid phosphatase and the calcitonin receptor and their survival/function is dependent on colony stimulating factor (CSF-1, also known as macrophage colony stimulating factor, MCSF-1) and RANK ligand (see *Figure 4.7*).

Osteoblasts: these comprise 5% of bone cells. They are derived from pluripotent mesenchymal stem cells that have the potential to differentiate into adipocytes, myocytes, chondrocytes and osteoblasts under the direction of different transcription factors. Osteoblasts are responsible for bone formation but when they become engulfed by osteoid during this process they are destined to become osteocytes. In general, increased mechanical stress stimulates local osteoblastic bone formation, whereas reduced loading (e.g. immobility) or microdamage results in osteoclastic bone resorption. They also express receptors for PTH and vitamin D.

Osteocytes: these comprise 90-95% of all adult bone cells. They derive from osteoblasts following mineralization of bone matrix (osteoid). These cells form a network throughout mineralized bone forming long dendrite-like processes that extend through canaliculi (tunnels) within the mineralized matrix. This enables them to interact with other osteocytes within the mineralized bone via gap junctions and also to interact with osteoblasts on the bone surfaces. They can sense mechanical load or stress as well as localized damage within bones and, through the release of cytokines and chemotactic signals, they can stimulate local bone remodeling.

Bone remodeling

Bone remodeling (see *Box figure 4.1*) occurs over several weeks and involves osteoblasts and osteoclasts which form a temporary anatomical structure known as a basic multicellular unit (BMU). Essentially this comprises a leading front of bone-resorbing osteoclasts which will break down bone, followed by a tail of osteoblasts which will deposit new bone osteoid followed by hydroxyapatite crystals (mineralization). It is a highly spatial and temporal arrangement of cells within the BMU and ensures coordination of the sequential process of bone remodeling: activation, resorption, reversal, formation, and termination.

Activation: prior to activation the bone surface is covered with bone lining cells including pre-osteoblasts and osteomacs (tissue macrophages). B cells within the bone marrow secrete osteoprotogerin (OPG) which inhibits the differentiation of osteoclasts (see *Figure 4.7*). In response to PTH, or signals from osteocytes that detect mechanical stress or damage to the bone matrix, osteoclast precursors are recruited to the remodeling site.

Resorption: PTH acts on osteoblasts and stimulates the production of the chemokine, monocyte chemoattractant protein (MCP-1) which attracts osteoclast precursors (hematopoietic stem cells or stromal cells). It also stimulates the production of RANK ligand and CSF-1 whilst inhibiting the production of OPG (see *Figure 4.7*). CSF-1 and RANK-L work in concert to promote proliferation and differentiation of osteoclast precursors to mature osteoclasts.

Reversal: mononuclear cells remove any collagen debris left in the lacunae of demineralized bone and prepare the surface for osteoblast-mediated bone formation.

Box 4.1 | continued

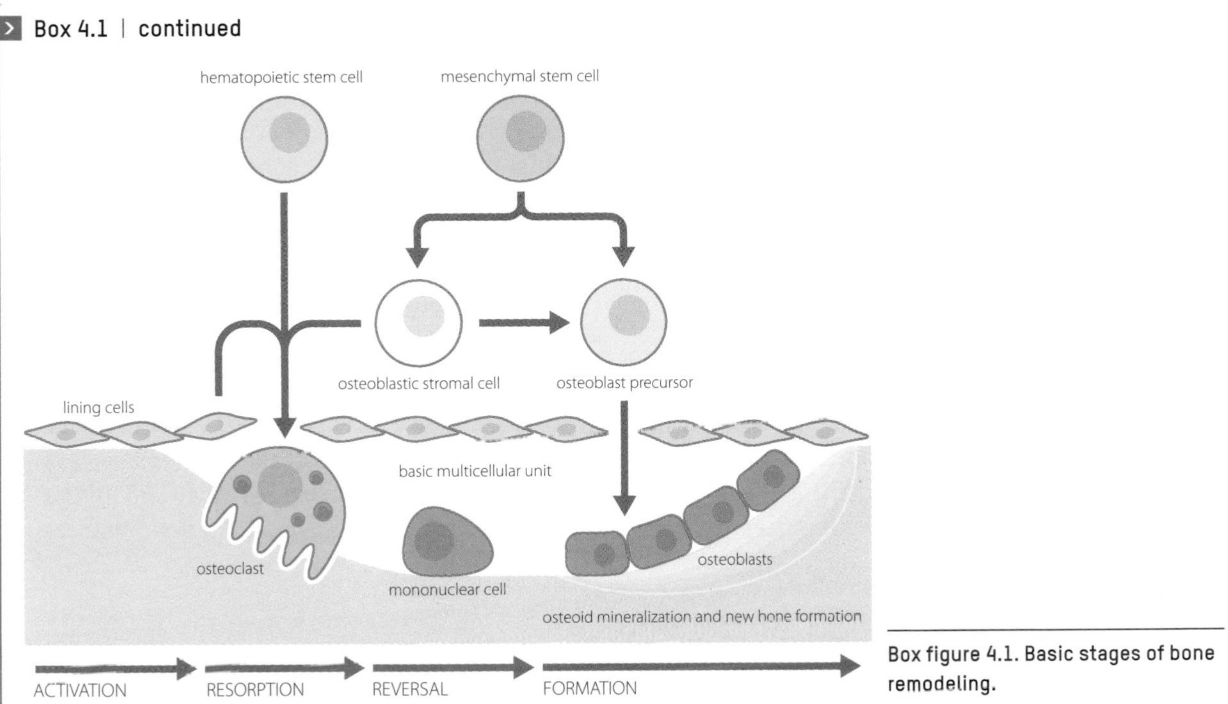

Box figure 4.1. Basic stages of bone remodeling.

Formation: mechanical stimulation and PTH activate bone formation signals via the osteocytes. Quite how these mechanical and hormonal factors exert the opposing effects on resorption and formation of bone remains to be determined, although bone formation is linked to their inhibitory effects on sclerostin expression in osteocytes. Ultimately, mesenchymal stem cells or early osteoblast progenitors return to the lacunae, they differentiate and form the bone osteoid, and finally hydroxyapatite is incorporated into the newly formed osteoid. This involves alkaline phosphatase.

Termination phase: following mineralization, mature osteoblasts either undergo apoptosis, revert back to a bone-lining phenotype, or become embedded in the mineralized matrix and become osteocytes.

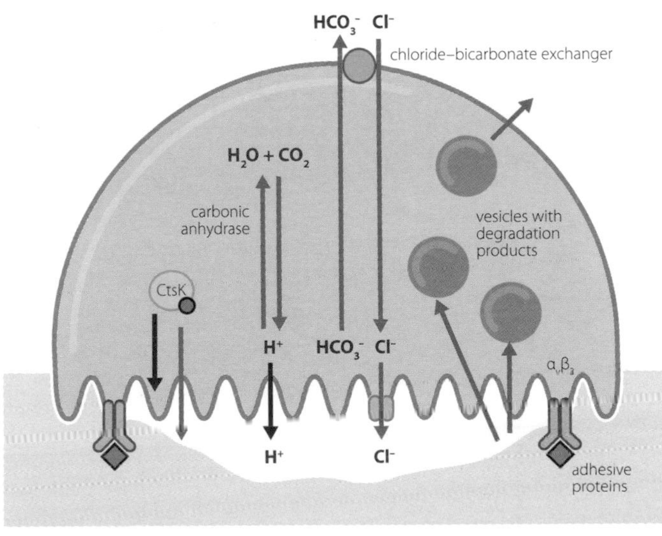

Box figure 4.2. Bone resorption.
Through integrin proteins ($\alpha_V\beta_3$), mature osteoclasts anchor themselves to adhesive proteins in the extracellular matrix of the bone surface creating an isolated microenvironment beneath the cells known as the sealed zone. The repeatedly folded plasma membrane creates a ruffled border. Under the action of carbonic anhydrase, H^+ and HCO_3^- are formed within the osteoclast. The H^+ is pumped into the sealed zone by an osteoclast-specific H^+ ATPase pump whilst the HCO_3^- is exchanged for Cl^- at the basolateral surface of the osteoclast. The hydrogen ions dissolve the mineralized matrix to release calcium and phosphate and the organic bone matrix is degraded by enzymes that break down collagen, particularly cathepsin K (CtsK). These degradation products are endocytosed at the ruffled border, transported across the cytoplasm in vesicles and released at the basolateral membrane by exocytosis.

(RANK-L) by the osteoblasts and, in turn, RANK-L binds avidly to a RANK receptor (receptor of activation of nuclear factor kappa B ligand) on osteoclast precursors, thus activating the transcription factor, nuclear factor (NF)-κB (*Figure 4.7*). In the presence of granulocyte monocyte colony stimulating factor (GM-CSF), this process results in an increase in the proliferation and maturation of osteoclast precursors (*Box 4.1*); this proliferation may be blocked by another osteoblast product, osteoprotogenin (OPG) which acts as a decoy receptor for RANK-L. Indeed RANK-L has become a target for treating osteoporosis (see *Section 4.7.1*) and a monoclonal antibody that binds to and inhibits the action of RANK-L is a potent inhibitor of bone turnover and decreases bone resorption in a dose-dependent manner.

In contrast, intermittent exposure to PTH increases bone formation by the preferential anabolic activation of osteoblasts rather than osteoclasts. A once daily subcutaneous injection of PTH stimulates bone formation and can improve bone mass and bone strength. Finally, PTH can indirectly raise serum calcium levels by stimulating the synthesis of the active form of vitamin D in the kidney and this, in turn, leads to an increased absorption of calcium in the gut (see *Section 4.4.4*).

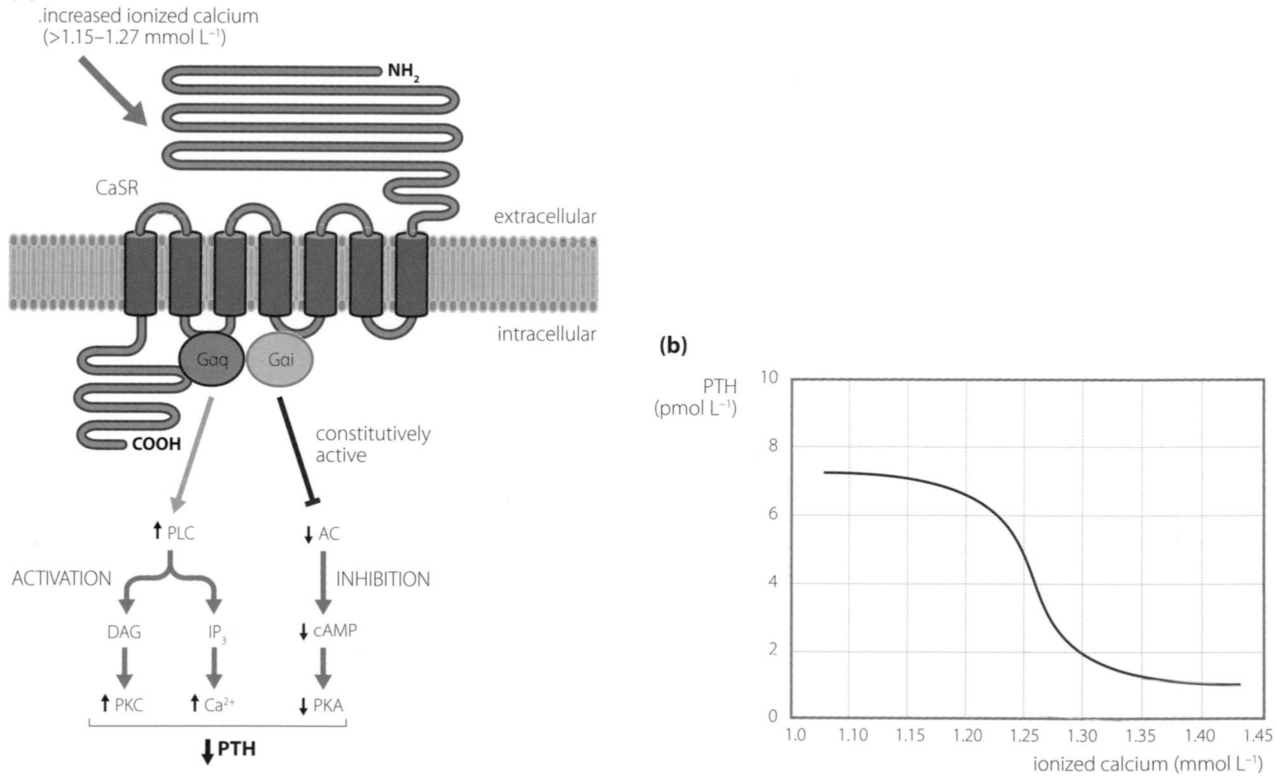

Figure 4.8. Control of PTH secretion in response to increased serum levels of ionized calcium (a) and the relationship between PTH secretion and serum calcium concentrations (b).
The calcium-sensing receptor (CaSR) is a unique GPCR. The adenyl cyclase (AC)/cAMP/protein kinase A (PKA) pathway is constitutively active, releasing PTH at relatively high levels when unbound levels of serum calcium are below 1.15–1.27 mmol/L. When levels of serum calcium are above this set point the CaSR is activated and this inhibits the AC/cAMP/PKA pathway via Gαi and Gαq protein activates phospholipase C (PLC) which produces diacyl glycerol (DAG) and inositol triphosphate (IP_3). In turn these activate protein kinase C (PKC) and increase intracellular levels of Ca^{2+}, respectively, resulting in decreased synthesis and release of PTH and a lowering of serum calcium levels.

4.4.2 Synthesis and control of parathyroid hormone secretion

PTH is synthesized as a 115 amino acid pre-pro-peptide containing a 25 amino acid signal sequence and a 6 amino acid pro-sequence. Both are cleaved off in the endoplasmic reticulum and a mature full-length PTH (of 84 amino acids) is stored in secretory vesicles in the chief cells of the parathyroid gland. Further cleavage of PTH into inactive fragments can occur either in the parathyroid gland or the circulation, but it is known that residues 1–6 are required for receptor activation and residues 18–34 are required for receptor binding. Thus truncated analogs (e.g. PTH 7–34) can bind to the receptor but cannot activate it and so these truncated analogs serve as competitive antagonists of PTH action. Once in the circulation the half-life of intact PTH is less than 5 minutes because it is rapidly broken down to other fragments with varying degrees of activity.

The control of PTH secretion is through a unique G-protein linked calcium-sensing receptor (CaSR) which detects the levels of circulating calcium (*Figure 4.8*). When the levels of ionized serum calcium rise above 1.15–1.2 mmol/L the CaSR is activated and PTH secretion is inhibited. This receptor is coupled to the Gq/PLC pathway which raises intracellular calcium via IP_3 and activates PKC via diacylglycerol (see *Figure 1.8*). The receptor is also coupled to an inhibitory GPCR, Gi, which simultaneously suppresses the activity of adenylate cyclase/cAMP, a signaling pathway thought to be involved in the constitutive release of PTH.

The release of stored cellular calcium by IP_3, coupled with an influx of calcium into the cell, activates calcium-sensitive proteases in the secretory vesicles of the chief cells. This induces the breakdown and inactivation of PTH. At the same time activation of the CaSR inhibits transcription and synthesis of PTH and also its release. Transcription of the *PTH* gene is additionally regulated by vitamin D such that high levels of 1,25-dihydroxycholecalciferol (the biologically active form of vitamin D (see *Section 4.4.5*) inhibit PTH synthesis. This is one of the many ways in which these two hormones cooperatively regulate calcium homeostasis.

4.4.3 The calcium sensing receptor

The CaSR is best known and understood for its role in suppressing the secretion of PTH. However, CaSRs are also expressed in the C cells of the thyroid gland, the kidney, intestine, bone, and focal areas of the brain. In the C cells of the thyroid gland the CaSR detects raised levels of calcium and, in contrast to PTH which is inhibited by raised calcium, it stimulates calcitonin secretion which lowers serum calcium levels. In the kidney tubule, activation of the CaSR increases urinary calcium and magnesium secretion and thus opposes the action of PTH, minimizing the possibility of calcium precipitation within the nephron. The CaSR also increases the excretion of Na^+, K^+, Cl^-, and H_20 and may be involved in sodium balance. The role of CaSR in the intestine is less well understood but it may regulate calcium absorption with varying loads of dietary calcium.

Interestingly, antibodies directed against the parathyroid CaSR have recently been identified in the serum of patients with autoimmune hypoparathyroidism and in some patients they have been shown to produce functional activation of the receptor inhibiting PTH secretion. This indicates a direct pathogenic role in the development of hypocalcemia. Conversely, antibodies that inhibit CaSR activation, thus raising PTH secretion, have been identified in hypercalcemic patients with autoimmune hyperparathyroidism. Both loss of function and gain of function mutations in the CaSR have also been identified:

- loss of function mutations (increased PTH secretion) are associated with familial hypocalciuric hypercalcemia (FHH, see *Box 4.5*)
- gain of function mutations (decreased PTH secretion) are associated with hypercalciuric hypocalcemia.

Novel drugs that target the CaSR have recently been developed and are collectively known as calcimimetics. They bind to the CaSR and inhibit the secretion of PTH. They are used in the treatment of primary hyperparathyroidism (see *Section 4.5*).

4.4.4 Actions of vitamin D

Vitamin D acts like a hormone and increases serum calcium levels (like PTH) but, unlike PTH, it is a steroid hormone, the precursor of which is mainly synthesized in the skin and it raises serum phosphate levels rather than lowering them. Being a steroid hormone, vitamin D binds to the nuclear vitamin D receptor (VDR) which generally functions as a heterodimer with the retinoid X receptor. This heterodimer, in conjunction with co-activators or co-repressors, regulates the transcription of vitamin D target genes. There are, however, responses to vitamin D that occur too rapidly for a genomic action such as a rapid increase in intestinal calcium absorption, insulin secretion and opening of Ca^{2+} channels in osteoblasts. As a consequence, VDRs have now been identified in association with caveolae present in the plasma membrane and these are thought to be responsible for the rapid actions of vitamin D.

The primary action of the active form of vitamin D (1,25-dihydroxycholecalciferol) is to increase intestinal absorption of both calcium and phosphate. The transport of calcium across epithelial cells (*Figure 4.9*) of the intestine, and also the kidney,

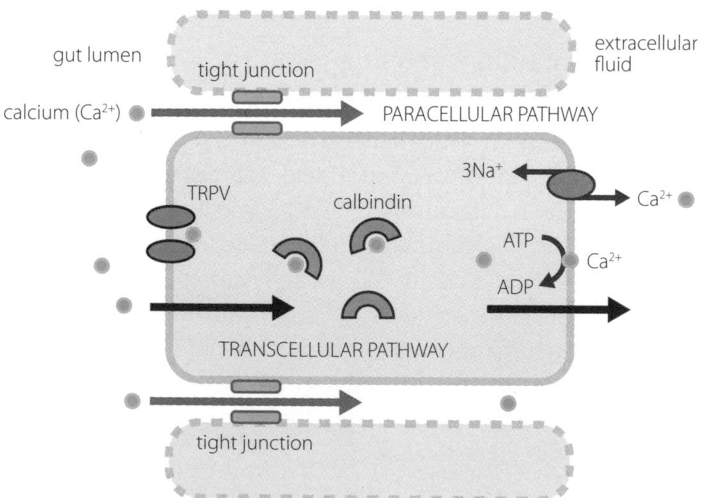

Figure 4.9. Transport of calcium across the epithelial cells of the intestine.
Paracellular transport. Diffusion through tight junctions is dependent on the concentration gradient between the gut lumen and extracellular fluid and does not require energy.
Transcellular transport. At the apical region calcium enters the cell through a selective calcium transporter (TRPV), binds to calbindin and is transported across the epithelial cell. It is extruded at the basolateral membrane by a sodium–calcium exchanger and a Ca^{2+}/ ATPase transporter.

mammary glands, and placenta, basically involves two mechanisms, paracellular and transcellular transport.

- The paracellular route is a process which does not require energy and is concentration-dependent. Calcium diffusion, which takes place along the length of the intestine, simply involves ions diffusing through tight junctions at the luminal surface of the epithelial cells, passing between two adjacent cells and out into the extracellular space.
- Transcellular transport requires energy and is regulated by vitamin D in the intestine. In this process calcium enters the epithelial cells via a selective Ca^{2+} transporter, TRPV (transient receptor potential of the vanilloid type), and then moves across the epithelial cell (this may involve the calcium-binding protein, calmodulin) to the basolateral membrane. Here it is extruded by a Ca^{2+}-ATPase transporter and a Ca^{2+}/Na^+ exchanger.

Vitamin D increases calcium absorption by increasing the expression of TRPV6 and the Ca^{2+}-ATPase which facilitates the transcellular transport of calcium. The mechanism through which vitamin D increases phosphate absorption in the gut has not been fully elucidated.

The VDR is also expressed in osteoblasts (*Figure 4.7*) and vitamin D has been reported to stimulate both bone resorption and formation, although some evidence suggests that its primary action is to deliver calcium and phosphate to bone. In the kidney vitamin D can enhance the effect of PTH by increasing expression of the calcium transporters.

Vitamin D has two further important actions in the homeostatic control of both calcium and phosphate. It can inhibit the synthesis of PTH and stimulate the synthesis of FGF23 (see *Section 4.4.6*), which has an important role in phosphate homeostasis. Whilst the net endocrine effect of vitamin D on the gut, bone, and kidney is to raise calcium and phosphate levels it also has other functions including regulation of immune function and cellular proliferation and differentiation. Indeed vitamin D deficiency has been related to several adverse health outcomes (see *Box 4.2*).

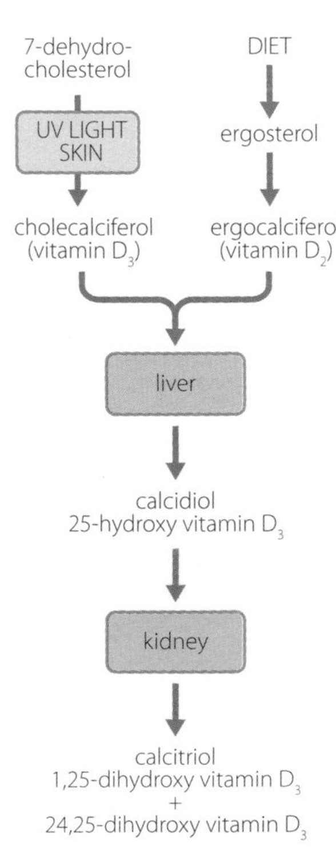

Figure 4.10. Synthesis of the active form of vitamin D_3.

4.4.5 Synthesis, transport, and metabolism of vitamin D

The major endogenous source of vitamin D_3 (cholecalciferol) is the skin where, under the photolytic action of UVB, 7-dehydrocholesterol (the precursor to cholesterol) is converted to pre-vitamin D_3. This is subsequently converted to vitamin D_3 through a thermal, non-enzymatic isomerization reaction. Once in the circulation vitamin D_3 is transported to the liver bound to a vitamin D binding protein (VDBP). In the liver vitamin D_3 is hydroxylated at the C-25 position by one of several cytochrome P450 enzymes to become 25-hydroxyvitamin D_3; the microsomal CYP2R1 enzyme seems to have the highest affinity for this vitamin. Vitamin D_2 (plant sources) and vitamin D_3 (animal sources, particularly oily fish) may also reach the liver after dietary intake and are also hydroxylated.

From the liver 25-hydroxyvitamin D is transported to the kidney where it undergoes a further hydroxylation either at C-1 or C-24 (*Figure 4.10*). 1,25-dihydroxyvitamin D (calcitriol) is the active form of the vitamin whilst 24,25-dihydroxyvitamin D, to which most of the 25-hydroxyvitamin D is shunted, is inactive and is the

Box 4.2 | Actions of vitamin D: beyond the endocrine control of calcium and phosphate metabolism

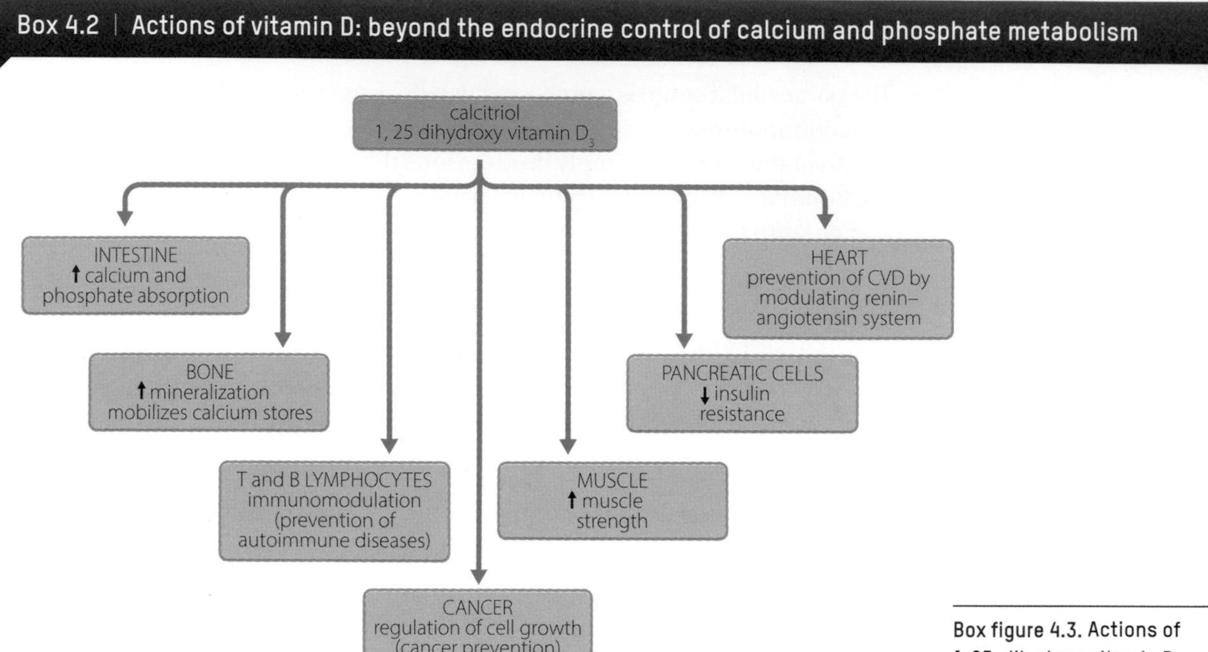

Box figure 4.3. Actions of 1,25-dihydroxyvitamin D.

Vitamin D receptors (VDRs) are widely distributed outside of the intestine, bone, and kidney axis and research has identified more than 30 different cell types that possess VDRs and respond to 1,25-dihydroxyvitamin D. Tissues that express VDRs include, amongst a large range, lymphocytes (T and B cells), monocytes and macrophages, adipose tissue, pancreatic β cells, lung, cardiac muscle, pituitary, placenta, prostate, ovary, testis, and skin. In addition, several tissues express 1α-hydroxylase (encoded by *CYP27B1*) and can convert circulating 25-hydroxyvitamin D to the active 1,25-dihydroxyvitamin D. Such tissues include macrophages and dendritic cells, endothelial cells, colon, breast tissue, pancreatic islets, parathyroid glands, placenta, prostate, and keratinocytes in the skin.

It is now recognized that both the circulating levels and the local production of 1,25-dihydroxyvitamin D have important biological actions beyond calcium and phosphate homeostasis, and that these actions may be responsible for the many health benefits associated with vitamin D sufficiency and adverse health effects in vitamin D deficiency. Broadly speaking, 1,25-dihydroxyvitamin D acts as an important modulator of immune function and a potent regulator of cellular differentiation and proliferation (*Box figure 4.3*).

Regulation of immune function

Innate immunity: this response involves the activation of toll receptors (TLRs) on monocytes and macrophages that recognize specific membrane patterns shed by infectious pathogens. Activation of TLRs leads to the production of antimicrobial peptides including cathelicidin. These polymorphonuclear cells are capable of responding to and producing 1,25-dihydroxyvitamin D because they have both CYP27B1 and VDRs. Stimulation of TLR2 by certain pathogens in macrophages/monocytes and stimulation of TLR2 in keratinocytes by wounding the epidermis increases the expression of CYP27B1 which, in the presence of adequate 25-hydroxyvitamin D, stimulates the expression of cathelicidin. Lack of substrate blunts the ability of these cells to produce cathelicidin.

Adaptive immunity: this response involves the ability of T and B lymphocytes to produce cytokines and immunoglobulins, respectively. 1,25-dihydroxyvitamin D suppresses B cell proliferation, differentiation, and antibody production and inhibits T cell proliferation, particularly T helper cells. At least part of these immunosuppressive actions stem from actions of 1,25-dihydroxyvitamin D on dendritic cells to reduce their antigen presenting capability. The ability of this hormone to suppress the adaptive immune system may be beneficial in protecting against autoimmunity such as inflammatory arthritis, type 1 diabetes and inflammatory bowel disease.

Regulation of proliferation and differentiation

Epidermis and hair follicle: 1,25-dihydroxyvitamin D promotes differentiation of keratinocytes in addition to its action on the innate immune response to wound healing.

Box 4.2 | continued

It also stimulates hair cycling but this mechanism remains unclear. Finally, analogs of 1,25-dihydroxyvitamin D are effective therapy for moderate forms of psoriasis and this is likely to be the result of its immunosuppressive effects on adaptive immunity.

Malignant cells and cancer: many malignant cells express VDRs and their potential benefits in the prevention and treatment of cancer are attributed to the ability of 1,25-dihydroxyvitamin D to stimulate the expression of cell cycle inhibitors and inhibit the expression of the cell adhesion molecule, E-cahedrin, and the transcriptional activity of β-catenin.

Other actions of vitamin D

Vitamin D deficiency has been associated with insulin resistance, decreased insulin production and an increased risk of developing type 2 diabetes mellitus. A deficiency of vitamin D has also been linked with an increased risk of developing hypertension as 1,25-dihydroxyvitamin D decreases renin production in the kidney and thus reduces activity of the renin–angiotensin–aldosterone system. Finally, researchers have suggested that fetal deprivation of vitamin D could be associated with adverse neuropsychiatric outcomes.

first step in the degradation process. The conversion of 25-hydroxyvitamin D to 1,25-dihydroxyvitamin D is stimulated by 1-alpha hydroxylase (or CYP27B1) which is principally expressed in the proximal tubular cells of the kidney. Its activity is a tightly regulated process and is stimulated by PTH and inhibited by FGF23. In addition, the active hormone not only feeds back to inhibit its own production (by suppressing PTH and thus 1-alpha hydroxylase activity), but also enhances its own degradation by up-regulating transcription of 24 hydroxylase.

No routine clinical assay is available for determining the serum concentration of either vitamin D_3 or D_2 and generally the total circulating concentration of 25-hydroxyvitamin D_3 is an acceptable functional measurement of vitamin D status because it is the most plentiful and stable metabolite of vitamin D in the circulation. It is generally agreed that levels of 25-hydroxyvitamin D >50 nmol/L represent vitamin D sufficiency, whilst levels less than this represent either insufficiency, deficiency, or severe deficiency (see *Table 4.1*). However, other researchers have suggested that a minimum serum concentration of >75 nmol/L represents vitamin

Table 4.1. **Circulating concentrations of key vitamin D metabolites**

Vitamin D metabolite	Vitamin D concentration	Vitamin D status
Vitamin D	Not routinely measured	–
25-hydroxyvitamin D	60–105 nmol/L >50 or >75 nmol/L 30–50 nmol/L *12–30 nmol/L <12 nmol/L	Normal range Sufficiency Insufficiency Deficiency Severe deficiency
1,25-dihydroxyvitamin D_2	50–125 pmol/L	
24,25-dihydroxyvitamin D	5–12 nmol/L	

*Patients with a 25-dihydroxyvitamin D_2 concentration <20 nmol/L probably have rickets or osteomalacia.

D sufficiency. *Table 4.1* therefore gives ranges for sufficiency, insufficiency, and deficiency to reflect these slight differences of opinion.

Whatever values are acceptable, there is no doubt that vitamin D deficiency is increasing; it is estimated that one billion people worldwide have either insufficient vitamin D or are deficient. There are several reasons to explain this:

- aggressive campaign to use sun screen which can absorb up to 99% of UVB photons, thereby reducing vitamin D_3 synthesis
- reduced intake of milk fortified with vitamin D
- obesity, through many possible mechanisms including sequestration in excess fat (vitamin D is fat soluble) and possible reduced exposure to sunlight in the obese population
- latitude
- seasonal variation
- skin pigmentation, because melanin absorbs UVB light
- reduced exposure to sunlight

The consequences of vitamin D deficiency are raised levels of PTH (secondary hyperparathyroidism), increased bone resorption, and osteomalacia (lack of bone mineralization). The latter occurs because PTH increases P_i excretion and thus the calcium phosphate product which is essential for bone mineralization (formation of hydroxyapatite crystals) is reduced.

4.4.6 Fibroblast growth factor 23

FGF23 is a new hormone that was discovered in 2000 and is part of the hormonal bone–parathyroid–kidney axis and it plays an important role in phosphate homeostasis. It is a 251 amino acid glycoprotein released mainly from osteoblasts and osteocytes in the skeleton and its synthesis is stimulated in response to dietary phosphate and serum levels of 1,25-dihydroxyvitamin D. The receptors for FGF23, of which four have been identified (FGFR 1–4), are typical tyrosine kinase receptors with a single transmembrane domain. However, for FGF23 to bind to its receptor a co-receptor, alpha-Klotho, is also required. In the kidney, activation of FGFR increases phosphate excretion by reducing the expression of the renal sodium–phosphate co-transporters. In the proximal tubules activation of FGFR inhibits CYP27B1 and thus vitamin D synthesis.

The control and actions of FGF23 can be summarized (*Figure 4.11*) as follows.

- An increase in circulating levels of P_i increases FGF23 leading to an increase in phosphate excretion.
- 1,25-dihydroxyvitamin D increases FGF23 secretion.
- FGF23 inhibits the synthesis of 1,25-dihydroxyvitamin D.
- FGF23 synergizes with PTH to increase P_i excretion.
- FGF23 may regulate the secretion of PTH.

Several diseases have been found to be caused by aberrant actions of FGF23. Excess FGF23 action (over-expression or resistance to proteolytic cleavage) can

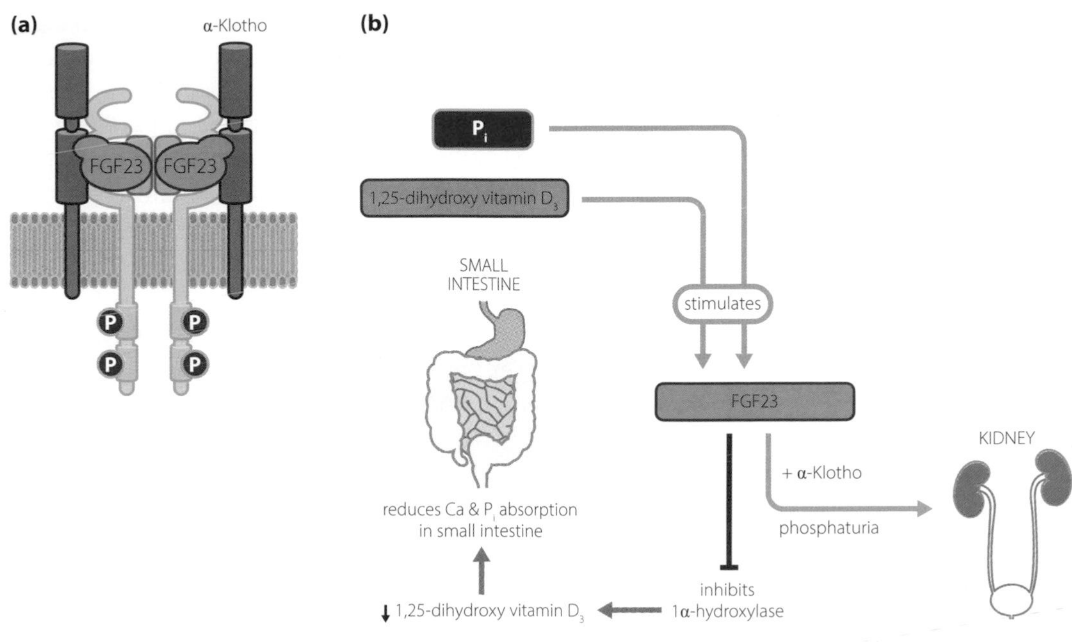

Figure 4.11. The FGF23 receptor (a) and overall actions of FGF23 (b) in calcium and phosphate homeostasis.
(a) The FGF23 receptor is a typical tyrosine kinase receptor with a single transmembrane domain that becomes activated (phosphorylated) by binding FGF23. This binding requires a co-receptor, alpha-Klotho. (b) FGF23 release is stimulated by rises in serum phosphate (P_i) and 1,25-dihydroxyvitamin D, and vitamin D increases phosphate excretion and inhibits 1α-hydroxylase. In turn, the reduced production of 1,25-dihydroxyvitamin D reduces calcium and phosphate absorption in the gut. Together these actions of PTH lower serum P_i levels.

cause hypophosphatemic rickets and osteomalacia, whilst impaired FGF23 action (increased susceptibility to proteolytic cleavage or resistance to the hormone) results in hyperphosphatemic tumoral calcinosis.

4.4.7 Calcitonin, PTH-related peptide, and other hormones in calcium homeostasis

Calcitonin is a 32 amino acid peptide secreted by the parafollicular C cells of the kidney in response to hypercalcemia and gastrin. The hormone's main action is to decrease bone resorption and, at pharmacological doses, the hormone effectively decreases bone turnover. The role of calcitonin in normal calcium homeostasis is unclear and calcitonin insufficiency (post-thyroidectomy) or excess (medullary thyroid carcinoma, see *Section 3.8.3*) has no marked effect on calcium regulation or on bone mineral density. At best calcitonin only plays a minor role in calcium homeostasis.

Several other hormones may affect calcium metabolism and bone turnover and these include estradiol, testosterone, glucocorticoids, growth hormone, and thyroid hormone. In addition, several local factors may affect bone and calcium homeostasis including interleukins, tumor necrosis factor-α (TNFα), and PTH-related peptide (PTHrP, see *Section 4.5.3*).

PTHrP is so named because its first 13 amino acids show striking homology to the first 13 amino acids of PTH (*Figure 4.12*). It is encoded by a gene which is distinct from the *PTH* gene, although probably from the same gene family originally. The structural resemblance to PTH enables PTHrP to bind to PTH type 1 receptors even though it is a 141 amino acid peptide compared to PTH which has 84 amino acids. PTHrP is widely expressed in tissues and in bone it plays a critical role in embryogenesis to prevent premature ossification of forming bone. In certain malignancies PTHrP may be so over-expressed that it is detectable in blood; it acts as an endocrine hormone, in a similar manner to PTH, with the exception that PTHrP does not stimulate CYP27B1 and the synthesis of 1,25-dihydroxyvitamin D in the kidney. However, patients with PTHrP-secreting tumors may present with hypercalcemia (*Figure 4.13* and *Section 4.5.3*).

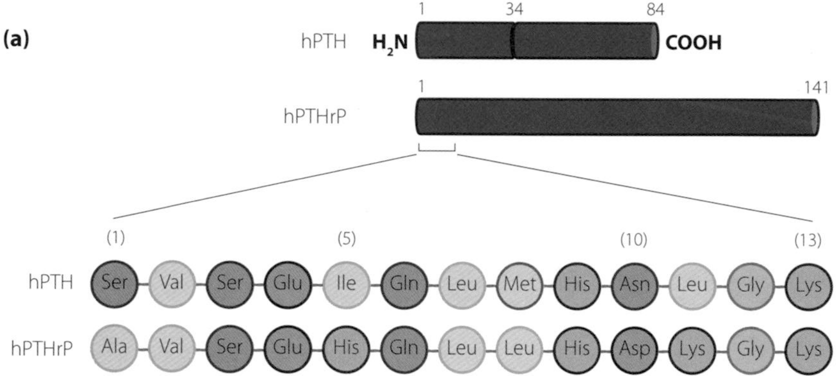

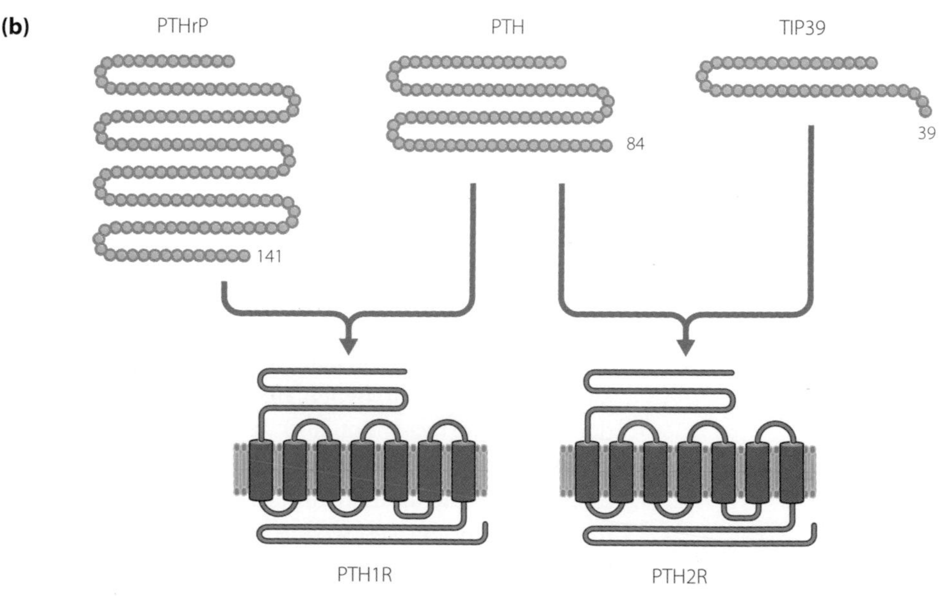

Figure 4.12. PTH and PTH-related peptides.
(a) PTHrP is the second member of the PTH family to have been discovered and although it is larger than PTH (141 amino acids compared to 84 for PTH), the first 13 amino acids show a striking degree of homology to PTH. (b) A hypothalamic peptide (tuberoinfundibular peptide) of 39 residues (TIP39) appears to represent a third member of the PTH gene family and can interact at a second PTH receptor termed the type II receptor to which PTHrP does not bind. The physiologic role of TIP39 and of the type II receptor have not yet been elucidated. PTH can interact with both the PTH1 and PTH2 receptors.

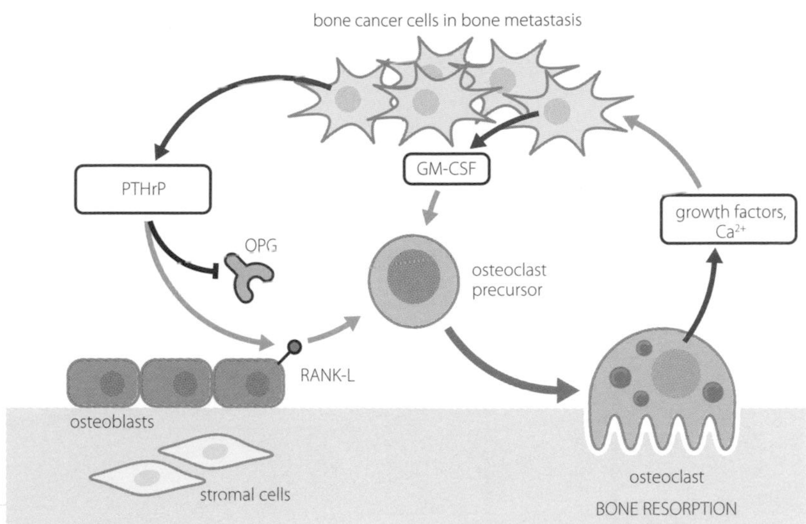

Figure 4.13. Pathologic roles of PTHrP.
In embryonic and early postnatal life locally produced PTHrP regulates cartilage growth in developing long bones, but it has no known role in adult life. Certain tumors produce high levels of PTHrP which stimulate calcium reabsorption in the kidney and also bone resorption. Granulocyte macrophage colony stimulating factor (GM-CSF) increases the pool of osteoclast precursors and PTHrP increases the expression of RANK ligand (RANK-L) and decreases osteoprotogerin (OPG). RANK ligand interacts with the RANK receptor on the osteoblast precursors and this stimulates their differentiation into mature osteoclasts which can cause severe bone loss because a vicious cycle is initiated. The PTHrP-stimulated osteoclast resorption releases bone-derived growth factors (such as TGFβ), which further stimulates tumor cells to synthesize more PTHrP. Thus, PTHrP is the principal factor in cancer-induced bone disease and is responsible for hypercalcemia of malignancy.

4.4.8 Integrated calcium and phosphate homeostasis

The endocrine control of serum levels of calcium and phosphate are shown in *Figures 4.5* and *4.6*. As the preceding text has explained, the endocrine control of phosphate and calcium to some extent involves wheels within wheels, with one hormone controlling the synthesis and secretion of another, complex feedback mechanisms and close interactions between dietary intake, the skeleton, and the kidney. Perhaps one of the best ways to illustrate these complex interactions is to look at what happens in hypocalcemia and in vitamin D deficiency and these are outlined in *Figures 4.14* and *4.15.*

CASE 4.2 179 182 187 191

- Woman of 58 years with somnolence, confusion, and dehydration
- High calcium, normal phosphate, and undetectable PTH

A 58 year old female teacher was admitted with somnolence, confusion, and dehydration. Further history from her relatives revealed that she had a fear of hospitals since the death of her mother from breast cancer at the age of 46. She had ignored a breast lump for some time and this had now developed into a fungating lesion on her left breast. She was a non-smoker, did not drink alcohol and was on no medication apart from over-the-counter analgesia (non-steroidal anti-inflammatories). On examination she was severely dehydrated with low blood pressure and a postural drop of 20 mmHg. Initial investigations revealed:

- total calcium: 3.8 mmol/L (NR 2.2–2.58)
- phosphate: 1.0 mmol/L (NR 0.8–1.5)
- PTH: undetectable

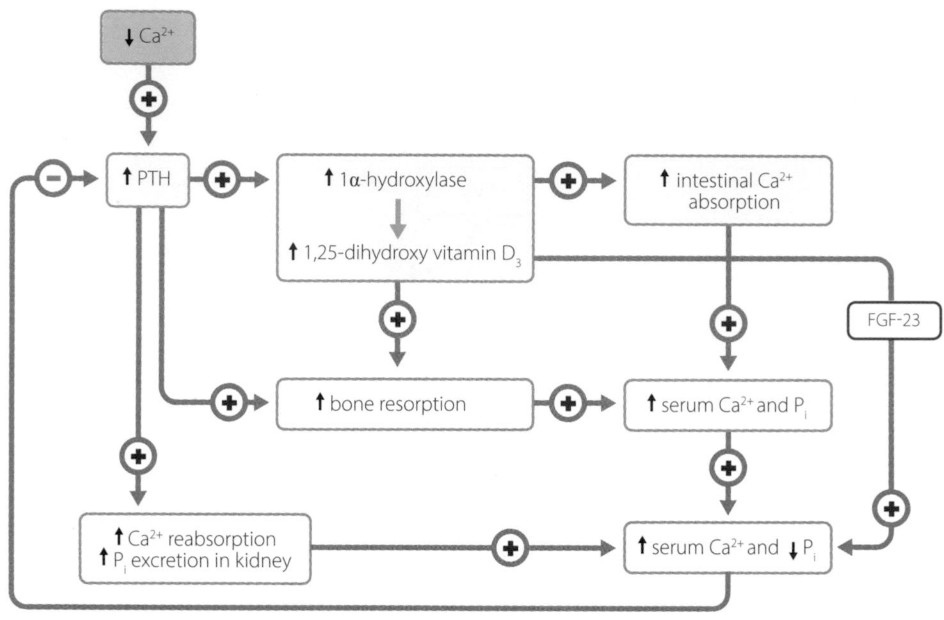

Figure 4.14. Endocrine responses to hypocalcemia.
A decrease in circulating free calcium, Ca^{2+}, stimulates a rise in PTH which increases Ca^{2+} reabsorption in the kidney, bone resorption, and the synthesis of active vitamin D (1,25-dihydroxyvitamin D). 1,25-dihydroxyvitamin D increases calcium absorption in the intestine, synergistically acts with PTH on bone, and stimulates the production of FGF23, which then increases phosphate excretion and thus lowers serum levels of phosphate (P_i).

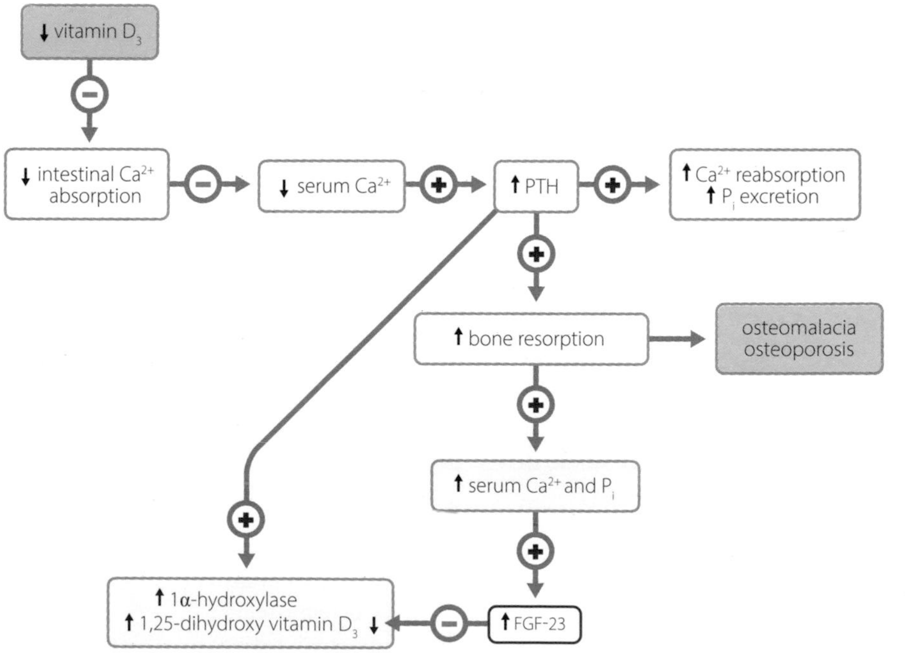

Figure 4.15. Endocrine responses to vitamin D deficiency.
A deficiency of vitamin D reduces Ca^{2+} absorption in the gut, resulting in hypocalcemia. This stimulates a rise in PTH secretion (secondary hyperparathyroidism) which acts to raise serum calcium and phosphate levels by its action on bone, and increasing Ca^{2+} retention and P_i excretion through its action on the kidney. The increase of serum P_i due to bone resorption stimulates release of FGF23 from bone which can counteract the synthesis of active vitamin D (1,25-dihydroxyvitamin D) stimulated by PTH.

4.5 Hypercalcemia

Hypercalcemia is an elevated calcium level in the blood and it can be caused by an excessive release of PTH or be independent of PTH (*Box 4.3*). Whatever the cause (and these are numerous), hypercalcemia results from increased skeletal calcium release, increased intestinal calcium absorption and/or decreased renal calcium excretion. As we have seen above, these functions are regulated by PTH and vitamin D (1,25-dihydroxyvitamin D) but hypercalcemia can also result from other causes such as malignancy and increased bone turnover (as can occur, for example, in immobilization, hyperthyroidism and excess ingestion of vitamin A).

Box 4.3 | Causes of hypercalcemia

Mediated by PTH

Primary hyperparathyroidism (sporadic)

Familial

- MEN-I and MEN-2A (*Section 8.5*)
- FHH (levels of PTH may be normal or high; *Box 4.5*)

Tertiary hyperparathyroidism secondary to acute renal failure

Independent of PTH

Hypercalcemia of malignancy

- PTHrP
- Activation of extra-renal 1α-hydroxylase (increased calcitriol)
- Osteolytic bone metastases and local cytokines

Vitamin D intoxication

Chronic granulomatous disorders

- Activation of extra-renal 1α-hydroxylase (increased calcitriol)

Medications

- Thiazide diuretics
- Lithium
- Teriparatide
- Excessive vitamin A
- Theophylline toxicity

Miscellaneous

- Hyperthyroidism
- Acromegaly
- Pheochromocytoma
- Adrenal insufficiency
- Immobilization
- Parenteral nutrition
- Milk alkali syndrome

Hypercalcemia can often be an asymptomatic laboratory finding, but symptoms (*Figure 4.16*) are more common at high blood calcium levels, i.e. >3 mmol/L. When levels rise above 3.75–4 mmol/L it is considered a medical emergency due to the high risk of cardiac arrest and coma resulting from calcium's ability to stabilize membrane potentials.

Measuring serum PTH levels is a useful way of differentiating the causes of hypercalcemia.

- If PTH is raised in association with hypercalcemia this indicates abnormal secretion of PTH due to primary or tertiary hyperparathyroidism.
- If PTH levels are suppressed in association with hypercalcemia this is due to the feedback effects of Ca^{2+} on the CaSRs in the parathyroid gland (see *Section 4.4.3* and *Figure 4.8*).

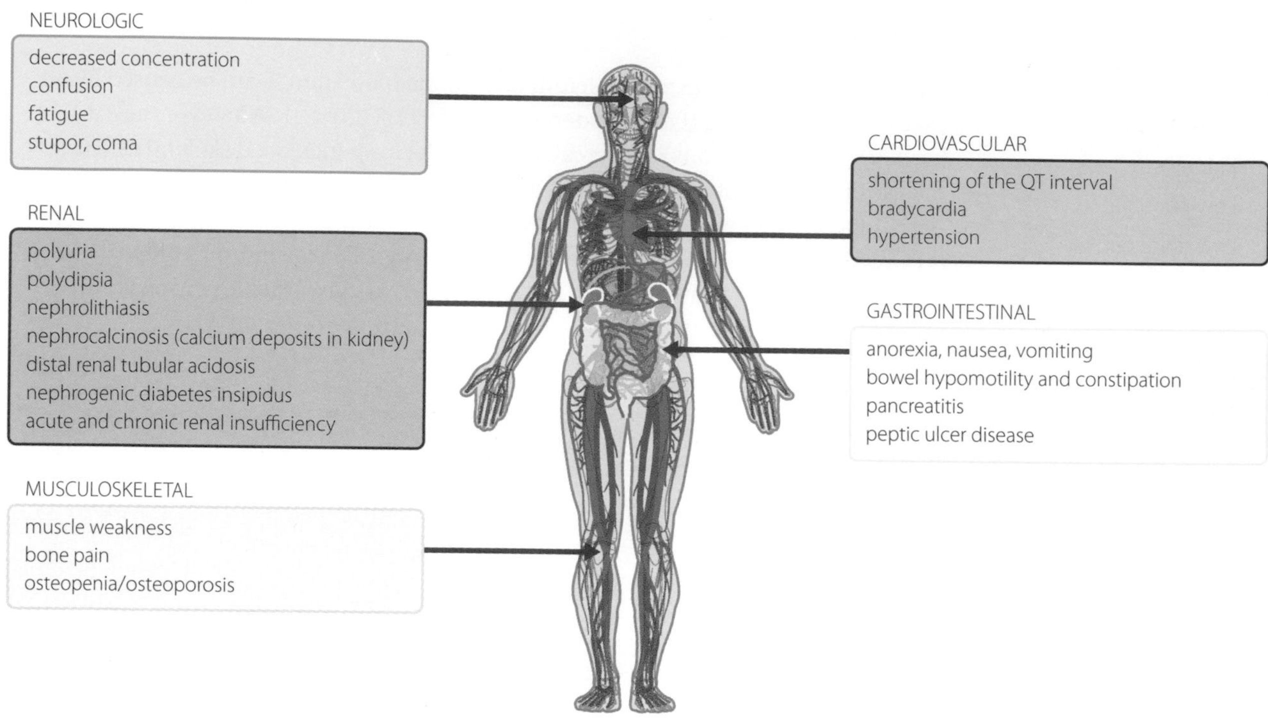

Figure 4.16. Symptoms of hypercalcemia.

CASE 4.1 AND 4.2 165 179 182

Subsequent investigations carried out for the patient in Case 4.1 revealed an elevated PTH level of 28 pmol/L (NR 1.0–6.8) suggesting a diagnosis of primary hyperparathyroidism.

In contrast, the unfortunate patient in Case 4.2 had an undetectable PTH result and, along with the history and physical findings, this suggested that her hypercalcemia was associated with malignancy.

4.5.1 Primary hyperparathyroidism

Primary hyperparathyroidism remains the most frequent cause of hypercalcemia in non-hospitalized patients. It is difficult to give an accurate estimate of its true incidence because numbers of cases are rising rapidly with the increasing ease of obtaining calcium estimates on routine blood tests. A reasonable estimate of incidence is around 40–50 per 100 000, with a female preponderance of about 3:1. It usually presents in or after the fifth decade – earlier presentations raise the possibility of a familial cause (e.g. multiple endocrine neoplasia (MEN)-1 or MEN-2A (see *Section 8.5*). In the majority of cases (80–85%), primary hyperparathyroidism is due to an adenoma of one (or very rarely more) parathyroid glands. Less frequently it may be due to multiple gland hyperplasia, and very rarely (<0.5%) to parathyroid cancer.

Many cases of primary hyperparathyroidism are asymptomatic and diagnosed by routine screening for non-specific symptoms or as part of a health check. Many patients will, however, have rather subtle symptoms (fatigue, mild cognitive

Box 4.4 | Symptoms and signs of excess PTH secretion

Bone disease
Kidney stones (nephrolithiasis)
Low phosphate
Low magnesium
High calcitriol
High uric acid (with or without gout)
Proximal renal tubular acidosis
Anemia

Box 4.5 | Familial hypocalciuric hypercalcemia (FHH)

FHH is usually asymptomatic and does not require treatment, hence its pseudonym, familial benign hypercalcemia. However, it is an important condition because it is often mistaken for the more common primary hyperparathyroidism leading to unnecessary and inappropriate surgical intervention. FHH is usually due to a loss of function mutation (autosomal dominant) in the CaSR and genetic testing is available to support the diagnosis and to screen family members.

The CaSR is a GPCR expressed in the parathyroid glands and the kidneys, among other tissues. It mediates the feedback inhibition of parathyroid hormone release from the parathyroid glands in response to a rise in serum calcium concentration (see *Section 4.4.3*). A loss of function mutation will inhibit this feedback pathway and so higher calcium levels are necessary to inhibit release of PTH, resulting in hypercalcemia associated with inappropriately normal or mildly elevated levels of parathyroid hormone. The degree of hypercalcemia is dependent on the mutation and its degree of effect on the CaSR function.

In the kidneys CaSR mediates feedback inhibition of PTH-independent calcium reabsorption. Loss of function of the CaSR will result in continued reabsorption of calcium in the kidneys despite relative hypercalcemia and so renal excretion of calcium will be low.

FHH presents with a combination of hypercalcemia, hypocalciuria, normal to high levels of PTH and hypermagnesemia. Although hypercalcemia is present from birth, it is often noticed later in life during a routine serum biochemistry screen. As suggested above, it is usually asymptomatic and requires no treatment, although occasional cases of FHH associated with renal stones or nephrocalcinosis, gallstones or pancreatitis have been reported.

Diagnosis and treatment of FHH

The diagnosis is based on moderate hypercalcemia associated with inappropriately normal or elevated PTH and a low urinary calcium clearance (calcium/creatinine clearance ratio <0.01). In some cases there is overlap between features of primary hyperparathyroidism and FHH and so genetic testing for CaSR mutations may be useful in these cases. In contrast to most cases of primary hyperparathyroidism, FHH does not require any treatment, indeed parathyroidectomy is ineffective.

Interestingly, a gain of function mutation in the CaSR gene can lead to the exact opposite condition, hypercalciuric hypocalcemia, also known as autosomal dominant hypocalcemia.

impairment) on close questioning. The symptoms of hyperparathyroidism may be due to excess levels of PTH directly (see *Box 4.4*) or may result from the effects of hypercalcemia mediated by uncontrolled excess of PTH (*Box 4.3*).

Diagnosis requires the demonstration of an elevated calcium level in the presence of a high level of PTH. Urinary calcium excretion measurement is useful and may help to differentiate true primary hyperparathyroidism from the less common FHH (*Box 4.5*). In true primary hyperparathyroidism, 40% of patients will have a high urinary calcium (>7.5 mmol/L, NR 2.5–7.5 mmol/L); some physicians believe that a markedly elevated level (>10 mmol/L) is an indication for early parathyroid surgery in view of the risk of nephrolithiasis (formation of kidney stones). Frequently urinary calcium excretion is reported as a calcium creatinine excretion ratio: [(24 hour urine calcium × serum creatinine) / (24 hour urine creatinine × serum calcium)] – a value of less than 0.01 makes FHH more likely than primary hyperparathyroidism.

A diagnosis of primary hyperparathyroidism (particularly in the younger age group or where there is evidence of gland hyperplasia) should raise the possibility of a familial syndrome such as MEN-1 or MEN-2A. MEN-1 (see *Section 8.5*) is due to loss of function mutations in the *MENIN* gene, a putative tumor suppressor, and more than 90% of patients with MEN-1 will have hyperparathyroidism; this is nearly always the first manifestation of the disease. Hyperparathyroidism also exists as part of MEN-2A and is related to loss of function of the *RET* proto-oncogene. Because this is associated with development of pheochromocytomas, patients should be screened with estimations of urinary or plasma catecholamines. Familial hyperparathyroidism can occur without other manifestations of, or gene mutations associated with, MEN. A rare but important condition is hyperparathyroidism jaw tumor syndrome (HPT-JT) which is an autosomal dominant condition associated with fibromas in the mandible or the maxilla and occasionally with tumors in the kidneys and the uterus. HPT-JT syndrome is associated with mutations of the *HRPT2* gene (which encodes a protein called parafibromin). The condition is important because parathyroid carcinoma is more common in HPT-JT syndrome (unlike FHH or in MEN-I and MEN-2A), occurring with an incidence of about 1 in 5.

Imaging in primary hyperparathyroidism

The diagnosis of hyperparathyroidism is purely on the history and biochemistry and imaging is really only useful to plan surgical intervention. A number of imaging modalities may be used (see *Box 4.6*).

- Ultrasound is cheap and non-invasive, although operator dependent. It can highlight co-existing thyroid pathology.
- Nuclear medicine scans using technetium-labeled MIBI (2-methoxy-isobutyl-isonitrile), which is taken up by overactive parathyroid glands but not by normal glands, are useful and have a sensitivity of around 80–85%. Such scans may be useful in detecting ectopic parathyroid glands prior to exploratory surgery.
- CT scanning of the neck and mediastinum can delineate parathyroid anatomy.
- MRI with contrast can be of value for lesions in the mediastium and for those individuals who have persistent disease following parathyroidectomy.
- Arteriography and selective venous sampling are invasive techniques but may occasionally be valuable where other imaging techniques have failed to help in identification of abnormal parathyroid tissue, particularly in recurrent disease.

4.5.2 Secondary and tertiary hyperparathyroidism

Secondary hyperparathyroidism

Secondary hyperparathyroidism is not a cause of hypercalcemia but is an appropriate response to a chronic stimulus for PTH production, most commonly chronic renal failure or vitamin D deficiency. In chronic renal failure (now known as chronic kidney disease or CKD) the development of secondary hyperparathyroidism usually pre-dates a worsening of CKD to a level requiring treatment with dialysis. It occurs as a response to hypocalcemia, impaired production of biologically active

Box 4.6 | Imaging of the parathyroid gland in primary hyperparathyroidism

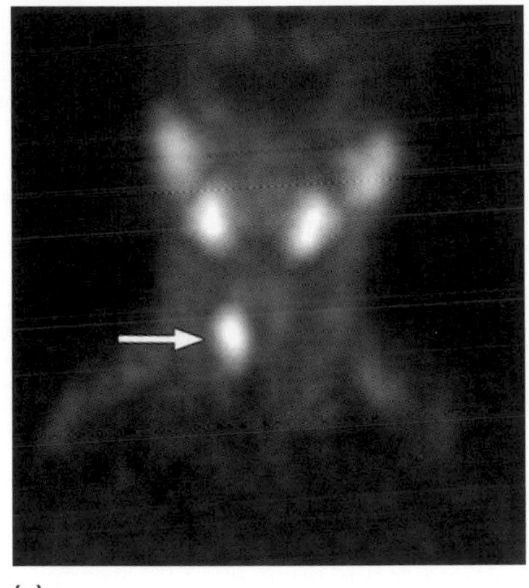

(a)

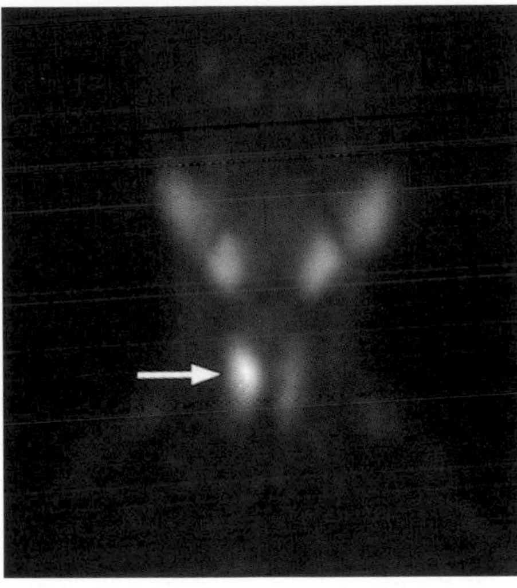

(b)

Box figure 4.4. SPECT images of a right superior parathyroid adenoma. (a) Early-phase ^{99m}Tc-sestamibi SPECT image shows physiologic uptake in salivary glands and thyroid gland, with focus of more intense uptake overlying superior pole of right thyroid lobe (arrow). (b) SPECT image taken 2 hours later shows radiotracer retention in adenoma (arrow) but clearing of tracer from overlying thyroid.

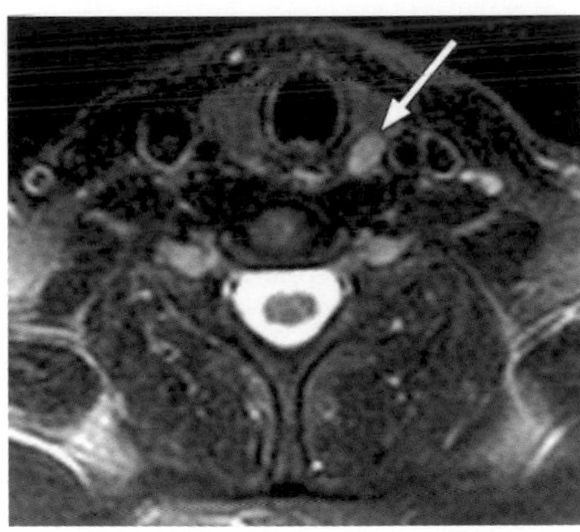

Box figure 4.5. MRI of a left parathyroid adenoma. Gadolinium-enhanced T1-weighted image with fat suppression shows intense enhancement typical of parathyroid adenomas (arrow).

1,25-dihydroxyvitamin D in the kidney, and hyperphosphatemia. High levels of phosphate can directly stimulate both PTH synthesis and parathyroid hyperplasia. Secondary hyperparathyroidism is important because it leads to development or worsening of a number of the symptoms and signs of CKD, including renal bone disease (uremic osteodystrophy and osteitis fibrosa cystica), cardiovascular disease, impaired red blood cell production, and non-specific behavioral changes.

Diagnosis of secondary hyperparathyroidism is usually straightforward; patients with CKD will have a low or just normal calcium level but an elevated PTH level. Vitamin D levels are usually low and phosphate high (although in secondary hyperparathyroidism due to vitamin D deficiency with normal renal function, phosphate levels will be low). Parathyroid imaging is unnecessary unless there is a suspicion of primary hyperparathyroidism. Skeletal X-rays may be useful especially at sites of bone pain.

The treatment of secondary hyperparathyroidism contrasts with that of primary because it is mainly medical rather than surgical. The aim is to normalize calcium and vitamin D and reduce levels of PTH to prevent ectopic calcification and normalize bone turnover. In the absence of renal failure this can often be achieved by correcting vitamin D deficiency (50 000 IU vitamin D_2 weekly for 8 weeks, or longer if necessary). If secondary hyperparathyroidism is due to advanced CKD, other options include:

- phosphate restriction
- phosphate binders (e.g. calcium carbonate or acetate; sevelamer hydrochloride; or lanthanum carbonate)
- limiting calcium supplementation
- vitamin D and analogs (of activated vitamin D) – calcitriol, paricalcitol, doxercalciferol, maxacalcitol.

If secondary hyperparathyroidism remains severe despite medical intervention, surgery may be considered. If surgery is undertaken, all glands need to be identified and removed with an autotransplantation of parathyroid tissue into the forearm musculature. This allows easy re-exploration should hyperparathyroidism recur post-operatively.

Tertiary hyperparathyroidism

Tertiary hyperparathyroidism is essentially the progression of secondary hyperparathyroidism (low calcium, high PTH) to an autonomous overproduction of PTH by the parathyroid glands in the setting of hypercalcemia (high calcium, high PTH). Usually this involves all glands, and it can occur after renal transplantation. It differs from primary hyperparathyroidism in that the phosphate levels often remain elevated (they are low in primary hyperparathyroidism) increasing the risk of calcinosis (formation of calcium deposits in soft tissue). The only treatment of benefit is surgical removal of all four glands with autotransplantation as above.

4.5.3 Other causes of hypercalcemia

In simple terms, hypercalcemia can occur as a result of any process where the amount of calcium getting into the bloodstream exceeds that which can be excreted by the kidneys (*Box 4.3*). This may be due to increased bone turnover or excessive gastrointestinal absorption of calcium. Both these processes are mediated by PTH, vitamin D, and PTHrP. Additionally, hypercalcemia can be caused by a variety of drugs and several endocrine and non-endocrine conditions may also be associated with raised levels of calcium.

Vitamin D excess

High serum concentrations of either 25-hydroxyvitamin D (calcidiol) or 1,25-dihydroxyvitamin D (calcitrol) can cause hypercalcemia by increasing both bone resorption and gut absorption. Although intestinal transport of calcium is primarily regulated by the biologically active 1,25-dihydroxyvitamin D, hypercalcemia does occur in patients with markedly elevated serum 25-hydroxyvitamin D concentrations; for example, those who ingest high doses of either vitamin D (which is converted to calcidiol in the liver) or calcidiol itself, or use vitamin D analogs for the treatment of some skin conditions. High serum 1,25-dihydroxyvitamin D concentrations are usually due to ingestion of calcitrol as treatment for hypoparathyroidism or for the hypocalcemia and secondary hyperparathyroidism of renal failure. The biological effects are short lived and normocalcemia can usually be restored by stopping treatment for 48 hours or so.

Endogenous production of 1,25-dihydroxyvitamin D can occur in patients with malignant lymphoma, chronic granulomatous disorders (especially sarcoidosis), and occasionally in other illnesses characterized by granuloma formation, such as Wegener's granulomatosis. In these situations, extra-renal conversion of 25-hydroxyvitamin D occurs in the granulomas themselves and is unregulated by PTH. The hypercalcemia in these situations is usually amenable to treatment with glucocorticoids (e.g. prednisolone).

Malignancy

Malignancy is the commonest cause of hypercalcemia in patients in hospital, occurring in patients with both solid tumors (typically breast and lung) and hematologic malignancies (particularly malignant myeloma). It is a poor prognostic marker and usually occurs in patients with known malignancy, although it may occasionally be the first manifestation.

Malignancy causes hypercalcemia by increasing bone resorption and calcium release from bone through three major mechanisms.

- Osteolytic metastases with local release of cytokines such as tumor necrosis factor and interleukin-1. In myeloma, osteoclast activating factors (lymphotoxin, hepatocyte growth factor, Il-6 and RANK ligand) are released.
- Tumor secretion of PTHrP, particularly in non-metastatic solid tumors (*Figure 4.13*).
- Tumor production of 1,25-dihydroxyvitamin D by activated macrophages occurs in patients with lymphoma.

The levels of hypercalcemia seen (often above 3.25 mmol/L) are usually higher than those associated with hyperparathyroidism. Occasionally tumors may secrete biologically active PTH rather than PTHrP.

CASE 4.2 179 182 187 191

This case was unusual in that the patient presented with hypercalcemia, whereas this is usually a later manifestation in solid tumors. Nevertheless it was clear that she had long-standing disease for which she had not sought medical advice. Breast cancer is associated with hypercalcemia and osteolytic bone metastases – those patients with hypercalcemia will often have elevated levels of PTHrP in the absence or presence of bone metastases.

Drugs

- Thiazide diuretics lower urinary calcium excretion (useful for the treatment of hypercalciuria and recurrent renal stones). This effect rarely causes hypercalcemia in normal individuals, but can lead to hypercalcemia in patients with concomitant hyperparathyroidism.

- Lithium may cause increased PTH release by altering the set-point at which serum calcium levels inhibit PTH secretion. The hypercalcemia usually, but not always, subsides when the lithium is stopped.
- Theophylline toxicity has been associated with mild hypercalcemia which usually responds to treatment with beta-blockers.

Other conditions related to hypercalcemia

Many miscellaneous endocrine and non-endocrine conditions may cause modest elevations of calcium. In thyrotoxicosis, thyroid hormone excess mediates an increase in bone resorption. In adrenal insufficiency, the generation of hypercalcemia is probably multifactorial and caused by increased proximal tubular reabsorption and increased bone resorption (possibly mediated by the action of thyroid hormones which are normally inhibited by physiological glucocorticoid concentrations). Pheochromocytomas are occasionally associated with hypercalcemia, either as part of MEN-2A with hyperparathyroidism (see *Section 8.5*) or by tumor production of PTHrP *(Figure 4.13)*. Hypercalcemia is sometimes reported in patients with acromegaly.

The milk-alkali syndrome consists of the triad of hypercalcemia, metabolic alkalosis, and renal insufficiency and is due to ingestion of large amounts of calcium and alkali. This was a common condition before the advent of specific treatments for peptic ulcer disease (i.e. histamine-2 receptor antagonists and proton pump inhibitors), but had virtually disappeared by the mid-1980s. However, it is now making a resurgence and is probably the third most common cause of hypercalcemia after primary hyperparathyroidism and malignancy. Factors responsible for this increase in incidence include an increase in calcium therapy for the prevention and treatment of osteoporosis, several over-the-counter remedies containing high concentrations of calcium carbonate, and the increased use of calcium carbonate to minimize secondary hyperparathyroidism in patients with CKD.

4.5.4 Treatment of hypercalcemia

Although specific treatment is determined by the etiology of the hypercalcemia, some general principles apply. Most patients with a calcium level of 3 mmol/L do not usually require immediate therapy, but those with intermediate levels (3–3.5 mmol/L) may, depending on symptoms and clinical state.

High levels of calcium inhibit arginine vasopressin (antidiuretic hormone) resulting in polyuria as a consequence of DI, so fluid replacement is of paramount importance. In acute, severe hypercalcemia, hydration with normal saline (0.9% NaCl, 3–4 liters per 24–48 h) can correct the extracellular fluid deficit occurring as a result of vomiting and polyuria. Urinary calcium excretion increases as a result of the enhanced glomerular filtration of calcium and decreasing tubular reabsorption of sodium and calcium. This form of therapy must be used cautiously in patients with compromised cardiovascular or renal function. If hypercalcemia is secondary to excess PTH or PTHrP then renal calcium retention may be an important contributory factor, necessitating the addition of a loop diuretic such as furosemide. Loop diuretics inhibit both sodium and calcium reabsorption in the kidney and promote calciuria as well as mitigating effects of possible fluid overload.

Acute hypercalcemia is often due to accelerated bone resorption and in these cases a bisphosphonate is the treatment of choice for inhibition of bone resorption (*Box*

Box 4.7 | Bisphosphonates for inhibiting bone resorption

Several bisphosphonates are available, with all sharing a common core structure of two phosphate groups linked to a carbon atom. This is very similar to the structure of pyrophosphate and so bisphosphonates can competitively inhibit actions of enzymes that utilize pyrophosphate. Two main classes exist:

- nitrogen containing (e.g. pamidronate and alendronate); these inhibit osteoclast induced bone resorption by affecting the HMG Co-A reductase pathway
- non-nitrogen containing (e.g. etidronate); these are incorporated into a non-functional analog of ATP which can compete with endogenous ATP and inhibit cellular metabolism, ultimately causing osteoclast apoptosis.

Oral bisphosphonates must be taken on an empty stomach with the patient sitting upright for at least 30 minutes before other medications or food to reduce the risk of gastroesophageal reflux and esophageal ulceration. Long-term bisphosphonate use is associated with a risk of osteonecrosis of the jaw, although this is most commonly seen in patients with malignancies who are using bisphosphonates for the management of hypercalcemia.

4.7). In acute severe hypercalcemia, following rehydration, pamidronate (90 mg) or zoledronate (4 mg) may be given intravenously. This will often normalize calcium levels and the effect may last for many weeks.

Calcitonin (4–8 IU/kg, i.m or s.c.) can also inhibit osteoclastic bone resorption and increase calcium excretion, but tachyphylaxis develops within a few days. It has a rapid onset of action and can be used as adjunctive therapy with a bisphosphonate to reduce the hypercalcemia more rapidly. Other alternative treatments designed to reduce osteoclast activity include plicamycin (a cytotoxic antibiotic) and gallium nitrate (a gallium salt of nitric acid which inhibits osteoclasts).

Patients with hypercalcemia due to hematologic malignancies such as lymphoma or myeloma and those with vitamin D intoxication or granulomatous disease may benefit from treatment with glucocorticoids (e.g. hydrocortisone 200–300 mg i.v. over 24 hours for 3 to 5 days).

Severely hypercalcemic patients refractory to other therapies and those with significant renal impairment may need either peritoneal or hemodialysis. After management of the acute hypercalcemic episode, treatment should be directed to the underlying cause.

4.5.5 Treatment of primary hyperparathyroidism

There is little consensus at present as to who should receive definitive treatment for hyperparathyroidism. Some endocrinologists advocate a 'watch and wait' philosophy in mild to moderate disease, but others are more aggressive. While it is probably reasonable to keep some patients with mild disease (calcium <3 mmol/L, urinary calcium excretion <10 mmol/day) under review without surgical intervention, this does not address the rather more subtle symptoms of mild cognitive impairment and quality of life, or the potential for worsening osteoporosis or risk of nephrolithiasis (kidney stones).

Surgical treatment

The mainstay of treatment of primary hyperparathyroidism remains surgical intervention. Pre-operative imaging (see *Box 4.6*) may be helpful but experienced surgeons still advocate exploratory surgery. It is essential to visualize all four parathyroid glands. Usually there will be a solitary adenoma which is macroscopically obvious: the other glands will be relatively atrophied (less than 5 mm in diameter and 50 mg in weight). In doubtful cases a frozen section biopsy can be taken. If there is evidence of gland hyperplasia, all four glands may be removed (with the inevitable outcome of post-operative hypoparathyroidism requiring life-long calcium and vitamin D supplementation). Alternatively, 3.5 glands can be removed (with the risk of recurrent hyperparathyroidism), but some surgeons continue to remove all glands and replace one in the forearm (an easier site for possible re-exploration if recurrent disease becomes apparent). Intra-operative measurements of PTH are available and may lead to greater therapeutic success because, once the source of excess PTH is identified and removed, PTH levels should fall to normal within about 15 minutes.

Alternatives to surgical treatment include doing nothing (i.e. applying a watch and wait philosophy and keeping patients under review to ascertain whether treatable symptoms have developed or whether there is worsening of renal function or osteoporosis) or medical treatments.

CASE 4.1

165 182

- Woman of 62 years with 4 month history of polyuria and polydipsia
- Poor appetite and weight loss of 6 kg
- Normal fasting blood sugar, slightly raised creatinine and raised calcium
- ? Hypercalcemia
- Imaging showed a solitary adenoma which was surgically removed

The biochemical diagnosis of hypercalcemia secondary to primary hyperparathyroidism was straightforward: the patient had high calcium, low phosphate, high PTH, normal vitamin D, and high urinary calcium excretion.

The primary treatment of hyperparathyroidism remains surgical – the patient underwent imaging studies with ultrasound and nuclear medicine MIBI scanning which revealed (*Case figure 4.1*) a solitary adenoma in association with the lower pole of the left thyroid lobe. She underwent targeted surgery as a day case and the adenoma was successfully removed. Within two weeks her calcium and PTH levels were completely normal. Her symptoms resolved rapidly and at review she mentioned that she had not realized how awful she felt pre-operatively – an indication of the insidious nature of hypercalcemia and the rather non-specific symptoms.

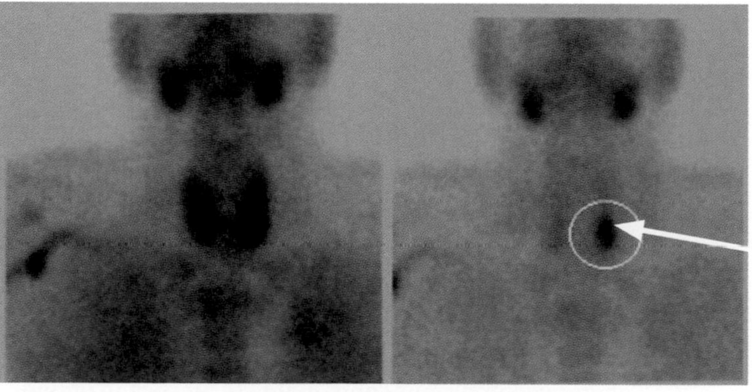

Case figure 4.1. Technetium 99m-sestamibi parathyroid scan.
The scan on the left (at 15 min) shows accumulation of tracer in the thyroid gland. On the right (at 2 h post-injection) the tracer is concentrated in a parathyroid adenoma clearly seen (arrow) in association with the lower left pole of the thyroid (left inferior parathyroid gland).

Medical treatment

- Bisphosphonates (*Box 4.7*) and hormone replacement therapy provide skeletal protection in patients with primary hyperparathyroidism. Neither of these classes of medications significantly lowers serum calcium or PTH levels.
- Cinacalcet is a novel calcimimetic drug which reduces PTH secretion by altering the function of parathyroid calcium-sensing receptors (see *Section 4.4.3*) and consequently reducing calcium and PTH levels and raising serum phosphorus. Cinacalcet does not, however, reduce bone turnover or improve bone mineral density (BMD). It is currently used in patients with primary hyperparathyroidism who are unsuitable for surgery, and also has a role in the management of parathyroid cancer and secondary hyperparathyroidism.

CASE 4.2

179 182 187 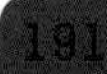

- Woman of 58 years with somnolence, confusion, and dehydration
- High calcium, normal phosphate, and undetectable PTH
- Advanced breast cancer discovered on biopsy

This patient had a less satisfactory outcome. She was reviewed by the surgical team who confirmed the diagnosis of breast cancer following a biopsy of the lesion. Her breast cancer was at an advanced stage; she had metastatic disease in the liver, lungs, and bones. Involvement of healthcare professionals from several disciplines established that she had a long-standing fear of doctors, medicine, and ill-health generally. She declined any further investigation or treatment (apart from palliative pain relief) and died 4 weeks after presentation.

4.6 Hypocalcemia

CASE 4.3

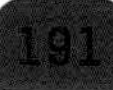 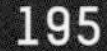

- Woman of 24 years unwell since thyroidectomy 3 weeks previously
- Low calcium, high phosphate, and low vitamin D

A 24 year old woman was admitted with severe pins and needles in both hands, associated with a perception of breathlessness and confusion. Although alert on admission there was a suggestion from an accompanying friend that she may have had a short-lived self-limiting seizure prior to admission. She had felt unwell, with other non-specific symptoms including muscle cramps, since a thyroidectomy operation 3 weeks previously. The thyroidectomy had been carried out for Graves disease associated with thyroid eye disease which had been difficult to treat due to non-compliance with medications. She had not attended a post-surgical follow-up and was not taking any medication. There was no family or other personal history of note. Initial blood tests revealed:

- Calcium: 1.6 mmol/L (NR 2.2–2.58)
- Phosphate: 1.8 mmol/L (NR 0.8–1.5)
- Vitamin D: 18 nmol/L (NR 60–105)
- Alkaline phosphatase: 65 IU/L (NR 36–126)

Hypocalcemia is a reduced serum level of ionized calcium and patients are usually considered to be hypocalcemic if the blood calcium level is less than 2.1 mmol/L or the ionized calcium level is less than 1.1 mmol/L. Serum ionized calcium concentrations are maintained within a very narrow range due to the close inter-relationship between serum ionized calcium, PTH, and vitamin D, and thus hypocalcemia is nearly always due to a deficiency of or resistance to PTH or vitamin D. If the parathyroid glands are functioning normally a deficiency or resistance to vitamin D will cause hypocalcemia, but this will result in elevated levels of PTH (secondary hyperparathyroidism) and so in this situation severe hypocalcemia is relatively unusual. Less commonly hypocalcemia may result from abnormal magnesium metabolism or to extravascular deposition of calcium, which can occur in several clinical situations. Mild hypocalcemia is frequently asymptomatic and is detected incidentally on routine testing.

The most common cause of hypocalcemia is post-surgical hypoparathyroidism which may result from the deliberate removal of parathyroid tissue for the treatment of hyperparathyroidism, or from the accidental removal of parathyroid tissue during a partial or total thyroidectomy. This was clearly the cause of hypocalcemia in Case 4.3. This patient had actually been started on calcium and vitamin D replacement post-operatively but had not taken the medication. Many patients will have transient hypocalcemia after thyroid surgery but far fewer will have long-standing hypocalcemia. Potential mechanisms for transient post-operative hypocalcemia include reversible damage to the parathyroids (peri-operative ischemia or hypothermia), release of calcitonin from the thyroid (calcitonin opposes the actions of PTH), or 'hungry bone syndrome' (in uncontrolled thyrotoxicosis there is increased bone turnover and hypercalcemia occurs frequently; once the thyroid hormone levels drop post-operatively this stimulus to increased bone turnover is removed and the bones, which are 'hungry' for calcium, avidly take up circulating calcium leading to humoral hypocalcemia). Autoimmune hypoparathyroidism and vitamin D deficiency are also encountered relatively frequently. The many causes of hypocalcemia are given in *Boxes 4.8* and *4.9* and the symptoms and signs are given in *Figure 4.17* and *Box 4.10.*

4.6.1 Hypoparathyroidism

Whilst post-surgical hypoparathyroidism is the commonest cause of hypocalcemia, there are numerous other causes of primary hypoparathyroidism (*Box 4.9*) including:

- autoimmunity
- developmental abnormalities
- hereditary metabolic disease
- infiltrative conditions
- metabolic disorders
- infectious causes

Figure 4.17. Symptoms of hypocalcemia.

COMMON SYMPTOMS	MANIFESTATIONS OF ACUTE HYPOCALCEMIA	CHRONIC MANIFESTATIONS
muscle cramps distal parasthesiae (pins and needles) shortness of breath (caused by bronchospasm) biliary and intestinal colic (caused by smooth muscle contraction) tetany confusion, hallucinations, and seizures are recognized Chvostek's and Trousseau's signs (see *Box 4.10*)	syncope (loss of consciousness) congestive heart failure	drying of the skin coarse hair pruritus (itching)

Box 4.8 | Causes of hypocalcemia

Low PTH (hypoparathyroidism)

- Post-surgery (thyroidectomy, parathyroidectomy, radical neck dissection)
- Radiation-induced destruction of the parathyroid glands
- Autoimmune polyglandular syndrome (associated with chronic mucocutaneous candidiasis and primary adrenal insufficiency)
- Isolated autoimmune hypoparathyroidism
- Abnormal parathyroid gland development
- DiGeorge syndrome
- Other genetic disorders (see *Box 4.9*)
- Hereditary metabolic disease: Wilson disease, hemochromatosis
- Hyper- or hypomagnesemia – (see below)
- Infiltration of the parathyroid gland (amyloidosis, granulomatous disease, iron overload, metastases)
- HIV infection
- Syphilis
- Abnormal PTH synthesis
- Isolated hypoparathyroidism due to activating antibodies to CaSR
- Activating mutations of CaSR (autosomal dominant hypocalcemia or sporadic isolated hypoparathyroidism)
- Hungry bone syndrome (post-parathyroidectomy)

High PTH (secondary hyperparathyroidism in response to hypocalcemia)

- Vitamin D deficiency or resistance
- PTH resistance
- Pseudohypoparathyroidism
- Hypomagnesemia (see below)
- Renal disease
- Hyperphosphatemia
- Tumor lysis
- Acute pancreatitis
- Osteoblastic metastases
- Acute respiratory alkalosis
- Sepsis or acute severe illness

Drugs

- Inhibitors of bone resorption (bisphosphonates, calcitonin), especially in vitamin D deficiency
- Cinacalcet (calcium mimetic)
- Calcium chelators (EDTA, citrate, phosphate)
- Foscarnet (due to intravascular complexing with calcium)
- Phenytoin (due to conversion of vitamin D to inactive metabolites)
- Fluoride poisoning

Disorders of magnesium metabolism

- Hypomagnesemia can reduce PTH secretion or cause PTH resistance and is therefore associated with normal, low, or high PTH levels

All of these causes result in low levels of PTH; the resultant biochemical abnormalities are therefore typically hypocalcemia and hyperphosphatemia.

Diagnosis, clinical features, and treatment of hypoparathyroidism

Diagnosis is biochemical: along with a low PTH level, patients will subsequently have low calcium and high phosphate levels which may be raised secondary to a decreased renal excretion, but alkaline phosphatase is typically normal. Hypocalcemia may manifest as a prolongation of the QT interval on the ECG. The clinical features are those of hypocalcemia (see *Figure 4.17*) although, like mild hypercalcemia, mild hypocalcemia is frequently asymptomatic and is detected incidentally on routine testing.

The mainstay of treatment in primary hypoparathyroidism centers around calcium and vitamin D replacement. Trials are taking place of a synthetic form of PTH called teriparatide, but this is not currently used in practice.

Box 4.9 | Genetic syndromes causing hypoparathyroidism

Autoimmune polyglandular syndrome

The occurrence of multiple autoimmune endocrinopathies in individuals has long been recognized and the genetics of some of these conditions is beginning to be understood.

Type 1 autoimmune polyglandular syndrome (APS-1) is an autosomal dominant condition caused by mutations in the *AIRE* (Autoimmune Regulator) gene. It is characterized by the development of Addison disease, autoimmune hypoparathyroidism, mucocutaneous candidiasis and ectodermal dysplasia.

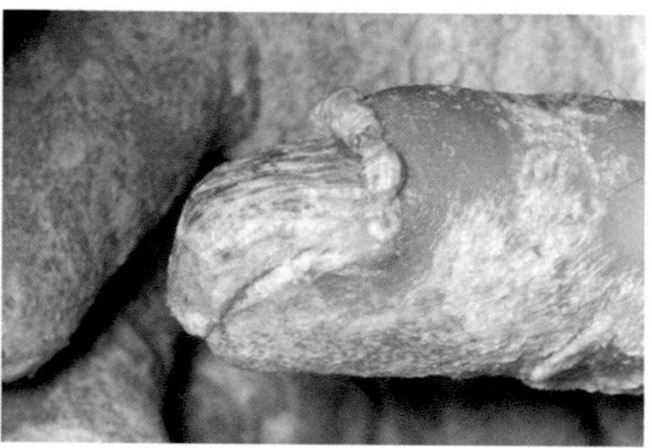

Box figure 4.6. Chronic infection of the skin with *Candida albicans* in a young patient with APS-1.

The condition develops in childhood and the major manifestations are normally apparent by the patient's twenties. In addition to the manifestations above, other autoimmune endocrinopathies can be seen including type 1 diabetes, pernicious anemia, vitiligo, and autoimmune hypogonadism.

APS-2 and APS-3 do not demonstrate monogenetic inheritance, although both show clear associations with HLA-DR3 and HLA-DR4. APS-2 describes the occurrence of autoimmune Addison disease in addition to either autoimmune hypothyroidism or type 1 diabetes. APS-3 describes the occurrence of autoimmune thyroid disease with one other autoimmune endocrinopathy in the absence of Addison disease. Autoimmune hypoparathyroidism may occur as a manifestation of either syndrome.

DiGeorge syndrome – 22q11.2 deletion syndrome, CATCH-22

The signs and symptoms of 22q11.2del syndrome are highly variable, even within affected members of the same family. Various names and descriptions (such as velo-cardio-facial syndrome, Shprintzen syndrome, DiGeorge syndrome, Sedlackova syndrome, and conotruncal anomaly face syndrome) are often used to describe what are almost certainly presentations of a single syndrome.

Features of 22q11.2del syndrome may include defects arising at birth including conotruncal heart defects, defects in the palate, most commonly related to neuromuscular problems with closure (velo-pharyngeal insufficiency), learning disabilities, mildly abnormal facial features, and recurrent infections (in some patients as a result of impaired T-cell mediated immune response due to an absent or hypoplastic thymus).

Developmental abnormalities of the neck may also cause hypoparathyroidism. The diagnosis of DiGeorge syndrome requires at least two of the following:

- cardiac abnormalities
- hypoparathyroidism and hypocalcemia
- thymic aplasia and immune deficiency.

22q11.2del syndrome may be first spotted when an affected newborn presents with hypocalcemia-induced convulsions associated with hypoparathyroidism.

The mnemonic CATCH-22 has been used to describe the features of DiGeorge syndrome, the 22 referring to the location of the genetic deletion abnormality:

Cardiac abnormality (especially tetralogy of Fallot)
Abnormal facies
Thymic aplasia
Cleft palate
Hypocalcemia.

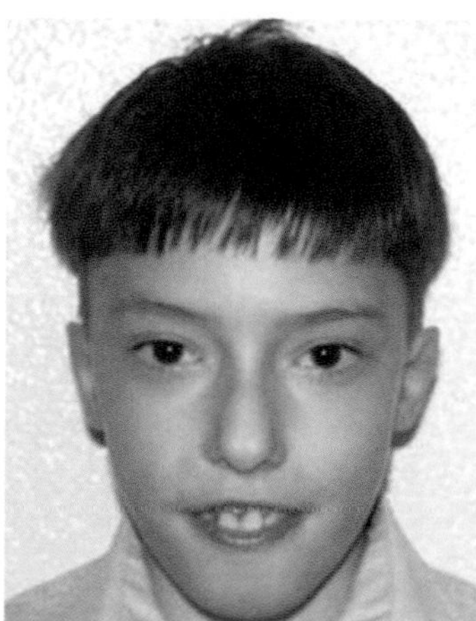

Box figure 4.7. Facial features of a patient with 22q11.2del syndrome.
Features include upslanted palpebral fissures, prominent nose with large tip and hypoplastic nares, small mouth with everted upper lip, and small dysmorphic ears. Reproduced from Digilio *et al.* (2005) *Images Paed. Cardiol.* with permission.

Box 4.10 | Neurological signs in hypocalcemia

Chvostek sign

Tapping over the area of the facial nerve anterior to the tragus results in twitching of the skin, initially at the angle of the mouth, then the nose, eye, and whole face as the calcium level falls.

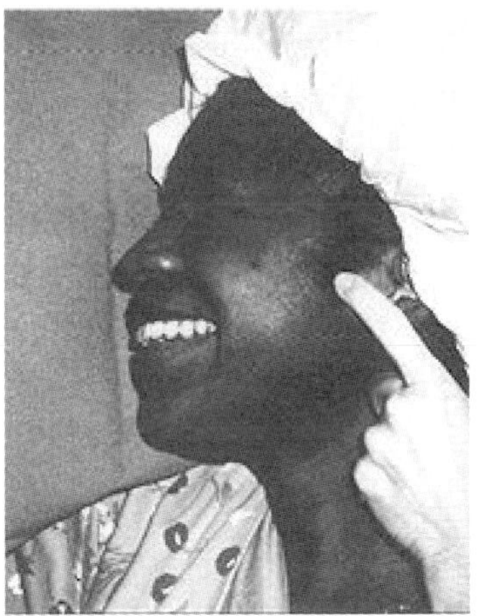

Box figure 4.8. Chvostek sign.

Trousseau sign

To elicit this sign, a blood pressure cuff is inflated to a pressure exceeding systolic blood pressure and held in place for about 3 minutes. Hypocalcemia-associated neuromuscular irritability will induce spasm of the muscles of the hand and forearm. The wrist and metacarpophalangeal joints flex, the distal interphalangeal (DIP) and proximal interphalangeal (PIP) joints extend, and the fingers adduct. The sign is also known as *main d'accoucheur* ('hand of the obstetrician') because it supposedly resembles the position of an obstetrician's hand in delivering a baby.

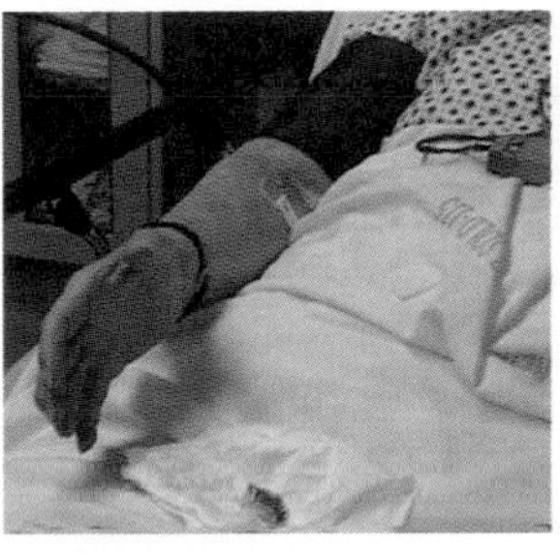

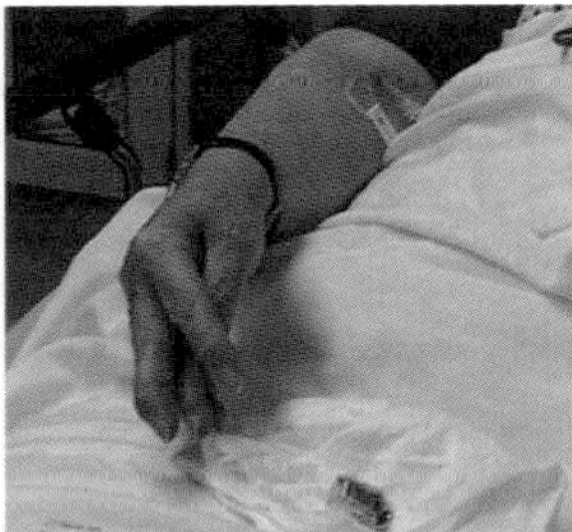

Box figure 4.9. Trousseau sign.

CASE 4.3 191 195

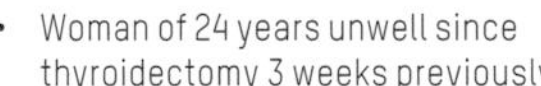

- Woman of 24 years unwell since thyroidectomy 3 weeks previously
- Low calcium, high phosphate, and low vitamin D
- Treatment was with calcium gluconate followed by calcium and vitamin D

The patient had presented acutely with severe symptomatic hypocalcemia secondary to acquired, post-surgical hypoparathyroidism. She was treated initially with 3 g of calcium gluconate given over 10 minutes, followed by an infusion of 5% dextrose containing 100 mL of 10% calcium gluconate. Once calcium levels were normalized, oral treatment with calcium and vitamin D was commenced (in this case as a combination tablet containing calcium 600 mg and vitamin D_3 400 IU; 4 tablets daily). Having had this frightening admission to hospital her compliance improved dramatically and she has remained normo-calcemic and asymptomatic since.

4.6.2 Pseudohypoparathyroidism

Mutations in the *GNAS1* gene encoding the PTH receptor (*Box 4.11*) result in resistance to the activity of circulating PTH. This gives rise to a biochemical picture similar to that seen in hypoparathyroidism, but with an elevated PTH secondary to the low serum calcium. The major presenting clinical features are those of hypocalcemia (*Figure 4.17*).

The syndrome can be divided into distinct subgroups dependent on the presence or absence of classical phenotypic abnormalities. Type 1a pseudohypoparathyroidism is

Box 4.11 | The *GNAS1* gene: pseudo- and pseudopseudo-hypoparathyroidism

In common with much of endocrinology, nomenclature seems designed to confuse. Pseudohypoparathyroidism describes a group of related disorders where there is end-organ (kidney/bone) resistance to the action of PTH; these disorders are characterized by low calcium, high PTH and high phosphate.

GNAS1 is a gene which encodes the alpha subunit of the G protein coupled to the PTH receptor. Mutations of *GNAS1* lead to an inability to activate adenyl cyclase on binding of PTH to the receptor and thus a lack of end-organ response.

The expression of the *GNAS1* gene is subject to imprinting, i.e. expression of the allele in a tissue is dependent on whether that allele is inherited from the mother or father. This is a form of epigenetic control of gene expression. In the case of *GNAS1* only the maternally inherited allele is expressed in the renal cortex. Inheritance of a maternal mutant allele results in type 1a pseudohypoparathyroidism (PHP type 1a) in which patients have the group of signs known as Albright hereditary osteodystrophy (AHO): round facies, obesity, short stature, developmental delay, short metacarpals, subcutaneous calcification, along with biochemical changes (high phosphate, low calcium, high PTH, hyperparathyroid bone disease). *GNAS1* is also expressed from the maternal allele in thyroid, gonads, and pituitary gland, so patients with PHP type 1a may also show resistance to TSH, LH, FSH, and GnRH.

Inheritance of a paternal mutant allele results in pseudopseudohypoparathyroidism, a clinical syndrome characterized by the same phenotypic abnormalities seen in PHP type 1a but in the absence of associated biochemical abnormalities. The explanation for this is that inheritance of the paternal mutant allele results in the characteristic phenotype, but the normal maternal allele maintains responsiveness in the kidneys to PTH so there is normal calcium homeostasis with normal levels of calcium, phosphate, and PTH.

Condition	Appearance	PTH levels	Calcium	Imprinting of *GNAS1* gene
Hypoparathyroidism	Skeletal defects	Low	Low	N/A
Pseudohypoparathyroidism type 1a	Skeletal defects	High	Low	Gene defect inherited from mother
Pseudopseudohypoparathyroidism	Skeletal defects	Normal	Normal	Gene defect inherited from father

PHP type 1b is characterized by hypocalcemia but no phenotypic abnormalities. It appears that the resistance to PTH here is confined to the kidneys and may be a result of mutations affecting the regulatory elements of *GNAS1* (rather than mutations of *GNAS1* itself). This is an autosomal recessive condition and is maternally inherited.

PHP type 2 does not have the phenotype of AHO. Patients have a normal (or elevated) urinary cyclic AMP response to PTH, but do not have the ability to excrete phosphate in response to PTH. The molecular defect has not been adequately described.

characterized by the presence of certain physical abnormalities (Albright hereditary osteodystrophy), most notably shortening of the 4th and 5th metacarpals and round facies. IQ can be mildly reduced. Type 1b pseudohypoparathyroidism is characterized by laboratory abnormalities in the absence of the classical phenotypic changes.

Patients have similar biochemical patterns to those with primary hypoparathyroidism, i.e. decreased serum and urinary calcium and increased serum phosphate. However, in pseudohypoparathyroidism the PTH is appropriately elevated in response to the hypocalcemia. Treatment of this disorder is similar to primary hypoparathyroidism and comprises vitamin D and calcium supplementation.

4.6.3 Vitamin D deficiency

Vitamin D deficiency is one of the most commonly occurring vitamin deficiencies. Biochemically it results in hypocalcemia whilst clinically it manifests as rickets in children and osteomalacia in adults. There are a variety of causes of vitamin D deficiency. The commonest causes result from a failure of the kidney to hydroxylate 25-hydroxyvitamin D to 1,25-dihydroxyvitamin D due to CKD and from inadequate formation of vitamin D in the skin due to limited sun exposure. These two causes explain the high incidence of vitamin D deficiency seen in patients with chronic kidney disease and in institutionalized individuals and in those from cultures (e.g. Islamic) where the body is kept covered. Less common causes of vitamin D deficiency are shown in *Box 4.12*.

Box 4.12 | Less common forms of vitamin D deficiency

- Malabsorption of dietary vitamin D
  - celiac disease
  - short bowel syndrome
  - cystic fibrosis
- Exclusive reliance on breast-feeding
  - occurs due to low amounts of vitamin D in breast milk
- Increased use of sunscreen
- Medications
  - phenobarbitol and rifampicin cause induction of cytochrome P450 enzymes which can result in increased catabolism of vitamin D
- Impaired C-25 hydroxylation (liver disease)
- Impaired C-1 hydroxylation (renal disease or type 1 vitamin D resistance)
- Target organ resistance (type 2 vitamin D resistance)

Diagnosis and treatment

Vitamin D deficiency is often detected following the incidental discovery of hypocalcemia. Biochemically, patients have decreased serum calcium, low vitamin D, and evidence of secondary hyperparathyroidism. Serum alkaline phosphatase is raised. Given the frequency of vitamin D deficiency in patients with CKD, serum creatinine and a calculated eGFR should be measured in all patients.

Vitamin D deficiency can be prevented by ensuring adequate sun exposure and sufficient dietary vitamin D intake. In certain groups (including breast-fed children, patients on drugs that adversely affect vitamin D metabolism, and patients with malabsorption) supplementation of the diet with exogenous vitamin D may also be necessary.

In developed vitamin D deficiency, high dose supplementation is needed to achieve adequate vitamin D replacement:

- in children 1000–2000 IU of vitamin D_3 in combination with calcium supplementation is normally adequate
- in adults with vitamin D deficiency secondary to inadequate sun exposure, 50 000 IU units of vitamin D weekly for a period of 8 weeks, followed by adequate daily oral supplementation to maintain the level, is usually sufficient
- in patients on drugs increasing catabolism of vitamin D, 50 000 IU of vitamin D should be given fortnightly for 8 weeks

- in patients with malabsorption, higher doses approaching 50 000 IU a day may be required.

Rickets

Vitamin D deficiency in children results in failure of developing skeletal tissue to ossify and this causes abnormal skeletal development. It has become uncommon in the developed world following the introduction of vitamin D supplementation for young infants. In the absence of malabsorption or infant-onset CKD, rickets is now usually seen only in children who are exclusively breast-fed or in children with dark skin and limited sun exposure. Rickets is still common in the developing world where access to vitamin D supplementation is limited.

The classical finding is bowing of the long bones in the legs, but abnormal development of all the major bones may occur including frontal bossing, kyphoscoliosis and chest wall deformities (*Figure 4.18*). Bone X-rays in patients with rickets demonstrate several classical abnormalities: radiographs of the metaphyses of long bones display characteristic widening and cupping, and a chest X-ray may show evidence of the classical rachitic rosary caused by prominent knobs of bone at the costochondral junctions as a result of failure of mineralization of the cartilage secondary to hypocalcemia.

Supplementation of calcium and vitamin D form the mainstay of the treatment of rickets, but surgical intervention may be necessary when severe abnormalities of skeletal growth have occurred.

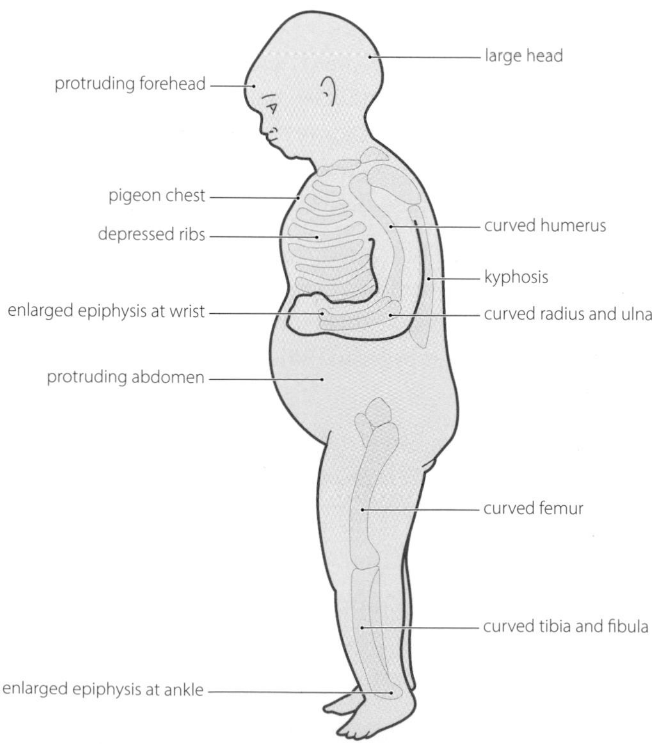

Figure 4.18. Abnormal development of bones in children with rickets.

Differential diagnosis. The following alternative causes of rickets in children should be considered:

- use of formula milk that is not fortified with appropriate minerals can result in severe phosphate deficiency which can manifest as rickets because phosphate is essential for bone mineralization
- hypophosphatemic vitamin D-resistant rickets is a genetic condition with an X-linked dominant pattern of inheritance. Mutations in the *PHEX* gene are thought to result in increased proteolysis of the MEPES extracellular matrix glycoprotein; the C-terminal peptide element of this glycoprotein causes excessive renal tubular phosphate excretion in the proximal renal tubule.

Osteomalacia

CASE 4.4 199 200

- European Caucasian woman of 44 years with 3 month history of bone pain and muscle weakness
- Mild anemia, low calcium, very high alkaline phosphatise and very low vitamin D
- DEXA scan revealed a T-score of -3.5
- Underlying celiac disease with high IgA/IgG antibodies resulting in impaired vitamin D absorption

A 44 year old Caucasian European woman presented with a 3 month history of diffuse, rather non-specific bone pain and proximal muscular weakness, mainly in the lower extremities and to a lesser extent in both shoulders. She now sought help because she was finding it increasingly difficult to get out of her chair, to hold her arms up to comb her hair (i.e. raising her hands above the level of her shoulders), and to walk upstairs.

Clinical examination showed evidence of bilateral, proximal muscle atrophy and weakness in the upper and lower extremities, and hypoactive reflexes in four extremities. Her hip range of motion was limited and painful. She had a waddling gait pattern. Laboratory workup revealed:

- Hb: 9.8 g/dL (NR 11.5–15) – a microcytic anemia
- MCV: 66 fL (NR 78–96)
- calcium: 1.8 mmol/L (NR 2.2–2.58)
- alkaline phosphatase: 650 U/L (NR 50–110)
- vitamin D (25-hydroxyvitamin D): 6 nmol/L (NR 60–105)

Other laboratory investigations were normal, including erythrocyte sedimentation rate (ESR), C-reactive protein (CRP), thyroid function tests, and creatinine kinase.

Bone mineral density using dual energy X-ray absorptiometry (DEXA) scan (*Box 4.15*) was requested and T-score measurements were low (3.5 SD below the mean at the femoral neck and 2.5 SD below the mean at the lumbar spine). A T-score compares bone density to the optimal peak bone density for gender. It is reported as number of standard deviations below the average: a T-score of greater than -1 is considered normal; a T-score of -1 to -2.5 is considered osteopenia, and at risk for developing osteoporosis; a T-score of less than -2.5 is diagnostic of osteoporosis.

A diagnosis of osteomalacia was made. Investigations for malabsorption were carried out and IgA antiendomysial antibody and antigliadin IgA and IgG antibodies were found to be elevated (high levels of these antibodies are highly suggestive of a diagnosis of celiac disease).

When vitamin D deficiency and subsequent failure to ossify bones occurs in adulthood the clinical syndrome of osteomalacia results. CKD and inadequate sun exposure are the commonest underlying pathologies, although malabsorption syndromes are also diagnosed. Unlike rickets, the metaphyseal growth plates are not affected and abnormalities arise instead from hypo-mineralization of trabecular and cortical bone. Vitamin D deficiency in patients with CKD contributes to the pathophysiology of renal osteodystrophy. Supplementation of vitamin D and calcium and treatment of the underlying cause of vitamin D deficiency are the mainstay of the treatment of osteomalacia.

The initial presentation is insidious with the development of non-specific bone pain, particularly in the back, pelvis and long bones of the leg. Further manifestations are a proximal myopathy, bowing of the legs, fractures, and features of hypocalcemia. The diagnosis may be made following a presentation with pathological fractures, whilst a significant number of patients are diagnosed incidentally where the only apparent symptom is fatigue. In addition to the biochemical changes seen in patients with vitamin D deficiency, several radiographic changes are seen in osteomalacia, particularly osteopenia and coarsening of trabecular bone. Looser zones may also be seen and these are pathognomonic of osteomalacia; they are pseudofractures which appear as thin, translucent bands, about 2 mm wide, running perpendicular to the surface of the bone extending from the cortex inwards (*Figure 4.19*) Essentially, Looser zones are incomplete stress fractures which heal with callus lacking in calcium; they are most frequently seen in the pubic rami, the necks of the humeri and femora and at the axillary edge of the scapulae.

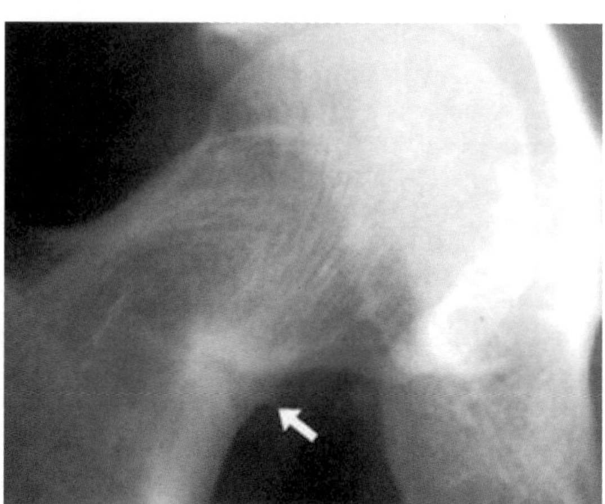

Figure 4.19. Looser zone (arrow) seen in the femoral neck of a patient with osteomalacia.

CASE 4.4 199 200

- European Caucasian woman of 44 years with 3 month history of bone pain and muscle weakness
- Mild anemia, low calcium, very high alkaline phosphatise and very low vitamin D
- DEXA scan revealed a T-score of -3.5
- Osteomalacia treated with vitamin D injections

The patient in Case 4.4 was somewhat unusual in that she had underlying celiac disease characterized by elevated IgA antiendomysial antibody and antigliadin IgA and IgG antibodies resulting in impaired vitamin D absorption.

In osteomalacia the treatment is aimed at normalizing vitamin D levels, usually with oral vitamin D replacement. In situations where absorption of vitamin D is impaired, intramuscular preparations are often used, and this patient was treated with an intramuscular injection of 300 000 U of ergocalciferol (vitamin D_2), repeated after 3 months.

Vitamin D excess

Excessive vitamin D supplementation can result in hypervitaminosis D and this is nearly always a result of either a prescribed or an over-the-counter medication rather than excessive dietary intake. An intake of greater than 15 000 μg/day (600 000 IU per day) for a period of weeks or months can result in hypervitaminosis D. Clinically the syndrome is manifested by the development of hypercalcemia and the attendant symptoms. Biochemically, patients demonstrate raised vitamin D levels and suppression of PTH secondary to the hypercalcemia. The immediate treatment is directed at lowering serum calcium: cessation of supplementation allows vitamin D levels to return to normal.

4.7 Metabolic bone disease

Metabolic bone disease is a term used to describe a range of conditions which cause bones to become fragile, increasing the risk of fracture. Osteomalacia, characterized by lack of bone mineralization resulting from vitamin D deficiency, was described above, and so this section will concentrate on the other metabolic bone diseases osteoporosis and Paget disease. An extremely rare inherited disorder known as osteopetrosis, literally meaning 'stone bone,' contrasts with the more common osteoporosis and osteomalacia in that patients with osteopetrosis have bones which harden and become more dense. They are, however, still prone to fracture because they become so brittle. Further details of this condition are given in *Box 4.13.*

Box 4.13 | Osteopetrosis

Osteopetrosis is a rare inherited condition caused by inadequate osteoclast mediated resorption and remodeling of bone (*Box 4.1*). In contrast to osteoporosis, the bones become extremely dense; however, the result is extremely brittle bone that is prone to fracture. Adult, infantile, and intermediate forms of the disease are described.

Infantile and intermediate onset osteopetrosis

Infantile osteopetrosis is normally diagnosed before the age of 1. The genetic defect causing infantile osteopetrosis has not been identified but the disease shows an autosomal recessive pattern of inheritance. It is associated with growth retardation, cranial nerve lesions caused by abnormal bone growth and bone marrow failure as the marrow space is replaced by abnormal osseous tissue. Bone marrow failure can result in extra-medullary hematopoiesis and the development of hepatosplenomegaly (enlargement of liver and spleen). The fracture risk is very high due to the abnormal structure of the bone and the overall prognosis is poor.

Intermediate disease occurs in childhood and also demonstrates an autosomal recessive pattern of inheritance. Although bone marrow failure does not occur, the overall prognosis remains poor.

Adult onset osteopetrosis

Adult osteopetrosis is inherited in an autosomal dominant fashion and follows a more benign course. It is often diagnosed incidentally following the discovery of abnormal-looking bone on radiographs. It is subdivided into type 1 and type 2 adult onset osteopetrosis. Type 1 adult onset osteopetrosis is caused by mutations in the *LPR5* gene and results in an increase in bone mass but without impairment of osteoclast activity. The skull vault is the main site of abnormal bone and the risk of fractures is low. In type 2 adult onset osteopetrosis the skull base, spine, and pelvis may be involved and the risk of fractures is high. Spinal X-rays of patients with type 2 adult onset osteopetrosis show a characteristic rugby jersey appearance. Bone marrow failure is not a feature of type 1 or type 2 adult onset osteopetrosis.

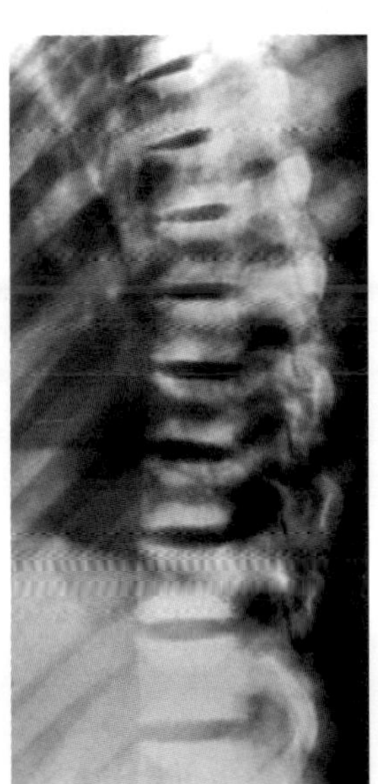

Box figure 4.10. Lateral spine X-ray in a young patient with osteopetrosis.
The X-ray shows vertebral end-plate thickening, referred to as rugby jersey spine – the vertebral bodies have broad stripes reminiscent of a rugby shirt.

Box 4.13 | continued

Diagnosis and treatment of osteopetrosis

Bone radiographs are normally diagnostic of osteopetrosis.

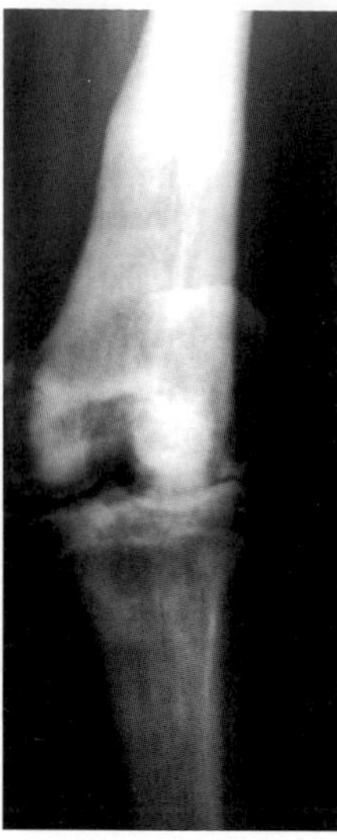

Box figure 4.11. Anteroposterior radiograph of the knee in a patient with osteopetrosis demonstrating generalized sclerosis and osteoarthritis.

Alkaline phosphatase is elevated in both infantile and type 2 adult onset osteopetrosis but may be normal in type 1 adult onset disease.

Adult onset disease requires no specific treatment, although supportive care is needed where complications such as fractures arise. A variety of treatments have been trialled in infantile osteopetrosis. High-dose vitamin D has been used to stimulate osteoclast activity and increase bone resorption. Interferon-γ has been used to stimulate white blood cell production and has been shown to significantly reduce the risk of infection. Erythropoietin has been used to reduce the incidence of anemia. Surgical intervention is sometimes necessary to treat fractures. A subset of patients with infantile osteopetrosis have disease caused by failure of the osteoclast lineage of cells to mature appropriately; such patients can be cured with bone marrow transplantation.

4.7.1 Osteoporosis

Osteoporosis is a disorder caused by loss of bone mass throughout the skeleton, accompanied by abnormal bone architecture and an increased risk of fractures. In contrast with osteomalacia, bone matrix (osteoid) is lost in addition to lack of bone mineralization. It is the commonest acquired bone disorder and the commonest cause of fractures in adults. Almost 33% of women and 20% percent of men over the age of 50 will have an osteoporotic fracture at some point in their lifetime. Vertebral and hip fractures are the most commonly encountered, with hip fractures a cause of significant morbidity and mortality.

Causes

The underlying cause of osteoporosis is excessive resorption of bone by osteoclasts at a rate that outstrips bone production by osteoblasts (*Box 4.1*). The excessive resorption results in decreased bone mass and, combined with incomplete remodeling, results in a distortion of bone architecture. Estrogen deficiency, normally as a result of the menopause, is the commonest underlying defect in osteoporosis, although other secondary causes (*Box 4.14*) must be sought and treated in all patients with osteoporosis.

Estrogen deficiency results in increased production of RANK ligand by osteoblasts (*Figure 4.7*). RANK ligand causes proliferation and maturation of osteoclast precursors and results in increased osteoclast activity and loss of bone mass. A wide variety of other factors can contribute to the pathogenesis of osteoporosis. Patients with low peak bone mass, impaired absorption of calcium, or other coexisting metabolic bone diseases such as hyperparathyroidism, are at higher risk of developing osteoporosis. Long-term use of steroidal anti-inflammatories (i.e.

Box 4.14 | Causes of secondary osteoporosis

- Endocrine disorders:
  - hyperparathyroidism
  - hyperthyroidism
  - hypogonadism
  - Cushing disease
  - adrenal insufficiency
  - vitamin D deficiency
- Gastrointestinal diseases:
  - inflammatory bowel disease
  - celiac disease
  - anorexia nervosa
  - chronic liver disease
- Chronic kidney disease
- Rheumatological diseases:
  - systemic lupus erythematosus
  - rheumatoid arthritis
- Hematological disease:
  - myeloma
  - thalassemia
- Inherited conditions:
  - cystic fibrosis
  - osteogenesis imperfecta
  - Marfan syndrome
  - Ehlers–Danlos syndrome
- Medication use:
  - oral steroids
  - phenytoin
  - heparin (long-term use)
  - hormonal therapies causing hypogonadism
  - excessive thyroxine replacement therapy
  - lithium
  - aromatase inhibitors

glucocorticoids) inhibits osteoblast activity and increases the risk of osteoporosis, so patients using oral glucocorticoids for prolonged periods should be given preventative therapy with bisphosphonates to lower this risk.

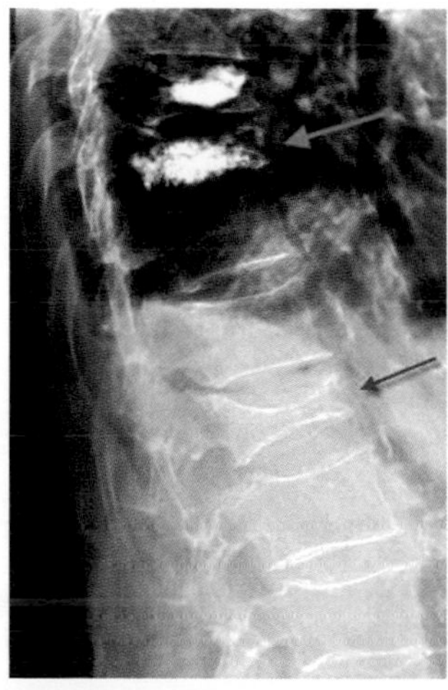

Figure 4.20. Crush fracture of the lumbar spine in osteoporosis. The red arrow indicates the lumbar vertebral crush fracture and the green arrow shows an area where treatment has been initiated; in this case a kyphoplasty where an inert filler material has been injected into the damaged vertebrae.

Symptoms

Osteoporosis is asymptomatic until complications occur. Fractures occurring following minimal trauma should raise the suspicion of underlying osteoporosis. The hip and vertebrae are the most common sites of significant fracture but fractures can occur at any site. Vertebral fractures may be asymptomatic or accompanied by the development of acute back pain which may resolve over 4–6 weeks. Multiple osteoporotic vertebral fractures can cause significant spinal deformities and patients may develop marked kyphoscoliosis (abnormal curvature of the spine).

Diagnosis

Measuring bone density by DEXA scanning (*Box 4.15*) is the mainstay of the diagnostic process. Routine practice is to measure bone density at the hip and vertebrae. T-scores (as explained in Case 4.4 in *Section 4.6.3*) between -1 and -2.5 establish the diagnosis of osteopenia and place the patient at risk of progression to established osteoporosis. A T-score below -2.5 establishes the diagnosis of osteoporosis. DEXA scanning should be undertaken in all women over 65 and men over 70, in patients aged over 55 with a significant risk factor for the development of osteoporosis, and in patients who present with fragility fractures. In severe osteoporosis bones may appear thin even on plain radiographs. Spinal radiographs may demonstrate osteoporotic vertebral crush fractures (*Figure 4.20*).

Laboratory testing is undertaken to look for evidence of secondary osteoporosis and should, routinely, include measurement of the bone profile, thyroid function tests, and PTH levels. Where appropriate, testing for other secondary causes (*Box 4.14*) should also be undertaken. In *primary* osteoporosis, measurements of calcium, PTH and alkaline phosphatase are all within normal ranges.

Box 4.15 | DEXA scanning

Dual-energy X-ray absorptiometry (DEXA) is an imaging technique which can be used to measure bone density. The hip and vertebrae are the most commonly assessed sites. Two results are generated at each site:

- Z-score – reports a patient's bone density relative to reference data for individuals of the same age and gender
- T-score – compares the patient's bone density to a population reference value of peak bone mass.

T-scores are used in making the diagnosis of osteoporosis and osteopenia. Normal bone density is considered to be a T-score greater than -1 (within 1 standard deviation of the population mean).

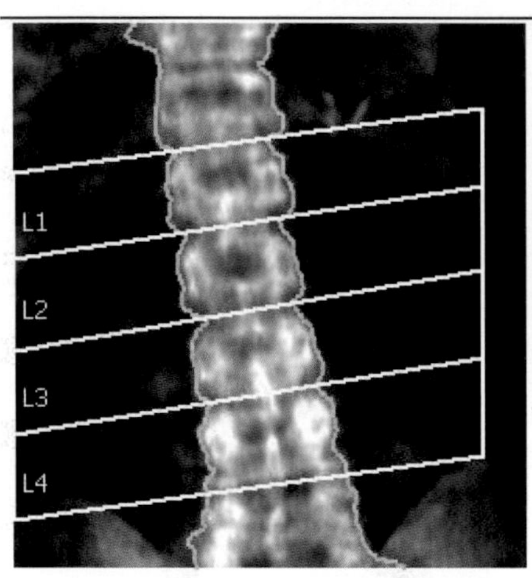

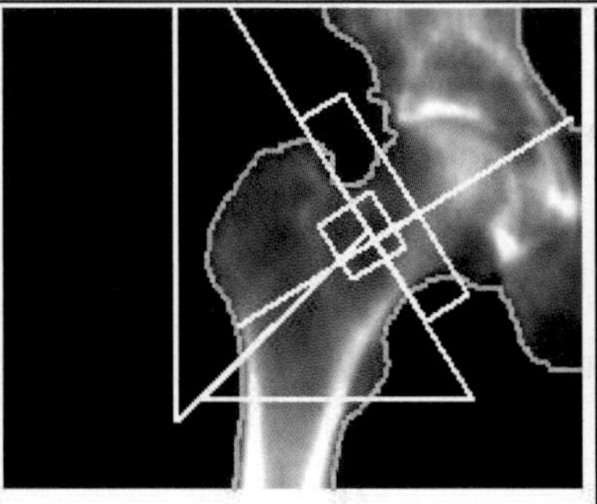

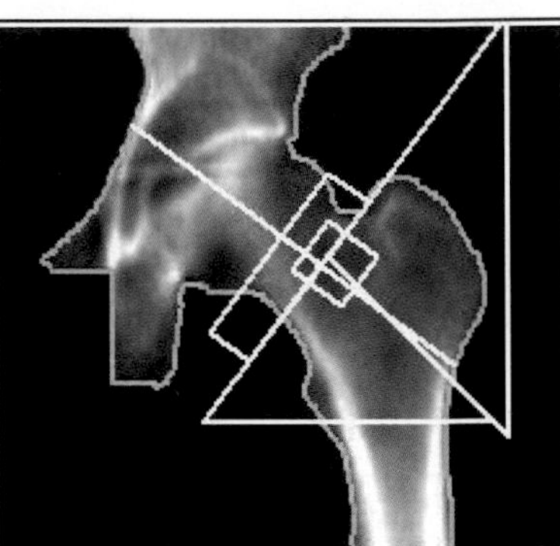

Image not for diagnosis

HAL chart results unavailable

Image not for diagnosis

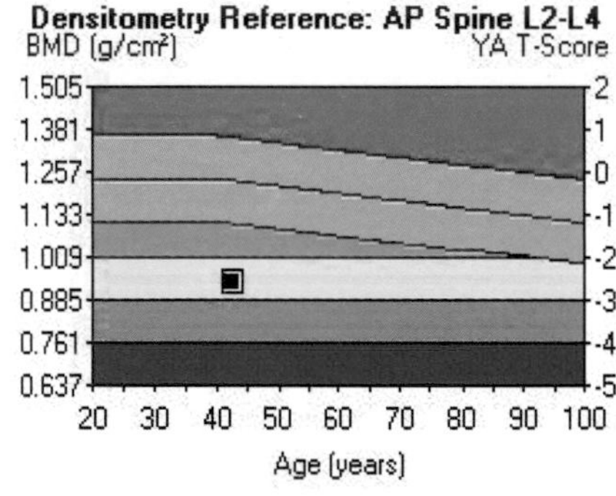

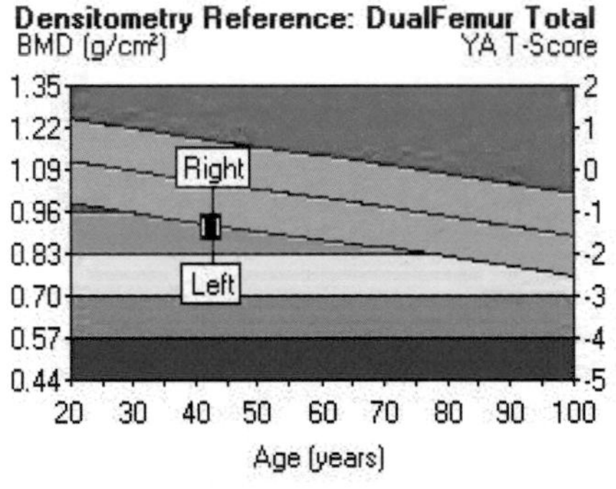

Region	BMD[1] (g/cm²)	Young-Adult[2,7] T-Score	Age-Matched[3] Z-Score	WHO Classification[11]
AP Spine L2-L4	0.937	-2.6	-2.5	-
DualFemur Total				
Left	0.913	-1.4	-1.1	-
Right	0.918	-1.3	-1.0	-
Mean	0.916	-1.3	-1.0	-
Difference	0.005	0.0	0.0	-

Box figure 4.12. DEXA scans of hip and spine.

In the spine the T-score is -2.6, indicative of osteoporosis.

Treatment of osteoporosis

Preventative treatment is indicated in all patients at risk of developing osteoporosis. Calcium and vitamin D should be measured and replaced if indicated. Patients should be encouraged to undertake regular weight-bearing exercise which promotes bone formation. Smoking and excessive alcohol intake are significant risk factors for development of osteoporosis and should be discouraged. Consideration should be given to prophylactic treatment of patients using long-term steroids with bisphosphonates.

Bisphosphonates (*Box 4.7*) are the major drug class used in the treatment of osteoporosis, with the most commonly used, risedronate and alendronate, being taken once weekly. Patients intolerant of oral therapy can be given an annual infusion of zolendronic acid. These three drugs have all been shown to reduce the risk of both hip and vertebral fracture. Bisphosphonates accumulate in the bone matrix where they subsequently enter osteoclasts and cause inhibition of binding to bone and early cell death. Vitamin D and calcium should be replaced in all patients initiated on bisphosphonate therapy.

In patients intolerant of, or with a contraindication to bisphosphonate therapy, a variety of other therapies are available (*Table 4.2*). Hormone replacement therapy (HRT) was once the treatment of choice in post-menopausal osteoporosis and is the only alternative class of therapy shown to reduce the incidence of both hip and vertebral fractures. However, several large scale trials have demonstrated significant cardiovascular risk as well as increased risk of cancer in patients using these therapies for a protracted period well after the menopause. Despite these risks HRT remains a treatment option for some patients, particularly those with marked coincident menopausal symptoms or those women who have had an early menopause; HRT is almost certainly safe in women until about 2 years after the mean age of the menopause (approximately 52 years in the USA and UK).

Selective estrogen receptor modulators (SERMs) cause an increase in bone mass without the attendant cardiovascular risks of HRT and the anabolic agent teriparatide (a recombinant form of PTH) also promotes an increase in bone mass. Both of these classes of agents have been shown to decrease the incidence of vertebral but not hip fracture. Calcitonin inhibits bone resorption through a direct effect on osteoclasts and has also been shown to reduce vertebral fracture rates, but with only a small effect on bone mineral density.

Other therapeutic agents used in osteoporosis include strontium and denosumab. Strontium inhibits bone resorption and also promotes bone formation; initial studies have shown a significant reduction in all fracture rates and an increase in bone mineral density after 1–3 years of treatment. Denosumab is a human monoclonal antibody directed against RANK ligand (*Figure 4.7*) that inhibits osteoclast activation in much the same way as the endogenous protein, osteoprotegrin. It must be given only 6-monthly and initial data suggest that it is more efficacious than bisphosphonates in increasing bone mineral density and reducing markers of bone turnover, further studies are awaited.

4.7.2 Paget disease of bone

Paget disease of bone (named after Sir James Paget, a surgeon from St Bartholomew's Hospital, London) results from excessive bone remodeling at specific sites, leading to

Table 4.2. **Prevention and treatment of osteoporosis**

Drug	Dosage	Osteoporosis indications	Effective in fracture reduction (+/–)		
			Vertebral	Hip	Non-vertebral
Estrogen	0.625 mg by mouth daily, variable dose patches, gels, and creams	Prevention of PMO*	+	+	+
Selective estrogen receptor modulators					
Raloxifene (Evista)	60 mg by mouth daily	Prevention and treatment of PMO*	+	–	–
Calcitonin (Miacalcin)					
Fortica	200 IU intranasally daily	Treatment of PMO*			
Calcima	100 IU subcutaneously daily	(>5 years past menopause)	+	–	–
	100 IU subcutaneously or intramuscularly daily				
Bisphosphonates					
Alendronate (Fosamax)	5 mg by mouth daily, **35 mg by mouth weekly,** 10 mg by mouth daily, or **70 mg by mouth weekly**	Prevention and treatment of PMO* and osteoporosis in men	+	+	+
Risedronate (Actonel)	5 mg by mouth daily, **35 mg by mouth weekly, 75 mg by mouth twice monthly**, or **150 mg by mouth monthly**	Prevention and treatment of PMO* and osteoporosis in men; Prevention and treatment of GIO†	+	+	+
Ibandronate (Boniva)	2.5 mg by mouth daily, 150 mg by mouth monthly, or 3 mg IV every 3 months	Prevention and treatment of PMO*	+	+	+
Zoledronate (Reclast)	**5 mg IV yearly**	Treatment of PMO*; in patients at high risk of fracture defined as a recent low-trauma hip fracture to reduce clinical fractures	+	+	+
Recombinant human parathyroid hormone (1-34)					
Teriparatide (Forteo)	20 mg subcutaneously daily	Treatment of PMO* and men with osteoporosis who are at high risk for fracture	+	NA	+

* PMO - post-menopausal osteoporosis.

†GIO - glucocorticoid-induced osteoporosis.

bone overgrowth and relative weakness of affected bone. After osteoporosis it is the second most common bone disease. True prevalence figures are difficult to ascertain because many cases remain asymptomatic, but it probably affects 1–2% of the population in the USA and UK. Sex distribution is equal and incidence increases with age. Diagnosis is extremely rare before the age of 40, although a juvenile form called idiopathic hyperphosphatasia has the same development of fragile and deformed bone as found in Paget's. The condition seems to have a predilection for Anglo-Saxon heritage, and is far less common in India and Asia.

The etiology is unclear, but population studies support a genetic cause (with first-degree relatives of an affected patient having about a ten-fold increased risk of developing the condition) and many families appear to show an autosomal dominant form of inheritance. Candidate genetic loci have been identified on chromosomes 5, 6, and 18, and mutations have been demonstrated in the *SQSTM1* gene which encodes a p62 protein (sequestosome 1). A viral etiology has also been postulated because viral material has been identified in osteoclasts from patients with Paget's, possibly from the paramyxoviridae family. Other studies suggest a link with the canine distemper virus and the measles virus.

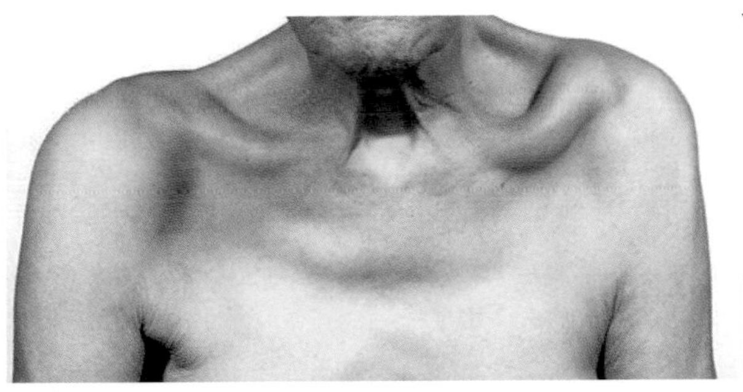

(a)

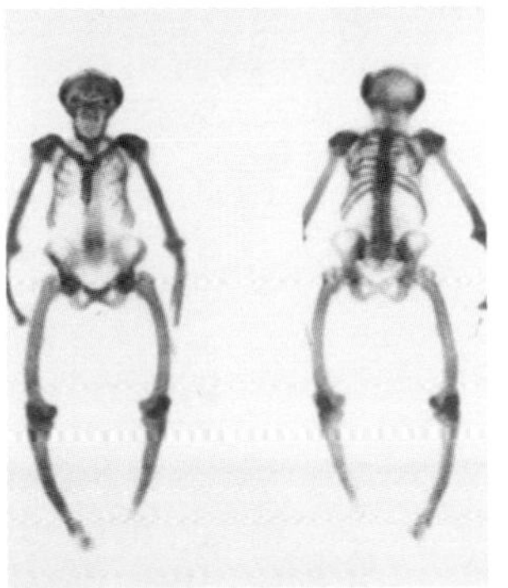

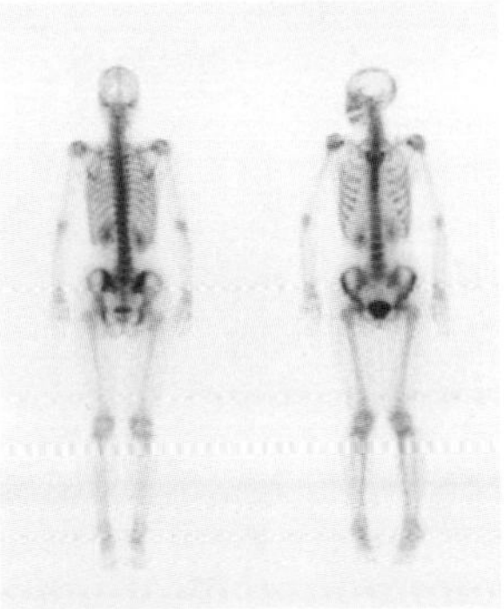

(b)

Figure 4.21. Skeletal deformities resulting from Paget disease.
(a) A patient with Paget disease. (b) A 67-year-old woman with a 20-year history of Paget disease of bone, resulting in conductive hearing loss, bone and joint pains, pathologic fractures, limb deformities, and difficulty walking. Treatment with calcitonin and etidronate had been unsuccessful. The left-hand panel shows anterior and posterior images from a bone scan obtained after the administration of [99m] technetium-labeled methylene diphosphonate. The markedly increased accumulation of radionuclide in almost the entire skeleton, sparing only the distal extremities, reflects the increased bone turnover in Paget disease. The bowing deformity of the long bones is typical of the disease. The right-hand panel shows a normal bone scan for comparison.

Clinical features

The majority of patients will be asymptomatic and diagnosed in the search for a reason behind a raised alkaline phosphatase or after an abnormality seen on an X-ray undertaken for an unrelated reason (*Figure 4.21*). Those patients who are symptomatic commonly present with pain and/or deformities in the affected areas (most commonly pelvis, spine, skull, and long bones). Other symptoms include fractures, bone tumors, bleeding from hypervascular bone (e.g. in orthopedic procedures), cardiac and neurological disease, and abnormalities of calcium/phosphate.

Diagnosis of Paget disease of bone

The diagnosis may be based on clinical suspicion of a patient presenting with a range of clinical features (*Table 4.3*). More frequently the diagnosis is made serendipitously after noting classical features on an X-ray or discovering an elevated alkaline phosphatase in someone without liver disease. Biochemical features include high

Table 4.3. **Clinical features of Paget disease of bone**

Pain
- may be due to periosteal stretching or microfractures
- may be due to associated nerve trapping, osteosarcoma, degenerative arthritis

Deformity
- long bones – resulting in bowing especially of tibia and fibula
- skull – 'osteoporosis circumscripta', leading to lucency on X-ray – followed by enlargement of the frontal and occipital areas

Fractures
- either traumatic or pathologic
- most commonly in femur, followed by upper third of tibia
- may be associated with excessive blood loss due to hyperemia of bone

Tumors
- occur in about 1% of Paget cases
- osteosarcomas are most common
- poor survival rate – approximately 15% five-year survival
- benign giant cell tumors may occur (osteoclastomas) – usually skull and facial bones

Neurological complications
- caused by nerve compression by enlarging bone
- 8th cranial nerve in the skull often affected – leads to hearing loss
- 2nd, 5th and 7th cranial nerves may also be affected (visual disturbance and facial palsy)
- spinal involvement may cause root impingement or ischemic myelitis as blood is diverted to hyperemic bone
- hydrocephalus may occur following blockage of the aqueduct of Sylvius in the skull base

Cardiac complications
- heart failure (high output)
- possible increased incidence of calcific aortic stenosis
- conduction defects

Defects of calcium and phosphate
- levels of calcium are usually normal in Paget disease but may increase on immobilization due to increased bone resorption.

alkaline phosphatase, normal calcium, and normal vitamin D (alkaline phosphatase levels are also high in osteomalacia, but with concurrent vitamin D deficiency). A nuclear medicine bone scan can accurately demonstrate 'hotspots', i.e. areas of affected bone with markedly higher radionuclide uptake, and X-rays of affected areas can help to differentiate these hotspots from areas of metastatic disease.

Treatment of Paget disease of bone

The aim of treatment is to reduce the rate of bone remodeling and to give adequate pain relief. The mainstay of treatment is with nitrogen-containing bisphosphonates (*Box 4.5*) which almost certainly prevent the development of a number of long-term complications of the condition, including bony deformity, pathological fractures, osteoarthritis, and some neurological deficits (e.g. deafness). Because of the risk of hypocalcemia with bisphosphonate therapy, additional calcium and vitamin D supplementation should be co-prescribed (about 800 IU of vitamin D per day, and 1200 mg of calcium). The efficacy of treatment can be monitored by serial measurements of alkaline phosphatase (which should drop toward the normal range) and, if indicated, by serial X-rays or bone scans. A second line therapy (if patients are intolerant of bisphosphonates) is calcitonin which may be given orally or by intranasal spray.

4.8 Further reading

Adams JS and Hewison M (2010) Update in Vitamin D. *Endojournals,* **95:** 471–8.

Adler JT, Meyer-Rochow GY, Chen H, *et al.* (2008) Pheochromocytoma: current approaches and future directions. *The Oncologist,* **13:** 779–93.

Bergwitz C and Juppner H (2010) Regulation of phosphate homeostasis by PTH, vitamin D, and FGF23. *Ann. Rev. Med.* **61:** 91–104.

Compston J (2009) Clinical and therapeutic aspects of osteoporosis. *Eur. J. Radiol.* **71:** 388–91.

Felger EA and Kandil E (2010) Primary hyperparathyroidism. *Otolaryngol. Clin. N. Am.* **43:** 417–32.

Fraser WD (2009) Hyperparathyroidism. *Lancet,* **374:** 145–58.

Iglesias P and Diez JJ (2009) Current treatments in the management of patients with primary hyperparathyroidism. *Postgrad. Med. J.* **85:** 15–23.

Lewiecki EM (2011) In the clinic. Osteoporosis. *Annals Int. Med.* **155:** 1–16.

Norman AW (2008) From vitamin D to hormones D: fundamentals of the vitamin D endocrine system essential for good health. *Am. J. Clin. Nutr.* **88:** 491S–9S.

Pearce SH and Cheetham TD (2010) Diagnosis and management of vitamin D deficiency. *Br. Med. J.* **340:** 142–6.

Poole KES and Compton JE (2006) Osteoporosis and its management. *Br. Med. J.* **333:** 1251–6.

Raggat LJ and Partridge NC (2010) Cellular and molecular mechanisms of bone remodeling. *J. Biol. Chem.* **285:** 103–8.

Razzaque MS (2009) The FGF23–Klotho axis: endocrine regulation of phosphate homeostasis. *Nature Rev. Endocrinol.* **5:** 611–9.

Riccardi D and Brown EM (2009) Physiology and pathophysiology of the calcium-sensing receptor in the kidney. *Am. J. Physiol. Renal Physiol.* **298:** 485–99.

Roodman GD (2010) Insights into the pathogenesis of Paget's disease. *Annals New York Acad. Sci.* **1192:** 176–80.

4.9 Self-assessment questions

(1) A 58 year old retired army officer has developed chronic kidney disease and as a consequence has impaired production of 1,25-dihydroxyvitamin D. Which of the following biochemical tests is most likely to be associated with his vitamin D deficiency?
- (a) Severe hypocalcemia
- (b) Raised levels of parathyroid hormone
- (c) Hypercalcemia
- (d) Hypercalciuria
- (e) Suppressed parathyroid hormone levels

(2) A 26 year old Asian lady presented with a marked peripheral myopathy, osteomalacia, mild hypocalcemia, hypophosphatemia, and hyperchloremic acidosis. Which of the following would best explain these clinical features?
- (a) Hypoparathyroidism and vitamin D resistance
- (b) Vitamin D excess
- (c) Malignancy
- (d) Vitamin D deficiency with secondary hyperparathyroidism
- (e) Pseudohyperparathyroidism

(3) Primary hyperparathyroidism:
- (a) Is a rare cause of hypercalcemia
- (b) Is always associated with a parathyroid adenoma
- (c) Is always associated with vitamin D deficiency
- (d) Is an important cause of osteoporosis
- (e) Is never familial

(4) What stimulates parathyroid hormone secretion?
- (a) Raised levels of serum calcium
- (b) Raised levels of 1,25-dihydroxyvitamin D
- (c) Hyperchloremic acidosis
- (d) Vitamin D deficiency
- (e) Increased phosphate excretion

(5) Which one of the following is contraindicated in the treatment of hypercalcemia associated with malignancy?
- (a) Fluid restriction
- (b) Bisphosphonates
- (c) Loop diuretics
- (d) Steroids
- (e) Hemodialysis

(6) RANK ligand
- (a) is induced on osteoclasts by parathyroid hormone
- (b) is inhibited by osteoprotogerin
- (c) is inhibited by 1,25-dihydroxyvitamin D
- (d) directly activates a transcription factor
- (e) stimulates RANK on osteoblasts

(7) Hypocalcemia causes
 (a) a decrease in 1,25-dihydroxyvitamin D
 (b) decreased bone resorption
 (c) reduced FGF23 secretion
 (d) increased phosphate excretion
 (e) decreased 1α-hydroxylase activity

(8) Which one of the following cause primary hyperparathyroidism?
 (a) Malignancy
 (b) Vitamin D intoxication
 (c) Multiple endocrine neoplasia type 1 (MEN-1)
 (d) Chronic granulomatous disorders
 (e) Milk alkali syndrome

(9) A 49 year old woman presented to her primary care physician with aches and pains, general malaise, anorexia, and weight loss over the last 4 months. The only other symptoms were polyuria and polydipsia. Subsequent results from blood tests showed that her fasting glucose concentrations were normal but her total serum calcium level was high at 4.1 mmol/L (NR 2.20–2.58).
 (a) Why might the physician have suspected diabetes mellitus?
 (b) What are the major causes of hypercalcemia?
 (c) What test would determine whether her hypercalcemia was due to primary hyperparathyroidism?

(10) A mother brought her 2 week old daughter to her family doctor because she had noticed her baby's right arm and leg had been twitching over the last few days. The baby was born naturally at 38 weeks after an uncomplicated pregnancy. She appeared healthy and normal. After various tests to investigate the symptoms, it was found that the baby had a low total serum calcium of 1.42 mmol/L (NR 2.20–2.58) and a high serum phosphate of 2.5 mmol/L (NR 0.8–1.5), but normal albumin levels.
 (a) What is the most likely cause of the infant's hypocalcemia?
 (b) What would be the next obvious tests to undertake?
 (c) Why would maternal hypercalcemia cause neonatal hypocalcemia?

CHAPTER 05 The endocrine pancreas

After working through this chapter you should be able to:

- Describe the metabolic actions of insulin and glucagon and how their secretions are controlled in the fed and fasted states
- Describe the differences between type 1 and type 2 diabetes mellitus and compare the etiologies and management of these two types of diabetes
- Outline the causes of secondary diabetes and other rare causes of this endocrinopathy
- Know the causes of diabetic complications and their possible outcomes
- Outline the diagnosis and management of diabetic complications
- Outline the classification of hypoglycemia and its causes

5.1 Introduction

The pancreas is a dual function organ with both exocrine and endocrine functions. Its exocrine function is to secrete a cocktail of digestive enzymes (pancreatic juice) into the duodenum via the pancreatic duct. Its endocrine function is to secrete hormones, principally insulin and glucagon, to control the metabolism of carbohydrate, protein, and lipid and the levels of circulating nutrients, notably blood sugar levels. The endocrine function of the pancreas is essential to life because the brain has an absolute requirement for glucose and in the absence of insulin no glucose is transported into nerve cells to maintain their energy requirements. Thus, complete loss of insulin secretion, as occurs in type 1 diabetes mellitus (see *Case 5.1*), can result in a diabetic coma and eventual death unless treated by insulin replacement. Type 1 diabetes mellitus has a prevalence of about 0.5% of the population, whereas type 2 diabetes mellitus, which is caused by defective insulin secretion and/or resistance (see *Case 5.2*), is more common and has a prevalence of about 5–10%. The prevalence of type 2 diabetes rises considerably with age and it is estimated to affect about 150 million people worldwide; this figure is expected to double in the next 20 years reflecting a global increase in obesity.

Whilst hyperglycemia can be treated, poor control of blood glucose levels leads to long-term diabetic complications such as cardiovascular disease, blindness, and kidney failure, and thus has very considerable health implications. To understand the etiology and consequences of both types of diabetes it is important to understand the basics of metabolism in the liver, muscle, and fat, how these are regulated by insulin and glucagon, and the control of insulin and glucagon secretion under different nutritional states.

5.2 Anatomy and embryology of the pancreas

5.2.1 Anatomy

Lying inferior to the stomach, the pancreas sits in the bend of the duodenum (*Figure 5.1a*), with a length of approximately 12–15 cm. The pancreas weighs less than 100 g, and over 98% of its rubbery mass is exocrine tissue composed of tiny blind-ending tubules surrounded by acinar cells that are arranged into lobules. Nestled amongst these lobules are the islets of Langerhans of which there are between 1 and 2 million in each adult pancreas (*Figure 5.1b*) – these provide the endocrine function of the pancreas. The size of each islet varies from 100 to 500 μm and comprises 1000–3000 cells; in total they constitute less than 2% of the mass of the pancreas and weigh about 1 g.

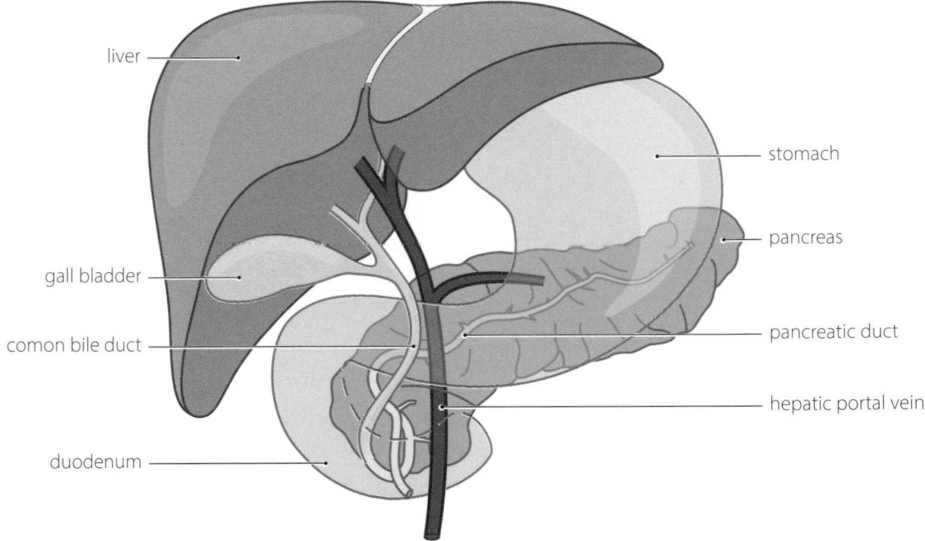

(a)

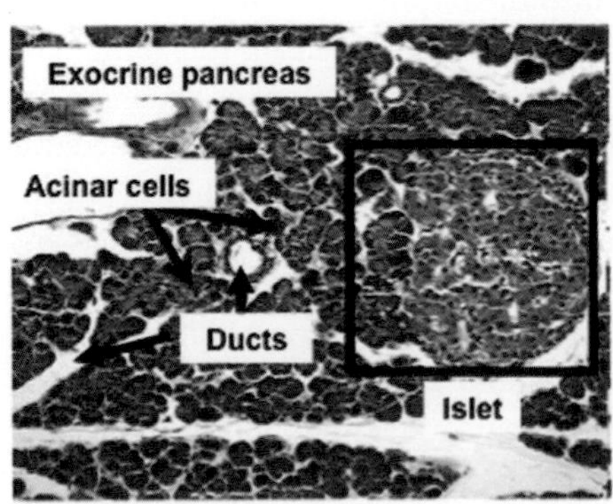

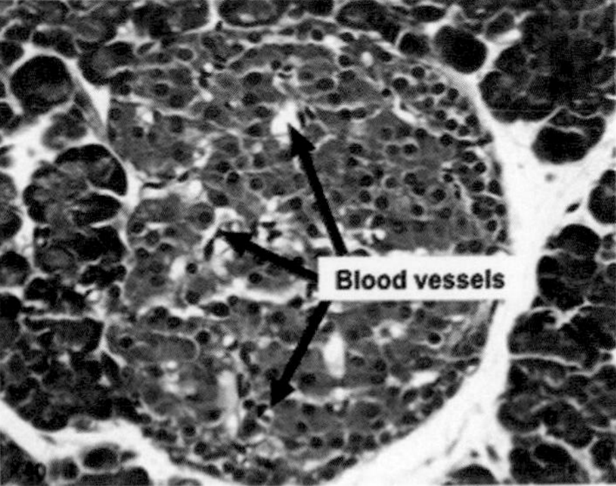

(b)

Figure 5.1. Gross anatomy and histology of the pancreas.
(a) Gross anatomy of the pancreas showing its anatomical relationship to the stomach, duodenum, and liver. The pancreatic duct joins the common bile duct and they both enter the duodenum where secretions from the exocrine pancreas aid digestion. The hepatic portal vein carries absorbed nutrients and the endocrine secretions of the pancreas (insulin and glucagon) directly to the liver.
(b) The left-hand image is a low-powered photomicrograph showing a pancreatic islet of Langerhans nestled in the exocrine pancreas which consists of acinar cells arranged in lobules around blind-ending tubules that drain into larger ducts which carry digestive enzymes to the duodenum. The right-hand image is a higher-powered photomicrograph (40x magnification) of the islet of Langerhans outlined in black in the left-hand image.

The pancreas is supplied by branches of the celiac and superior mesenteric arteries and the hepatic portal vein drains the gland. The liver is therefore the first organ to receive the endocrine signals secreted by the pancreatic islets and these have potent effects on hepatic metabolism.

In the human pancreatic islets there are four types of endocrine secreting cells:

- the alpha (α) cells producing glucagon
- the beta (β) cells producing insulin
- the delta (δ) cells producing somatostatin
- the F cells producing pancreatic polypeptide.

The hormones are all polypeptides and, whilst insulin is secreted exclusively by β cells, the other hormones or derivatives from the same prohormone are also secreted by the gastrointestinal mucosa. Somatostatin is also found in the brain and inhibits the release of growth hormone from the anterior pituitary gland (*Chapter 2*).

In rodent species the β cells are located mainly within the core of each islet and the other cells are towards the periphery, whereas in the human islet the different cell types secreting hormones are more randomly dispersed and the population of islet cell types varies considerably from one islet to the next. Blood flow to each islet is five to tenfold higher than that to the exocrine pancreas and the network of capillaries flows from the core to the mantel of the islet. The islets are richly innervated with both parasympathetic and sympathetic fibers. The parasympathetic vagal innervation stimulates the early phase of insulin secretion as well as optimizing post-prandial insulin secretion, whilst the sympathetic innervation from splanchnic nerve trunks stimulates glucagon secretion and inhibits somatostatin secretion.

5.2.2 Embryology

The pancreas develops initially from the ventral and dorsal buds of the gut endoderm but the ventral bud becomes displaced due to rotation of the gut and eventually fuses with the dorsal bud (*Figure 5.2*). When fully developed the broad right end of the

CASE 5.1 215 240

- Woman of 17 years with 24 hour history of vomiting, abdominal pain, and disturbed consciousness
- Mother reports daughter has 3 week history of polyuria, polydipsia, and weight loss
- Random glucose 23 mmol/L

A 17 year old woman presented to the Emergency Department with a 24 hour history of repeated vomiting, abdominal pain, and disturbed level of consciousness. She had a history of productive cough and fever for 2 days. A pregnancy test was negative. Her mother who accompanied her said that she had been troubled with polyuria, polydipsia, and unintentional weight loss for about 3 weeks prior to admission. She had no past medical history of note and was not on regular medications. Her mother had primary autoimmune hypothyroidism. She did not smoke and drank minimal alcohol. On examination she was drowsy, had a Glasgow Coma Scale score of 11/15, had dry mucous membranes, and her JVP was undetectable. Respiratory system examination revealed bronchial breathing in the right base, with a pulse rate of 100/min, blood pressure of 90/65 mmHg, a respiratory rate of 24/min and her oxygen saturations were 98% on air. Random glucose was 23 mmol/L.

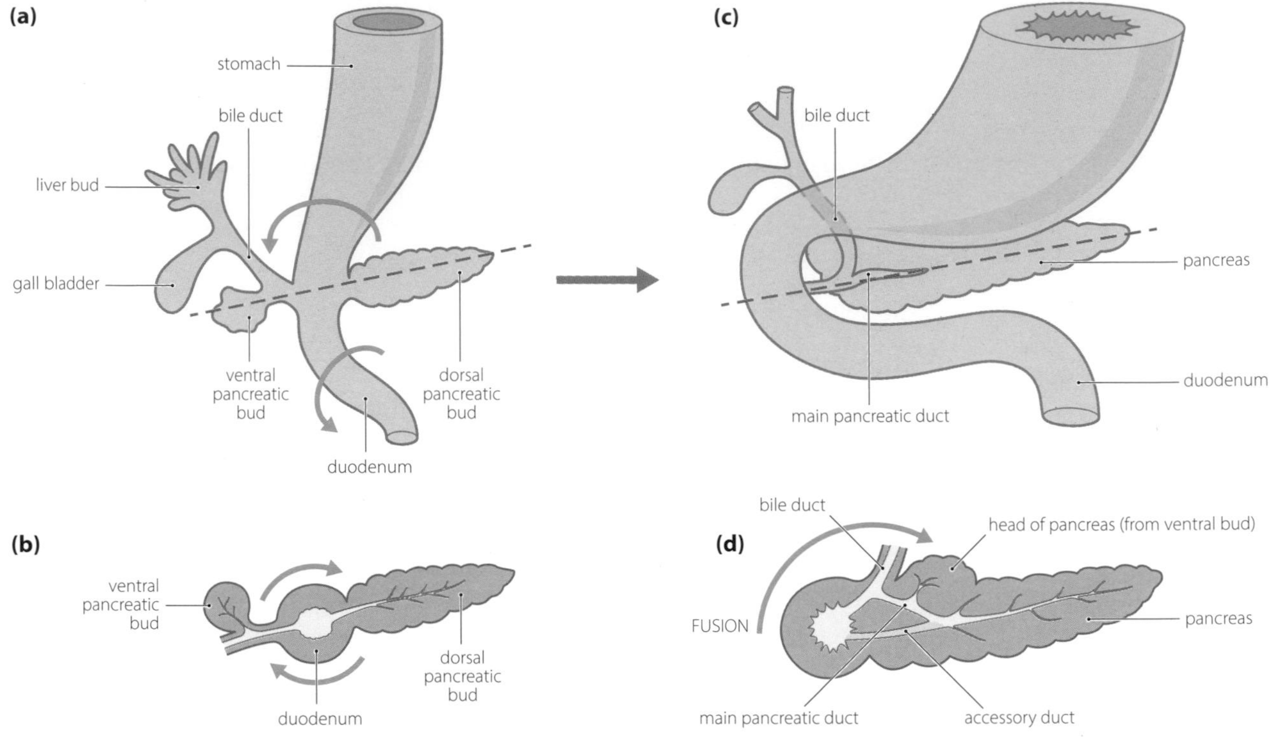

Figure 5.2. Embryology of the pancreas.
Schematic drawings of the development of the human pancreas at (a and b) 6 weeks, and (c and d) 8 weeks of gestation. Growth and rotation of the duodenum (indicated by arrows) cause movement of the ventral pancreatic bud towards the dorsal bud, allowing their eventual fusion (d). Union of the distal part of the dorsal pancreatic duct and the entire ventral pancreatic duct forms the main pancreatic duct. The proximal part of the dorsal pancreatic duct usually disappears, but it may persist as an accessory duct (d). Dotted lines indicate the level of the corresponding transverse sections shown on the right.

CASE 5.2

216 245

- Woman of 44 years with type 2 DM; now gaining weight
- Practice nurse concerned about management as HbA1c also rising

A 54 year old woman presented complaining of an inability to lose weight, fatigue, and low mood. She had been diagnosed with type 2 diabetes mellitus 15 years previously and had been managed by her primary care physician. The practice nurse was concerned about her management and referred her to the diabetes clinic. Initial investigations revealed an elevated glycated hemoglobin (HbA1c) at 9.5%/80 mmol/mol (NR 4–6.5%/20–48 mmol/mol) which represented a deterioration from last year's level of 8%/64 mmol/mol. She was taking:

- metformin (1 g orally tds)
- gliclazide (160 mg bd)
- simvastatin (40 mg od)
- ramipril (an antihypertensive ACE inhibitor; 10 mg od)
- aspirin (75 mg od)

She complained of significant weight gain (approximately 11 kg over the last year) and her BMI was now 42 kg/m^2 despite having a healthy diet and taking regular exercise. She was also known to have hypertension, mixed hyperlipidemia, pre-proliferative retinopathy, and chronic kidney disease (stage 2). There was no history of pancreatitis.

gland, the head, is derived from the ventral and dorsal buds. The main body of the organ which tapers to form the tail is formed from the dorsal bud. These differences in ontogeny between the ventrally derived head section and the dorsally derived head, body, and tail section are responsible for differences in innervation, blood supply, and endocrine composition.

5.3 Basic physiology

5.3.1 Actions of hormones secreted by pancreatic islets

Overall, insulin is an anabolic hormone promoting the uptake of glucose and other nutrients into liver, muscle, and fat, whereas glucagon is a catabolic hormone promoting the release of nutrients from the liver. Somatostatin, released from the δ cells of the islets, has inhibitory paracrine functions on the release of both insulin and glucagon, whilst the precise function of pancreatic polypeptide is unknown. It is important to understand carbohydrate, protein, and fat metabolism, to appreciate how insulin and glucagon control this metabolism in the liver, muscle, and adipose tissue, and so control the flow of nutrients.

5.3.2 Overview of glucose, amino acid, and fat metabolism

Glucose metabolism

Glucose is always present in the blood and is continually being removed and replaced so that the concentration remains relatively constant at around 5 mmol/L. Of all the nutrients in the circulation glucose is the most constant. Glucose enters blood by:

- absorption from the intestine; digestion of polysaccharides (starch) and disaccharides (e.g. sucrose) releases glucose
- breakdown of glycogen in the liver (glycogenolysis); however, note that glucose from glycogen breakdown in muscle does not enter the circulation because muscle lacks glucose-6-phosphatase which breaks down glucose-6-phosphate (*Figure 5.3*)

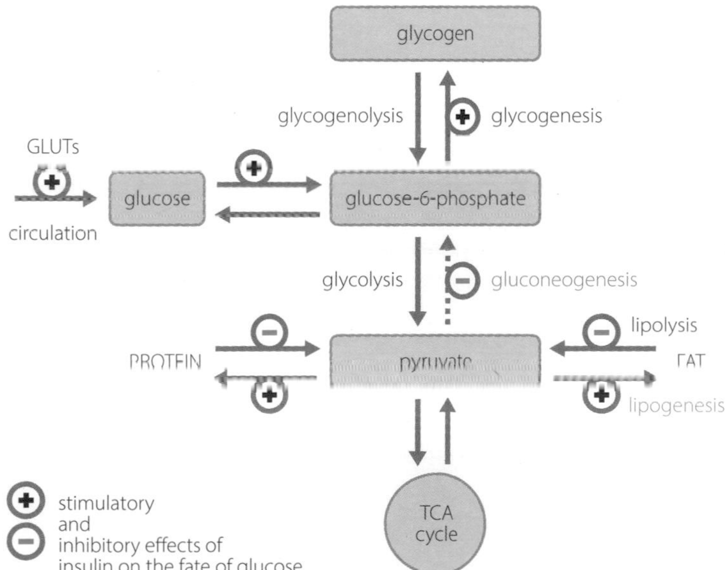

Figure 5.3. The flexible uses of glucose.
A highly simplified figure to illustrate the metabolic fate of glucose. Glucose, taken up from the circulation, can be stored in the form of glycogen, metabolized to pyruvate and used for the synthesis of proteins or *de novo* synthesis of lipids, or used as an energy substrate by entering the TCA cycle. These actions are reversible and the overall flow of fuel will depend on nutritional state and the insulin to glucagon ratio.

- gluconeogenesis in the liver; the substrates for gluconeogenesis, in order of importance, are smaller molecules, usually alanine (largely from muscle), lactate (from anaerobic glycolysis), and glycerol (from adipose tissue lipolysis), although other amino acids can also act as precursors (*Figure 5.3*).

Glucose is removed from blood by:

- uptake into tissues; the importance of glucose is such that there are specific glucose transporters (GLUTs) for the absorption and uptake of glucose into cells, each of which have distinct features and distribution (*Box 5.1*).

Glucose can be stored in liver and muscle in the form of glycogen (*Figures 5.4* and *5.5*) or converted to fatty acids and stored as triacylglycerol in adipose tissue, liver, and muscle (*Figures 5.5, 5.6,* and *5.7*). It is also oxidized to produce energy and these flexible uses of glucose are outlined in *Figure 5.3*.

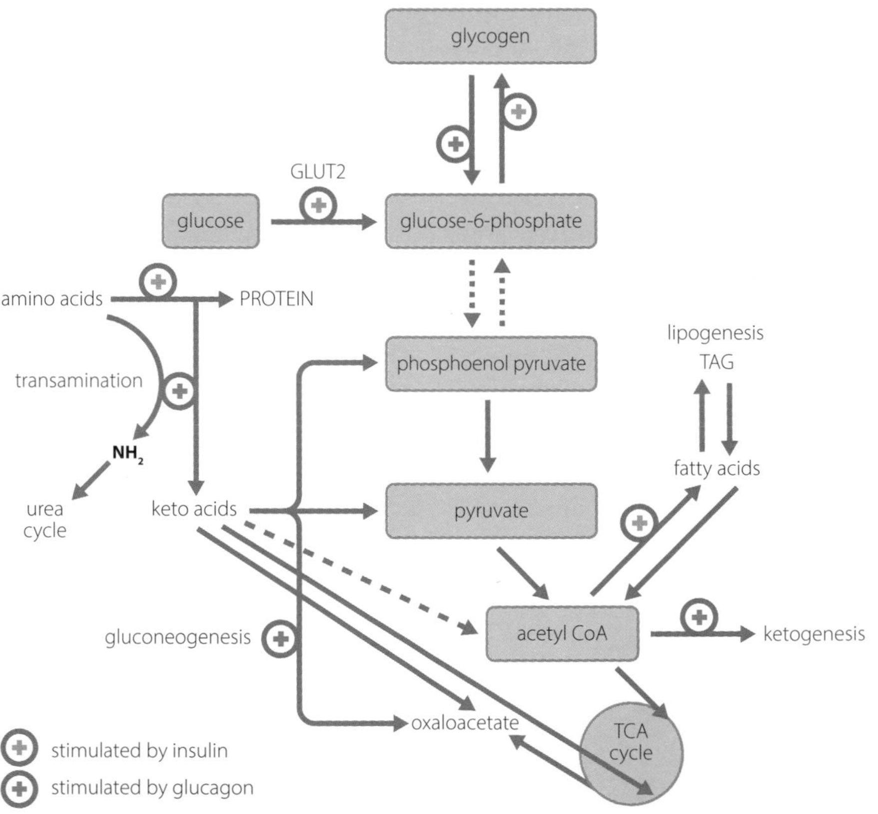

Figure 5.4. Glucose and amino acid metabolism in the liver.
The liver has a major role in balancing the actions of insulin and glucagon. Insulin stimulates uptake of glucose through GLUT2 transporters, the formation of glycogen, the formation of fatty acids and triacylglycerol (TAG) from acetyl CoA, and the uptake of amino acids and subsequent protein synthesis. Glucagon is an important regulator of the catabolism (transamination) of amino acids, which occurs predominantly in the liver. The keto acids may enter a catabolic pathway directly, e.g. the keto acid of alanine is pyruvate, that of glutamic acid is 2-oxoglutarate, and that of aspartic acid is oxaloacetate, the latter two being intermediates of the TCA cycle. Alternatively, keto acids undergo further metabolism to acetyl CoA. Glucagon stimulates the formation of keto acids from acetyl CoA and it also stimulates gluconeogenesis, the formation of glucose from oxaloacetate.

Box 5.1 | Glucose transporters (the GLUT and SGLT families of sugar transport proteins)

Facilitated diffusion of dietary sugar from the intestinal lumen into the circulation and uptake of glucose from the circulation into target cells involves specific transport proteins, of which there are two structurally and functionally distinct groups.

- **The Na^+-dependent glucose transporters** (SGLT1 and 2). These are members of a larger family of Na^+ transporters (encoded by the *SLC5A* gene). They utilize the electrochemical gradient of Na^+ set up by the Na^+–K^+ ATPase pump to transport glucose (and galactose) against a concentration gradient. They are responsible for transporting glucose from the lumen of the intestine across the brush border of the enterocytes of the gut and from the glomerular filtrate into the proximal tubule cells of the kidney. SGLT1 is a high affinity, low capacity transporter located both in the intestine and kidney, but SGLT2 is a low affinity, high capacity transporter predominantly expressed in convoluted proximal tubules. SGLT2 is considered to be the major transporter of glucose from the glomerular filtrate into the tubular cells, with SGLT1 recovering any remaining glucose and so preventing glucose loss in the urine.
- **The facilitative glucose transporters** (GLUTs). These utilize the diffusion gradient of glucose and other sugars to transport sugars. The GLUT family (GLUT 1–12, GLUT 14, and the H^+ myo-inositol transporter, HMIT) are structurally similar with 12 transmembrane helices and intracellular amino and carboxy termini (*Box figure 5.1*). N-linked glycosylation can occur in the extracellular loop between helices 1 and 2.

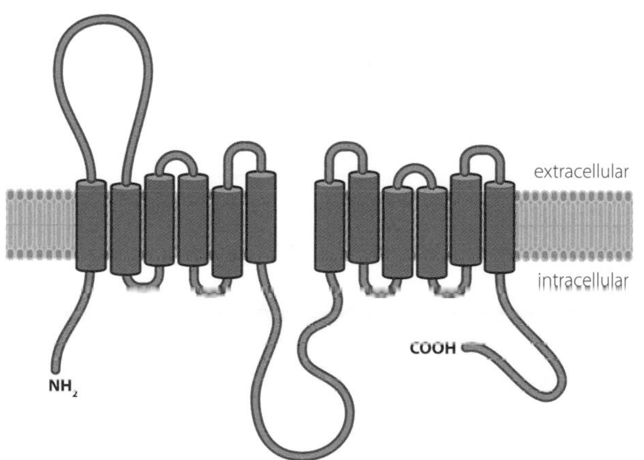

Box figure 5.1. Basic structure of the GLUTs.

Based on structural (sequence) similarities, three classes of GLUTs have been identified.

Class I: GLUTs 1–4

- GLUT1. High affinity transporter expressed mainly in brain (including the blood–brain barrier) and erythrocytes, but moderate levels in adipose tissue, muscle, and liver. Allows a relatively constant uptake of sugar.
- GLUT2. Low affinity transporter mainly expressed in pancreatic β cells, intestine, kidney, and hepatocytes. Allows extracellular and intracellular glucose concentrations to equilibrate across the membrane. This transporter is important in the glucose-sensing mechanisms of the β cells and in transporting glucose across the basolateral surface of enterocytes in the intestine and proximal tubule cells in the kidney.
- GLUT 3. High affinity for glucose and is present in tissues with a high demand for glucose, in particular the brain.
- GLUT 4. Medium affinity transporter found in liver, muscle, and adipose tissue where, in response to insulin, they are translocated from GLUT4-containing storage vesicles to the plasma membrane resulting in an immediate 10–20-fold increase in glucose transport into cells. These are responsible for the reduction in the postprandial rise in glucose levels.

Class II: GLUT5, 7, 9, and 11; the major one is GLUT5 which is important for fructose absorption in the small intestine and is also expressed in adipose tissue.

Class III: GLUT 6, 8,10,12, and HMIT.

Class II and III transporters are expressed in a variety of tissue including the brain, heart and skeletal muscle, liver, and adipose tissue. Their precise function in glucose homeostasis is ill-defined but some of these new transporters may be implicated in the development of T2DM

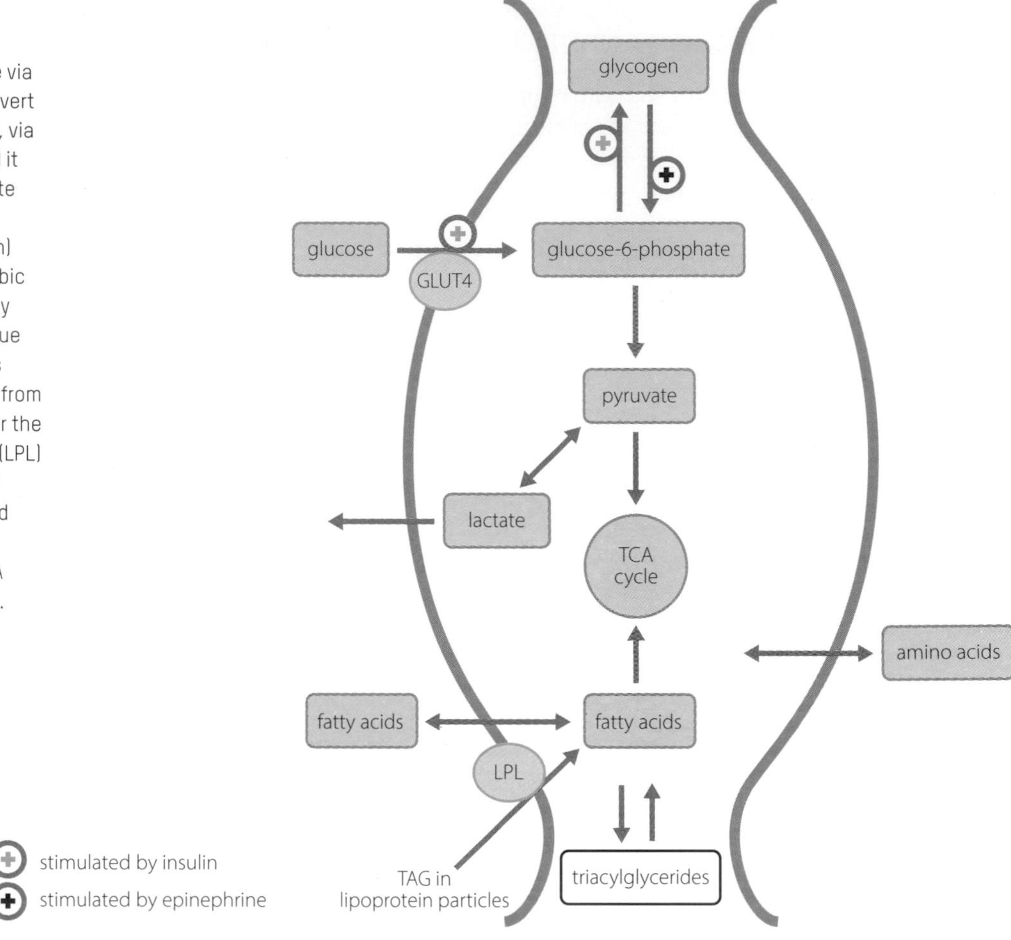

Figure 5.5. Major metabolic pathways in muscle. Muscle can take up glucose via GLUT4 transporters and convert it to glycogen. Alternatively, via glucose-6-phosphate (G6P) it can be converted to pyruvate which can be converted to lactate (anaerobic oxidation) or enter the TCA cycle (aerobic oxidation) to produce energy for contraction. Muscle tissue can also take up fatty acids once they are broken down from triacylglycerides (TAG) under the action of lipoprotein lipase (LPL) in the capillaries. Free fatty acids can then be converted back into TAG for storage in muscle or can enter the TCA cycle for energy production.

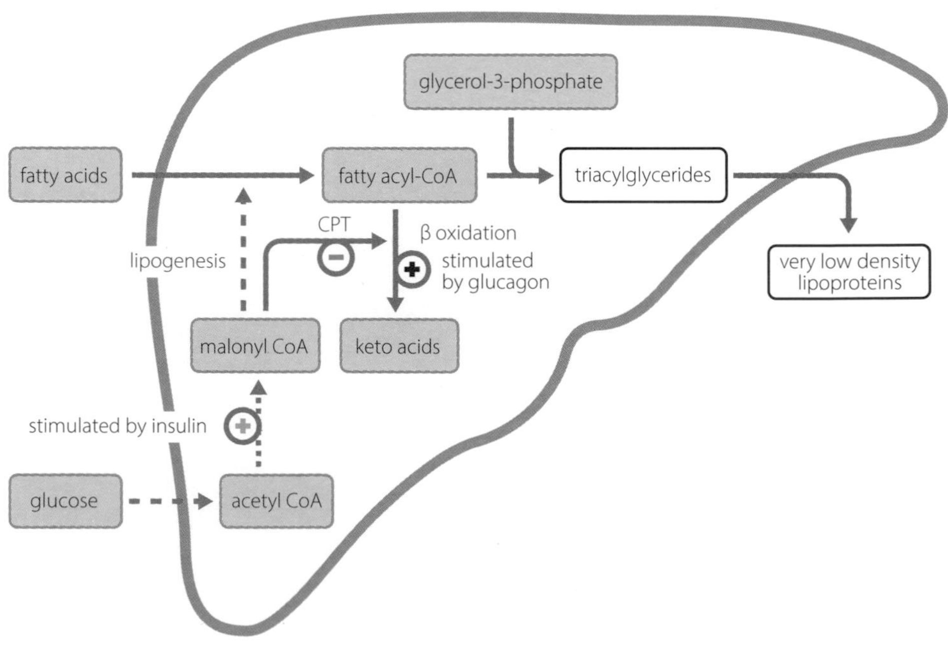

Figure 5.6. Fatty acid metabolism in the liver. Fatty acids are taken up by the liver and converted to fatty acyl-CoA esters. To enter the mitchondria the esters are converted to acyl-carnitine derivatives by the action of carnitine *o*-palmitoyltransferase (CPT). In the mitochondria they undergo β-oxidation to keto acids (see also *Figure 5.9*). CPT is inhibited by malonyl CoA, an intermediate in *de novo* lipogenesis. Glucagon stimulates β-oxidation whilst insulin promotes the formation of triacylglycerol (TAG) in hepatocytes which can be exported back into the circulation in the form of very low density lipoproteins (VLDLs).

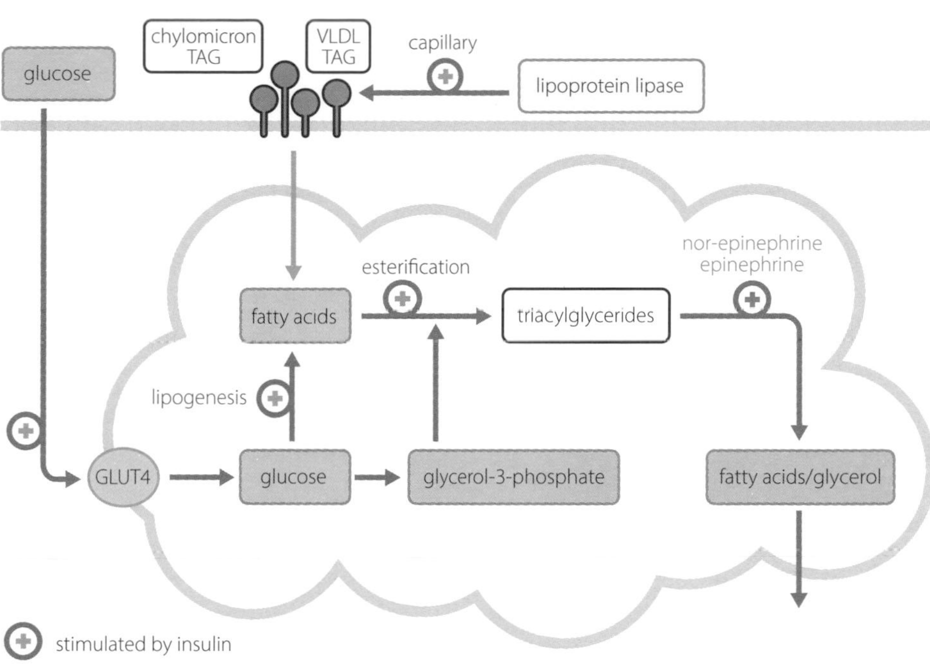

Figure 5.7. Major metabolic pathways in adipose tissue. Adipose tissue takes up fatty acids after the triacylglycerol (TAG) in chylomicrons or very low density lipoproteins (VLDLs) has been hydrolyzed to fatty acids by the action of lipoprotein lipase in the capillaries. The fatty acids are then re-esterified to form triacylglycerides for storage in adipose tissue. Glucose can also be taken up by adipose tissue through the GLUT4 transporters and, through *de novo* synthesis, converted to TAG either via fatty acids or glycerol-3-phosphate. These anabolic actions are stimulated by insulin whilst nor-epinephrine and epinephrine stimulate lipolysis.

Amino acid metabolism

There are 20 different amino acids that can be incorporated into proteins and several others that simply exist in the body. Each has a specific pathway for synthesis (except for essential amino acids that must be derived from the diet) and degradation, so the topic of amino acid metabolism is huge. Like glucose, amino acids can also be oxidized to produce energy and this oxidation contributes around 10–20% of the body's total oxidative metabolism under normal conditions. The total content of amino acids (in the form of protein and notably in muscle) could represent a large energy store; however, unlike glucose and fatty acids, proteins are not normally stored for energy and total body proteins do not fluctuate as, for example, glycogen stores do. Daily protein turnover is approximately 3% of our total protein, and total oxidation of amino acids roughly balances daily protein intake.

The liver has a particular importance in protein metabolism for several reasons:

- it is the first organ through which newly absorbed amino acids from the intestine pass
- it provides important links between carbohydrate and amino acid metabolism (*Figure 5.4*) and can convert amino acids into glucose (gluconeogenesis)
- it is the site of urea synthesis.

Fatty acid metabolism

Triacylglycerol (TAG) and non-esterified fatty acids (NEFAs) which are not attached to glycerol – also called free fatty acids (FFAs) – are always present in plasma and, like glucose, are constantly being used and replaced. Neither TAG nor FFAs are water soluble; FFAs are carried in plasma bound to albumin and TAG is carried in the plasma in specialized particulate structures known as lipoproteins (*Figure 5.8*). TAG can only be taken up into tissues after it has been hydrolyzed to FFAs by lipoprotein

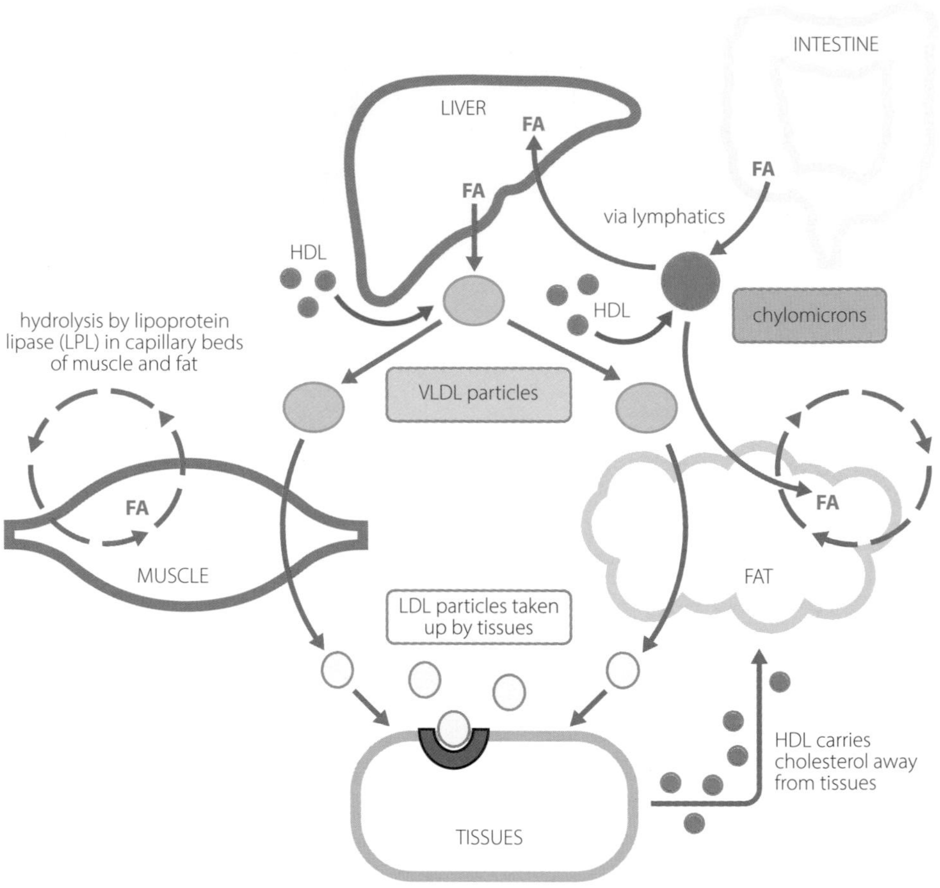

Figure 5.8. Overview of the transport and turnover of lipids in the body.
Fats are mainly transported round the body bound to lipoproteins. Dietary fats are taken up by the mucosal cells of the intestine in the form of fatty acids where they form triacylglycerides (TAG). Together with cholesterol and phospholipids they are packaged into chylomicrons (the largest of the lipoproteins) and enter the circulation via the lymphatic system. Chylomicrons are only found in the circulation after a meal. In the capillary beds of the liver and adipose tissue the TAGs in the lipoproteins are broken down to fatty acids under the action of lipoprotein lipase (LPL), and then taken up by these tissues where they will be re-esterified to TAG. In the post-absorptive state, the liver can export TAGs into the circulation in the form of very low density lipoproteins (VLDLs) where they can be taken up into adipose and muscle cells after their hydrolysis to fatty acids by LPL in the capillary beds. Depleted of TAG the VLDL particles, enriched with cholesterol, become low density lipoproteins (LDL) and these particles can be taken up by all tissues through an LDL receptor-mediated mechanism. This is important in the delivery of cholesterol to steroid synthesizing organs such as the adrenal gland and gonads. High density lipoproteins (HDLs), which contain a high proportion of protein, are important in the formation of chylomicrons and are also important in transporting cholesterol away from tissues. Thus HDLs are considered to be 'good' cholesterol, LDLs considered to be 'bad' cholesterol.

lipase present in capillaries. In adipose tissue and to some extent the liver and muscle, FFAs are re-esterified back to TAG and stored in this form (see *Figures 5.6* and *5.7*).

5.3.3 Actions of insulin and glucagon on liver, muscle, and adipose tissue metabolism

The three major target organs for the action of insulin are the liver, muscle, and adipose tissue, whereas glucagon only exerts its effects on the liver.

The major metabolic pathways in the liver are:

- glucose metabolism – glycogen formation, glycogenolysis, and gluconeogenesis (*Figure 5.4*)
- amino acid metabolism – synthesis of proteins, metabolism of amino acids to keto acids which can be shunted into lipogenesis, ketogenesis, and gluconeogenesis (*Figure 5.4*)
- fatty acid metabolism – lipogenesis and keto acid formation (*Figure 5.6*).

As would be predicted from the anabolic and catabolic actions of insulin and glucagon, respectively, insulin:

- stimulates glycogen formation and inhibits glycogenolysis
- promotes lipogenesis and inhibits lipolysis and ketogenesis
- stimulates the uptake of amino acids

whereas glucagon:

- stimulates glycogenolysis and gluconeogenesis (*Figure 5.4*)
- stimulates the formation of keto acids by promoting β-oxidation of acetyl-CoA to form ketones (*Figures 5.6* and *5.9*).

The major metabolic actions of insulin in muscle and adipose tissue are:

- increased uptake of glucose in both tissues by stimulating the synthesis and insertion of GLUT4 transporters into cell membranes (*Box 5.1*)
- increased glycogen formation and the esterification of FFAs into TAG in muscle (*Figure 5.5*)
- to promote storage of TAG in white adipose tissue, to inhibit the breakdown of TAG by inhibiting hormone sensitive lipase, and also to stimulate *de novo* lipogenesis from glucose (*Figure 5.7*).

5.3.4 Insulin: glucagon secretion and integrated metabolism

The differential secretion of these hormones depends on the nutritional state existing at any one time. The phrase *post-absorptive state* is used when all of the last meal has been absorbed from the intestinal tract but not much further time has elapsed, so 'starvation' is not apparent. In humans it is typically represented by the state after an overnight fast, but before breakfast is consumed. This is the time when blood glucose levels are usually measured and, if they are over 7.0 mmol/L (NR 4.5–5.0 mmol/L) diabetes mellitus is diagnosed.

Insulin secretion is stimulated by a rise in blood glucose concentrations as occurs after eating, but it is the ratio of circulating insulin to glucagon that determines the overall integrated metabolism at any one time. After an overnight fast, insulin levels are low as is the ratio of insulin to glucagon. At this point the rate at which glucose enters and leaves the circulation is about 130 mg/min and most of this (about 80 mg) comes from gluconeogenesis and the rest from glycogenolysis in the liver. In the fasted state, FFAs and glycerol are released from adipose tissue, as a result of lipase breaking down TAG, and these are then taken up by the liver and muscle for an energy substrate. In the liver, FFAs are either converted to TAG and exported back into the circulation as VLDLs (*Figure 5.8*), or they are shunted into the production

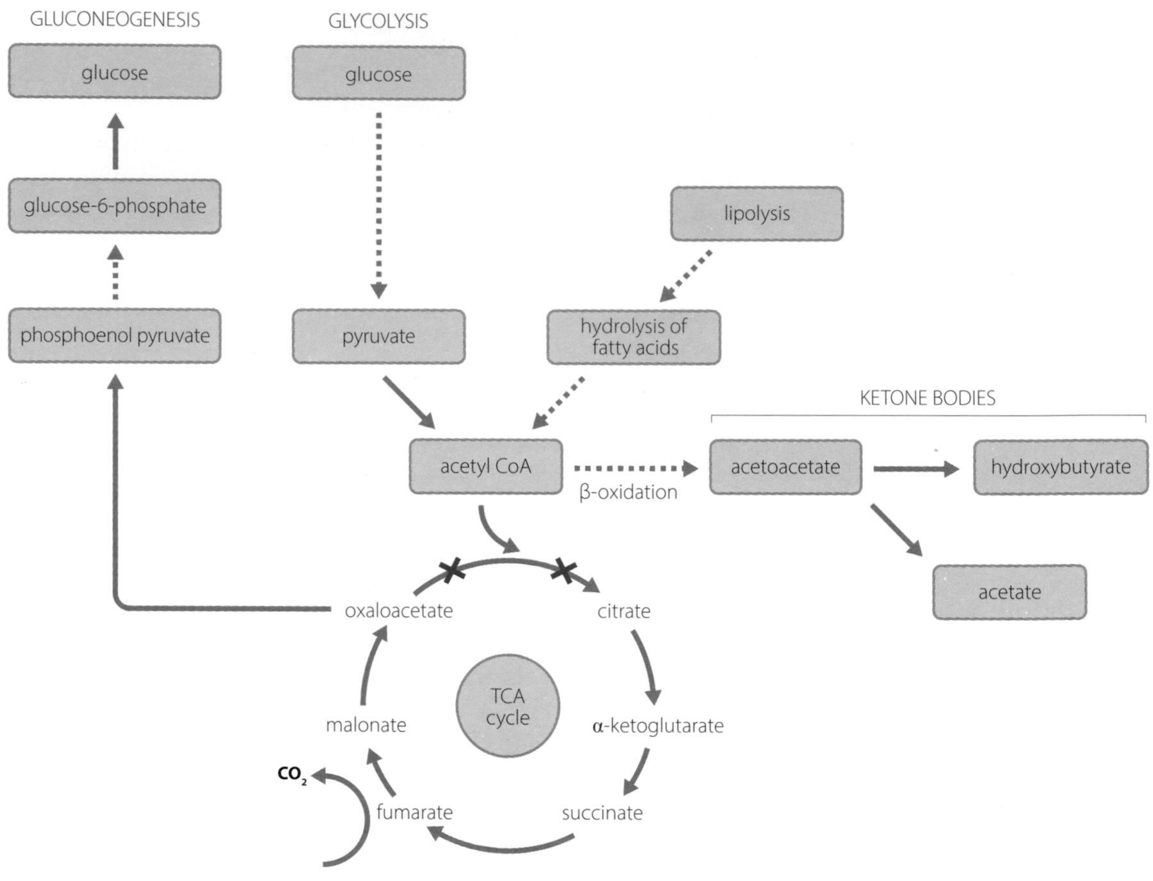

Figure 5.9. Keto acid formation in the liver.
The β-oxidation of fatty acids in the liver produces keto acids, otherwise known as ketone bodies, although they are dissolved substances, not particles. The keto acids are acetoacetate and 3-hydroxybutyrate, which are exported into the circulation. The rate of oxidation determines keto acid formation, a process stimulated by glucagon but inhibited by insulin. In addition, oxaloacetate is consumed by the gluconeogenic pathway because pyruvate cannot be directly metabolized back to glucose. This metabolic process is also stimulated by glucagon. As a consequence, the rate at which acetyl CoA enters the TCA cycle is reduced and is shunted into the formation of keto acids. When excess keto acids are released into the circulation and overcome the buffering capacity of the blood, ketoacidosis occurs – a typical consequence of untreated T1DM.

of ketone bodies. The turnover of ketone bodies is rapid and levels are generally low and they do not contribute much to the total resting energy expenditure. However, this contribution increases markedly during more prolonged starvation and in type 1 diabetes mellitus (see *Figure 5.9*).

After breakfast the metabolism changes from production to storage mode. Absorbed glucose from the intestine reaches the liver directly where it is taken up into the hepatocytes through the GLUT2 transporters. Stimulated by glucose, the insulin:glucagon ratio increases and glycogenolysis is switched to glycogen formation by activation of glycogen synthetase and inactivation of glycogen phosphorylase. Gluconeogenesis still continues, due to an increased lactate production after a meal, but this glucose is stored as glycogen (the 'indirect' pathway). About 1–2 hours after a carbohydrate meal there is almost no release of glucose from the liver. Simultaneously, glucose uptake into muscle and adipose tissue is also stimulated by insulin. The TAG entering the circulation, in the form of chylomicron particles formed after absorption of fats in the gut (*Figure 5.8*), is taken up by muscle and adipose tissue after its hydrolysis by lipoprotein lipase in the capillaries of the tissues.

5.3.5 Synthesis, release, and metabolism of insulin secretion

The gene for insulin codes for an RNA with two introns and two exons, and the mature RNA codes for a pre-prohormone consisting of a signal sequence and a B, C, and A chain (*Figure 5.10*). The signal sequence is rapidly cleaved during synthesis in the rough endoplasmic reticulum leaving a prohormone in which the A and B

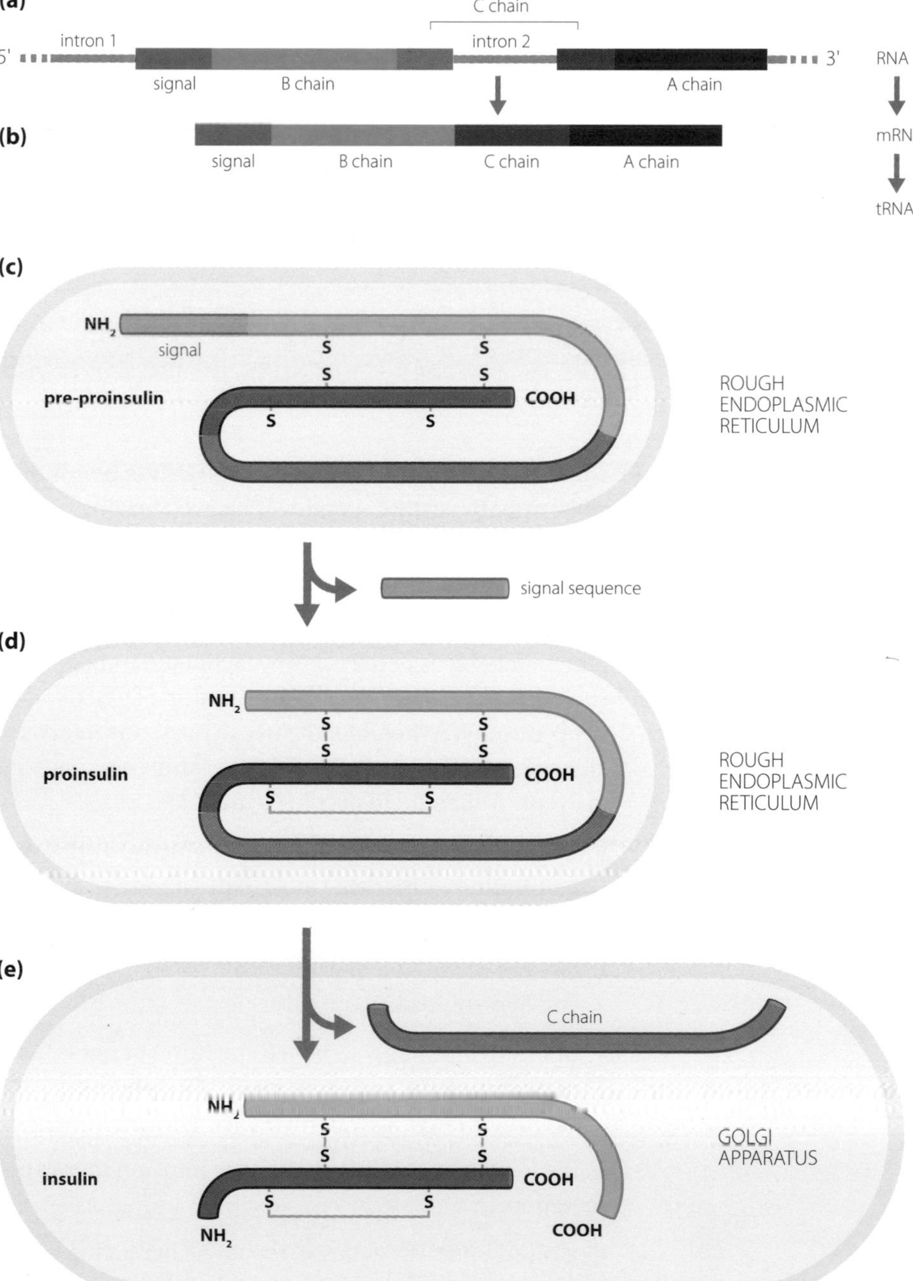

Figure 5.10. Synthesis of insulin.
The insulin gene codes an RNA with two exons and two introns (a), from which the introns are excised forming messenger RNA (b). Pre-proinsulin (comprising chains A–C) is synthesized in the rough endoplasmic reticulum (c) and, after cleavage of the signal sequence, proinsulin is formed with the formation of disulfide bonds between cysteine residues (d). In the Golgi apparatus the C-peptide is cleaved leaving mature insulin (e); the insulin and C-peptide are both then packaged into secretory granules.

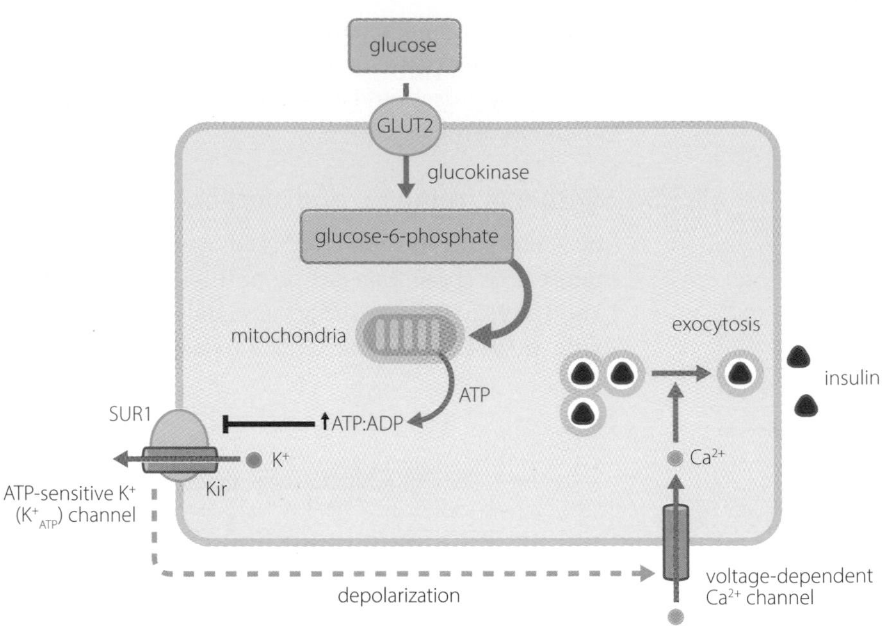

Figure 5.11. Control of insulin secretion.
The uptake of glucose through the GLUT2 transporter results in its oxidative metabolism in the mitochondria, increased formation of ATP and thus an increase in the ratio of ATP to ADP. This closes the ATP-sensitive potassium channel, resulting in depolarization of the cell membrane and opening of voltage-dependent calcium channels. The intracellular rise in Ca^{2+} concentrations stimulates the secretion of insulin from secretory granules.

chains become linked through two disulfide bonds on cysteine residues. In the Golgi apparatus the C-peptide is cleaved leaving biologically active insulin and the C-peptide, both of which are secreted simultaneously. The C-peptide has no established function.

A rise in blood glucose concentration stimulates insulin release. Glucose enters the pancreatic β cells of the islets by facilitated transport through GLUT2 transporters such that the extracellular concentration of glucose equilibrates with the intracellular concentration. When blood glucose rises, this increases the conversion of glucose to glucose-6-phosphate by glucokinase and, as a consequence, the following sequence of events is thought to occur (*Figure 5.11*):

- an increase in the metabolism of glucose-6-phosphate in the mitochondria generating an increase in ATP and an increase in the ATP:ADP ratio, which causes
- closure of the ATP-sensitive potassium channels causing a depolarization of the β cell, resulting in
- opening of voltage-sensitive calcium channels, a rise in intracellular Ca^{2+} concentrations, and the release of insulin; this is very rapid and occurs within minutes of exposure to increased glucose concentrations.

In response to a continuous glucose infusion there are two phases of insulin secretion:

- a rapid initial 'first phase' response occurring within the first 5 minutes – this represents the release of stored insulin

- a second phase which occurs later represents newly formed insulin which is released as soon as it is synthesized.

The half-life of insulin in the systemic circulation is about 4–6 minutes and approximately 50% of hepatic portal insulin is removed from the circulation by the liver during its initial transit. The kidney is the major site of insulin clearance in the systemic circulation, although other tissues can also degrade any residual insulin not degraded by the liver and kidney. The primary enzyme responsible for this degradation is now thought to be insulin-degrading enzyme (IDE) although other enzymes, including lysosomal enzymes, undoubtedly contribute to the cleavage and inactivation of insulin.

5.3.6 How does insulin exert its cellular effects?

The insulin receptor (IR) is a heterodimer and consists of two extracellular α subunits and two transmembrane β subunits (*Figure 5.12*). The α subunit contains the ligand binding domain and this regulates the tyrosine kinase activity of the intracellular domain of the β subunit. The insulin receptor gene contains 12 exons and, through alternate splicing of exon 11, two isoforms are produced:

- IRa retains exon 11 and has a moderate affinity for insulin as well as insulin growth factor 2 (IGF-2); this receptor is found mainly in fetal tissues, the adult central nervous system, and hematopoietic cells
- IRb omits exon 11 and has a high affinity for insulin and predominates in classical insulin-sensitive target tissues such as liver, muscle, and adipose tissue.

Insulin has multiple effects on its target tissues and these include:

- increasing glycogen synthase and thus the conversion of glucose-6-phosphate to glycogen
- increasing enzyme activity (esterification) involved in the conversion of FFAs to TAG
- increasing enzyme activity involved in protein synthesis from amino acids
- inhibiting carnitine palmitoyltransferase which is responsible for β-oxidation of fatty acyl-CoA to keto acids
- insertion of GLUT4 transporters (*Box 5.1*) into the membrane of muscle and adipose cells increasing glucose uptake in these tissues.

Signaling at the insulin receptor is complex (*Figure 5.13*) and involves:

- insulin binding to the extracellular β domains
- autophosphorylation of the tyrosine kinase domains on the β subunits and subsequent phosphorylation of the insulin receptor substrate (IRS) protein
- IRS then activating PI-3 kinase, resulting in the recruitment and activation of PDK 1 and then AKT at the plasma membrane
- AKT subsequently activating glycogen synthase resulting in increased glycogen synthesis
- AKT also phosphorylating the AS160/TBC1D1 kinase which leads to the transport of GLUT4 vesicles to the cell membrane by VAMP-2 SNARE proteins where they become tethered to t-SNARE complexes in the cell membrane

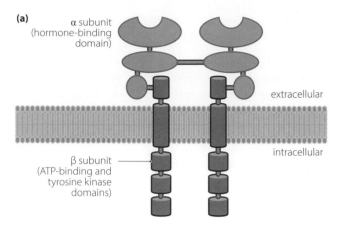

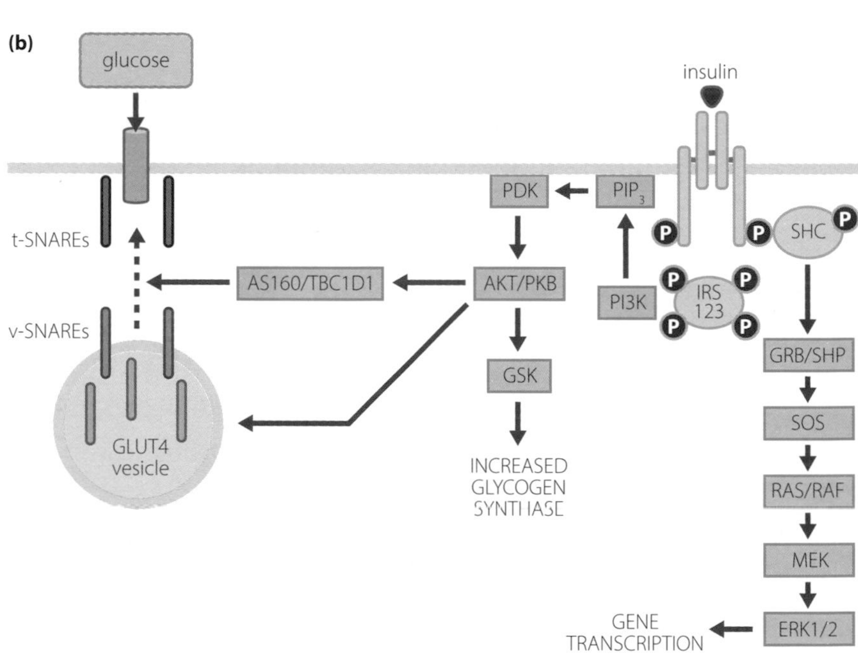

Figure 5.12. Structure of the insulin receptor (a) and insulin signaling (b) to regulate enzyme activity, gene expression, and cellular location of GLUT4 in muscle and adipose tissue.
The postprandial rise in insulin secretion stimulates the insertion of the GLUT4 tranporters into the plasma membrane of muscle and fat cells; an action that is vital in blood glucose homeostasis. Binding of insulin to the two extracellular α subunits of the receptor leads to activation of the intrinsic tyrosine kinase activity of the transmembrane β subunits and autophosphorylation of specific tyrosine residues. The activated receptor then phosphorylates a host of proteins including the insulin receptor substrate (IRS) family of proteins which, in turn, subsequently phosphorylate PI3 kinase (PI3K). Activated PI3K catalyzes the phosphorylation of phosphatidylinositol 4,5-bisphosphate (PI 4,5-P_2/PIP_2) to PI 3,4,5-P3 (PIP_3), resulting in subsequent phosphorylations of phosphoinositide-dependent kinases 1 & 2 (PDK) and subsequently AKT (protein kinase B, PKB). AKT is tightly associated with the GLUT4 containing vesicles as well as phosphorylating the AS160/TBC1D1 complex. Activation of these two pathways results in the physical insertion of GLUT4 proteins into the membrane which involves trafficking, docking, and fusion of the GLUT4 vesicles. This requires the vesicle-associated SNARE proteins (v-SNARES such as VAMP2/3) and target membrane SNARES (t-SNARES such as SNAP-23 and syntaxin 4). AKT may also activate glycogen synthase kinase (GSK) and insulin can activate other signaling pathways such as the MEK/ERK system.

- GLUT4 transporters therefore being inserted into the membrane allowing increased glucose uptake into muscle and adipose cells
- other cell signaling pathways are also activated by insulin and these include the MEK/ERK signaling pathway that may activate enzymes and induce gene transcription.

5.3.7 Synthesis, release, and metabolism of glucagon

Compared with the overwhelming information about the physiology of β cells, comparatively little is known about the function of the glucagon-secreting α cells (and most of this is derived from rodent species) despite the importance of glucagon in counteracting hypoglycemia by activating liver glycogenolysis and gluconeogenesis to release glucose into the bloodstream.

The proglucagon gene is expressed in the pancreatic islets, the distal ileum and the large intestine, as well as certain brain neuronal cells. It encodes a number of peptide hormones that are differentially expressed in these different organs (*Figure 5.13*). These hormones are important in controlling blood glucose homeostasis, intestinal cell proliferation, and satiety.

In the pancreatic α cells the predominant post-translational products are glicentin-related polypeptide (GRPP), glucagon, intervening peptide-1 (IP-1), and the major proglucagon fragment (MPGF). Glucagon is essential for maintaining glucose homeostasis in the fasting state by stimulating glycogenolysis and gluconeogenesis in the liver. To date no physiologic functions have been identified for GRPP, IP-1, or MPGF.

In the enteroendocrine L-cells of the intestine and the central nervous system, post-translational products of the proglucagon gene are glicentin, oxyntomodulin (OXM), GLP-1, IP-2, and GLP-2. OXM inhibits gastrointestinal secretion and motility and

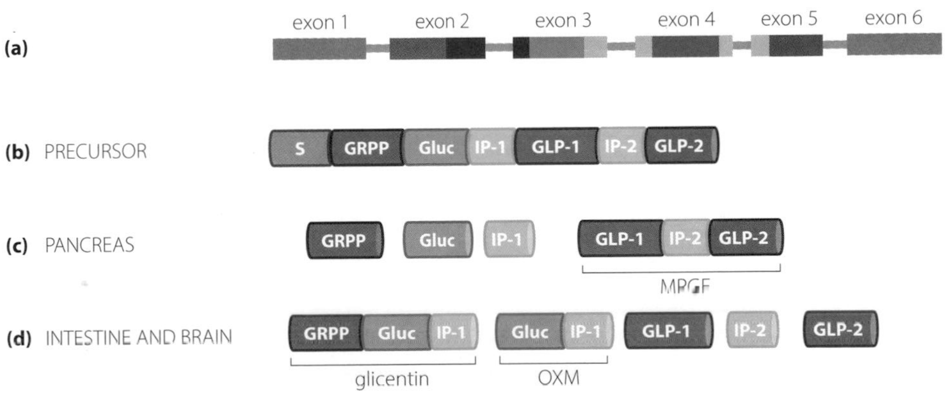

Figure 5.13. Structure of the proglucagon gene (a), the precursor protein (b), and the post-translational processing of the protein in the pancreas (c) and intestine and brain (d).
(a) The exons of the proglucagon gene.
(b) The 180 amino acid precursor protein.
(c) In the pancreatic α cells the predominant post-translational products are glicentin-related polypeptide (GRPP), glucagon (Gluc), intervening peptide-1 (IP-1), and the major proglucagon fragment (MPGF).
(d) In the enteroendocrine L-cells of the intestine and the central nervous system post-translational products are glicentin, oxyntomodulin (OXM), glucagon-like peptide (GLP)-1, intervening peptide (IP)-2, and GLP-2.

stimulates pancreatic enzyme secretion and intestinal glucose uptake. GLP-1 is an incretin (*Box 5.2*) which increases the release of insulin in response to oral ingestion of nutrients, whilst GLP-2 increases intestinal glucose transport and proliferation of intestinal cells. Both OXM and GLP-2 have also been associated with satiety and inhibition of food intake.

The release of glucagon requires the initiation of a cascade of ion channel activation which leads to a full depolarization of the glucagon-secreting cell. Glucose enters the

Box 5.2 | Incretins

Incretins are hormones secreted by the gastrointestinal tract that enhance glucose-stimulated insulin secretion in response to nutrient ingestion. In view of the fact that T2DM is associated with reduced insulin secretion, long-acting agonist drugs and inhibitors of the enzyme that degrades incretins are being developed as new treatment options for this disorder.

The first incretin to be discovered was gastric inhibitory peptide (GIP) because it inhibited gastric acid secretion, but only at pharmacologic doses. It was subsequently renamed glucose-dependent insulinotropic polypeptide to reflect its physiologic action yet retain the acronym. GIP is released from K cells, principally located in the more proximal regions (duodenum and jejunum) of the small intestine, in response to glucose or fat ingestion. Discovery of the second incretin followed the sequencing of mammalian proglucagon gene which was found to encode further peptides, including two that were similar to glucagon and thus aptly named glucagon-like peptide (GLP)-1 and GLP-2. GLP-1 and GLP-2 are released from L endocrine cells, located mainly in the distal ileum and colon, in response to nutrient ingestion, particularly nutrients rich in fats and carbohydrates. Both are liberated from proglucagon through specific post-translational proteolytic cleavage.

Both incretins act via GPCRs and activation of the GIP and GLP-1 receptors is associated with increases in cAMP and intracellular calcium and activation of various kinases. Both GIP and GLP-1 have similar actions on the pancreatic β cells, including inhibition of the ATP-sensitive potassium channel leading to depolarization of the β cell, and opening up of voltage-dependent calcium channels. Apart from stimulating insulin secretion, both hormones also stimulate insulin synthesis, increase β cell proliferation, and reduce β cell apoptosis, and GLP-1 also inhibits glucagon secretion. Their receptors are also widely distributed in peripheral tissues as well as the brain and various non-pancreatic effects of these incretins have been described. The half-lives of these hormones are between 2 and 7 minutes and they are both targets for the degrading enzyme dipeptidyl peptidase-4 (DPP-4) which renders them biologically inactive.

Due to rapid inactivation, degradation-resistant GLP-1 receptor agonists have been developed. The first, exendin-4, was isolated from lizard venom and, with 53% amino acids identical to native GLP-1, was shown to be a potent agonist at the GLP-1 receptor. A synthetic exendin-4, exenatide is now in common clinical use. Liraglutide is a long-acting GLP-1 analog that is 97% homologous to native GLP-1, and has a fatty acid acyl group which allows covalent binding to albumin which improves liraglutide's pharmacokinetic profile. Adding either of these two drugs to standard oral glucose-lowering medications shows improvements in glucose and insulin concentrations and decreases glycosylated hemoglobin (HbA1c). Four DPP-4 inhibitors, sitagliptin, vildagliptin, linagliptin and saxagliptin, are also available but the consequences of inhibiting DPP-4 for many years in susceptible patients is not known. There is interest in whether GLP-1 receptor agonists or DPP-4 inhibitors may modify the natural history of T2DM or prevent the transition from impaired glucose tolerance to frank T2DM.

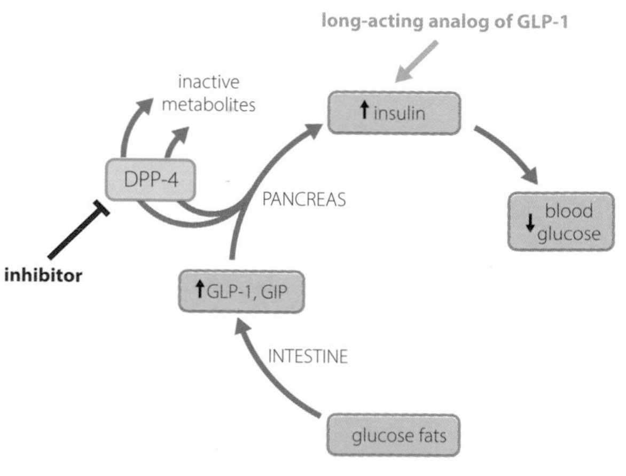

Box figure 5.2. The targets of incretins.

α cells of the islet by the GLUT1 (coded for by *SLC2A1*) transporter. At low levels of glucose there is moderate activity of ATP-sensitive potassium channels which sets the membrane potential to a point at which T-type calcium channels are activated. This induces further depolarization, leading to activation of voltage-dependent sodium channels and full depolarization of the cell. This then opens up L- or N-type calcium channels, leading to Ca^{2+} influx and exocytosis of glucagon granules. At high levels of glucose the ATP/ADP ratio rises in the cell and this closes the ATP-sensitive potassium channels and results in a depolarization of the cell membrane beyond a critical level, although some researchers have argued that glucose may be hyperpolarizing instead of depolarizing. Either way, inactivation of the ATP-sensitive potassium channels inactivates voltage-sensitive sodium channels involved in the depolarization cascade and thus glucagon secretion is inhibited.

Whilst glucagon secretion is regulated by circulating concentrations of glucose, other mechanisms regulating α-cell function have been elucidated, including:

- inhibition of glucagon secretion by somatostatin
- inhibition of glucagon release by GLP-1
- stimulation of glucagon release by fatty acids and amino acids
- inhibition of glucagon secretion by insulin

It should be noted that the last two regulatory mechanisms remain controversial in humans because most studies concerning glucagon secretion and its control have been carried out on rodents.

5.3.8 How does glucagon exert its cellular effects?

The glucagon receptor is a conserved GPCR with a large extracellular amino-terminal domain involved in ligand binding. The receptor is linked to a $G\alpha_s$ trimeric protein which, when activated by ligand binding, leads to the activation of adenylate cyclase, the generation of cAMP, and activation of protein kinase A (PKA), although the receptor can also activate the phospholipase C/inositol phosphate pathway via G_q proteins (see *Chapter 1*).

The glucagon receptor is present in many tissues including the liver, pancreatic β cells, adipocytes, heart, kidney, brain, and smooth muscles, although the regulation of glucose homeostasis through its action in the liver is the major function of glucagon. This is primarily achieved by up-regulating key enzymes such as glucose-6-phosphatase (glucose production from glucose-6-phosphate) and phosphoenolpyruvate carboxykinase (conversion of oxaloacetate into phosphoenolpyruvate (*Figure 5.4*); these actions stimulate gluconeogenesis. At the same time, glucagon inhibits the activity of glycogen synthase and an elevated glucagon:insulin ratio also accelerates fatty acid β-oxidation and formation of keto acids. Thus glucagon may also be involved in ketoacidosis (*Figure 5.9*), a medical complication of type 1 diabetes.

5.4 Diabetes mellitus

Diabetes mellitus is derived from the Greek word for siphon and *mellitus* meaning 'to do with honey'. The name pertains to frequent urination, urine sweet with glucose, and a consequent intense thirst – typical characteristics of untreated diabetic patients. The diagnosis of diabetes is simple and based on elevated fasting blood

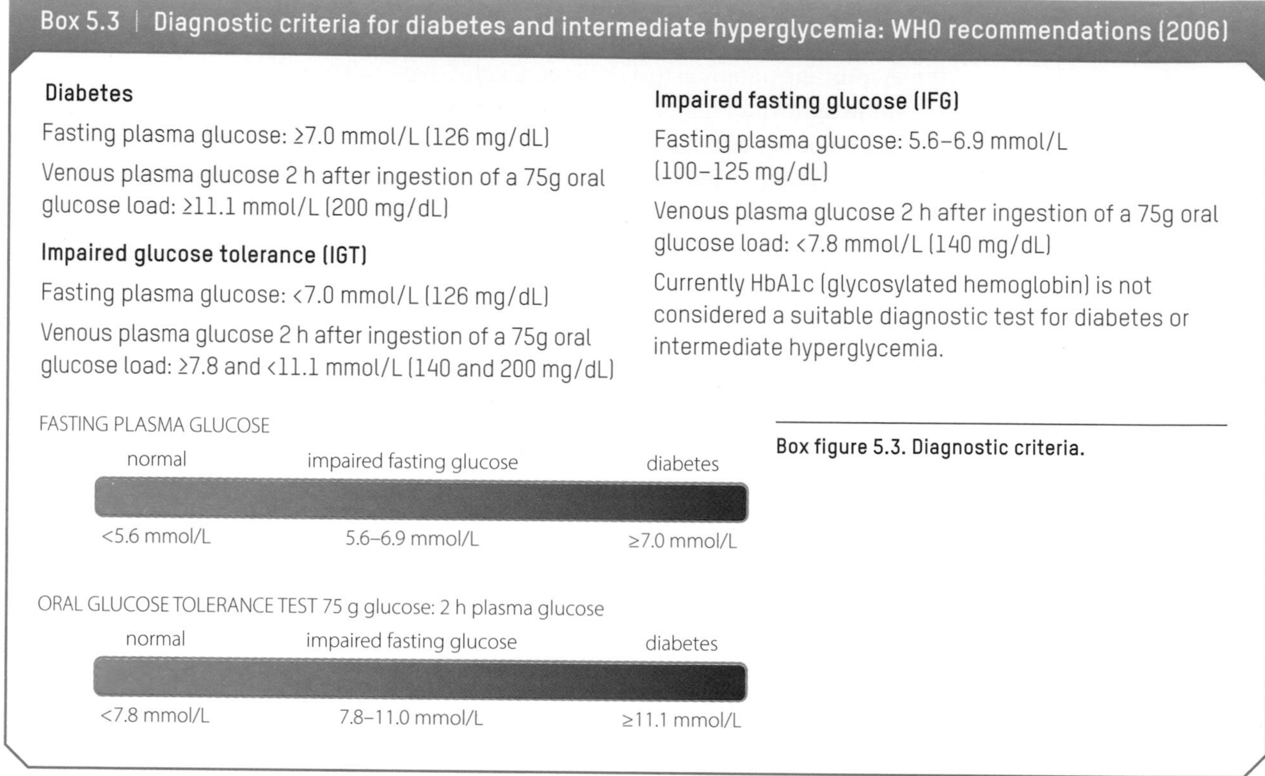

Box 5.3 | Diagnostic criteria for diabetes and intermediate hyperglycemia: WHO recommendations (2006)

Diabetes

Fasting plasma glucose: ≥7.0 mmol/L (126 mg/dL)

Venous plasma glucose 2 h after ingestion of a 75g oral glucose load: ≥11.1 mmol/L (200 mg/dL)

Impaired glucose tolerance (IGT)

Fasting plasma glucose: <7.0 mmol/L (126 mg/dL)

Venous plasma glucose 2 h after ingestion of a 75g oral glucose load: ≥7.8 and <11.1 mmol/L (140 and 200 mg/dL)

Impaired fasting glucose (IFG)

Fasting plasma glucose: 5.6–6.9 mmol/L (100–125 mg/dL)

Venous plasma glucose 2 h after ingestion of a 75g oral glucose load: <7.8 mmol/L (140 mg/dL)

Currently HbA1c (glycosylated hemoglobin) is not considered a suitable diagnostic test for diabetes or intermediate hyperglycemia.

Box figure 5.3. Diagnostic criteria.

glucose (>7 mmol/L) or a level of glucose 2 hours after a 75 g glucose load in excess of 11.1 mmol/L as specified by the World Health Organization (*Box 5.3*).

Patients with impaired fasting glucose concentrations (5.6-6.9 mmol/L) on a sample taken after an overnight fast, or impaired glucose tolerance (7.8-11.0 mmol/L) on a sample taken 2 hours after a 75 g glucose load, are at risk of the subsequent development of frank diabetes. A retrospective cohort study showed that approximately 25% of individuals with newly acquired impaired fasting glucose levels go on to develop type 2 diabetes, most within 2.5 years.

5.5 Type 1 diabetes mellitus

Type 1 diabetes mellitus (T1DM), alternatively known in the older literature as insulin-dependent diabetes mellitus (IDDM), is caused by autoimmune destruction of the β cells and an absolute loss of insulin secretion. Typically the disease presents in childhood or adolescence and patients tend to be on the lean side. The pathogenesis of the autoimmune destruction of the β cells of the islets of Langerhans is thought to involve both genetic and environmental factors, although the loss of a significant proportion of β cells is necessary before the clinical manifestations of diabetes are apparent (*Figure 5.14*).

5.5.1 Etiology of type 1 diabetes mellitus

Genetic factors

The human insulin gene is located on the short arm of chromosome 11. Genetic susceptibility is an important factor in the etiology of T1DM, but there are other factors that can trigger the disease. A rate of concordance of 30–40% has been

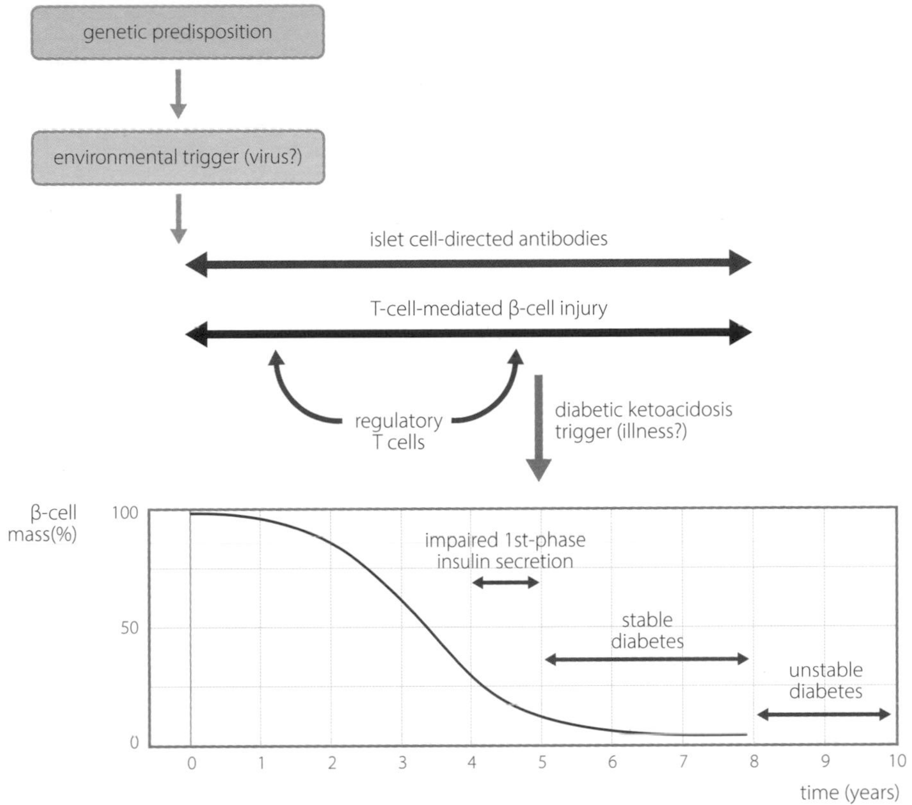

Figure 5.14. The natural history of T1DM.

shown in identical twins which supports the theory that genetic factors are not 100% implicated in the pathogenesis of T1DM. HLA genes, located on the short arm of chromosome 6, play a major role. In non-affected siblings, identical HLA gave them a 15–20% increased risk of developing T1DM, compared to 5% if they share one gene and <1% if HLA genes are not shared. Specific HLA haplotypes have been linked to T1DM. More than 90% of patients with T1DM have DR4, DQB*0302, and/or DR3*0201 haplotypes. Carrying other alleles can be protective such as in DQB*0301, DQB*0602, DRB*0403, or DRB*0406.

Environmental factors

A role for environmental triggers has been suggested in the development of T1DM in view of the rising incidence across the world (approximately 3% per year), with environmental changes being thought to affect the penetrance of T1DM gene alleles. Human and animal model studies seem to suggest that autoimmunity can be promoted or diminished by infections with viruses, including rubella virus, mumps virus, cytomegalovirus, retrovirus, rotaviruses, and enteroviruses (especially coxsackievirus B). Viruses can induce strong cellular responses and can cause local inflammation of the pancreas and ultimately β cell destruction.

Ineffective resolution of inflammation can result in 'misreading' of inflammatory signals and the development of chronic inflammatory disease or autoimmune diseases. T cells play a major role in the inflammatory pathogenesis of T1DM. The communication between the immune cells and the β cells can influence the amplitude of the insulitis through the local production of chemokines and cytokines as well as the danger signals from the dying β cells. The intensity of the early response depends on the genetic background of the individual. Cytokines contribute to long-

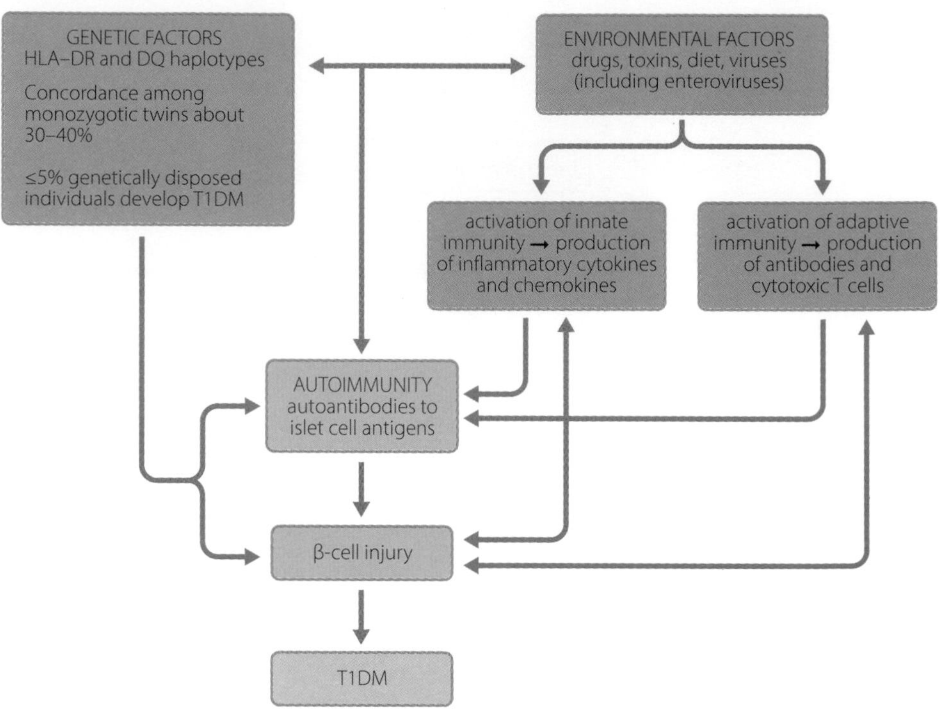

Figure 5.15. Factors involved in the etiology of T1DM.
There are genetic linkages in the human leukocyte antigen (HLA) complex of genes and specific HLA genes have been linked with the development of T1DM, particularly the HLA-DR and HLA-DQ alleles. Such genetic factors may predispose an individual to the development of autoantibodies and/or their response to environmental factors.

The role of enteroviruses in the etiology of T1DM has been investigated widely. The production of inflammatory cytokines and chemokines may trigger an autoimmune response as well as directly damaging β cell function. Similarly, activation of the adaptive immune system by the inflammatory response may directly damage β cell function, which may contribute to β cell antigen release. There is a dialog between β cells and the immune system that is mediated by cytokines and chemokines.

Disturbed immune tolerance and molecular mimicry between viral and self-antigens may lead to a chronic autoimmune attack on β cells. Islet cell antibodies are strongly associated with the development of T1DM. Autoantibodies to islet antigens indentified so far: glutamate decarboxylase (GADA), islet antigen (IA)-2A (IA-2A/ICA512) and IA-2B (phogrin), insulin autoantibodies (IAA), and zinc transporter-8 (ZnT8A). All the major antibodies are directed against the secretory apparatus of the β cells.

The genetic background of an individual and the interaction with environmental cues probably modulates the induction, amplification, and maintenance or resolution of β cell function.

term suppression of β cell function and can have an effect on their modulation and regeneration which can result in insulin resistance. In contrast, some inflammatory mediators might promote β cell survival and proliferation. *Figure 5.15* outlines the genetic and environmental factors that may contribute to the eventual destruction of β cells both through inflammatory mediators and the production of autoantibodies against islet antigens. These antibodies are directed against the secretory apparatus of the β cells and are strongly associated with the development of T1DM. Almost all patients with T1DM have multiple antibodies which are present before the clinical symptoms of diabetes are apparent.

5.5.2 Metabolic disturbances in type 1 diabetes mellitus

As would be predicted from the actions of insulin and glucagon, the metabolic pattern of untreated T1DM is:

- increased lipolysis resulting in increased circulating levels of FFAs
- esterification of FFAs in the liver increasing VLDL–triacylglycerol secretion
- loss of uptake of TAG into adipose tissue
- increased proteolysis
- loss of uptake of glucose into muscle (normally this accounts for ~75% of whole body insulin-stimulated glucose uptake)
- increased gluconeogenesis
- formation of excess ketone bodies (keto acids) resulting in diabetic ketoacidosis.

These overall effects are summarized in *Figure 5.16*.

Glucagon secretion is increased in T1DM and this is thought to be due to the general 'stress' state which stimulates the sympathetic and adrenomedullary system. This fuels gluconeogenesis and the formation of keto acids (3-hydroxybutyric acid and acetoacetic acid) and acetone (together these are called ketone bodies). The accumulation of ketone bodies and glucose in the blood, together with dehydration, leads to an increased osmolality of body fluids and, in combination with the acidosis,

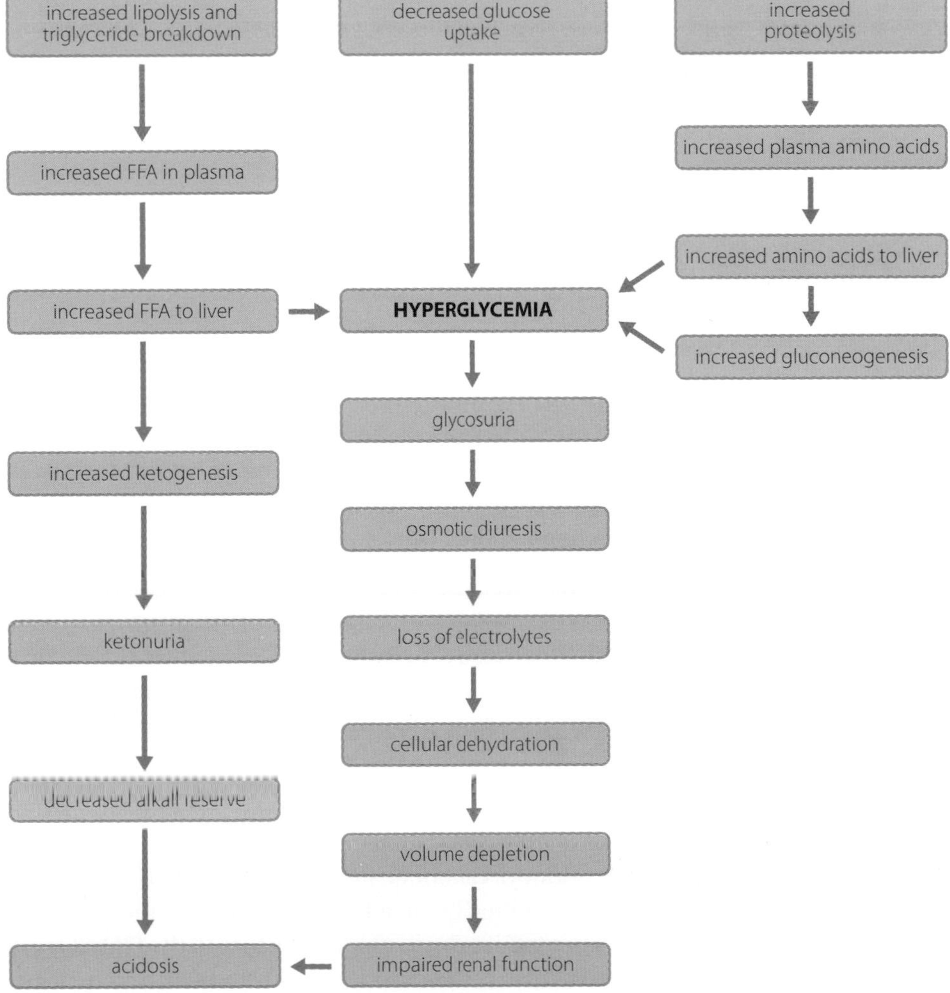

Figure 5.16. Overview of the metabolic disturbances in diabetes mellitus.

Box 5.4 | Diabetic emergencies: diabetic ketoacidosis

Diabetic ketoacidosis (DKA) is a medical emergency defined by the combination of hyperglycemia, ketonemia, and acidosis. It results from the absolute or relative deficiency of insulin in the presence of an increase in the counter-regulatory hormones (i.e. glucagon, cortisol, growth hormone, epinephrine). This causes increased gluconeogenesis and glycogenolysis resulting in worsening hyperglycemia. Alternative energy is provided by breakdown of free fatty acids which result in ketogenesis.

The incidence of DKA is difficult to ascertain but some population studies estimated approximately 4.6–8 episodes per 1000 patients with diabetes. It is a significant cause of morbidity and mortality. Mortality is about 5–10% overall and is much higher in the elderly. DKA can typically occur in patients with T1DM but is also recognized in patients with T2DM with significant β cell loss.

Criteria for diagnosis:

- raised blood ketone level >3 mmol/L and/or significant ketonuria (2+ or more)
- blood glucose >11 mmol/L or known diabetes mellitus
- bicarbonate <15 mmol/L and/or pH less than 7.3

Precipitants:

- new diagnosis of diabetes (10%)
- infection (30%)
- management errors/concordance issues (15%)
- no cause identified (40%)
- other, e.g. myocardial infarction (5%)

Clinical features:

- secondary to hyperglycemia: excessive thirst, polyuria, polydipsia, dehydration, altered consciousness (drowsiness, confusion), or coma
- secondary to ketonemia: abdominal pain, vomiting, Kussmaul respiration

Management

The objectives of management are to:

1. restore circulatory volume with intravenous fluids; the average fluid loss in DKA is 3–6 L
2. achieve clearance of ketones
3. correct hyperglycemia with intravenous insulin infusion
4. correct the electrolyte imbalance
5. identify the cause of DKA

Complications:

- hypo / hyperkalemia
- cerebral edema
- hypoglycemia
- pulmonary edema

can eventually lead to diabetic coma (or hyperglycemic coma) progressing to death if not treated. The tendency to develop ketoacidosis is one feature that distinguishes type 1 from type 2 diabetes, presumably because the insulin that remains in T2DM is sufficient to prevent ketoacidosis. If ketoacidosis does develop it is a medical emergency and the features and management of diabetic ketoacidosis (DKA) are outlined in *Box 5.4*.

The only treatment for this form of the disease is insulin replacement and, prior to its discovery in 1921, sufferers of this disease would have a short, painful life. Described by a Greek physician in the first century AD 'it consists in the flesh and bones running together into urine; the patients are tortured with an unquenchable thirst; the whole body wastes away'. These effects are due to lack of glucose uptake into tissues and organs, loss of lipogenesis, and utilization of muscle proteins for gluconeogenesis.

The frequent urination is due to the fact that the excess plasma glucose filtered in the kidneys cannot be totally reabsorbed (as normally occurs) because the glucose concentration in the tubules exceeds the tubular maximum (12 mmol/L) for reabsorption. The remaining glucose in the filtrate creates an osmotic effect which prevents water reabsorption in the tubules and hence an osmotic diuresis.

5.5.3 Management of type 1 diabetes mellitus

Treatment with subcutaneous insulin injections

Insulin is the mainstay of treatment for T1DM because of the absolute deficiency of insulin. The objective of this treatment is to maintain blood glucose levels in the normal range and to mimic, as far as possible, the endogenous pattern of insulin secretion (*Figure 5.17*). Maintaining optimal glycemic control has been shown to reduce the risk of developing long-term complications. The Diabetes Control and Complications Trial (DCCT) demonstrated that with intensive glycemic control the rates of retinopathy, nephropathy, and neuropathy (see *Section 5.8*) were reduced in patients with T1DM. In the EDIC trial (a follow-up study of the DCCT trial), intensive glycemic control decreased fatal and non-fatal cardiovascular events. Intensive glycemic control can be associated with an increased incidence of hypoglycemia. In the DCCT trial, an inverse relationship between HbA1c (glycosylated hemoglobin) and the frequency of hypoglycemia was shown. The risk of severe hypoglycemia, requiring the help of another person, was higher in males, adolescents, and those with previous episodes of severe hypoglycemia. Education plays a major role in preventing those episodes.

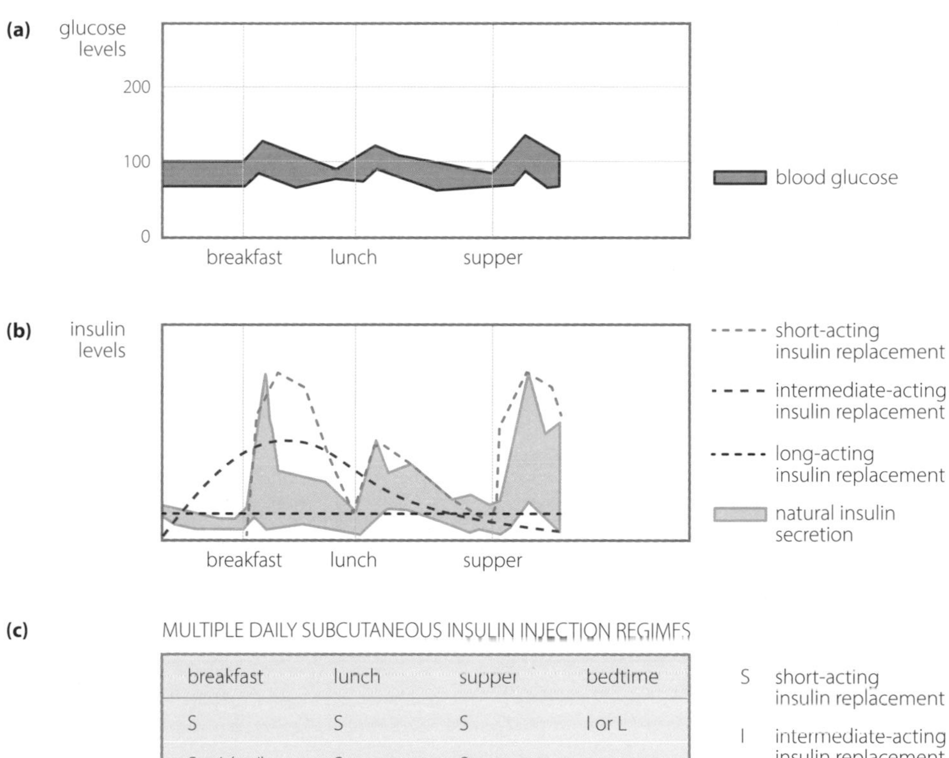

breakfast	lunch	supper	bedtime
S	S	S	I or L
S + L(or I)	S	S	
S + I	S	S	I

Figure 5.17. Management of T1DM with subcutaneous insulin injections.
(a) Typical profile of glucose levels over a 24 hour period
(b) Profile of insulin levels over a 24 hour period. Short-acting insulin (e.g. aspart, lispro, glulisine) works within 30 minutes of the injection, reaches a peak at 2–4 hours and lasts about 6 hours. Intermediate-acting insulin (e.g. NPH or Humulin/Novolin) works within 2–4 hours, peaks 4–12 hours later and lasts up to 18 hours. Long-acting insulin (e.g. detemir, glargine) remains stable over 24h.
(c) Possible insulin injection regimes.

The insulins available for use can be classified according to their source (animal, human, analog) or action profile (short-, intermediate-, long-acting). Insulin may be administered using the conventional multiple daily injections (MDI) or continuous subcutaneous infusion; the choice depends on the clinical condition and patient's preference. *Figure 5.17* shows comparisons between natural insulin release and that which can be achieved with insulin replacement, along with different injection regimes combining short- with intermediate-/long-acting insulin preparations. The targets for successfully managing T1DM are shown in *Box 5.5* and *Box 5.6* outlines

Box 5.5 | Targets for management of T1DM

Glycemic control

- HbA1c <7.5%/58 mmol/mol (<6.5%/48 mmol/mol if increased cardiovascular risk)
- Glucose monitoring:
  - preprandial glucose: 4–7 mmol/L
  - postprandial glucose: <9 mmol/L
  - avoid pursuing tight targets if quality of life is affected or if there is a risk of significant hypoglycemia or hypoglycemia unawareness

Blood pressure: intervene if:

- above 135/85 mmHg, **or**
- above 130/80 mmHg with abnormal albumin excretion rate or in the presence of features of the metabolic syndrome

Lipid and antithrombotic control

- see *Box figure 5.4*

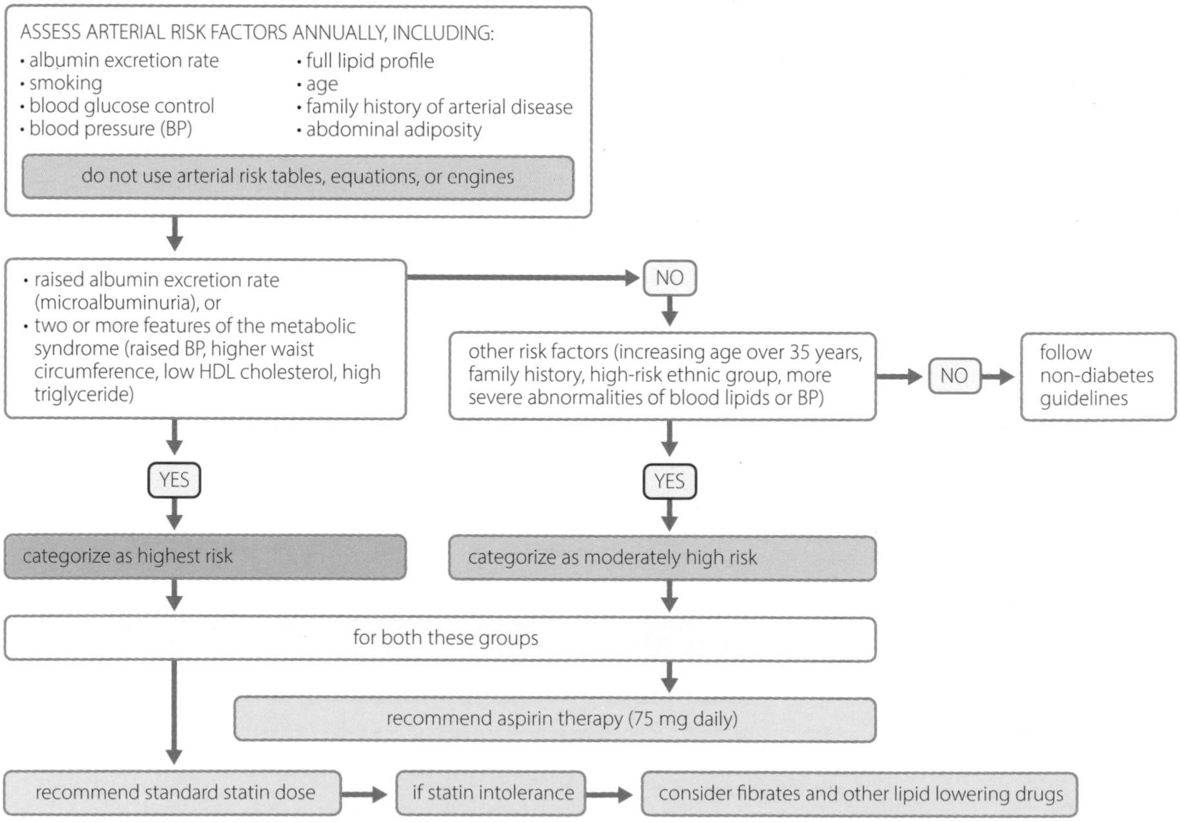

ASSESS ARTERIAL RISK FACTORS ANNUALLY, INCLUDING:
- albumin excretion rate
- smoking
- blood glucose control
- blood pressure (BP)
- full lipid profile
- age
- family history of arterial disease
- abdominal adiposity

do not use arterial risk tables, equations, or engines

↓

- raised albumin excretion rate (microalbuminuria), or
- two or more features of the metabolic syndrome (raised BP, higher waist circumference, low HDL cholesterol, high triglyceride)

→ NO → other risk factors (increasing age over 35 years, family history, high-risk ethnic group, more severe abnormalities of blood lipids or BP) → NO → follow non-diabetes guidelines

YES → categorize as highest risk

(other risk factors) YES → categorize as moderately high risk

for both these groups → recommend aspirin therapy (75 mg daily)

→ recommend standard statin dose → if statin intolerance → consider fibrates and other lipid lowering drugs

Box figure 5.4. Lipid and antithrombotic management.
Reproduced from NICE guideline CG15: Type 1 diabetes: diagnosis and management of type 1 diabetes in adults (updated March 2010).

Box 5.6 | Annual review for people with T1DM

Annual assessment of:

- education and skills
- arterial risk factors against targets: glycemic control, blood pressure, lipids, smoking
- developing complications: retinopathy, nephropathy, neuropathy, erectile dysfunction

Education

Learning to live with diabetes is a continual process which involves all aspects of life. A multi-disciplinary approach to education helps people with T1DM cope with various aspects of diabetes management.

Diet

Carbohydrates are the main factors controlling blood glucose levels. However, paying attention to other aspects of diet such as salt and fat intake is important because this would help maintain blood pressure and plasma lipid levels. The aim is to lead a healthy lifestyle. The general guidelines for diet in people with T1DM are as follows:

- have regular meals
- aim to include more starchy carbohydrate foods (such as bread, pasta, rice, cereals, etc.) and limit sugar and sugary food
- cut down fat intake in general, particularly saturated fat
- eat more fruit and vegetables
- include more beans and pulses
- eat oily fish at least twice a week
- daily salt intake of 6 g or less
- alcohol intake within recommended levels: 2 units/day for women and 3 units/day for men
- avoid 'diabetic' foods and drinks; they can still affect blood glucose levels and contain as much fat and calories as the ordinary ones

Exercise

Exercise helps to control weight and improve well-being in general. It is worth noting that during exercise muscles utilize glucose without the need for insulin. Therefore, this can have an effect on glycemic control. Patients are advised to check their glucose level before, during, and after exercise. Insulin dose (around the time of exercise) needs to be decreased by 20–30% to avoid hypoglycemia. Quickly absorbed carbohydrate should be taken 15–30 minutes before and then every 30 minutes during the exercise to prevent hypoglycemia. There is also a risk of late hypoglycemia (4–8 hours after the end of the exercise) because of the replenishment of depleted glycogen stores. This can be prevented by ingestion of slowly absorbed carbohydrates immediately after the exercise.

the broad objectives for annual review of patients with stable T1DM and highlights the importance of reiterating the need for education, diet, and exercise.

Continuous subcutaneous insulin infusion (CSII)

This is achieved by the attachment of an insulin pump to a catheter on the outside of the body. The pump delivers short-acting insulin at a programmed basal rate with a facility to administer a bolus of insulin to cover meals and also correct blood glucose fluctuations. According to NICE guidelines in the UK, CSII is indicated in patients with T1DM whose attempts to achieve target HbA1c result in disabling hypoglycemia, or whose HbA1c levels remained high despite a high level of care using multiple daily injections (MDI).

Islet cell transplantation (ICT)

Following the success of islet cell transplantation by the Edmonton group in Canada in 2000, many groups worldwide adopted the technique and started to offer this type of therapy. However, it is still an experimental therapy and its availability is currently limited to people with T1DM who have extreme problems with glycemic control and severe disabling hypoglycemia which may be life-threatening or have drastically reduced quality of life. Around 500 000 or more islets are infused into the portal vein of the recipient. Data from the Collaborative Islet Transplant Registry (CITR) indicated insulin independence for 71% of adults who received the therapy at 1 year. This figure goes down to 52% at 2 years and 23% at 3 years. Patients are required to remain on immunosuppression after the procedure.

CASE 5.1

215 240

- Woman of 17 years with 24 hour history of vomiting, abdominal pain, and disturbed consciousness
- Mother reports daughter has 3 week history of polyuria, polydipsia, and weight loss
- Random glucose 23 mmol/L
- Diagnosed with severe diabetic ketoacidosis after further tests
- T1DM treated with MDIs of subcutaneous insulin

The patient underwent further investigations; arterial blood gas assessment on room air revealed:

- pH 7.24 (NR 7.35–7.45)
- pCO_2 3.1 kPa (NR: 4.7–6.0)
- pO_2 8 kPa (NR: 9.3–13.3)
- bicarbonate 5 mmol/L (NR: 22–26)
- base excess -18 mmol/L (NR: -3 to +3)
- potassium 3.5 mmol/L (NR: 3.5–5.2)

Urine dipstick was strongly positive for ketones (4+) but otherwise unremarkable. Further blood tests including U&Es, LFTs, plasma glucose, glycated hemoglobin, and full blood count were requested. Chest X-ray revealed a right lower lobe consolidation.

A diagnosis of severe diabetic ketoacidosis was established based on the hyperglycemia, metabolic acidosis and ketonemia. The patient was transferred to a high dependency unit and a central venous access was established. She was started on intravenous fluids with 0.9% saline, intravenous insulin infusion, and appropriate antibiotics for pneumonia. Potassium chloride was added to the 0.9% saline infusion. Over the next 24 hours her consciousness level improved and her vomiting stopped by the next morning.

The diabetes team reviewed her the following morning and the diagnosis of T1DM was explained to her. They had a discussion about the implications of the diagnosis and treatments available. She was started on MDIs of subcutaneous insulin. The diabetes specialist nurse trained her to monitor her blood glucose levels and how to recognize and avoid hypoglycemia. She learned to self-administer insulin with an insulin pen and how to manage blood glucose levels during intercurrent illnesses. She was also made aware of 'sick day rules' – essentially, the need to continue insulin injections even if not well enough to eat, and indeed to increase the dose of insulin by injection should self-documented sugar levels increase. She was also reviewed by the dietician.

The insulin infusion and intravenous fluids were stopped after 24 hours and she was converted to subcutaneous insulin alone. After the diabetes team review, she was discharged from hospital on oral antibiotics and an MDI insulin regimen. An early follow-up was organized by the diabetes nurse specialist. Following discharge she was referred to the intensive education programme DAFNE (Diabetes Adjustment For Normal Eating) and on review in the diabetes clinic 4 weeks later she was doing well. She will remain on insulin therapy for the rest of her life and have an annual review of her condition (*Box 5.6*).

5.6 Type 2 diabetes mellitus

T2DM usually develops later in life, from the mid-thirties onwards, and patients are very often overweight. It should be noted, however, that T2DM is being diagnosed more frequently at earlier ages, and even in children, due to the rising prevalence of obesity in many countries. This form of the disease is not life-threatening in the short term and treatment does not usually require insulin; blood sugar levels can be controlled with diet and insulin-secreting or insulin-sensitizing drugs. Though one might perceive T2DM to be a milder form of the disease, in fact the long-term consequences of diabetic complications in poorly controlled diabetics are just as severe as in T1DM.

T2DM is characterized by insulin resistance coupled with loss of β cell function and insulinopenia with a similar metabolic profile to that seen in T1DM, but without ketoacidosis because of the presence of insulin to suppress lipolysis and hence ketogenesis. Insulin resistance has been attributed to several defects in the insulin signaling pathway, including dysfunction of the insulin receptor substrate (IRS) protein, the downstream PI-3 kinase/AKT signaling activity (*Figure 5.12*), and inactivation of GLUT4 (*Box 5.1*). The decline in β cell function frequently observed in T2DM patients has been attributed to glucose toxicity and lipotoxicity as a result of high blood glucose concentrations, or hyperlipidemia. More recently evidence has focused on oxidative stress because elevated glucose concentrations increase reactive oxygen species and, because islets appear to have intrinsically low antioxidant enzyme defenses, this leads to their loss of function.

The loss of insulin secretion and resistance to insulin is usually accompanied by a relative or absolute increase in glucagon secretion in the fasting and postprandial states, thereby potentiating glucose mobilization from the liver and maintaining the hyperglycemic state. Interestingly, and conversely, the secretion of glucagon in response to hypoglycemia in type 1 and long-lasting type 2 diabetes is impaired, increasing the risk of hypoglycemia, especially in patients treated with insulin. Thus diabetes is also associated with defects in the glucagon secretory response of α cells to both hyper- and hypoglycemia. If hyperglycemia becomes severe a hyperosmolar hyperglycemic state (HHS) – previously known as hyperosmolar non-ketotic coma (HONK) – can develop and this is a medical emergency (*Box 5.7*).

5.6.1 Management of type 2 diabetes mellitus

The present goal of T2DM therapy is to reduce glycosylated hemoglobin (HbA1c) to 7.5% (58 mmol/mol) or lower. Circulating glucose binds to hemoglobin irreversibly forming HbA1c, and levels of HbA1c directly reflect prevailing glucose levels over the preceding 2–3 months (i.e. the life of a red cell). Studies such as the Diabetes Control and Complications Study (DCCT) and the UK Prospective Diabetes Study (UKPDS) have shown that the increase in HbA1c is directly related to the risk of complications and hence there is a need to set targets for HbA1c for patients which is usually in the range of 6–7.5% (42–58 mmol/mol). Note that HbA1c has traditionally been reported as a percentage, but since 2009 the measurement has been standardized by the International Federation of Clinical Chemistry and reported as mmol/mol. There is not an easy conversion between the two units, the simplest being: mmol/mol = 10.93 x % – 23.5. Using this, an HbA1c of 6% would be 42 mmol/mol, and the average patient target range would become 42–58 mmol/mol rather than 6–7.5%.

Box 5.7 | Diabetic emergencies: hyperosmolar hyperglycemic state

HHS (previously known as hyperosmolar non-ketotic coma: HONK) occurs less frequently than diabetic ketoacidosis (DKA) but it carries a higher mortality. It usually occurs in patients with T2DM and patients tend to be older. Hyperglycemia results from impaired utilization of glucose, increased glycogenolysis, and gluconeogenesis. Osmotic diuresis further complicates the hyperglycemic state. Glucose values are higher than in DKA. Ketogenesis does not occur in HHS as a result of the presence of sufficient insulin to prevent lipolysis and subsequent ketogenesis. However, it is not sufficient to control hyperglycemia.

HHS can be precipitated by:

- inadequate treatment or non-concordance (21–41%)
- acute illness/infection (32–60%)
- endocrine: acromegaly, thyrotoxicosis, Cushing syndrome
- drugs, e.g. steroids, beta-blockers, clozapine, total parenteral nutrition, nasogastric feeding
- previously undiagnosed diabetes

Clinical features

HHS develops more insidiously than DKA. Symptoms include polyuria, polydipsia, and weight loss. Lethargy, focal neurological signs (hemiplegia/hemiparesis), seizures, and even coma in later stages are more common in HHS. Neurological deterioration is linked to the rise in plasma osmolality (occurs with plasma osmolality around 320–330 mosmol/kg). The fluid loss in HHS is about 8–10 liters.

Management

The aim of the therapy is to restore the extracellular fluid volume. Rapid correction of plasma osmolality can result in the development of cerebral edema. The fluid of choice is isotonic saline (i.e. 0.9% sodium chloride). The optimal rate of infusion depends on the patient's clinical state. Correction of potassium is important and patients should be closely monitored. Because hyperosmolality and hypernatremia can contribute to a hypercoagulable state, prophylactic anti-coagulation may be considered. Fluid management in HHS is essential to correct the fluid loss and hyperglycemia. Intravenous insulin infusions can facilitate the correction of hyperglycemia. As in DKA, identifying and treating the underlying cause of HHS is an integral part in the management.

Despite the abundance of available anti-diabetes therapies, a considerable number of people with T2DM continue to have relatively poor glycemic control and are at risk for macrovascular and microvascular disease (see *Section 5.8*). There are many choices for the treatment of T2DM and one common approach is shown in *Figure 5.18*. The following are the options which can be considered.

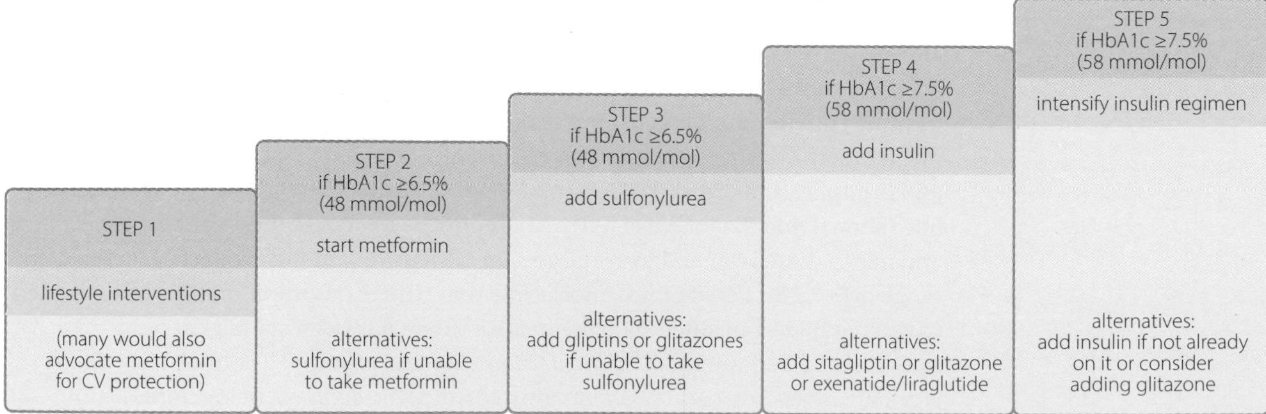

Figure 5.18. An approach to treatment of patients with type 2 diabetes mellitus.
Reproduced from *GP Update Handbook* (www.gp-update.co.uk) with permission.

Diet

Energy intake must be controlled to maintain as low a body weight as possible because excess weight is linked with insulin resistance. Drugs may be used to treat any underlying obesity. In addition, the intake of simple sugars (mono- and disaccharides) should be low to slow down the rate of absorption of carbohydrate and thus minimize the postprandial rise in blood glucose concentration. Simple sugars are more rapidly absorbed than more complex carbohydrates.

Acarbose

This is an inhibitor of α-amylase, the pancreatic enzyme that digests starch. When taken with meals it slows down carbohydrate digestion and absorption and thus minimizes the postprandial rise in glucose.

Insulin secretagogues

Sulfonylureas are drugs that combine with the SUR protein associated with the ATP-sensitive potassium channel in β cells. Like glucose they close potassium channels, depolarize the β cell, and ultimately increase the secretion of insulin (see *Figure 5.12*). In healthy type 2 diabetic subjects they also inhibit glucagon secretion. These drugs reduce glycosylated hemoglobin (HbA1c) by 1–2% (11–22 mmol/mol) and fasting blood glucose concentrations by around 3.5 mmol/L. Hypoglycemia is the most common side-effect of these agents although other well-recognized side-effects include an increased appetite and weight gain, so these may not be the first drug of choice in obese patients.

Meglitinides, otherwise known as glinides, are newer insulin secretagogues that have a faster onset and shorter duration of action than the sulfonylureas and reduce HbA1c by 0.5–2.0% (6–22 mmol/mol). They are associated with a reduced risk of hypoglycemia and cause less weight gain, though they must always be taken immediately before meals to avoid hypoglycemia.

Insulin sensitizers

A widely used sensitizer is the biguanide drug, metformin, which increases glucose utilization, decreases hepatic gluconeogenesis, inhibits glycogenolysis and improves insulin sensitivity, particularly in skeletal muscle. Its precise mode of action is unclear but may be via adenosine monophosphate protein kinase (*Box 5.8*). It is the first choice treatment in obese patients because it is associated with lack of weight gain and even weight loss in some patients. Because it does not affect insulin release (as occurs with sulfonylureas) it does not cause hypoglycemia, unless it is used in combination with insulin secretagogues.

More recently, a group of drugs known as thiazolidinediones, commonly referred to as glitazones, have been introduced to treat T2DM. In contrast to metformin, these agents increase insulin sensitivity by increasing the efficiency of glucose transporters in muscle and adipose tissue. They can reduce HbA1c by 1–2% (11–22 mmol/mol). Glitazones activate the transcription factor PPARγ (*Box 5.9*) in adipose tissue resulting in altered gene transcription, modulation of fatty acid metabolism, and a reduction in circulating FFAs. They do not cause hypoglycemia when used as a single agent, but may do so when used in conjunction with other agents.

Glucagon-like peptide-1 (GLP-1) therapies

GLP-1 agonists: endogenous GLP-1 increases insulin secretion and inhibits glucagon secretion (*Box 5.2*). GLP-1 agonists are the most recently developed drugs used

Box 5.8 | AMP-activated protein kinase

AMP-activated protein kinase (AMPK) is an energy sensor (can be thought of as a fuel gauge) and is activated when there is a cellular decrease in high energy phosphate, resulting in an increase in the AMP:ATP ratio. AMPK is an enzyme and an important mediator of cellular metabolism. It stimulates glucose uptake and lipid oxidation to produce energy whilst turning off energy (ATP)-consuming processes such as gluconeogenesis, protein synthesis, and lipogenesis, thus rebalancing cellular energy. Binding of AMP to this heterotrimeric protein makes it more susceptible to phosphorylation by upstream kinases and less susceptible to phosphatase activity, resulting in activation of the protein. Altered cellular calcium levels can also result in phosphorylation of AMPK, a process which is independent of changes in the AMP:ATP ratio. Phosphorylated AMPK stimulates insulin-independent glucose uptake in contracting muscle, increases lipid β-oxidation in liver (ketone formation), reduces both lipolysis and lipogenesis in adipose tissue (hence reducing circulating lipids), and increases insulin sensitivity. Collectively, activation of AMPK in skeletal muscle, liver, and adipose tissue results in a favorable milieu for prevention of T2DM, i.e. reduced circulating glucose concentrations, reduced plasma lipids and fat accumulation, as well as increased insulin sensitivity. Interestingly, the antidiabetic action of thiazolidinediones (e.g. rosiglitazone, suspended for treatment in 2010) and biguanides (metformin) involves activation of AMPK, probably by impairing mitochondrial function and so resulting in changes in the AMP:ATP ratio, although other unknown mechanisms may exist.

Box 5.9 | Peroxisome proliferator-activated receptors

Peroxisome proliferator-activated receptors (PPARs) are ligand-activated transcription factors belonging to the nuclear receptor superfamily which includes steroid receptors. Three receptor subtypes have been identified and cloned, PPARα, PPARγ, and PPARβ/δ and overall they are sensors of altered lipid metabolism, particularly intracellular fatty acid levels.

- Activation of PPARα promotes lipid metabolism and increases HDL cholesterol synthesis. It is highly expressed in tissues with high fatty acid oxidation, such as liver, kidney and heart muscle and also in vascular endothelial cells, smooth muscle cells, macrophages and T lymphocytes.
- Activation of PPARγ, the most widely investigated subtype of these receptors, is important in the differentiation of adipocytes and in regulation of genes involved in glucose and lipid metabolism. It is mainly expressed in white and brown adipose tissue and in other tissues including endothelial cells, vascular smooth muscle cells and, to a lesser extent, immune cells such as macrophages.
- Activation of PPARβ/δ promotes fatty acid metabolism and suppresses macrophage-derived inflammation. It is the most ubiquitously expressed of these receptor subtypes.

Drugs targeting the PPARs

- Drugs that activate PPARα are the fibrate class of hypolipodemic drugs, including clofibrate, fenfibrate and bezafibrate. They lower serum triglycerides and increase HDL cholesterol in hyperlipidemic patients.
- Drugs that activate PPARγ are the thiazolidinediones, commonly referred to as glitazones. They enhance insulin sensitivity in target tissues and lower glucose and fatty acid levels in type 2 diabetics. Pioglitazone is currently marketed as a first-line drug for the treatment of T2DM.
- Drugs that activate PPARβ/δ are currently being investigated as potential cardioprotective drugs.
- PPARα and γ dual agonists are currently under development for the potential treatment of T2DM and provide an option for treating cardiovascular disease. Their reported pro-inflammatory and pro-atherogenic effects require further investigation.

for the treatment of T2DM. Exenatide is a pure GLP-1 agonist acting at the GLP-1 receptor and resistant to protease degradation (by DPP-4). It is usually administered as a twice daily injection and used in conjunction with metformin or a sulfonylurea. Clinical trials have demonstrated a reduction in fasting and postprandial blood sugars, a reduction of HbA1c of 1–2% (11–22 mmol/mol) and a weight loss of 2–5 kg. Liraglutide is a once daily human GLP-1 analog. It is effective in reducing blood sugar and weight. Liraglutide is a derivative of human GLP-1 (97% homology) which is protected against DPPIV degradation. Being bound to serum albumin protects it from elimination by the kidneys, resulting in a prolonged half-life (around 24 hours).

Dipeptidyl peptidase-4 (DPP-4) inhibitors: the alternative target to the GLP-1 receptor is the DDP-4 enzyme (*Box 5.2*) that rapidly inactivates endogenous GLP-1 giving it a circulating half-life of <2 minutes. DPP-4 inhibitors (e.g. sitagliptin, vildagliptin, and saxagliptin) prolong the activity of endogenously secreted GLP-1. These drugs, like GLP-1 agonists, are also effective in controlling hyperglycemia, improving pancreatic β cell function and reducing HbA1c by ~1% (11 mmol/mol). They have a low risk of hypoglycemia and can be used as monotherapy or in combination with other treatments for hyperglycemia. In contrast to long-acting GLP-1 therapies, these drugs are available orally, have a longer duration of action and only require a daily dosing. They do not, however, reduce appetite or cause weight loss (in contrast to GLP-1 agonists). A comparison of the action of GLP agonists and DDP-4 inhibitors is shown in *Table 5.1*.

Table 5.1. **Comparison of action of GLP-1 receptor agonists and DPP-4 inhibitors**

Impact on:	GLP-1 receptor agonist	DPP-4 inhibitor
Insulin secretion	Increased	Increased
Glucagon secretion	Stopped	Stopped
Postprandial hyperglycemia	Reduced	Reduced
Appetite	Reduced	Unaffected
Satiety	Induced	Unaffected
Body weight	Reduced	Unaffected
β cell function	Preserved	Preserved
Gastric emptying	Reduced	Unaffected
Adverse GI effects	Common	Rare

Adapted from Triplitt *et al.* (2007; *J. Manag. Care Pharm.* **13**: S2–S16) with permission from the Academy of Managed Care Pharmacy.

CASE 5.2 216 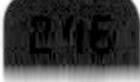 245

- Woman of 44 years with type 2 DM; now gaining weight
- Exenatide started: HbA1c improved and weight lost

The patient was started on exenatide, a GLP-1 agonist. HbA1c improved to 7.2% (55 mmol/mol) within 4 months and she dropped 12 kg in weight. Nausea was the main side-effect initially but this subsided eventually. Her lipid profile also markedly improved. She continues under review at the diabetes clinic.

5.7 Rarer forms of diabetes mellitus

CASE 5.3 246 247

- Afro-Caribbean man of 38 years with 4 week history of polyuria, polydipsia, and blurred vision
- Mother and paternal grandfather had T2DM
- BMI 40 kg/m^2, random glucose 27 mmol/L, 3+ ketonuria
- Low pH, low pCO_2, low bicarbonate
- Diabetic ketoacidosis diagnosed and treatment started with insulin infusion – HbA1c was 13% (119 mmol/mol)
- T1DM suspected and subcutaneous insulin continued with addition of metformin

A 38 year old man, originally from Jamaica, presented to the Emergency Department with a 4 week history of polyuria, polydipsia, and blurred vision. He started to vomit in the 24 hours leading to his presentation. He had no significant past medical history. His mother and paternal grandfather had type 2 diabetes mellitus. He smoked 20 cigarettes per day and drank about 25 units of alcohol per week.

Clinically he was dehydrated, tachypneic, pulse rate 102/min, blood pressure 110/70 mmHg. Physical examination revealed central obesity (BMI 40 kg/m^2), no signs of cortisol excess, and was otherwise unremarkable. Random glucose was 27 mmol/L and he had significant (3+) ketonuria. Arterial blood gases revealed:

- pH 7.2 (NR 7.35–7.45)
- pCO_2 3.6 kPa (NR: 4.7–6.0)
- pO_2 11.4 kPa (NR: 9.3–13.3)
- bicarbonate 14 mmol/L (NR: 22–26)

A diagnosis of diabetic ketoacidosis was made and he was started on intravenous fluids and insulin infusion. As soon as the acidosis had resolved and the vomiting had stopped he was switched to subcutaneous insulin.

HbA1c was 13% (119 mmol/mol). Fasting lipids showed mixed hyperlipidemia with low HDL. Otherwise LFTs and U&Es were unremarkable.

Anti-GAD and anti-islet cell antibodies were requested in view of the discordant body habitus and clinical presentation of diabetic ketoacidosis. A presumed diagnosis of T1DM was made based on the fact that he developed diabetic ketoacidosis. Insulin requirements were 120 units during the 24 hours he needed intravenous insulin. This seems to suggest insulin resistance. He was therefore continued on subcutaneous insulin with the addition of metformin.

The patient received education about the diagnosis, diet, home blood glucose monitoring, hypoglycemia awareness, and insulin administration prior to discharge. He was discharged home on MDIs of subcutaneous insulin.

Diabetes can be associated with a number of other endocrinopathies which all have in common the generation of insulin resistance, usually by excess of gluco-regulatory hormones.

- Cushing syndrome/disease (see *Chapter 6*) and exogenous glucocorticoid-induced diabetes. Excess cortisol increases hepatic gluconeogenesis and glucose formation due to the catabolic effects (proteolysis and lipolyis) of this hormone.
- Acromegaly (see *Chapter 2*). Excess growth hormone which stimulates fat mobilization, hepatic gluconeogenesis and glycogenolysis and increases insulin resistance.
- Pheochromocytoma (see *Chapter 6*). Excess epinephrine and nor-epinephrine from the adrenal medulla which inhibits insulin secretion, increases glycogenolysis in liver and muscle and lipolysis in fat via activation of α-adrenergic receptors.

- Thyrotoxicosis (see *Chapter 3*) increases gluconeogenesis and can result in insulin resistance.

Other subtypes of diabetes include:

- ketosis-prone diabetes ('Flatbush' diabetes, J type diabetes)
- monogenic diabetes
- post-transplant diabetes.

Ketosis-prone diabetes

Ketosis-prone diabetes is an emerging type of diabetes increasingly described among non-Caucasian individuals. It has been described in individuals of African, Caribbean, and Hispanic origin and, to lesser extent, in Native American, Chinese, and Japanese individuals. Patients usually present with diabetic ketoacidosis or unprovoked ketosis, but they do not necessarily match the phenotype of autoimmune T1DM. The Aβ classification system is used to classify ketosis-prone diabetes based on the presence or absence of antibodies (A) and β cell function (β) into four types:

- A+β+ (positive islet cell antibodies but with maintained β cell function)
- A-β- (negative antibodies but impaired β cell function)
- A+β- (positive antibodies and impaired β cell function)
- A-β+ (negative antibodies and normal β cell function, although presenting with ketoacidosis).

All patients need to be started on insulin and treated along the recommended guidelines for the management of diabetic ketoacidosis. Before discharge from hospital they are started on a twice daily regime of pre-mixed insulin and then closely followed-up in clinic after discharge to classify them and decide on a future management plan. Depending on the type of ketosis-prone diabetes some of those patients will be weaned off insulin and continued on oral hypoglycemic agents and lifestyle management. Patients with β-subtype must not be weaned off insulin because they are at risk of ketoacidosis due to lack of β cell function. β cell function is determined most accurately by assessing the C-peptide response to a glucagon load (1 mg).

CASE 5.3

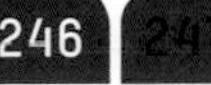

- Afro-Caribbean man of 38 years with 4 week history of polyuria, polydipsia, and blurred vision
- 3 months later HbA1c was down to 6% (42 mmol/mol) and insulin was stopped 1 month later

On subsequent reviews in the diabetes clinic the patient's insulin requirements plummeted in the next 8 weeks as he started to develop hypoglycemia. Three months after discharge HbA1c improved to 6% (42 mmol/mol). Anti-GAD and anti-islet cell antibodies were both negative. Insulin was stopped 4 months after discharge from hospital.

Case 5.3 demonstrates a patient who initially presented with what appeared to be classical T1DM but it became clear that he could be managed appropriately and effectively with insulin sensitization by metformin alone. This is a typical presentation of ketosis-prone diabetes.

Monogenic diabetes

The term maturity onset diabetes of the young (MODY) is obsolete. It was historically used when diabetes was described as either juvenile-onset (type 1) or maturity-onset (type 2). It described patients with autosomal-dominant inherited diabetes in young patients (diagnosed before 25 years of age) who do not require insulin. The term MODY implies resemblance to type 2 diabetes; however, this is not accurate. The term monogenic diabetes (1–2% of diabetes cases) is increasingly used to describe a group of genetic subtypes with different ages of onset, hyperglycemia patterns, response to treatment, and the presence of extra-pancreatic features. *Table 5.2* describes how to differentiate type 1 and 2 diabetes from monogenic diabetes.

Table 5.2. **Differentiation of monogenic diabetes from type 1 and type 2 diabetes**

			Monogenic diabetes (associated mutation given)			
Features	**T1DM**	**T2DM**	**Glucokinase**	**TNF**	**K^+_{ATP}**	**Maternally inherited**
Insulin dependence	Yes	No	No	No	Yes	Yes or No
Parent affected	2–4%	Yes	Yes	Yes	15%	Mother
Age of onset	6m–20y	13–20y	Birth	13–20y	<6m	18–22y
Obesity	No	Increased	No	No	No	Rare
Acanthosis nigricans	No	Yes	No	No	No	No
Glycemia	High	Variable	Mild	High	High	Variable
β cell autoantibodies	Yes	No	No	No	No	No
C-peptide (nmol/L)	<0.33	0.5–>1	0.1–0.7	0.1–0.7	<0.2	0.1–0.7

Adapted by permission from Macmillan Publishers Ltd: Murphy *et al.* (2008; *Nature Clin. Pract. Endo. Metab.* 4: 200–13). © 2008.

Post-transplant diabetes

An increasing number of patients are undergoing organ transplantation with an increased graft survival rate and increased longevity. Many post-transplant patients are developing diabetes largely as a result of chronic immunosuppressive drug regimes. This has been linked to higher rates of cardiovascular disease and infection. The diagnostic criteria are similar to those in non-transplant patients, using the existing WHO and ADA criteria. In renal transplant patients, it occurs in about 25% of patients in the first 3 years after transplantation. Risk factors include older patients (>40 years), obesity, non-Caucasians (particularly Afro-Caribbeans, Asians, Hispanics), use of glucocorticoids and calcineurin inhibitors, and hepatitis C infection. Patients undergoing pre-transplant evaluation should be screened for diabetes because they are at increased risk of cardiovascular morbidity and mortality. The immunosuppression regimen should take the risk of post-transplant diabetes into account and be adjusted accordingly, taking into consideration the concern for rejection.

5.8 Diabetic complications

Complications of diabetes mainly affect either the macrovasculature or the microvasculature.

Macrovascular complications, as the name suggests, are a result of disease in major arteries and may result in stroke, myocardial infarction, and peripheral artery disease. Microvascular complications are a result of disease in smaller vessels and predictably affect organs which are dependent on a functional microvasculature, i.e. the kidney, nervous system, and retina.

Atherothrombosis is the major cause of cardiovascular morbidity and mortality in the industrialized world and diabetes mellitus is a major risk factor. Atherothrombosis is defined as the disruption of an atherosclerotic plaque in a major conduit artery and the formation of a platelet-rich thrombus. The major clinical manifestations of atherothrombosis are sudden cardiac death, myocardial infarction, ischemic stroke, and peripheral arterial ischemia, particularly limb ischemia. Atherothrombosis accounts for nearly 80% of deaths amongst patients with diabetes. Microvascular disease affects arterioles, capillaries, and venules, and pathological changes in the diabetic microvasculature can alter organ perfusion. Organs heavily dependent on their blood supply, namely the retina, kidney, and peripheral nervous system, are particularly vulnerable and damage to their microvasculature leads to diabetic retinopathy, nephropathy, and neuropathy. Taken together these diabetic complications are the most common cause of blindness in adults of working age, of end-stage renal failure, and of non-traumatic limb amputation.

Many of the earliest pathological responses to hyperglycemia are manifest in the vascular cells that directly encounter elevated blood glucose levels and have poor control of regulating intracellular glucose concentrations, i.e. endothelial cells and vascular smooth muscle cells in the macrovasculature, and endothelial cells, pericytes (retinopathy) and podocytes (nephropathy) in the microvasculature. The pathogenesis of diabetic macrovascular and microvascular disease is complex (see *Box 5.10*) and involves the interaction of multiple mechanisms, but to date there is no single unifying scheme to explain all of the changes. Five major mechanisms have been proposed to contribute to the development of microvascular complications, with the most consistent modification being the thickening of the basement membrane (adjacent to the endothelium) in capillary and pre-capillary arterioles in the retina, glomeruli, myocardium, skin, and muscle. The thickening of the basement membrane alters vessel function directly, promoting clinical problems such as hypertension, reduced wound healing, and tissue hypoxia and, ultimately, frank loss of microvasculature. In the retina and the kidney microvascular complications lead to the loss of pericytes and podocytes surrounding the basement membrane eventually leading to blindness and renal failure.

5.8.1 Common diabetic complications resulting from macro- and microvascular disease

Although distinction can be made between macro- and microvascular damage, many of the long-term consequences of diabetic complications result from vascular damage, both in major conduit arteries as well as in pre-capillary arterioles, capillaries and venules.

Heart disease and stroke

The vast majority of deaths in people with diabetes are due to myocardial infarction and stroke, and the risk for these complications is 2 to 4 times higher amongst people with diabetes compared to matched controls. High blood pressure is also more common in diabetics.

Box 5.10 | Etiology of diabetic complications

Macrovascular

The process of atherogenesis

It has been difficult to separate the relative effects of hyperglycemia and dyslipidemia in atherogenesis associated with diabetes and to determine the precise factors predisposing diabetic patients to plaque formation. Plaque formation involves the following mechanisms (*Box figure 5.5*):

- endothelial injury or inflammatory activation
- recruitment of monocytes to the activated endothelial layer and their infiltration into the innermost layer of the arterial wall (tunica intima)
- in the tunica intima the monocyte acquires characteristics of a tissue macrophage
- macrophages bind and internalize lipoprotein particles (LDLs) that have been modified by oxidation or glycation
- these process give rise to the arterial foam cells, a hallmark of atherogenic plaques
- foam cells form a lipid core, and some die in this location forming a necrotic core and releasing their lipids; foam cells also stimulate proliferation of smooth muscle cells of the artery
- as the atherosclerotic plaque matures it develops a fibrous cap made of dense extracellar matrix
- activated mononuclear phagocytes can degrade the extracellular matrix resulting in rupture of the plaque, exposure of the blood to macrophage-derived prothrombic factors and hence the formation of a platelet-rich thrombus

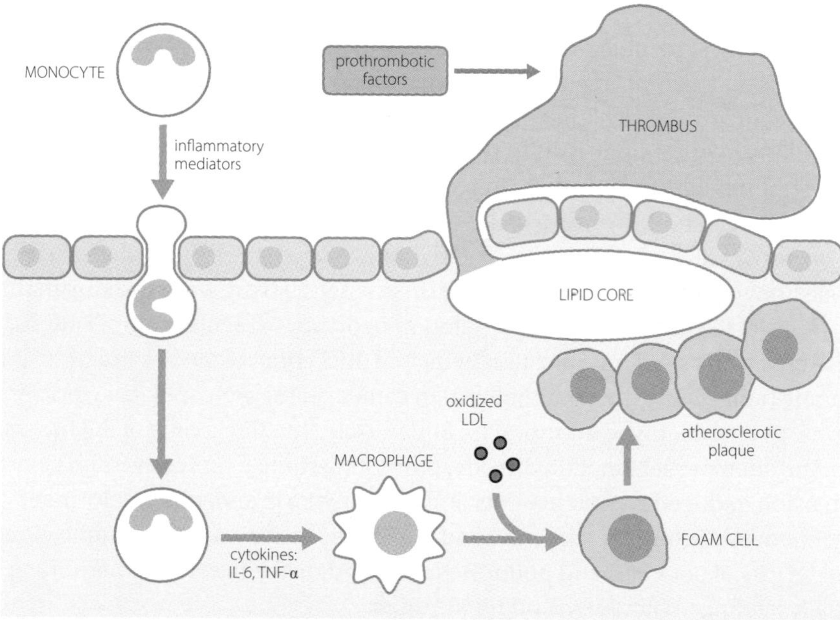

Box figure 5.5. The stages of atherogenesis.

Summary of the factors implicated in the pathogenesis of macrovascular complications

These involve endothelial cells, macrophages, and vascular smooth muscle cells and some of their actions are briefly described.

Endothelial cells:

- activation of the transcription factor NF-κB stimulating the production of pro-inflammatory molecules
- increased production of reactive oxygen species
- decreased production of the vasodilator, nitric oxide
- increased lipid peroxidation products

Monocyte-derived macrophages:

- increased production of pro-inflammatory cytokines and monocyte chemoattractant protein-1 (MCP-1)
- induction of protein kinase C which increases the expression of pro-inflammatory genes and other genes coding for proteins involved in blood flow abnormalities, vascular occlusion, and angiogenesis

Box 5.10 | continued

Vascular smooth muscle cells:

- increased proliferation and migration into tunica intima
- increased matrix degradation
- increased production of non-enzymatic glycation proteins (advanced glycation end products, AGE) which can modify extracellular matrix molecules such as collagen through their actions on specific receptors for AGE, termed RAGE.

Microvascular

Five major mechanisms have been proposed to contribute to the development of microvascular complications, although it should be noted that the most consistent microvascular modification is the thickening of the basement membrane (adjacent to the endothelium) in capillary and pre-capillary arterioles in the retina, glomeruli, myocardium, skin, and muscle. This can lead to the loss of cells surrounding the basement membrane, e.g. pericytes in the retina, podocytes in the kidney causing increased blood flow and capillary permeability, and small hemorrhages due to the breakdown of the endothelial cells. These structural changes subsequently cause capillary closure and, as a result of ischemia and the production of growth factors, induce the growth of new, but fragile, microvessels – angiogenesis. These microvessels can rupture and hemorrhages in the retina or vitreous humor can result in blind spots or blindness, respectively. In the kidney, damage to the basement membrane and podocytes (the glomerular filtration barrier) causes kidney dysfunction and, eventually, kidney failure.

The thickening of the basement membrane alters vessel function directly, promoting clinical problems such as hypertension, reduced wound healing, and tissue hypoxia, and ultimately frank loss of microvasculature.

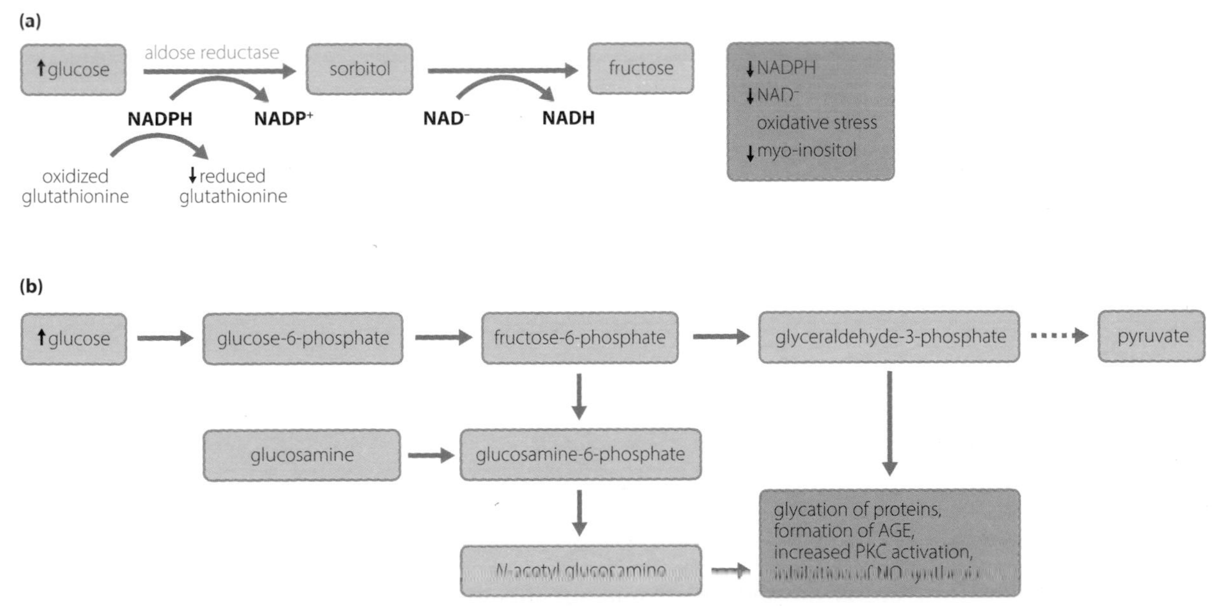

Box figure 5.6. Outline of the polyol (a) and hexosamine (b) pathways that are increased in diabetes and implicated in the development of diabetic complications.

The five mechanisms implicated in microvascular disease as a result of hyperglycemia are

1. Increased flux through the polyol pathway (see *Box figure 5.6a*). This focuses on the enzyme aldose reductase (present in retina, lens, kidney nervous tissue, and blood vessels) which normally reduces toxic aldehydes to inactive alcohols. In hyperglycemia it also reduces glucose to sorbitol which is subsequently oxidized to fructose. The formation of sorbitol consumes the co-factor NADPH which is essential for regenerating a critical intracellular antioxidant, reduced glutathione, and thus the polyol pathway increases the susceptibility to intracellular oxidative stress. Sorbitol also accumulates and

Box 5.10 | continued

increases the susceptibility of osmotic cellular damage.

2. Increased activity of the hexosamine pathway (see *Box figure 5.6b*). Glucose is normally metabolized to glucose-6-phosphate, fructose-6-phospate and through the normal glycolytic pathway to pyruvate. In hyperglycemia, some of the fructose-6-phosphate gets diverted into the formation of glucosamine-6-phosphate and finally to *N*-acetyl glucosamine which is capable of modifying the activity of transcription factors and hence the expression of genes promoting microvascular complications.
3. Increased intracellular production of AGE precursors. This non-enzymic production of glycated proteins not only alters the function of intracellular proteins involved in gene transcription but the glycated proteins can also diffuse out of the cell and modify extracellular matrix proteins causing changes in signaling between the matrix and cell and hence cellular dysfunction.
4. Increased synthesis of diacyl glycerol which activates protein kinase C. In turn, protein kinase C has numerous actions on the transcription of genes that promote microvascular complications such as angiogenesis, capillary occlusion and expression of pro-inflammatory peptides.
5. Over-production of superoxide radicals by the mitochondrial electron transport chain. High intracellular glucose concentrations increase the activity of the TCA cycle pushing more electron donors into the electron transport chain and increasing the donation of electrons to oxygen and the generation of superoxide radicals. It has been proposed that these superoxides can activate the polyol pathway, increase the activation of the hexosamine pathway, the formation of AGE and activation of protein kinase C. Thus, generation of reactive oxygen species (oxidative stress) may underlie all the mechanisms implicated in the pathogenesis of macrovascular and microvascular complications of diabetes.

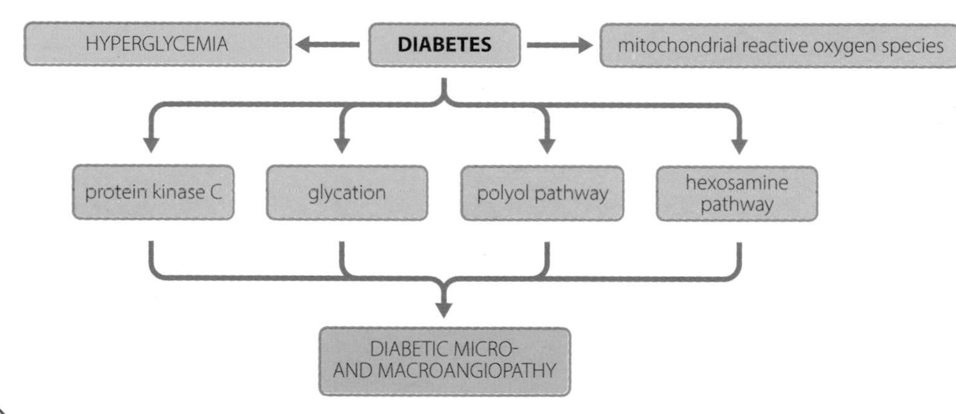

Box figure 5.7. Overview of the different factors involved in diabetic macro- and microangiopathy in diabetes.

Retinopathy and blindness

The loss of pericytes surrounding endothelial cells in the retina causes increased blood flow, increased capillary permeability, and small hemorrhages due to the breakdown of the endothelial cells. These structural changes subsequently cause capillary closure and, as a result of ischemia and the production of growth factors, induce the growth of new, but fragile, microvessels – a process known as angiogenesis. Hemorrhages on the retina can cause 'blind' spots, but those into the vitreous humor can cause blindness. Indeed, diabetic retinopathy is the leading cause of new cases of blindness in adults aged 20–74 years.

Nephropathy and renal failure

In the kidney endothelial cells, the basement membrane and podocytes constitute the glomerular filtration barrier; any structural changes that occur increase glomerular filtration rate and this allows entry of macromolecules, including proteins, into the glomerular filtrate. Diabetic nephropathy is the leading cause of kidney failure.

Neuropathy and loss of neural function

Vascular changes cause damage to neural function and about 30% of people with diabetes have a peripheral neuropathy which affects distal sensory, motor, and/or autonomic nerves. Diabetes, however, can cause nerve damage in every organ system including the digestive tract, heart, and sex organs. Thus symptoms of nerve damage can be widespread and include:

- numbness, tingling, or pain in the toes, feet, legs, hands, arms, and fingers
- wasting of the muscles of the feet or hands
- indigestion, nausea, or vomiting
- diarrhea or constipation
- dizziness or faintness due to a drop in blood pressure after standing or sitting up
- problems with urination
- erectile dysfunction in men and vaginal dryness in women
- weakness.

The diabetic foot and lower limb amputations. Sensory neuropathy may be painful or painless and patients with reduced sensation in their limbs may not notice minor injuries. It is important that patients with diabetes have a regular review which includes assessment of their feet; a workable approach to the care of the diabetic foot is summarized below.

- Patients and professionals should share decision making.
- Patients should have a regular foot examination that tests foot sensation with a 10 g monofilament or tuning fork, investigates foot pulses, looks for foot deformity, and checks footwear.
- Foot risk and care guidelines are as follows:
  - low current risk (normal sensation, palpable pulses): requires education and annual review
  - increased risk (neuropathy or absent pulses): refer to specialist foot team and review every 3–6 months
  - high risk (neuropathy or absent pulses plus deformity, skin change, or previous ulcer): review by foot protection team every 1–3 months
  - foot ulcer: urgent assessment within 24 hours by multidisciplinary team

Any injury coupled with poor blood supply (ischemia) can lead to ulcers and infections which can penetrate into deep soft tissues and into the bone (osteomyelitis). Ulcers and infections of the foot are considered a medical emergency and patients should be referred to a specialist medical team within 24 hours because an untreated or poorly treated diabetic foot can lead to amputation of the lower limb; diabetic patients are the largest group of people who undergo non-traumatic lower-limb amputations.

Diabetic complications in pregnancy

Poorly controlled diabetes prior to conception or during the first trimester can lead to birth defects in 5–10% of pregnancies, or spontaneous abortions in 15–20% of pregnancies. During the second and third trimesters of pregnancy, poorly controlled maternal diabetes can lead to excessively large babies (macrosomia) (*Box 5.11*).

Other complications

Periodontal (gum) disease is more common in people with diabetes as is their susceptibility to many illnesses including pneumonia and influenza. Uncontrolled diabetes often leads to biochemical imbalances causing diabetic ketoacidosis (*Box 5.4*) and HHS/HONK (*Box 5.7*).

5.8.2 Preventing diabetic complications

One of the most important preventative measures is good glycemic control and several studies have shown that reducing glycosylated hemoglobin by just one percentage point (e.g. from 8 to 7%) can reduce the risk of microvascular complications by 40%. Good blood pressure control and control of blood lipids can reduce the risk of heart disease and stroke. Good foot care plans are important for the care and treatment of the diabetic foot and detecting and treating early diabetic kidney disease can help reduce the decline in kidney function.

5.9 Hypoglycemia

CASE 5.4 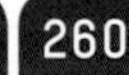 260

- Woman of 32 years with dizziness and blackouts preceded by hunger and tremor – relieved with sugary drinks
- All initial tests normal, except for a low random glucose

A 32 year old woman presented with recurrent episodes of dizziness and blackouts preceded by hunger and tremor. Drinking sugary drinks tended to relieve the episodes. There was no past medical history of note and she was not on regular medication. A family history was unremarkable. She worked as a teacher and was finding it difficult to cope at work.

- Physical examination was unremarkable.
- Full blood count, U&Es, LFTs, and thyroid function were unremarkable.
- 9 am cortisol 320 nmol/L (NR 140–690) associated with a normal ACTH.
- She was not able to do a fasting blood glucose because she had to eat to stop the dizziness; a random glucose was 3.1 mmol/L.

She was admitted for a supervised fast. Capillary blood glucose monitoring was started. She began to develop the same symptoms about 2 hours into the fast. Blood glucose was 2.1 mmol/L. The samples were analyzed for insulin, pro-insulin, C-peptide, and sulfonylurea. The fast was ended and her hypoglycemia was corrected.

Hypoglycemia is defined as abnormally low blood sugar resulting in symptoms which are secondary to a lack of glucose supply to the brain (neuroglycopenic) and an activation of the sympathetic nervous system (adrenergic/cholinergic) (*Figure 5.19*).

Absolute values that determine 'an abnormally low blood sugar' are difficult and may vary from person to person. The lower limit of the 'normal range' of blood sugar

Box 5.11 | Diabetes in pregnancy

The incidence of diabetes in pregnancy is rising, partly as a result of identification of more women with pre-existing T2DM and changes in diagnostic criteria for gestational diabetes (88% of pregnant women with diabetes have gestational diabetes, 8% have pre-existing T2DM, and 4% have T1DM). During pregnancy there is a state of insulin resistance and hyperinsulinemia. Overt diabetes develops when the pancreatic function is not able to counteract the state of insulin resistance.

Pre-conception counseling

For women with pre-existing diabetes, who are contemplating pregnancy it is important to conduct pre-conception counseling including optimization of glycemic control (HbA1c <7%/53 mmol/mol) and of blood pressure. Thyroid function, renal function including albumin:creatinine excretion, and a psychological assessment to establish the readiness for pregnancy should also be undertaken. An assessment of medication used is crucial in order to stop the ones with potential teratogenic effects (e.g. ACE inhibitors, statins, etc.).

Folic acid supplementation needs to be started 1 month prior to conception and continued throughout the first trimester. The American College of Obstetricians and Gynecologists recommend supplementation with a minimum of 0.4–0.8 mg of folic acid daily.

Detection and diagnosis

The American Diabetes Association (ADA) recommendations (2011) are as follows.

- Pre-natal detection of undiagnosed T2DM using the standard diagnostic criteria.
- Screen for gestational diabetes at 24–28 weeks of gestation using a 75 g oral glucose tolerance test. The diagnosis is made when any of the thresholds is exceeded: fasting glucose ≥5.1 mmol/L, 1 hour ≥10.0 mmol/L, and 2 hours ≥8.5 mmol/L.
- Post-partum oral glucose tolerance test at 6–12 weeks for screening of persistent diabetes.
- Life-long screening (at least every 3 years) for women with history of gestational diabetes.

Management

Glucose monitoring

Achieving good glycemic control during pregnancy has been shown to reduce fetal and neonatal complications; however, this is potentially at the expense of increasing the frequency of hypoglycemic episodes. Close monitoring of blood glucose aims to prevent those episodes. Self blood glucose monitoring is recommended before and 1 hour after meals, at bedtime and during the night if nocturnal hypoglycemia is suspected. The ADA recommended the following targets for blood glucose self-monitoring (which need to be achieved without excessive hypoglycemia):

- Gestational diabetes:
  - preprandial ≤5.3 mmol/L, **and either**
  - 1 hour postprandial ≤7.8 mmol/L, **or**
  - 2 hours postprandial ≤6.7 mmol/L
- Pre-existing type 1 or type 2 diabetes:
  - preprandial, bedtime, and overnight glucose of 3.3–5.4 mmol/L
  - peak postprandial glucose of 5.4–7.1 mmol/L
  - HbA1c <6.0%/42 mmol/mol

Nutritional therapy

Dietary input is essential in order to achieve adequate nutrition, taking into account the carbohydrate intake and distribution of meals throughout the day. The aim is to achieve good glycemic control, avoid ketosis, provide adequate nutrition to the fetus and mother, and maintain adequate weight gain.

Medication

Some pregnant women with gestational diabetes and pre-existing T2DM may be able to achieve good glycemic control with diet alone; however, some may require pharmacological therapies.

Insulin. Insulin remains the mainstay of treatment to achieve a good glycemic control. As a result of the state of insulin resistance and hormonal changes during pregnancy, pregnant women with pre-existing diabetes will require higher doses of insulin to achieve adequate glycemic control. This needs to be carefully managed in order to prevent episodes of hypoglycemia. Insulin can be administered using a subcutaneous MDI regime or a continuous subcutaneous insulin infusion via an insulin pump.

Oral hypoglycemic tablets. Oral hypoglycemics are commonly used in non-pregnant women with T2DM; however, there are concerns about their safety during pregnancy. Metformin has recently been recommended by NICE in the UK for use in women with pre-existing diabetes in the preconception period and during pregnancy as an alternative or an adjunct to insulin. The ADA and NICE recommend discontinuation of other oral hypoglycemics and to achieve glycemic control using insulin.

Complications

- Fetal: macrosomia, miscarriage, stillbirth, intrauterine death, prematurity, polyhydramnios, congenital malformations.
- Neonatal: hypoglycemia, hyperbilirubinemia, hypocalcemia, respiratory distress, birth trauma, neonatal death.
- Maternal: pre-eclampsia, operative complications.

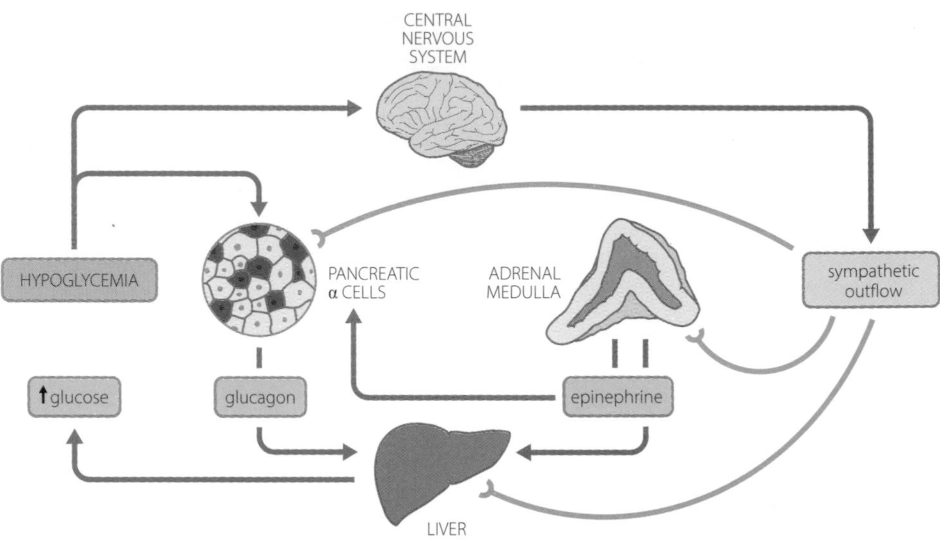

Figure 5.19. Metabolic responses to hypoglycemia.
Hypoglycemia is detected by the brain resulting in activation of the sympathetic nervous system. It is also detected directly by glucagon-secreting α cells in the pancreas. The net result is a stimulation of gluconeogenesis in the liver to correct the hypoglycemia.

is usually taken as 3.9 mmol/L and a reasonable consensus limit for biochemical hypoglycemia uses a value of 2.2 mmol/L. A confident diagnosis of hypoglycemia can only be made if the three parts of the so-called Whipple's triad are fulfilled:

- the symptoms may be due to low blood sugar
- the blood sugar is low at a time that symptoms occur
- the symptoms are relieved by administration of glucose.

5.9.1 Physiological responses to hypoglycemia

The brain can neither synthesize nor store the glucose on which it depends almost exclusively as a fuel. To recap the basic physiology, glucose concentrations are predominantly regulated by insulin and glucagon. Insulin is released (in response to a series of events initiated by sensing of glucose entry into the pancreatic β cells) and acts to normalize blood sugar by decreasing hepatic glucose production (through inhibition of glycogenolysis and gluconeogenesis) and by increasing glucose uptake by skeletal muscle and adipose tissue (by translocation of glucose transporters to the cell surface). Insulin also acts to inhibit glucagon secretion by direct gene inhibition leading to a further reduction in glucose production.

Where fuel sources are not available (i.e. in the fasting state), a series of mechanisms are activated to prevent significant falls in glucose levels; these counter-regulatory mechanisms are activated long before the normal individual starts to become symptomatic. Initially, insulin secretion is prevented (at a normal level of fasting glucose of about 4.4 mmol/L) and this is followed by an increase in glucagon secretion (at a glucose level of about 3.6–3.9 mmol/L), leading to an increase in hepatic glucose production. Subsequently, epinephrine secretion is increased. Epinephrine restores blood glucose through a number of mechanisms including a direct glucagon-like effect on the liver, inhibition of insulin secretion (through α-2

Box 5.12 | Symptoms of hypoglycemia

Neuroglycopenic	**Adrenergic/cholinergic**
Confusion and unusual behavior	Sweating
Fatigue, drowsiness	Tremor
Blurred vision	Hunger
Weakness	Palpitations
Dizziness	Anxiety
Seizures	
Coma	
Death	

receptors), inhibition of glucose utilization, and enhanced delivery of gluconeogenic substrates from the periphery to the liver (*Figure 5.19*). If low sugar levels persist, growth hormone and cortisol secretion are increased which act to enhance hepatic glucose production and inhibit peripheral glucose uptake and usage. As glucose continues to fall (3.1–3.5 mmol/L) increased sympathetic activity leads to sweating, anxiety, palpitation, and tremor and, in turn, a triggering of behavioral defense, i.e. eating. As hypoglycemia progresses it leads to confusion, seizures, coma, and ultimately death. Symptoms of hypoglycemia are summarized in *Box 5.12*.

This hierarchy of defense mechanisms is impaired in type 1 and long-standing (insulinopenic) type 2 diabetes. Counter-regulation is compromised – β cell failure results in a loss of insulin and glucagon responses and recurrent hypoglycemia attenuates the epinephrine response through a process of hypoglycemia-associated autonomic failure (HAAF). In HAAF the glycemic threshold for sympathetic activation occurs at increasingly lower glucose levels, in conjunction with a reduction in neuroglycopenic symptoms, ultimately leading to a reduction in efficacy of behavioral defense mechanisms.

5.9.2 Classification and causes of hypoglycemia

Hypoglycemia is common in patients receiving treatment for diabetes, particularly those with T1DM on insulin replacement. Patients early on in the course of T2DM experience fewer episodes, although the number of episodes increases as the disease progresses, due to increasing α and β cell dysfunction and increasing requirements for exogenous insulin and/or insulin secretagogues. Drugs used to increase the efficacy of endogenous insulin (metformin, thiazolidindiones, GLP-1 agonists, DPP-4 inhibitors and glucosidase) should not result in hypoglycemia. In contrast, insulin, insulin analogs and insulin secretagogues (meglitinides, sulfonylureas) can cause a state of relative or absolute insulin excess and result in hypoglycemia.

The diagnosis and delineation of the etiology of hypoglycemia is often a little more complicated in the patient without diabetes (possible causes are listed in *Box 5.13*). Overall, the commonest cause is probably drugs (including insulin/insulin secretagogues which may have been taken accidentally or surreptitiously or even administered maliciously) and alcohol. Well over 100 drugs have been implicated in hypoglycemia, many with a low quality of supporting evidence. The most commonly cited are salicylate, quinolones, ACE inhibitors, β-blockers and indomethacin.

Box 5.13 | Causes of hypoglycemia

- Drugs: insulin, insulin secretagogues, alcohol, salicylates, and numerous others.
- Critical illnesses including hepatic, cardiac, renal failure, extreme starvation, malaria.
- Deficiency of counter-regulatory hormones: cortisol, growth hormone, glucagon, epinephrine.
- Endogenous hyperinsulinemia: insulinoma, activating insulin, or insulin receptor antibodies.
- Following gastric bypass surgery.
- Rare congenital deficiencies of enzymes of carbohydrate metabolism (e.g. galactosemia).

Causes of hypoglycemia in children/infants

- Pre-term or small for gestational age babies.
- Cortisol deficiency.
- Infant of diabetic mother/maternal drugs.
- Hyperinsulinemic hypoglycemia of infancy.
- Glycogen storage diseases (types 1, 3, and 6).
- Disorders of protein metabolism.
- Disorders of fat metabolism.

Alcohol inhibits gluconeogenesis but has no effect on glycogenolysis, so the hypoglycemia associated with alcohol often follows an alcohol binge with little or no food ingestion where liver stores of glycogen are used up and new glucose formation is ineffective.

Hypoglycemia is also commonly encountered in many hospitalized patients with severe or critical illness. Trauma (including burns) and severe sepsis result in development of a hypercatabolic state with high glucose turnover. Eventually, increased glucose utilization cannot be matched by increased glucose production (as gluconeogenesis is inhibited by cytokines) and, once glycogen stores are depleted, hypoglycemia follows.

Liver and kidney disease are often complicated by hypoglycemia. In the former, once about 80% of the liver is compromised, failure of gluconeogenesis may result in fasting hypoglycemia. In renal disease up to 50% of hospitalized patients will suffer hypoglycemia. The mechanisms are not entirely clear but again probably involve reduced gluconeogenesis in association with reduced renal clearance of insulin. In tropical countries malaria is a very common cause of hypoglycemia (and many of the drugs used in its treatment are also implicated).

A deficiency of hormones that are glucose counter-regulatory (i.e. that help maintain euglycemia) occasionally causes or contributes to hypoglycemia. Removal of a catecholamine-secreting pheochromocytoma can result in sudden hypoglycemia (see *Chapter 6*). Cortisol deficiency (due to primary adrenal disease or ACTH deficiency) may lead to hypoglycemia; deficiency of adrenal-derived regulatory hormones leading to hypoglycemia is more common in infants and children. Some patients with diabetes (either type 1 or type 2) may develop adrenal insufficiency or ACTH deficiency leading to significant reduction in insulin requirements to maintain euglycemia. Primary glucagon deficiency is extremely rare, but acquired deficiency (after long-standing diabetes, pancreatectomy, or chronic pancreatitis) may result in profound hypoglycemia following insulin administration.

Box 5.14 | Hypoglycemia related to endogenous hyperinsulinism

Autoimmune hypoglycemia

Antibodies may be directed to insulin itself (where they bind insulin which is released appropriately in response to glucose, and then dissociate resulting in uncontrolled insulin release) or to insulin receptors (where they may be stimulatory leading to uncontrolled receptor activation and signaling).

Nesidioblastosis

This is a term originally coined in 1938 to describe the neo-differentiation of islets of Langerhans from pancreatic ductal epithelium which leads to diffuse islet cell hyperplasia. This results in an unregulated elevation of serum insulin, C-peptide, and proinsulin leading to recurrent hypoglycemia. The disorder is now usually termed persistent hyperinsulinemic hypoglycemia of infancy (PHHI), or occasionally congenital hyperinsulinism (CHI). PHHI is the commonest cause of hyperinsulinemic hypoglycemia in neonates and infants. It may be transmitted as an autosomal dominant or recessive trait, and mutations in genes encoding the sulfonylurea receptor, the inwardly rectifying potassium channel and other genes have been described. If left untreated, PHHI can lead to brain damage or death secondary to severe hypoglycemia. Although PHHI was initially thought to affect only infants and children, numerous cases have been reported in adults of all ages, but at a much lower incidence, although some would contest that this is an entity in adults and there is no known genetic link. PHHI is often poorly responsive or unresponsive to medical management, necessitating 95% or near-total pancreatectomy.

Insulinomas

Insulinomas are rare (incidence about 4 per million) but despite this are the most common cause of endogenous hyperinsulinemia in adults. There is a slight female preponderance (about 60%) with most cases being diagnosed before the age of 50. Around 5–7% are malignant and about 7–10% occur in association with MEN-1 (where the tumors tend to be multiple; see *Chapter 8*). Tumors may be very small (one-third are less than 1 cm in diameter) and difficult to identify using standard imaging techniques. The symptoms are those of hypoglycemia (see *Box 5.12*) and are usually significantly worsened by prolonged fasts and exercise. The diagnosis is based on the demonstration of a low sugar (glucose <2.2 mmol/L) at the same time as an inappropriately high insulin and C-peptide. In about 70–75% of cases, symptoms and diagnostic biochemistry can be obtained after an overnight fast of about 18 h. In less clear-cut cases a prolonged fast of up to 72 h may need to be carried out under observation and in hospital. The fast is continued (with blood taken regularly) until the glucose reaches about 2.2 mmol/L and a sample taken at that point for insulin and C-peptide. The sensitivity of the test may be increased by measuring β-hydroxybutyrate (which will be low in insulinoma because unregulated insulin excess will lead to anti-ketogenesis, despite the low sugar) and/or assessing the glucose response to 1 mg of glucagon given intravenously (which will be high). Once the diagnosis is confirmed it is necessary to try to localize the tumor, sometimes a frustrating exercise: at least 99% of insulinomas occur in the pancreas so that is a reasonable place to start the hunt. There is no single procedure which is ideal and no real consensus as to whether pre-operative localization is still necessary given the success of intra-operative ultrasound in expert hands. Localization studies are summarized in *Box table 5.1* below.

Treatment of insulinomas

Surgical. Surgery remains the mainstay of treatment and, where pre-operative localization has been unhelpful, surgical exploration with intra-operative ultrasound can be useful. Enucleation of the insulinoma is often possible, but a formal pancreatectomy may be necessary if there is suspicion of malignancy. Success rates are between 75 and 95% in experienced hands.

Malignant insulinomas are rare (see above) but difficult to deal with and the diagnosis is usually made peri-operatively. The malignant tumors are often rather larger (>5 cm as opposed to <2 cm) and radical resection is recommended which may achieve survival rates of up to 25% at 10 years. Metastatic disease is best dealt with by resection or laparoscopic radiofrequency thermal ablation.

Medical. Small frequent meals may help, as may continuous glucose infusion using implantable pumps. Diazoxide (which suppresses insulin secretion by direct action on β cells and which promotes glycogenolysis indirectly) is useful prior to surgery or in those in whom surgery is contraindicated or has failed. Side-effects include hirsutism, nausea, weight gain, and edema. Calcium channel blockers (e.g. nifedipine) are sometimes used but are more effective in patients with nesidioblastosis. Somatostatin analogs can produce relatively modest symptomatic relief.

Box 5.14 | continued

Box table 5.1. **Options for localization of insulinomas**

Trans-abdominal ultrasound

- Operator dependent
- Difficult in obese patients
- Success rate of 9–70% claimed
- No ionizing radiation

Endoscopic ultrasound

- Invasive
- Success rate of 60–95%
- Needs experienced operator

Intra-operative ultrasound

- Needs experienced operator
- Success rate of 85–100%
- Identifies non-palpable lesions
- Good for head of pancreas

Selective venous sampling

- Calcium stimulation (insulinomas secrete more insulin in response to a rise in calcium)
- Invasive and expensive
- Only used if re-operation necessary

Trans-hepatic portal vein sampling

- Only capable of regionalization
- Invasive and difficult

MRI

- 40–100% sensitivity
- No ionizing radiation

CT scanning

- Non-invasive
- Good resolution
- Inexpensive
- Sensitivity 20–40%
- Good for larger tumors and/or hepatic metastases

Octreotide scanning

- Sensitivity up to 50%
- Good for metastases

Non-islet cell tumor hypoglycemia

Many tumors can result in hypoglycemia without producing excess insulin. Large tumors of mesenchymal or hepatic origin, which may be intra-abdominal, intra-thoracic, or retroperitoneal, can increase skeletal usage of glucose by production of incompletely processed insulin-like growth factors (usually a form of 'big' IGF-2). Insulin and C-peptide levels are low or undetectable.

CASE 5.4

254 260

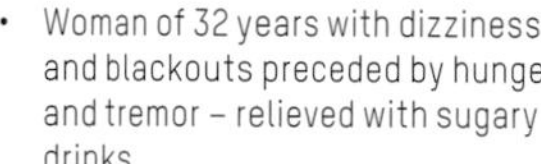

- Woman of 32 years with dizziness and blackouts preceded by hunger and tremor – relieved with sugary drinks
- All initial tests normal, except for a low random glucose
- High levels of insulin, pro-insulin, and C-peptide were found, consistent with endogenous hyperinsulinemic hypoglycemia
- Diazoxide treatment started to reduce insulin secretion and control hypoglycemia
- An insulinoma was suspected and located in pancreas on endoscopic ultrasound

The patient underwent further investigation. A blood and urine sulfonylurea screen was negative. Insulin, pro-insulin, and C-peptide levels were markedly elevated in the presence of hypoglycemia, consistent with endogenous hyperinsulinemic hypoglycemia. She was started on diazoxide initially to diminish insulin secretion and control the hypoglycemia. The co-existence of hyperinsulinemia in the light of hypoglycemia and after the exclusion of exogenous insulin or sulfonylurea therapy is highly suspicious of an insulinoma, and in view of this the diazoxide treatment was changed to octreotide (the somatostatin analog) given in a dose of 100 μg tds by subcutaneous injection.

CT and MRI scans did not demonstrate a lesion in the pancreas or show evidence of liver metastasis. Subsequent endoscopic ultrasound revealed a 1 cm lesion in the tail of the pancreas. A distal pancreatectomy was carried out. The patient was given reducing levels of octreotide until complete withdrawal and has not reported symptoms since the operation.

5.9.3 Hypoglycemia related to endogenous hyperinsulinism

Endogenous hyperinsulinism occurs when insulin levels do not reduce once glucose concentrations fall back to normal (or low) levels. This may occur as a result of:

- autoimmune hypoglycemia
- a functional β cell disorder – 'nesidioblastosis'
- a tumor of the β cells (e.g. insulinoma – sometimes associated with multiple endocrine neoplasia (MEN) type 1 (see *Chapter 8*)
- overuse or accidental (or malicious) use of insulin or insulin secretagogues.

Details of disorders related to endogenous hyperinsulinism are given in *Box 5.14.*

5.10 Further reading

American Diabetes Association (2011) Executive summary: standards of medical care in diabetes. *Diabetes Care,* **1:** S4–S10.

Brownlee M (2005) The pathobiology of diabetic complications: a unifying mechanism. *Diabetes,* **54:** 1615–25.

Cheer K, Shearman C, and Jude EB (2009) Managing complications of the diabetic foot. *Br. Med. J.* **339:** 1304–7.

de Kort H, de Koning EJ, Rabelink TJ, Bruijn JA, and Bajema IM (2011) Islet transplantation in type 1 diabetes. *Br. Med. J.* **342:** d217.

Ekeblad S (2010) Islet cell tumours. *Adv. Exp. Med. Biol.* **654:** 771–89.

Gallagher EJ, Leroith D, and Karnieli E (2011) The metabolic syndrome – from insulin resistance to obesity and diabetes. *Med. Clinics N. Am.* **95:** 855–73.

Gallwitz B (2011) GLP-1 agonists and dipeptidyl-peptidase IV inhibitors. *Handbook Exp. Pharmacol.* **203:** 53–74.

Lautz D, Halperin F, Goebel-Fabbri A, and Goldfine AB (2011) The great debate: medicine or surgery: what is best for the patient with type 2 diabetes? *Diabetes Care,* **34:** 763–70.

Lin Y and Sun Z (2010) Current views on type 2 diabetes. *J. Endocrinol.* **204:** 1–11.

McCarthy MI (2010) Genomics, type 2 diabetes, and obesity. *New Engl. J. Med.* **363:** 2339–50.

Nauck M (2009) Unraveling the science of incretin biology. *Am. J. Med.* **122:** S3–S10.

Niswender KD (2011) Basal insulin: physiology, pharmacology, and clinical implications. *Postgrad. Medicine,* **123**(4)**:** 17–26.

Oberg K (2010) Pancreatic endocrine tumors. *Seminars Oncol.* **37:** 594–618.

Quesada I, Tudurí E, Ripoll C, and Nadal A (2008) Physiology of the pancreatic α-cell and glucagon secretion: role in glucose homeostasis and diabetes. *J. Endocrinol.* **199:** 5–19.

Savage MW (2011) Management of diabetic ketoacidosis. *Clinical Med.* **11:** 154–6.

Stolar M (2010) Glycemic control and complications in type 2 diabetes mellitus. *Am. J. Med.* **123:** S3–S11.

Wood S and Trayhurn P (2003) Glucose transporters (GLUT and SGLT): expanded families of sugar transport proteins. *Br. J. Nutr.* **89:** 3–9.

Useful websites

American Diabetes Association: www.diabetes.org

CDC – Diabetes Public Health Resource: www.cdc.gov/diabetes

Diabetes UK: www.diabetes.org.uk

National Diabetes Statistics, 2011: http://diabetes.niddk.nih.gov/dm/pubs/statistics

5.11 Self-assessment questions

(1) Which one of the following statements about insulin is true? It:
  (a) Stimulates lipolysis
  (b) Inhibits amino acid uptake
  (c) Stimulates gluconeogenesis
  (d) Inhibits glycogenolysis
  (e) Stimulates the insertion of GLUT-2 transporters into the cell membrane

(2) The actions of glucagon include which one of the following?
  (a) Inhibition of GLUT-4 transporters
  (b) Promotion of β-oxidation of acetyl CoA
  (c) Stimulation of glycogen synthase
  (d) Inhibition of ketone formation
  (e) Promotion of fatty acid uptake into adipose tissue

(3) Sulfonylureas act by which one of the following mechanisms?
  (a) Binding to ATP-dependent potassium channels on β-cell membranes
  (b) Suppressing hepatic gluconeogenesis
  (c) Activating PPARγ receptors in adipocytes
  (d) Hyperpolarizing β-cells
  (e) Stimulating glycogenolysis

(4) Diagnosing diabetes requires which one of the following results?
  (a) An elevated fasting venous blood glucose ≥7.0 mmol/L
  (b) Blood glucose levels >10 mmol/L 2 hours after an oral glucose tolerance test (OGTT)
  (c) A random venous blood glucose of >14 mmol/L
  (d) HbA1c levels >5.8% (40 mmol/mol)
  (e) A fasting plasma glucose of <7.0 mmol/L and a 2 hour post-OGTT of >11 mmol/L

(5) Which one of the following targets for the treatment of type 1 diabetes mellitus is correct?
  (a) HbA1c <9.2% (77 mmol/mol)
  (b) Preprandial glucose between 6 and 10 mmol/L
  (c) Blood glucose levels <11 mmol/L 2 hours after an OGTT
  (d) Postprandial glucose <9 mmol/L
  (e) Blood pressure <110/70 mmHg

(6) Which one of the following is a cause of hyperglycemia rather than hypoglycemia?
  (a) Gastric bypass surgery
  (b) Insulinoma
  (c) Cortisol excess
  (d) Glycogen storage diseases
  (e) Alcohol excess

(7) Hyperinsulinemic hypoglycemia is associated with which one of the following?
  (a) Insulinomas
  (b) Metformin ingestion
  (c) Starvation
  (d) Severe burns
  (e) Chronic liver disease

(8) A 34 year old woman of Indian origin with a BMI of 33 kg/m^2 and who has a family history of type 2 diabetes mellitus books into a prenatal clinic at 8 weeks of gestation. This is her second pregnancy and her previous child was a healthy boy weighing 4.7 kg. Which one of the following factors would exclude her from having an oral glucose tolerance test to screen for gestational diabetes?
  (a) Her BMI
  (b) Her age
  (c) Her ethnicity
  (d) Previous birth weight
  (e) Positive family history of type 2 diabetes

(9) A young woman attends her family doctor complaining that she had been drinking a lot of water recently and passing a lot more urine than normal. Otherwise she is feeling healthy, although she has lost some weight even though her appetite has increased.
  (a) Based on the symptoms above, what is the most likely diagnosis and why?
  (b) What test would confirm her diagnosis and what measurements would be accepted?
  (c) What are her treatment options?

(10) Four years ago a 14 year old schoolgirl was diagnosed with type 1 diabetes mellitus. She injected herself twice a day with human insulin and had to keep to a strict diet, both of which she found difficult. On her 18th birthday, after a light supper, she went out clubbing with her friends who kept buying her drinks. She had been dancing for an hour or so and had consumed four vodka and Cokes before she began to feel sweaty, shaky, and dizzy and finally had a fit and collapsed. She was taken to hospital.
  (a) What is the most likely explanation for her collapse and fit?
  (b) Why did the alcohol have an effect?
  (c) What caused her symptoms?

CHAPTER 06 The adrenal glands

After working through this chapter you should be able to:

- Identify the different steroid hormones secreted by the adrenal cortex and describe their synthesis, transport, and metabolism
- Describe how their hormones' secretions are controlled, how they act on their target cells and their physiological roles
- Know the signs and symptoms of excess and insufficient adrenocortical hormones, the diagnosis of their causes and their treatments
- Know the catecholamines secreted by the adrenal medulla and describe their synthesis and metabolism
- Outline the diagnosis and treatment of pheochromocytoma

6.1 Introduction – adrenal cortex and medulla

The two adrenal glands sit on the top of each kidney (hence the terms *ad*renal or *supra*renal) and each weighs approximately 4 g. The cortex forms about 90% of the mass, with the remainder being the medulla (*Figure 6.1*). The two parts of the gland are distinct in that the adrenal cortex synthesizes and secretes steroid hormones (cortisol, aldosterone, and androgens) derived from cholesterol, whilst the medulla secretes epinephrine (adrenaline) and nor-epinephrine (nor-adrenaline) derived from the amino acid tyrosine. The cortex and medulla also differ both embryologically and physiologically, although their hormones often act in a concerted manner.

The glands are supplied by blood from branches of the aorta, phrenic and renal arteries and the blood vessels drain from the outer cortex inwardly to the adrenal medulla. This is important in developing and maintaining the functional zonation of the adrenal cortex and allows high levels of cortisol (produced in stress) to stimulate the synthesis of phenylethanolamine *N*-methyl transferase in the medulla, which converts nor-epinephrine to epinephrine.

The adult adrenal cortex produces the steroid hormones in three distinct layers.

- The outer zona glomerulosa layer synthesizes the mineralocorticoid, aldosterone, and this hormone is important in the control of sodium

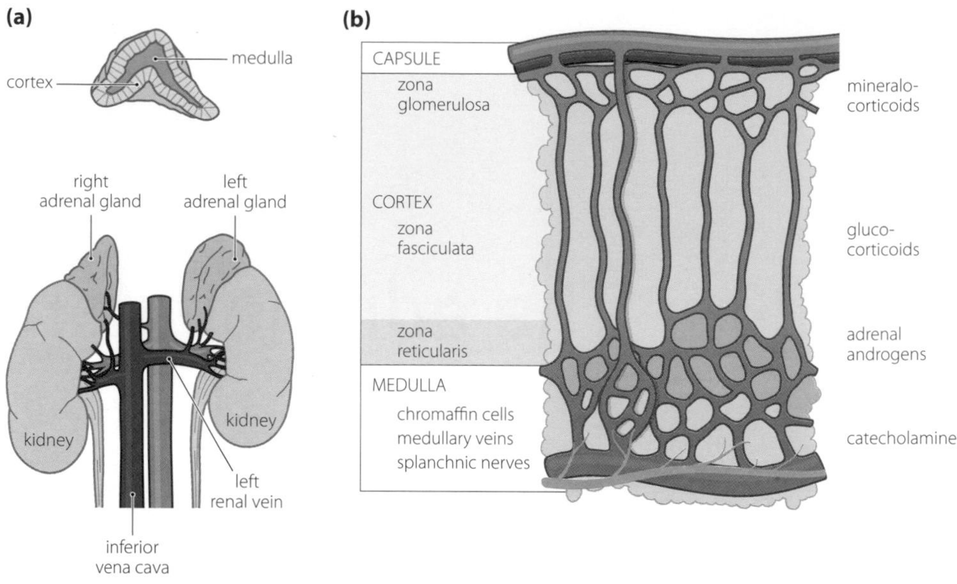

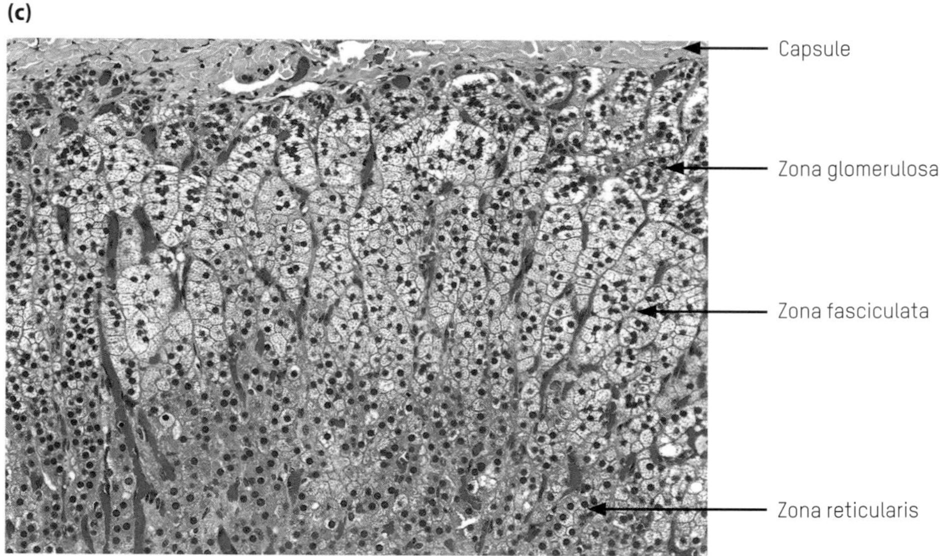

Figure 6.1. Anatomy and histology of the adrenal glands.
(a) Location of the two adrenal glands sitting on top of each kidney. The venous drainage of the right adrenal gland is into the inferior vena cava and the left adrenal gland drains into the left renal vein.
(b) Cross-section showing the functional zonation of the adrenal gland and the direction of blood flow within the gland.
(c) Histological section through the adrenal gland. Reproduced from http://webpathology.com with permission from Dr Dharam M. Ramnani.

reabsorption in the kidney. Along with other hormones aldosterone is important in the homeostatic control of blood volume and blood pressure.

- The middle zona fasciculata layer synthesizes the glucocorticoid, cortisol, and this hormone has widespread effects on the body. It not only has major metabolic actions but also has effects on other systems and tissues, including the cardiovascular system, immune system, skin and connective tissue, bone, and fetal lungs.

- The innermost zona reticularis layer produces adrenal androgens. These are less important, but are a precursor for estrogen synthesis in post-menopausal women.

Secretions of catecholamines from the adrenal medulla support functions of the sympathetic nervous system. Thus, in functional terms, the adrenal gland is not a single endocrine gland but secretes different steroids, with widely differing activities, in addition to catecholamines. Disorders of adrenocortical and adrenomedullary function are relatively rare compared with those of the pancreas (diabetes mellitus) and thyroid but their effects can be profound.

6.2 Embryology and development of functional zonation of the adrenal glands

The cells which form the adrenal cortex originate from the mesoderm and are initially part of the adrenogonadal primordium within the urogenital ridge. By embryonic week 8 the adrenocortical primordium is separate from the gonadal primordium (*Figure 6.2*) and consists of an outer definitive zone and an inner fetal zone. Transcription factors GL13, SF-1, and DAX1 appear to be central to this

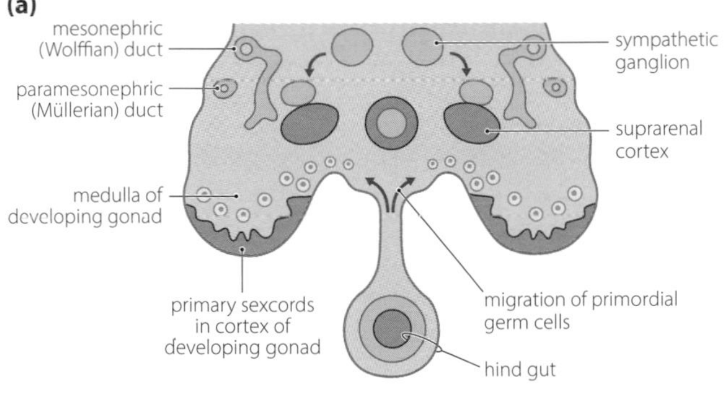

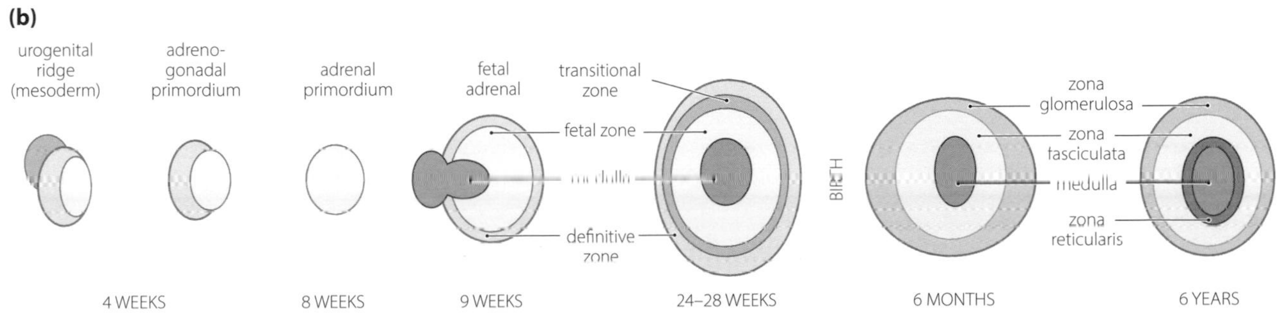

Figure 6.2. Embryology of the adrenal glands.
(a) Transverse section of the caudal region of a 6 week embryo. The diagram also shows the development of the reproductive tracts (see *Chapter 7*).
(b) The kidneys, gonads, and adrenal glands develop from the mesoderm in the urogenital ridge which then separate to become the adrenogonadal primordium and finally the adrenal primordium (suprarenal cortex). Cells from the adjacent sympathetic ganglion derived from the neural crest invade the fetal adrenal premordium and form the adrenal medulla. Subsequently, different layers develop secreting distinct steroids and it is not until around 6 years of age that the gland reaches its final maturation and the zona reticularis is formed (see text for further details).

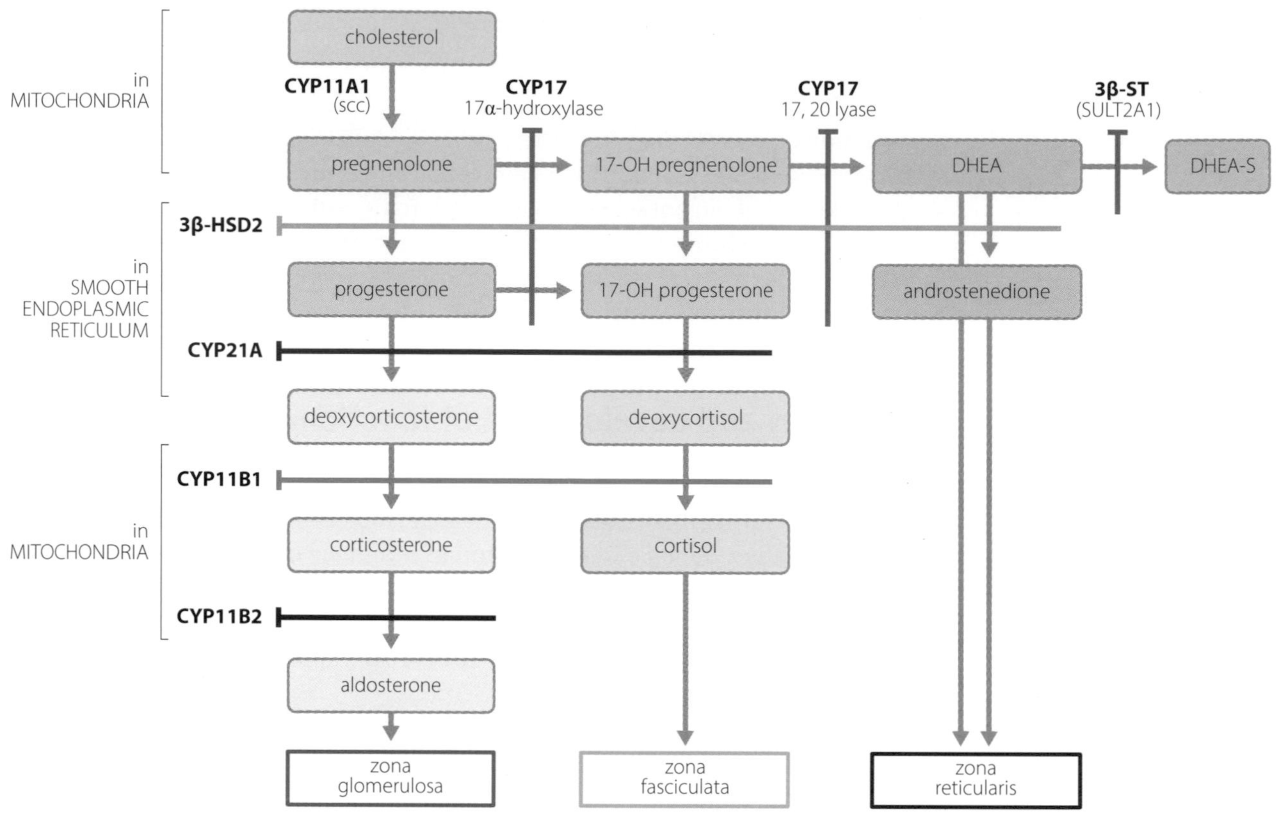

Figure 6.3. Steroid synthesis in the adrenal cortex.
Cholesterol is taken up into the mitochondria by steroidogenic acute regulatory (StAR) protein and converted to pregnenolone by the side chain cleavage (SCC) enzyme CYP11A1. 3β-hydroxysteroid dehydrogenase (HSD) oxidizes the OH group on carbon 3 converting pregnenolone to progesterone in the smooth endoplasmic reticulum. Other reactions involve P_{450} enzymes and, like the SCC enzyme, the genes coding for these enzymes and the enzymes themselves are abbreviated to CYP. In the zona reticularis dehydroepiandrosterone is sulfated by 3β-sulfatase (ST). The synthesis of steroid hormones involves trafficking between the mitochondria and smooth endoplasmic reticulum as indicated.
Abbreviations/alternative names:
CYP11A1: P_{450}scc; CYP17: P_{450}c17; 3β-HSD: 3β-hydroxysteroid dehydrogenase; CYP21: 21-hydroxylase/P_{450}c21; CYP11B1: 11β-hydroxylase/P_{450}c11; CYP11B2: aldosterone synthase/P_{450}c18; 3β-ST: DHEA-sulfotransferase/SULT2A1. The genes coding for the P_{450} heme-containing enzymes are abbreviated to CYP.

development. Around week 9 of gestation, cells from the neural crest migrate into the adrenal primordium to form the adrenal medulla. These cells are modified sympathetic neurons and become encapsulated within the adrenocortical cells. At this time the fetal adrenals are huge in proportion to other organs and are destined to become an androgen 'factory'. However, between embryonic weeks 7 and 12 there is a transient expression of 3β-hydroxysteroid dehydrogenase type 2 (3β-HSD2) (*Figure 6.3*) which shunts steroid synthesis away from producing the androgen, dehydroepiandrosterone (DHEA), and thus preventing virilization of a female fetus. This time is critical for the sexual development of the reproductive tracts and in the male is dependent on testosterone secreted by the fetal testes (see *Chapter 7*). Beyond 12 weeks of gestation, 3β-HSD2 synthesis is suppressed and there is an increased expression of CYP17/20 lyase activity, increasing the synthesis of DHEA and its sulfated form, DHEA-S, from the fetal adrenal; these are converted to estrogens in the placenta.

In the third trimester of pregnancy a transitional zone appears and is thought to produce cortisol after 24–28 weeks of pregnancy. At birth each fetal adrenal gland weighs 8–9 g, twice the weight of an adult gland. Postnatally the fetal zone begins to involute and has disappeared by about 6 months of life. The definitive zone expands to form the zona glomerulosa and the zona fasciculata (*Figure 6.2*). The zona reticularis only begins to develop after 4 years of age and starts producing androgens after 6–8 years of age (the 'adrenarche') which precedes the pubertal activation of the gonadal axis (*Chapter 7*). This could result from an increase in 17,20-lyase expression of *CYP17* and modulation by other factors such as growth hormone, insulin-like growth factor, and insulin, and high levels of estradiol. Whilst the synthesis of both mineralocorticoids and glucocorticoids remain relatively constant throughout life, adrenal androgen secretions begin to decline after 30 years of age (the 'adrenopause').

The origin of the stem cells of the cortical zones, which become morphologically distinct (*Figure 6.1*), is not clearly defined although it is thought that cortical cells originate from the outer layers of the cortex and move inwards. Functionally, in terms of steroid synthesis, it is due to the zone-specific expression of enzymes involved in steroid biosynthesis. The zona glomerulosa does not express CYP17 (17α hydroxylase) and so cannot synthesize cortisol or androgens, and aldosterone synthase (CYP11B2) is only expressed in the glomerulosa layer. In the zona reticularis, 17α-hydroxyprogesterone cannot be converted to cortisol but is shunted into the formation of androgens (*Figure 6.3*).

6.2.1 Steroid synthesis in the adrenal glands

In the adrenal cortex, about 80% of the cholesterol required for steroid synthesis is captured by receptors which bind LDLs. The adrenal glands may also use HDL following uptake through a putative HDL receptor, SR-B1. The remaining 20% of cholesterol is synthesized from acetate within the adrenal cells by the normal biochemical route. The cholesterol can be stored as esters in lipid droplets or utilized directly.

The synthesis of adrenal steroids involves:

- Hydrolysis of cholesterol esters and the active transfer of free cholesterol to the outer membrane of the mitochondria by a sterol transfer protein.
- The transfer of hydrophobic cholesterol to the inner mitochondrial membrane chaperoned by the **st**eroidogenic **a**cute **r**egulatory (StAR) protein (*Figure 6.3;* see also *Figure 1.5*).
- On the inner side of the membrane the first enzymatic process in steroid hormone synthesis occurs. This involves the conversion of cholesterol to pregnenolone by an enzyme known as side chain cleavage enzyme, P_{450}scc.
- Pregnenolone is then shuttled from the mitochondria to the smooth endoplasmic reticulum where it is converted to progesterone or to 17α-hydroxypregnenolone.

- Through subsequent hydroxylations between mitochondria and smooth endoplasmic reticulum, progesterone can be converted to corticosterone (another glucocorticoid only released in small amounts in humans) and then aldosterone, whilst 17α-hydroxypregnenolone can be converted to androgens and cortisol (*Figure 6.3*). There is, however, considerable interconversion between these two pathways.

6.3 Basic science

6.3.1 Glucocorticoids and their actions

In humans, the major glucocorticoid synthesized and released from cells in the zona fasciculata is the C21 steroid, cortisol, although smaller amounts of corticosterone are also produced. They are multi-functional hormones (see *Box 6.1*) affecting nearly every cell in the body and modulating the expression of approximately 10% of our genes. Glucocorticoids are essential for life; they maintain homeostasis and enable the body to cope with physical and emotional stress.

They have potent metabolic effects which are essentially catabolic in muscle and fat (proteolysis and lipolysis) and anabolic in the liver. The overall effect is to increase

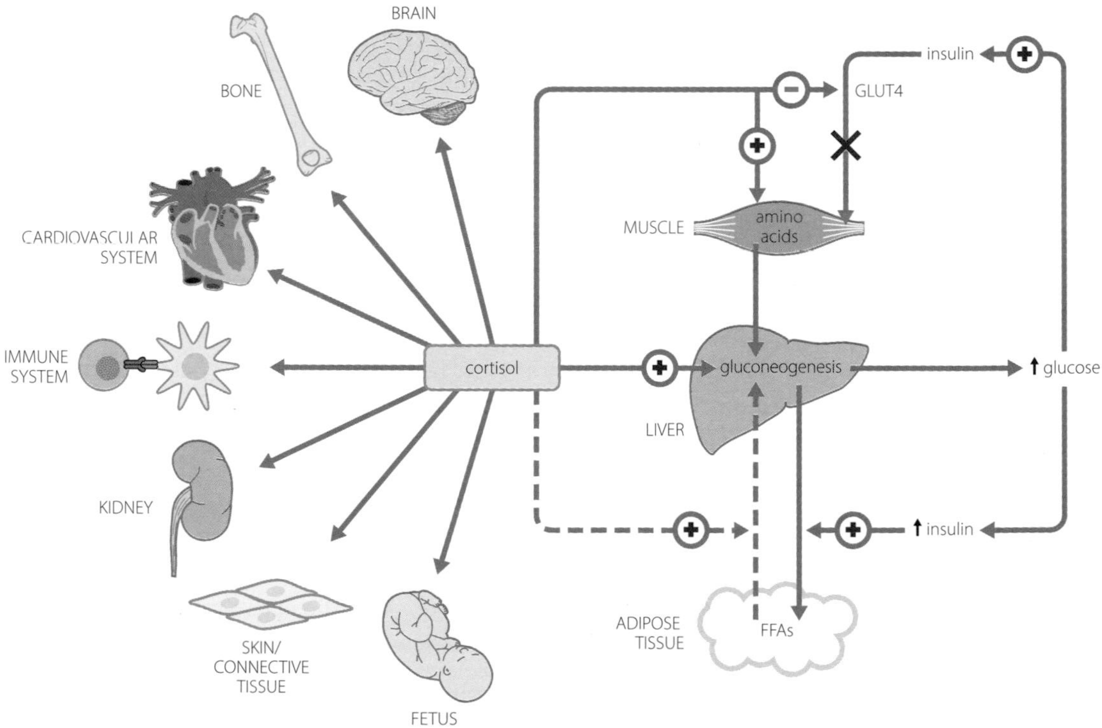

Figure 6.4. The major actions of cortisol on metabolism and other targets of cortisol action.

- Cortisol stimulates the release of amino acids from muscle. These are taken up by the liver and converted to glucose (gluconeogenesis).
- The increased circulating concentration of glucose stimulates insulin release. Cortisol inhibits the insulin-stimulated uptake of glucose in muscle via the GLUT4 transporter.
- Cortisol has mild lipolytic effects. These are overpowered by the lipogenic action of insulin secreted in response to the diabetogenic action of cortisol.
- Cortisol also has varied actions on a wide range of other tissues (see text for details).

Box 6.1 | Major biological actions of cortisol

System	Specific target	Physiological function
Metabolic	Liver	Increased glycogen synthesis and gluconeogenesis.
	Skeletal muscle	Increased proteolysis, decreased protein synthesis, increased glycogenolysis, decreased GLUT4 mediated glucose uptake.
	Adipose tissue	Increased lipolysis, decreased lipogenesis.
Plasma glucose		Fasting state cortisol contributes to maintenance of plasma glucose. In stress, cortisol increases blood glucose at expense of muscle protein. Permissive effect on lipolytic actions of epinephrine and GH in adipose tissue.
Cardiovascular	Heart	Increased contractility.
	Blood vessels	Maintenance of vascular tone. Increased vascular reactivity to catecholamines.
Kidney		Increases GFR, decreases calcium reabsorption. In excess has mineralocorticoid action (Na^+ retention).
Skin/connective tissue	Fibroblasts	Inhibits proliferation.
	Collagen	Inhibits formation.
	Bone, cartilage	Increases bone resorption, inhibits bone-forming activity of osteoblasts.
Immune	Inflammatory response	Inhibits phospholipase A_2, a key enzyme in prostaglandin, leukotriene, and thromboxane synthesis. Stabilizes lysosomes.
	Immune response	Inhibits monocyte proliferation, decreases circulating T lymphocytes.
Central nervous	Psychiatric parameters	Maintains emotional balance, decreases REM sleep, induces hippocampal atrophy.
Fetus	Development	Normal development of CNS, retina, skin, GI tract, and lungs.
	Lung	Stimulates production of surfactant.

blood glucose concentrations and so, like growth hormone, epinephrine, and glucagon, cortisol is also considered to be diabetogenic. It does this by opposing the stimulatory action of insulin on the GLUT4 transporters (*Figure 6.4*) in muscle and fat which decreases glucose uptake in these tissues and at the same time increases glucose production and release from the liver. The latter is accomplished through gluconeogenesis using amino acids (from the catabolic actions on muscle) as the primary carbon source. They also have complex actions on lipid deposition, as is observed in Cushing disease (see *Section 6.4* and Cases 6.1 and 6.2).

Glucocorticoids are important modulators of immune and inflammatory responses (*Box 6.2, Figures 6.5* and *6.6*) that are essential for host defense against infection and

Box 6.2 | Anti-inflammatory and immunosuppressant actions of glucocorticoids

The anti-inflammatory and immunosuppressant actions of glucocorticoids are diverse and are the result of increasing or decreasing the transcription of genes involved in inflammation and immunosuppression.

Activated glucocorticoid receptors (GRs) **stimulate** the expression of many proteins including:

- annexin-1/lipocortin-1 which inhibits formation of inflammatory prostaglandins and leukotrienes (see also *Figure 6.5*)
- an IL-1 receptor antagonist which inhibits immune responses
- Iκβ-α, an inhibitor of nuclear factor-κβ (NFκβ) which is a transcription factor that regulates genes that code for pro-inflammatory proteins
- the β_2-adrenergic receptor.

Activated GRs also **inhibit** the expression of numerous proteins and these include:

- the immunoregulatory cytokines (e.g. the family of interleukins (ILs) and tumor necrosis factor (TNF)-α
- chemokines
- adhesion molecules
- inflammatory enzymes (e.g. inducible nitric oxide, COX-2 and phospholipase A_2)
- inflammatory receptors such as the tachykinin and bradykinin receptors
- the vasodilator, endothelin-1.

Whilst switching on anti-inflammatory/immuno-suppressant genes involves the association of activated GRs with co-activators, the acetylation of histones and trans-activation of gene transcription, switching off pro-inflammatory genes does not appear to involve recruitment of co-repressors with histone deacetylase activity. Instead, activated GRs may bind to and inhibit the activity of transcription factors (e.g. NFκβ) and/or their co-activators such as CREB binding protein which have been activated by inflammatory stimuli such as IL-1 and TNF-α (*Figure 6.8*).

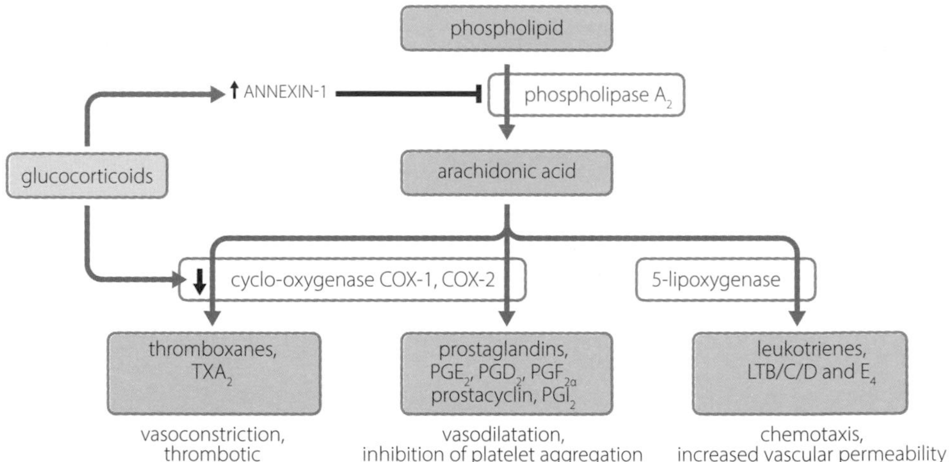

Figure 6.5. The effects of glucocorticoids on inflammatory mediators derived from arachidonic acid. The synthesis of inflammatory mediators derived from arachidonic acid and an outline of their actions. Glucocorticoids inhibit the inflammatory response by inducing annexin-1 which inhibits phospholipase A_2 and inhibits the induction of COX-2.

injury. It is these actions which led to the development of a huge range of synthetic steroidal anti-inflammatory drugs with a huge profit for the pharmaceutical industry.

Glucocorticoids also have a spectrum of other actions (*Box 6.1*). They raise blood pressure partly by their ability to alter the sensitivity of the cardiovascular system to catecholamines and through their ability to have aldosterone-like effects, thereby increasing sodium and water retention. In the central nervous system cortisol

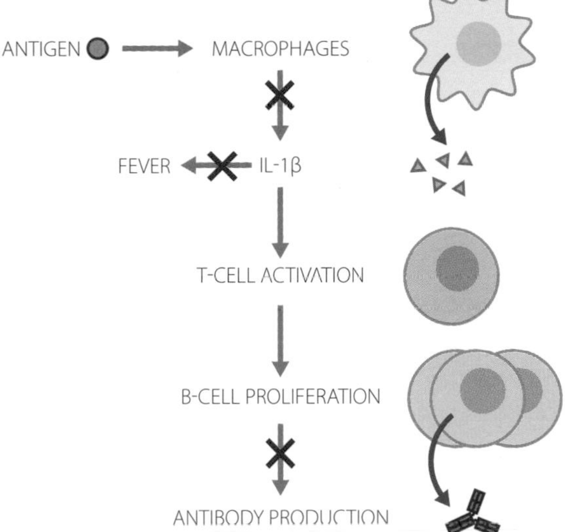

Figure 6.6. Immunosuppressant actions of glucocorticoids. Glucocorticoids inhibit the immune response by inhibiting the expression of interleukin (IL)-1β and other cytokines, stimulating the expression of an interleukin receptor antagonist and ultimately inhibiting antibody production.

is important in organizational effects during development and in the adult can contribute to neuronal plasticity as well as neurodegeneration. Glucocorticoids can also have effects on mood and behavior and in depression cortisol levels may be raised and its secretion does not show a daily rhythm.

In the fetus, cortisol facilitates maturation of several organs and tissues (including the central nervous system) and is particularly important in the synthesis of alveolar surfactant during the final weeks of gestation. Babies born prematurely may therefore suffer from respiratory distress syndrome.

Other less well-defined actions include complex effects on bone, positive and negative effects on cell growth, induction of pro-apoptotic signals in cells, and an increase in the glomerular blood flow/filtration rate in the kidney.

6.3.2 How do glucocorticoids exert their cellular effects?

Many of the actions of glucocorticoids are mediated through classic steroid receptors which are ubiquitously expressed throughout the body. The human glucocorticoid receptor (hGR) is the product of one gene (located on chromosome 5) that contains 9 exons (*Figure 6.7*). The 5′ promoter region contains three different transcription sites, each of which produces a different first exon that is fused to the common exon 2 after excision of the introns. Alternate splicing of exon 9 gives rise to two distinct mRNAs coding for hGRα and hGRβ. In addition, other splice variants have been identified such as hGR-A (lacking exons 5, 6, and 7) and hGR-B (lacking exons 8 and 9) and these have been detected at high levels in glucocorticoid-resistant myeloma patients. Each hGRα and hGRβ mRNA also produces additional isoforms depending on the site at which translation of the mRNA into the protein is initiated. Thus multiple splice variants and isoforms of the hGR exist, all of which are derived from a single gene and result from different transcriptional and translational activities. However, the most ubiquitous and predominant form is hGRα with 777 amino acids whilst hGRβ (typically 742 amino acids) is generally expressed at much lower levels (*Figure 6.7*). Like all steroid receptors, they can also undergo post-translational modification such as phosphorylation, sumoylation, and ubiquitination (*Section 1.6*).

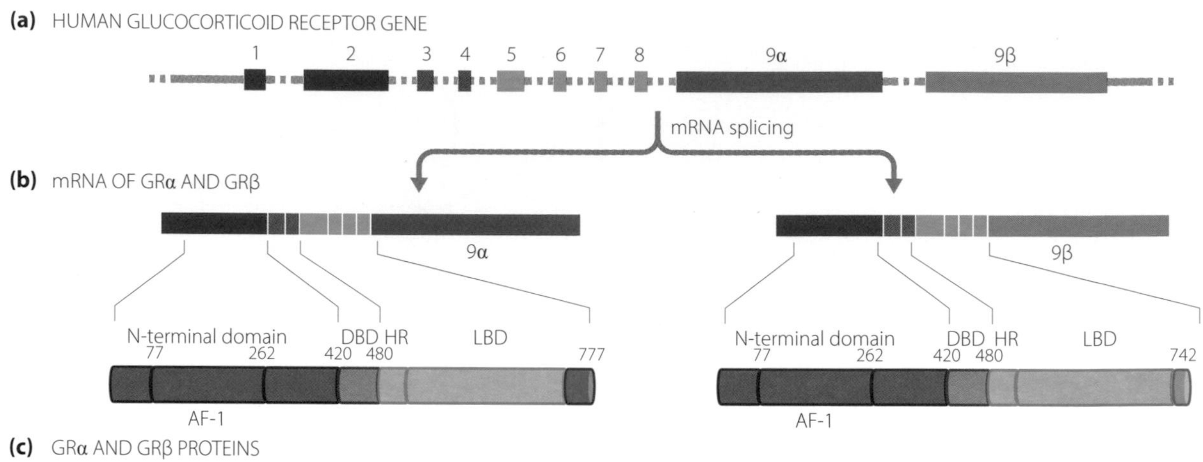

Figure 6.7. Glucocorticoid receptors.
(a) Structure of the gene coding for the glucocorticoid receptor (GR). Exon 1 has alternative start sites for the transcription of RNA.
(b) Alternative splicing of the 9th exon in pre-mRNA gives rise to two different mRNAs coding for GRα and GRβ. Only exons 2–9 are translated into the receptor proteins.
(c) Structure of the major GRα and GRβ proteins indicating the activating function-1 (AF-1), DNA binding domain (DBD), hinge region (HR), and ligand-binding domain (LBD) of each receptor.
Additional variation in the structure and function of the protein results from alternative start sites for the initiation of translation within exon 2 and post-translational modifications of the protein, e.g. phosphorylation, ubiquitination and sumoylation. Different translational start sites give rise to several shorter isoforms of both receptors (these are not shown in the diagram). GRα, located in the cytoplasm, is considered to be the predominant receptor and is transcriptionally active, whilst GRβ, located in the nucleus, is an inhibitor of the transcriptional activity of GRα.

hGRα exists in the cytoplasm in association with heat shock proteins, Hsp90 and Hsp70. These are essential chaperones which induce a conformational change in the glucocorticoid receptor, opening up the hydrophobic pocket of the ligand-binding domain and allowing cortisol to enter and bind. Dissociation of the heat shock proteins and phosphorylation of the receptors facilitates translocation of the hormone–receptor complex into the nucleus, where it forms a homo- or heterodimer with another hormone–receptor complex. The effects of heterodimeric forms may differ from those of the homodimers.

Unlike hGRα, hGRβ is localized in the nucleus of cells, it does not bind glucocorticoids and is transcriptionally inactive. hGRβ has been shown to be a dominant inhibitor of the transcriptional activity of hGRα and recently this activity has been attributed to the formation of hGRα/hGRβ heterodimers. It is thought that hGRβ may be involved in the regulation of tissue-specific sensitivity to glucocorticoids and be a contributing factor to glucocorticoid resistance. Thus an imbalance of hGRα and hGRβ may underlie the pathogenesis of various clinical conditions associated with glucocorticoid resistance, such as rheumatoid arthritis, systemic lupus erythematosus, and ulcerative colitis.

There are several ways in which activated hGRs induce a particular cellular response (*Figure 6.8*). First, they may bind directly to a glucocorticoid response element (GRE) on the DNA, attract co-activators and either initiate gene transcription (e.g. the expression of enzymes required in gluconeogenesis) or repress gene

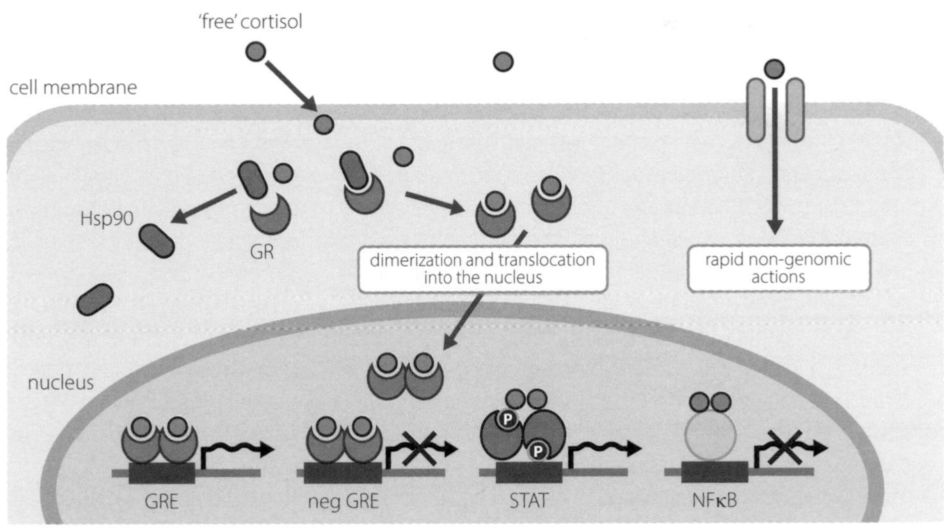

Figure 6.8. Regulation of genomic and non-genomic effects in target cells by glucocorticoid receptors. Unbound 'free' cortisol diffuses across the cell membrane and releases a heat shock protein (Hsp) from the glucocorticoid receptor (GR) and then binds with the receptor in the cytoplasm. This then dimerizes with another cortisol/receptor complex. After translocation to the nucleus the dimers may either bind to glucocorticoid response elements (GRE) to stimulate or, less frequently, inhibit (neg) transcription. Alternatively they may bind to other transcription factors such as STAT or NFκB to stimulate or inhibit their transcriptional activity. Cortisol may also stimulate membrane/cytosolic receptors to activate non-genomic events (see text for further details).

transcription. Secondly, they may activate other transcription factors such as STAT-5 (activated, for example, by growth hormone via JAK (see *Chapter* 1)) and this does not require binding of the hGR to DNA. Similarly, the activated hGR may inhibit activity of another transcription factor such as AP-1 and nuclear factor (NF)-κB. The inhibition of NF-κB represses the expression of pro-inflammatory cytokines; this is an important anti-inflammatory mechanism of glucocorticoids. Thus a drug that would target specifically the transcriptional activity of NFκB (*Figure 6.8*) could act as a potent anti-inflammatory drug and avoid the use of glucocorticoids which have mainly trans-activational activity in many target cells. Glucocorticoid anti-inflammatory therapy has many systemic side-effects, as indicated by the widespread actions of these steroids.

Although the majority of endocrine and metabolic actions of glucocorticoids appear to be mediated by direct binding of hGR dimers to DNA (i.e. trans-activational rather than trans-repressional) a few actions of glucocorticoids are too rapid to involve gene transcription. There is increasing evidence that glucocorticoids have non-genomic actions either via membrane receptors or via cytosolic receptors that can interact with classic cell signaling pathways. One of the most notable non-genomic effects is the rapid phosphorylation of annexin-1 (lipocortin-1, encoded by *ANXA1*) which inhibits the activation of phospholipase (PL) A2 via the EGF receptor. PLA2 stimulates the synthesis of arachidonic acid, the precursor to the pro-inflammatory prostaglandins, thromboxanes, and leukotrienes (*Figure 6.5*). The glucocorticoid regulation of T-cell activity and the rapid feedback effect of glucocorticoids is also mediated by a non-genomic action involving *ANXA1* (*Box 6.3*). Other examples of rapid non-genomic effects include activation of the PI3 kinase signaling pathway

Box 6.3 | Annexin-1

Annexin-1 (ANXA1), formerly known as lipocortin-1, was first identified as a protein with calcium and phospholipid binding properties. It is a mediator in the glucocorticoid inhibition of phospholipase A2 and cyclooxygenase 2, thus inhibiting the synthesis of pro-inflammatory eicosanoids (see *Figure 6.5*). Since its initial discovery, a family of 13 calcium or calcium and phospholipid binding proteins have been identified and this family of proteins have high biological and structural homology. Apart from its anti-inflammatory actions on the innate immune system, ANXA1 has been shown to be a positive regulator of T-cell regulation in the adaptive immune system and has been implicated in playing a role in T-cell-driven immune diseases. It also has a wide range of other biological effects contributing to processes as diverse as cell adhesion and migration, cell growth and differentiation, cell signaling, apoptosis, lipid metabolism, and cytokine expression.

ANXA1 is abundantly expressed in the anterior pituitary gland and to a lesser extent in the hypothalamus and other parts of the brain. Experimental studies have shown that ANXA1 not only mediates anti-inflammatory actions of glucocorticoids but also the early onset (non-genomic) negative-feedback actions of glucocorticoids on the hypothalamic–pituitary axis. ANXA1 is not expressed in either the CRH/VP neurosecretory cells in the hypothalamus or corticotrophs in the anterior pituitary gland; instead it is expressed in non-endocrine cells of the hypothalamus and folliculostellate cells in the pituitary gland. Further evidence revealed that the rapid actions of glucocorticoid feedback involved the translocation of ANXA1 to the cell surface and the release of this protein which may then act in a paracrine manner on adjacent neurosecretory cells and pituitary corticotrophs to inhibit the release of CRH and ACTH. The ANXA1 receptor has recently been identified as a GPCR belonging to the formyl peptide receptor (FPR) family.

(see *Chapter 1*), stimulation of GABA release, and inhibition of voltage-gated calcium channels.

6.3.3 Transport and metabolism of glucocorticoids

Cortisol binds to the high affinity corticosteroid-binding globulin (CBG or transcortin) and this transport protein normally carries approximately 90% of the circulating hormone. A smaller percentage (~6%) is bound to albumin that has a low affinity but a high capacity for the hormones and the remaining 4% is unbound or 'free'. Like thyroxine-binding globulin (TBG), these proteins are synthesized by the liver and their concentrations in blood are altered by a number of factors. For example, pregnancy and estrogen administration increases CBG synthesis 2–3-fold, increasing total cortisol with a normal unbound fraction. Conversely, reduced CBG concentrations are observed in states such as cirrhosis, hyperthyroidism, and nephritic syndrome.

The uptake of steroids by cells from capillary blood occurs by diffusion from the free hormone pool although, as with thyroid hormones, there is experimental evidence for specific transport mechanisms. In the circulation, cortisol is in equilbrium with its biologically inactive 11-keto analog, cortisone (*Figure 6.9*).

Cortisol has a circulating half-life of 70–120 minutes and is metabolized mainly in the liver by reductase and hydrogenase enzymes: cortisol is metabolized to allo-tetrahydrocortisol (allo-THF) and tetrahydrocortisol (THF), and cortisone to tetrahydrocortisone (THE) (*Figure 6.9*). These reduced metabolites are conjugated and excreted in the urine as glucuronides and only 1% of the total cortisol excretion is accounted for by the free unmetabolized cortisol. Thus measurement of cortisol metabolites in the urine provides a useful clinical index of cortisol secretion.

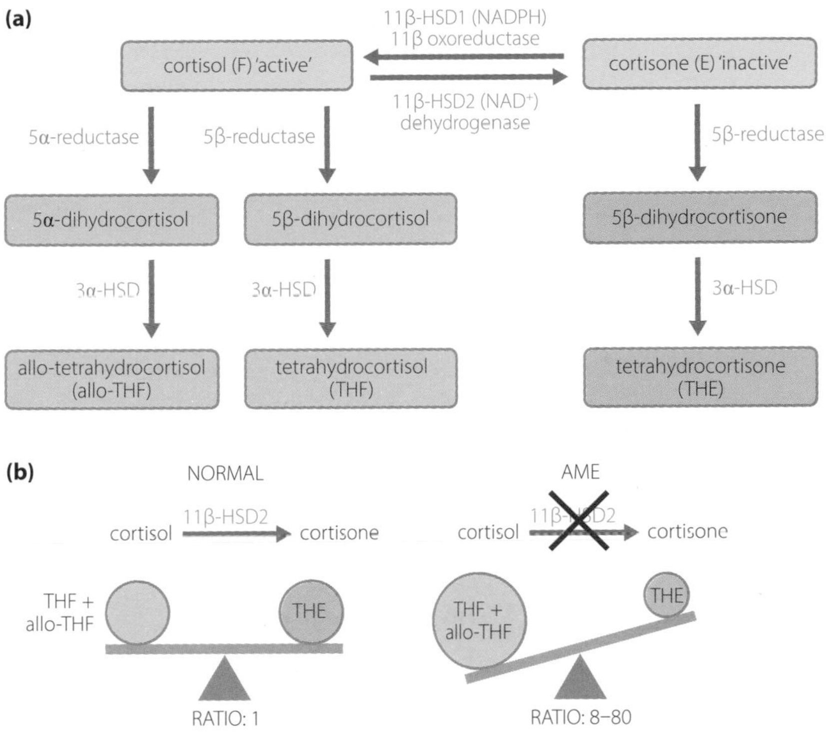

Figure 6.9. Metabolism of cortisol.
11β-hydroxysteroid dehydrogenase (HSD)1 is widely distributed in the body and its predominant activity is to convert inactive cortisone to active cortisol. 11β-HSD2 has a distinct tissue-specific expression in classic mineralocorticoid target tissues and rapidly inactivates cortisol to prevent its interaction with the aldosterone receptor.
Cortisol is metabolized to tetrahydrocortisol (THF) and allo-THF and cortisone is metabolized to tetrahydrocortisone (THE). Normally the ratio for these metabolites in the urine is 1:1 but in the very rare cases of apparent mineralocorticoid excess (AME) this ratio changes and excess cortisol acts with the aldosterone receptors (see *Section 6.7* and *Figure 6.14* for further details).

6.3.4 Availability of cortisol at the glucocorticoid receptor and its metabolism

At a pre-receptor level, glucocorticoid activity is regulated by two isoenzymes, 11β-hydroxysteroid dehydrogenase1 (11β-HSD1) and 11β-HSD2 that interconvert active cortisol and inactive cortisone. 11β-HSD1 has bidirectional activities interconverting cortisol and cortisone, although *in vivo* the enzyme predominantly has 11-oxoreductase activity and so converts cortisone to cortisol using NADPH as a co-factor (*Figure 6.9*). It thus increases the availability of cortisol at the glucocorticoid receptor. 11β-HSD2 has only unidirectional dehydrogenase activity, converting cortisol to inactive cortisone using NAD^+ as a co-factor. Unlike 11β-HSD1, which is widely distributed in the body, 11β-HSD2 exhibits a distinct tissue-specific expression in classical mineralocorticoid target tissues such as the distal tubule of the kidney, colon, and salivary glands. In these tissues this enzyme rapidly inactivates cortisol and thus prevents cortisol from interacting with the mineralocorticoid receptor for which it has equal affinity.

The ratio of the urinary excretion of cortisol and cortisone metabolites is normally 1:1, but patients with inactivating mutations of 11β-HSD2 have dramatically reduced, or absent, excretion of THE (*Figure 6.9*). Such mutations are very rare (fewer than 100 cases have been reported worldwide) and give rise to a rare form of severe hypertension and hypokalemic metabolic alkalosis known as apparent mineralocorticoid excess. This is because cortisol, which circulates at a concentration 100 times higher than that of aldosterone, inappropriately interacts with the aldosterone receptor.

6.3.5 Adrenal androgens

The major androgens secreted by the reticularis zone of the adrenal cortex are DHEA and its sulfated form DHEA-S, and to a lesser extent androstenedione. Once in the circulation these androgens are mainly transported bound to albumin, which contrasts with the transport of testosterone which is extensively bound to the specific sex hormone binding globulin (SHBG). Although their direct biological activity is minimal they serve as precursors for peripheral conversion to active androgenic hormones, testosterone and dihydrotestosterone, and subsequently to estrogens (*Figure 6.10*). They may also be metabolized directly to androstenediol and its sulfate and are excreted either as conjugates with glucuronide or as sulfates. DHEA-S can be excreted directly by the kidneys.

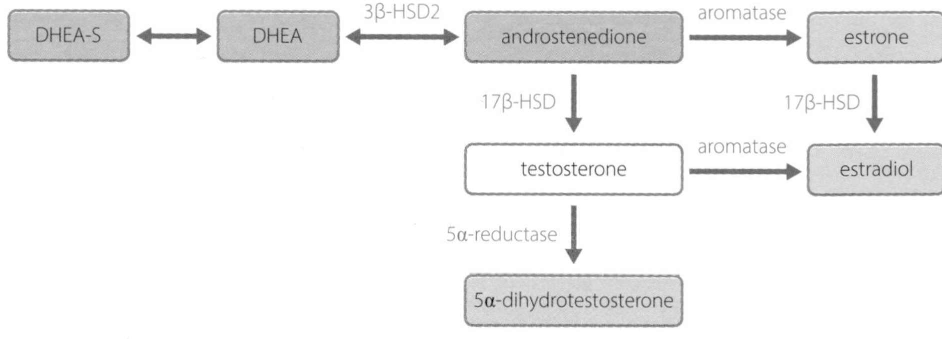

Figure 6.10. Peripheral metabolism of adrenal androgens to more potent androgens and estradiol. Dehydroepiandrosterone (DHEA) and its sulfated (S) form can be converted to androstenedione by 3β-hydroxysteroid dehydrogenase (HSD)2 and then to testosterone and 5α-dihydrotestosterone by the enzymes indicated. Alternatively, androstenedione and testosterone can be converted to estrone (a weak estrogen) or estradiol, respectively, by the action of aromatase. Subsequently estrone can be converted to estradiol.

In males with normal gonadal function the conversion of androstenedione and DHEA/DHEA-S (via androstenedione) to testosterone accounts for less than 5% of the circulating concentrations of this hormone. Thus in adult males adrenal androgen secretion is of no clinical consequence, although in prepubertal boys excess adrenal androgen secretion may cause penile enlargement and early development of secondary sex characteristics (see *Chapter 7*). In women, adrenal androgens contribute substantially to circulating concentrations of androgens, and adrenal-derived testosterone is important in maintaining normal pubic and axillary hair. When secreted in excess as, for example, in congenital adrenal hyperplasia (CAH) (Case 6.4) these androgens cause hirsutism (*Box 6.4*) and acne. In post-menopausal women, adrenal androgens provide the main source of precursors for estrogen synthesis in peripheral tissues. This is clinically significant in estrogen-dependent cancers such as those of the breast and endometrium.

The secretion of adrenal androgens begins around the age of 4–6 years, reaches a peak between 20 and 25 years and thereafter declines with age so that at 70–80 years of age, peak DHEA/DHEA-S concentrations are less than 20% those of young adults. This age-related decline has been termed 'andropause' and there is continuing debate as to whether DHEA should be considered as potential hormone replacement therapy both in ageing men and women. Such replacement would provide a precursor for peripheral testosterone and estrogen synthesis.

Box 6.4 | Hirsutism

Low concentrations of androgens are required for terminal hair growth in the axillae, lower abdomen and upper thighs but higher concentrations cause growth at distances away from these areas (hirsutism). The majority of androgens in women originate from steroid precursors synthesized in the adrenal cortex and excess androgens, such as occurs in CAH, cause hirsutism. In clinical practice attention should also be paid to the ovaries in addition to the adrenal glands because they both may produce excess androgens as, for example, in polycystic ovary syndrome (see *Chapter 7*). In extreme cases, excess of androgens leads to loss of female characteristics and masculinization. Assessing mild hyperandrogenism and hirsutism can be problematic. It is important to distinguish the fine vellus hair that covers most of the body from the stiffer and thicker terminal hair whose growth and distribution is dependent on androgens (*Box figure 6.1*). Pale skins with dark vellus hairs and ethnic variation in the amount of body hair should also be taken into account when assessing mild hirsutism. The severity of hirsutism can be assessed by the Ferriman and Gallwey scoring system (see *Box figure 6.2*).

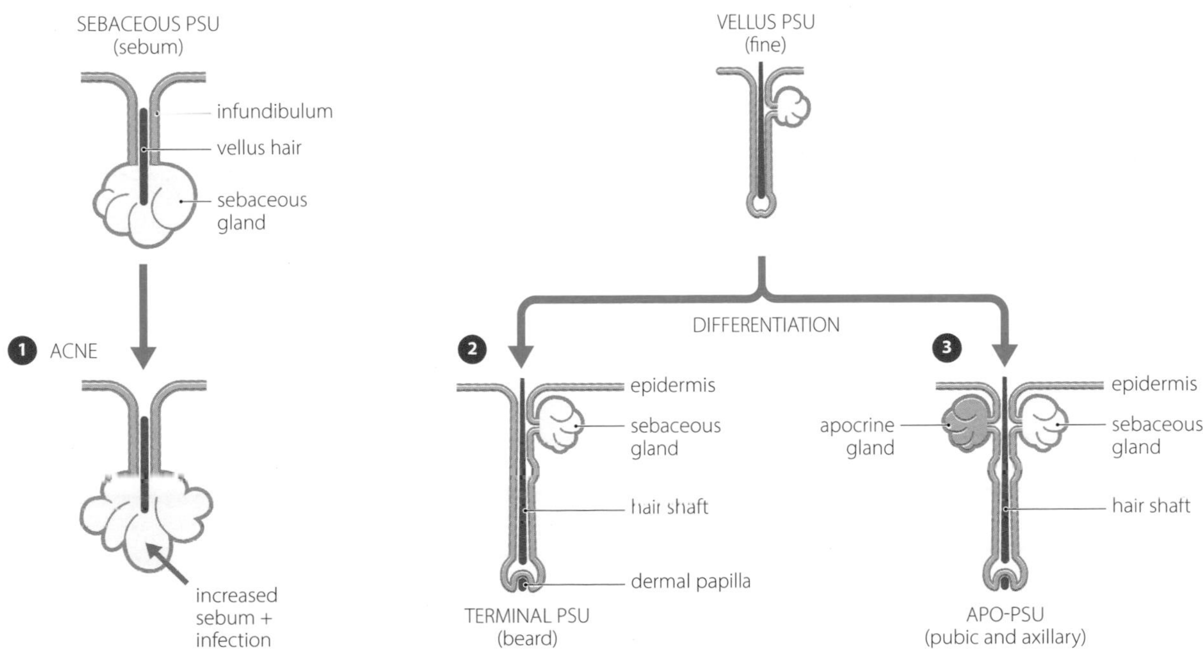

Box figure 6.1. Different classes of pilosebaceous units.

(1) Androgens (indicated by blue arrows) stimulate sebum secretion and together with infection this can cause acne.

(2) Androgens stimulate differentiation of vellus pilosebaceous units (PSUs) to terminal PSUs encouraging mustache and beard growth.

(3) Androgens stimulate differentiation of vellus hairs to apo-PSUs encouraging increased growth in areas of pubic and axillary hair.

Box 6.4 | continued

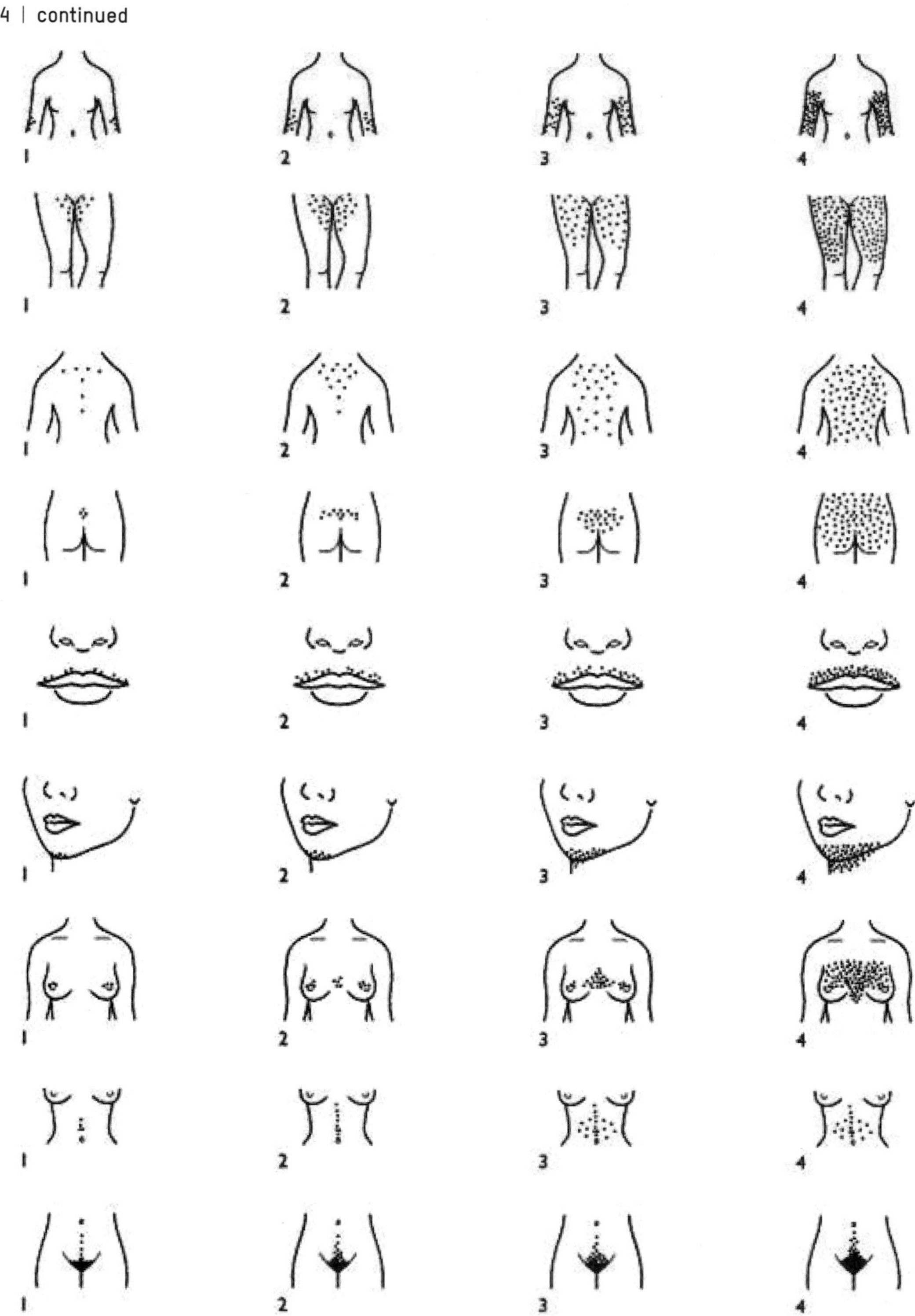

Box figure 6.2. The Ferriman and Gallwey system for assessing hirsutism resulting from excess androgen secretions in females. Nine body regions are evaluated for their degree of hair growth from 0 to 4. A total score >8 is a sign for hirsutism.
Originally described by Ferriman DM and Gallwey JD (1961) Clinical assessment of body hair growth in women. *J. Clin. Endocrinol.* **21**: 1440–7. Reproduced with permission from The Endocrine Society.

6.3.6 CRH, ACTH, and the control of glucocorticoid and androgen production

The synthesis and secretion of ACTH is stimulated by CRH, a 41 amino acid peptide that is secreted by neurosecretory cells predominantly located in the paraventricular nucleus of the hypothalamus. Released from nerve terminals in the median eminence, CRH is transported to the anterior pituitary corticotrophs in the hypophyseal portal capillaries where it acts on a GPCR to stimulate an increase in cAMP. The subsequent signal transduction pathways stimulate both the synthesis and release of ACTH (*Figure 6.11*). The action of CRH on pituitary corticotrophs is potentiated by AVP, also known as antidiuretic hormone (ADH). AVP is secreted by neurosecretory cells in the supraoptic and paraventricular nuclei of the hypothalamus and though their axons classically terminate in the posterior pituitary, some terminate on the capillaries of the median eminence.

CRH is widely distributed throughout the central nervous system and it exerts its action through two CRH receptor subtypes, CRHR1 and CRHR2; these have different expression patterns within the brain. Both CRHR1 and CRHR2 are present in the anterior pituitary gland, although CRH has a low affinity for CRHR2. CRH in the brain appears to act as a neuromodulator, and hyperactivity of CRH neurons both

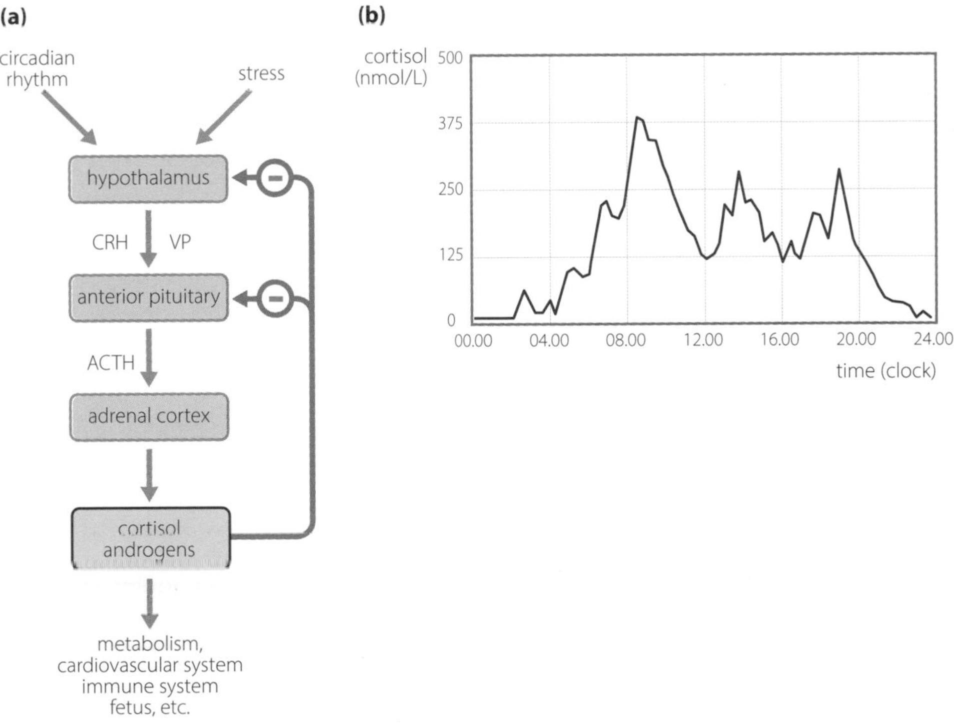

Figure 6.11. Control of glucocorticoid and androgen production.
(a) Corticotropin-releasing hormone (CRH), together with vasopressin (VP), stimulate the corticotrophs of the anterior pituitary gland to synthesize and secrete adrenocorticotropin hormone (ACTH). In turn, ACTH stimulates the adrenal cortex to synthesize and release cortisol and androgens. Cortisol exerts negative feedback effects on the hypothalamic–pituitary axis so when levels of cortisol rise the synthesis and release of CRH and ACTH are reduced. These feedback effects can be over-ridden by stress (physical or emotional) and the 'biological' clock.
(b) Circadian rhythm in cortisol secretion.

Box 6.5 | Synthesis of adrenocorticotropic hormone (ACTH) and related peptides

The pro-opiomelanocortin (POMC) gene codes for a large prohormone that is subsequently cleaved into biologically active fragments by peptidases (*Box figure 6.3*). This processing is tissue specific. ACTH and the three melanocyte hormones (shaded) act on the family of G-protein coupled melanocyte receptors (MCR) of which there are five subtypes (*Box table 6.1*).

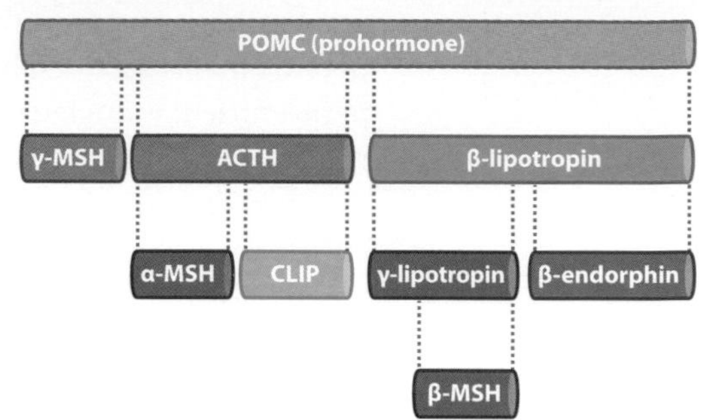

Box figure 6.3. Processing of the POMC prohormone.

Box table 6.1. **Distribution and functions of MCR subtypes and affinity of different ligands**

MCR subtype	Ligand affinity	Prevalent tissue expression	Functions
MC1R	γ-MSH ≥ ACTH >> γ-MSH	Melanocytes Immune/inflammatory cells; keratinocytes; endothelial cells; glial cells	Pigmentary effects Antipyretic/anti-inflammatory
MC2R	ACTH	Adrenal cortex	Steroidogenesis
MC3R	γ-MSH = ACTH ≥ α-MSH	CNS Macrophages	Autonomic functions Anti-inflammatory
MC4R	α-MSH = ACTH >> γ-MSH	CNS	Control of feeding and energy homeostasis; erectile activity
MC5R	α-MSH ≥ ACTH > γ-MSH	Exocrine glands, lymphocytes	Regulation of exocrine secretions, immunoregulatory functions

Reproduced from Catania *et al.* (2004) Targeting melanocortin receptors as a novel strategy to control inflammation. *Pharmacological Reviews*, **56**: 1–29, with permission from ASPET.

in the hypothalamus and other brain regions may not only activate the increased ACTH/adrenal activity associated with stress, but also certain associated behavioral symptoms such as depression, sleep, appetite disturbances, and psychomotor changes.

ACTH is derived from a large precursor molecule pro-opiomelanocortin (POMC) that is cleaved by the action of specific peptidase enzymes (*Box 6.5*). Whilst this prohormone can give rise to numerous hormones, including opioid peptides and MSH, the main product of POMC cleavage in the pituitary corticotrophs is ACTH. In the brain, other products predominate.

The ACTH receptor is one of a family of GPCRs of melanocortin of which 5 subtypes have been identified: MC1R to MC5R (*Box 6.5*). MC2R is the receptor expressed in the adrenal glands. Other melanocortin receptors are expressed in the brain and all melanocortin receptors are widely expressed in peripheral tissues and cells. Both ACTH and the MSHs α, β, and γ bind to these receptors with different affinities and such ligand binding controls various functions including skin pigmentation, inflammation, energy homeostasis, body weight regulation, penile erections, and sebum secretion. The ability of ACTH to bind with melanocortin receptors explains the skin pigmentation so frequently observed in Addison disease (Case 6.3).

ACTH has a half-life of 4–8 minutes and its binding to the ACTH/MC2R stimulates adenyl cyclase and cAMP production. The early actions of ACTH on the synthesis of glucocorticoids and androgens include the induction of StAR protein to increase transport of cholesterol across the mitochondrial membrane and an increased conversion of cholesterol to pregnenolone by the side chain cleavage enzyme $P_{450}scc$ (see *Figure 6.3*). Subsequent actions include the induction of steroidogenic enzymes and increased corticosteroid production. Whether or not androgen synthesis and secretion are under some other control mechanism remains uncertain. ACTH also stimulates conspicuous structural changes in the adrenal cortex characterized by hypervascularization, cellular hypertrophy, and hyperplasia. This is particularly notable when excess ACTH is secreted over prolonged periods of time and accounts for the increased adrenal size observed in pituitary-dependent Cushing disease or CAH (Case 6.4). Conversely, adrenal atrophy occurs in ACTH-deficient states such as through loss of pituitary function or exogenous immunosuppressant glucocorticoids that suppress endogenous ACTH release (negative feedback).

6.3.7 Feedback control of glucocorticoids

The production of glucocorticoids is controlled by a classical negative feedback loop in which neurons in the hypothalamus detect circulating concentrations of glucocorticoids and consequently stimulate or inhibit the release of CRH and AVP (*Figure 6.11*). Raised glucocorticoids down-regulate CRH and AVP mRNA in the hypothalamus, reducing the peptide concentrations in the paraventricular nucleus and CRH secretion. Other effects include diminished ACTH secretion via suppression of POMC gene transcription.

The feedback loop can, however, be over-ridden by both internal and external factors. Human biological clocks (normally entrained to the light–dark cycle) produce a circadian rhythm in the release of ACTH and, consequently, cortisol with peak concentrations of these hormones occurring in the early morning and a nadir in the evening (*Figure 6.11*). Thus, for patients requiring cortisol replacement therapy a larger dose of the steroid is given in the morning with lower doses at other times of the day to simulate the normal endogenous rhythm (Case 6.3). Stress, whether generated by physical or emotional trauma, is also a potent stimulus to cortisol secretion and can over-ride negative feedback effects. In addition to the ACTH drive of the adrenal cortex, there is also evidence for non-ACTH-mediated regulation that could partly explain why, in some clinical situations, there is a dissociation between ACTH and cortisol secretions.

Historically, the steroid-producing cells of the adrenal cortex and the catecholamine-producing chromaffin cells of the adrenal medulla were regarded as two independent endocrine systems. It is now known that there is functional cortical–chromaffin cross-talk and that multiple contact zones exist between the cortex and medulla. Consequently, disorders of the adrenal cortex affect chromaffin cell function and vice versa. For example, patients with Addison disease (Case 6.3) or CAH (Case 6.4) show reduced catecholamine synthesis. In addition, the nerve supply of the adrenal cortex can modulate adrenocortical function and immunomodulatory peptides, such as cytokines which are released within the gland or derived from circulating leukocytes, can stimulate cortisol secretion. The latter could, in part, account for the rise in cortisol seen during chronic infection and sepsis.

6.4 Excess glucocorticoids – Cushing syndrome

CASE 6.1

284 292

- Woman of 45 years with PCOS, presents with amenorrhea, weight gain, hirsutes, and hypertension
- Metformin and oral contraceptive pill used for treatment but stopped; currently on bendroflumethiazide and ramipril
- Tests showed high fasting sugar, undetectable ACTH, and failure to suppress cortisol, confirming Cushing syndrome

A 45 year old woman presented to the endocrine clinic with amenorrhea, weight gain, hirsutes and hypertension. She had previously been diagnosed with PCOS (*Chapter 7*) and had been treated with metformin and the oral contraceptive pill. The oral contraceptive pill was stopped by her family doctor when her blood pressure was recorded at 165/105 mmHg and she had been started on bendroflumethiazide and ramipril. It was noted that she was overweight (with central adiposity), with mild hirsutes and acne and rather plethoric facies. She had purple striae across her abdomen and prominent supraclavicular fat pads. There was no bruising or myopathy. She had stopped metformin some 9 months before the consultation and her fasting sugar measured in primary care was 8.2 mmol/L (NR 3.5–6.1).

Initial screening investigations reported:

- an overnight (1 mg) dexamethasone suppression test which showed failure to suppress cortisol
- ACTH was undetectable (<5 pg/mL)
- normal electrolytes
- moderately high 24-hour urine free cortisol at 425 nmol/L (NR 50–300)

These results confirmed Cushing syndrome and further investigations to delineate the cause were initiated.

CASE 6.2

293

- Man of 31 years with features highly suggestive of Cushing syndrome
- Tests showed no diurnal variation in cortisol, high ACTH, and no cortisol suppression on dexamethasone testing

A 31 year old man presented to the clinic with a constellation of symptoms including peripheral edema, poor libido, weight gain, acne, pigmentation, and myopathy. On examination he was profoundly Cushingoid with thinning of the skin, plethoric facies, supraclavicular and intrascapular fat pads, striae, and significant myopathy (he could not stand from a squatting position unsupported).

Screening investigations were carried out:

- salivary cortisol measurements taken at 09.00h and 00.00h on three occasions showed no diurnal variation
- ACTH measurements (at 0900h) were consistently high on two occasions (50 and 60 pmol/L; NR <26 pmol/L)
- no suppression of cortisol on a low dose dexamethasone suppression test

Further investigations were commenced.

Cushing syndrome is used to describe a range of signs and symptoms occurring as a result of prolonged exposure to glucocorticoids. Traditionally, Cushing syndrome refers to the condition initially described by Harvey Cushing in 1932 and published as "The basophil adenomas of the pituitary body and their clinical manifestations" in the Bulletin of The Johns Hopkins Hospital. Interestingly, Cushing had previously won the coveted Pulitzer prize for his biography of Sir William Osler. His original description was of hyper-cortisolemia resulting from an ACTH-secreting pituitary adenoma (now known as Cushing **disease**). Cushing **syndrome** refers to all causes of hypercortisolism which can be usefully divided into those that are ACTH-dependent (pituitary adenomas and ectopic ACTH) and those that are independent of ACTH control (autonomous adrenal adenomas, carcinomas, and other rare causes).

6.4.1 Causes of Cushing syndrome

Exogenous corticosteroid exposure

Prescribed or over-the-counter steroid-containing remedies are by far the commonest cause of features of cortisol excess and account for over 98% of all cases of Cushing syndrome. It is usually termed iatrogenic Cushing syndrome to distinguish it from endogenous causes. The history can usually help to distinguish this from endogenous causes – particularly when the patient describes long-term airways disease treated with inhaled or parenteral steroids, or of dermatological conditions such as eczema treated with long-term topical steroids. Diagnosis can sometimes be more challenging when patients occasionally neglect to mention (or indeed realize) that they may be exposed to significant levels of exogenous steroids from over-the-counter treatments (e.g. hydrocortisone creams, skin-whitening preparations, or some traditional Chinese medicines).

Endogenous Cushing syndrome

This is rare with an estimated incidence in Europe of approximately 2–3 cases per million per year; 60–70% of cases are due to pituitary ACTH-secreting adenomas (strictly Cushing disease), 20–30% are caused by cortisol-secreting adrenal tumors (adenomas or carcinomas), and 5–10% of cases result from an ectopic source of ACTH – usually a lung or bronchus tumor.

- ***ACTH-secreting adenomas (Cushing disease) and ectopic ACTH.*** Excess ACTH stimulates bilateral adrenal hyperplasia and an excess of cortisol, adrenal androgens, and 11-deoxycorticosterone. In contrast with some other endocrine disorders, the excess ACTH does not induce a desensitization state in the adrenal cortex; indeed the opposite occurs so that the adrenocortical response to ACTH is amplified. The rise in cortisol levels is paralleled by increased DHEA, DHEA-S, and androstenedione secretion, and their peripheral transformation to testosterone and dihydrotestosterone may result in a state of androgen excess in females. Hirsutism (*Box 6.4*) is extremely common in women with this disease (see Case 6.1) and contrasts with patients who are taking exogenous anti-inflammatory glucocorticoids; in these cases patients will have suppressed ACTH levels due to the feedback effects of the drugs and the endogenous secretion of both glucocorticoids and androgens will be suppressed (*Figure 6.12*). Thus features of excess androgen secretion will not be observed.
- ***ACTH-independent Cushing syndrome – adrenal adenomas and carcinomas.*** These tumors autonomously produce excess cortisol secretion which suppresses the endogenous release of ACTH (*Figure 6.12*). Most cases involve benign adenomas although carcinomas, which are very rare, often secrete both excess androgens and glucocorticoids.
- ***Familial Cushing syndrome and other rare causes.*** Familial Cushing syndrome is seen in some individuals due to an inherited tendency to develop tumors of one or more endocrine glands such as MEN-1 (see *Chapter 8*). Other rare causes

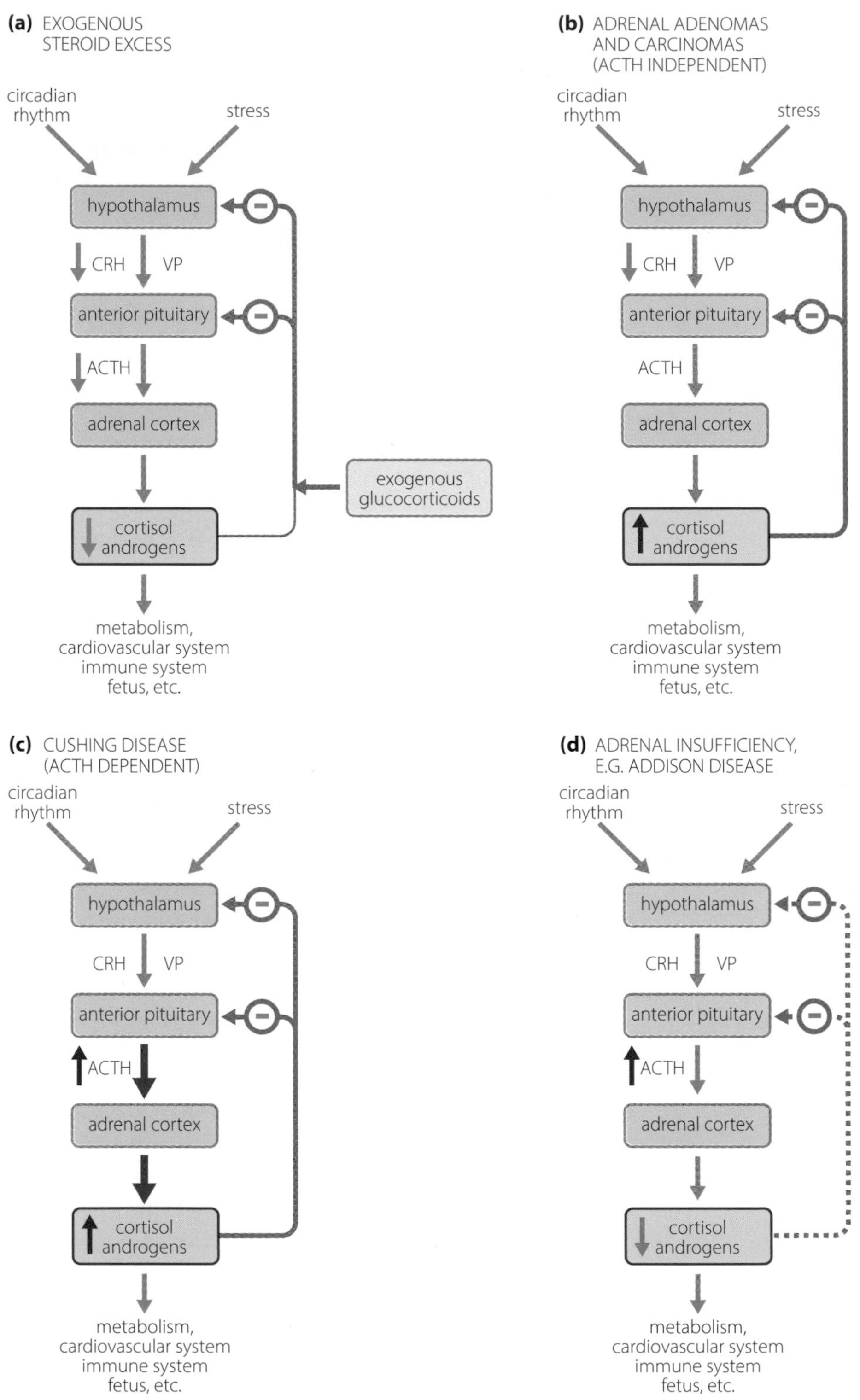

Figure 6.12. Activity of the hypothalamic–pituitary–adrenal axis in various disorders of adrenocortical function.

(a) Exogenous steroid excess.
(b) Adrenal adenomas and carcinomas (ACTH independent).
(c) Cushing disease (ACTH dependent).
(d) Adrenal insufficiency, e.g. Addison disease.

include McCune–Albright syndrome, adrenal macronodular hyperplasia, and food-induced Cushing's. McCune–Albright is a rare syndrome characterized by polyostotic fibrous dysplasia, café au lait spots, and sexual precocity. It may rarely lead to Cushing syndrome secondary to ACTH-independent macronodular adrenal hyperplasia as a result of activating mutations of Gs-α. Food-induced Cushing's can be due to aberrant adrenal receptors for GIP (gastric inhibitory peptide) which, when stimulated, cause ACTH-independent release of cortisol from the adrenals in response to food intake.

Patients with classic full-blown Cushing syndrome are usually clinically obvious, but a number of patients may have some features without others and some may have a constellation of symptoms which might suggest Cushing's (and indeed may have tests pointing towards abnormal cortisol secretion), but which may be explained by some other pathology (e.g. depression, alcoholism, poorly controlled diabetes, or obesity).

The signs of Cushing syndrome are many and varied and not usually of great specificity or sensitivity (*Box 6.6*). The syndrome, however, is associated with increased morbidity and mortality. Chronic hypercortisolism is associated with reduced life expectancy such that patients with a persistent abnormality of cortisol secretion, despite treatment, will have a standardized mortality ratio of up to 5 compared with a normal age/sex matched population. Moderate immunosuppression, osteoporosis, and subtle defects of cognition and mood often persist.

6.4.2 Diagnosis of Cushing syndrome

The biochemical diagnosis of Cushing syndrome is divided into two phases:

- confirmation of cortisol excess (*Box 6.7*)
- determination of cause of cortisol excess.

Again, the importance of exclusion of exogenous glucocorticoid usage is of paramount importance and cannot be over-emphasized.

The next aim should be to determine those patients that are at high risk and criteria should include:

- the presence of symptoms that are relatively discriminatory (striae, myopathy, easy bruising, plethoric facies)
- accumulation of physical signs and symptoms with time
- high risk groups ('atypical' PCOS, hypertension in the young, those with adrenal incidentalomas, unexplained osteoporosis in the young, poorly controlled diabetes with other suspicious features)
- children with obesity and reduced linear growth
- a family history of endocrinopathies such as MEN-1 (*Chapter 8*) or Carney complex (*Box 6.8*).

Confirmation of cortisol excess

The hallmark of Cushing syndrome is its resistance to the suppressive effects of exogenous synthetic glucocorticoids (e.g. dexamethasone) at doses that would normally completely suppress ACTH/glucocorticoid release. High doses of

Box 6.6 | Clinical features of Cushing syndrome

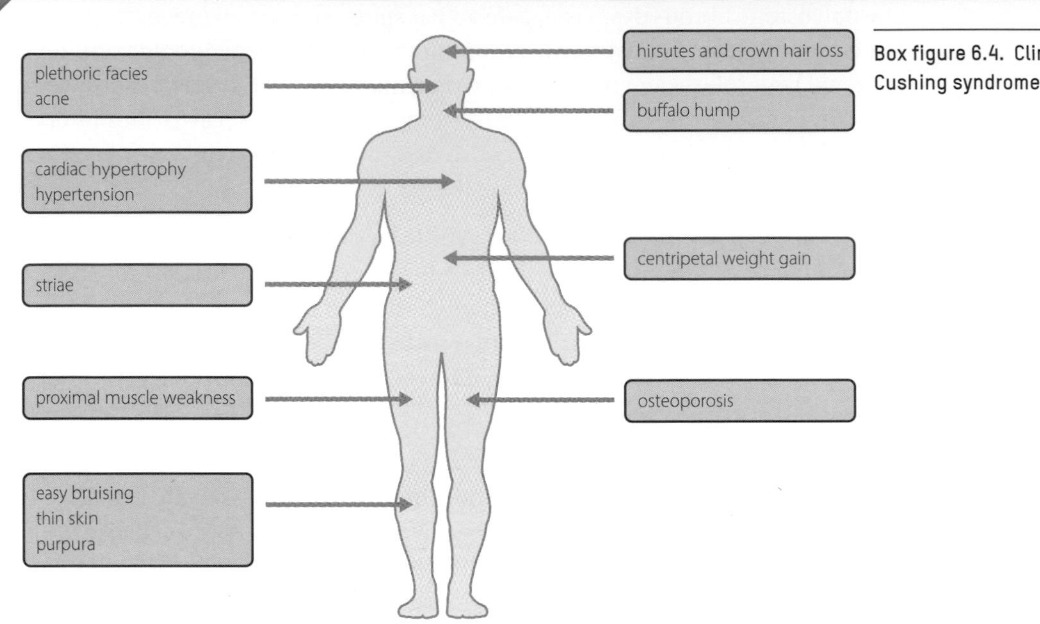

Box figure 6.4. Clinical features of Cushing syndrome.

Discriminatory (but low sensitivity)

- Striae (purple)
- Proximal muscle weakness
- Plethoric facies
- Easy bruising
- Weight gain with poor linear growth (in children and adolescents)

Other features

- Buffalo hump (a fat pad at the base of the neck)
- Obesity (classically central or centripetal with thin limbs)
- Thin skin and poor skin healing
- Peripheral edema
- Hirsutism with crown hair loss
- Acne
- 'Cushingoid facies' – round, full, reddened face
- Virilization, short stature, advanced or delayed puberty (in children)

Symptomatic

- Depression
- Difficulty with weight management
- Fatigue
- Psychotic features
- Decreased libido
- Menstrual abnormalities
- Back pain

Other conditions which may raise suspicion of Cushing's

- Diabetes mellitus
- Hypertension (especially in youth)
- PCOS
- Osteoporosis (especially in youth)
- Low potassium
- Adrenal incidentaloma
- Apparent immunosuppression

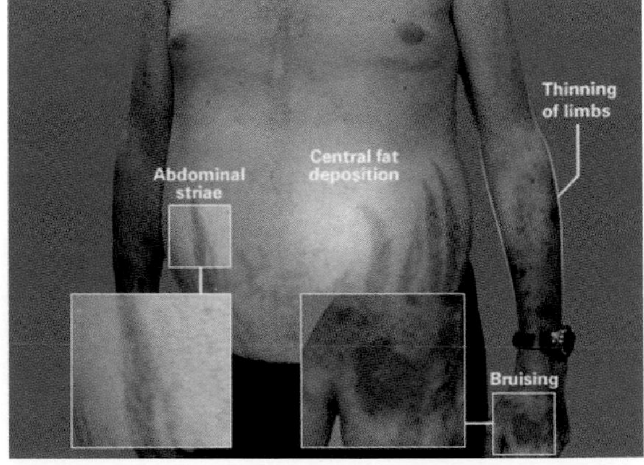

Box figure 6.5. Characteristic signs of Cushing syndrome. These include hyperpigmented abdominal striae, central fat deposition, thinning of limbs, and easy bruising. Note the sternotomy scar for coronary artery bypass grafting – coronary artery disease occurred at a relatively young age in this patient who had diabetes and hypertension.

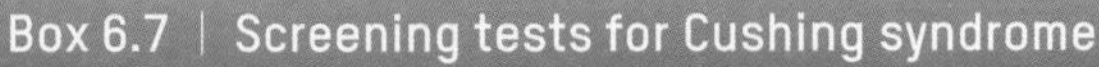

Box 6.7 | Screening tests for Cushing syndrome

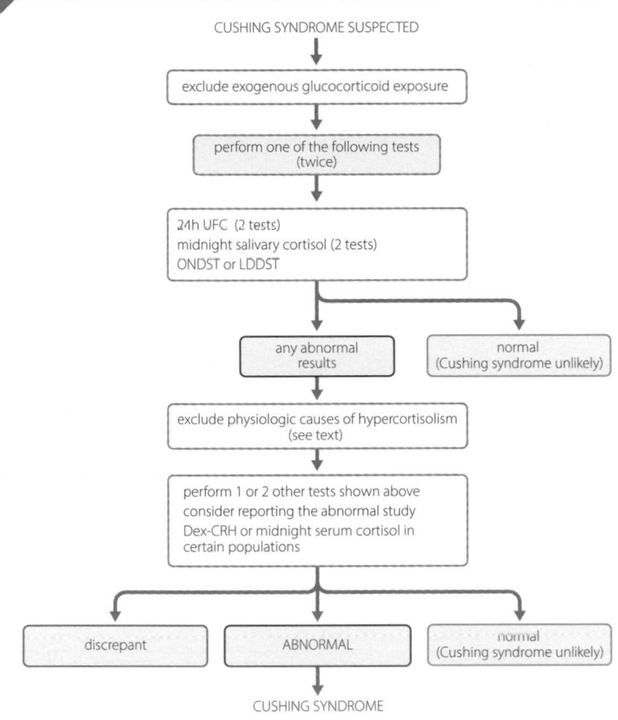

Box figure 6.6. Algorithm for Cushing syndrome diagnosis.

Urinary free cortisol test: 24h UFC

Measurement of urinary free cortisol (UFC) is simple and non-invasive. 10% of plasma cortisol is unbound ('free') and therefore biologically active. Diurnal variation in cortisol during the day is negated by the integrated nature of the 24h UFC. It has a sensitivity of approximately 95% for the diagnosis but there is significant day to day variation so multiple collections are required. The major drawback of the test is inadequacy of the 24-hour urine collection – minimized by giving the patient written instructions and measuring creatinine excretion (which should be around 1000 mg/day) to assess completeness.

Overnight and low dose dexamethasone suppression test: ONDST and LDDST

Normal individuals will respond to exogenous glucocorticoid administration by 'switching off' ACTH and endogenous cortisol production. Dexamethasone is a potent synthetic glucocorticoid with a long duration of action and little or no cross-reactivity in cortisol assays.

For the ONDST, a single dose of 1 mg dexamethasone is taken at midnight followed by measurement of a 09.00h plasma cortisol. Higher doses have no real value and may give false negative results in some patients with pituitary Cushing disease.

In the LDDST, dexamethasone is given in a dose of 0.5 mg 6 hourly for 48 hours, cortisol being measured at 09.00h, 6 hours after the final dose.

The sensitivities of the two tests are similar, but the LDDST has a higher specificity and therefore fewer false positive results.

Salivary cortisol measurements

Salivary cortisol measurements reflect free plasma cortisol. The test is simple and non-invasive, can be performed at home and samples remain stable for some time after collection. Local 'normal' ranges for midnight cortisol need to be determined – published data are highly variable, ranging from about 3.6 nmol/L (0.13 mg/dL) to 15.2 nmol/L (0.55 mg/dL). Nevertheless this is a potentially useful and relatively simple way of determining whether there is a loss of circadian rhythm of cortisol secretion which is a salient feature of Cushing's.

Midnight serum cortisol

Where there is still diagnostic uncertainty, a formal midnight serum cortisol may be helpful, but this is a more complex investigation that requires admission to hospital for a period of time prior to the test (to allow acclimatization). The patient needs to remain asleep (the blood is taken from a previously inserted cannula or within 5 minutes of waking the patient) and free of co-morbidities that may affect interpretation of the result (depression, infection, critical illness, etc.). A sleeping value of less than 50 nmol/L (1.7 μg/dL) effectively excludes Cushing's.

DEX–CRH test

In some cases of pseudoCushing's (e.g. depression, alcoholism, obesity) the phenotype of the patient may be strongly suggestive of Cushing syndrome and the ONDST or LDDST may be equivocal. In these cases some investigators advocate the use of a combined DEX–CRH test where the LDDST is followed by a CRH test. Patients are given dexamethasone (0.5 mg every 6 h for 8 doses) followed by intravenous administration of 1 μg/kg ovine CRH 2 h after the last dose of dexamethasone. A plasma cortisol value (measured 15 min after CRH administration) that is greater than 38 nmol/L has a 100% diagnostic accuracy for Cushing's.

Box 6.8 | Carney complex

There are three rather rare causes of Cushing syndrome associated with bilateral nodular adrenal disease:

- ACTH-dependent macronodular hyperplasia due to long term hypersecretion of pituitary or ectopic ACTH
- ACTH-independent macronodular adrenal hyperplasia
- ACTH-independent micronodular hyperplasia – primary pigmented nodular adrenocortical disease (PPNAD) – which may be sporadic or familial (as part of Carney complex).

PPNAD accounts for less than 1% of Cushing syndrome; the hypercortisolism results from pigmented autonomous adrenal nodules. It may occur as part of Carney complex, an autosomal dominant condition characterized by:

- skin pigmentation with lentigines on the neck, face, and trunk
- endocrine tumors including PPNAD, GH secreting pituitary adenomas, thyroid adenomas, ovarian cysts
- neuroendocrine tumors including atrial myxomas, schwannomas, osteochondromyxomas, breast ductal adenomas.

Mutations in at least four genes have been identified in association with Carney complex including the tumor suppressor gene *PRKAR1A* (mapping to 17q22–24) and the phosphodiesterase 11a isoform gene *PDE11A* (mapping to 2q31–35).

Carney complex (and indeed PPNAD) is interesting in that Cushing syndrome usually presents at an earlier age and may be cyclical in nature, with periods of apparent remission and relapse. Adrenal imaging may be unhelpful because the adrenal glands are often of normal size and with normal gross morphology on imaging. Some patients will have a paradoxical rise in urinary cortisol in response to a dexamethasone suppression test.

dexamethasone can suppress ACTH/cortisol in patients with Cushing syndrome, suggesting that the feedback loop remains intact but its sensitivity is very much reduced. This contrasts with patients with an ectopic source of ACTH in which no suppression is observed irrespective of the dose of dexamethasone (i.e. there is no feedback loop).

Initial tests (*Box 6.7*) should include one or more of the following:

- urinary free cortisol (on at least two occasions)
- overnight 1 mg dexamethasone suppression test (ONDST)
- midnight salivary cortisol
- low dose dexamethasone suppression test (LDDST); 0.5 mg dexamethasone 6 hourly with a blood test after the 8th dose
- low dose dexamethasone suppression test with CRH.

All of these tests are relatively easy to undertake on an outpatient basis without the disruption that an admission may cause. However, many of these tests are subject to producing false positive/negative results, largely as a consequence of assay precision, interference, actions of drugs that may be taken concomitantly, or incomplete urine collections. A common cause of error is in women using the oral contraceptive pill which leads to an increase in CBG and thus an increase in cortisol levels with an apparent failure to suppress cortisol in response to exogenous dexamethasone. Dexamethasone metabolism may be increased by drugs that induce hepatic Cyp3A4 enzymes (e.g. some anti-epileptics, barbiturates, rifampicin). Some patients may have 'cyclical' disease where they cycle in and out of periods of florid cortisol excess and where several baseline determinations may be necessary.

In addition, there are a number of clinical conditions which may mimic some of the clinical features of Cushing syndrome and/or be associated with a failure to fully suppress cortisol with low dose dexamethasone. In patients who show some features of Cushing's these clinical conditions include:

- pregnancy
- depression
- alcoholism
- diabetes mellitus
- obesity.

In patients without features of Cushing's these clinical conditions include:

- stress
- malnutrition
- anorexia
- excess of CBG (e.g. oral contraceptive).

Box 6.9 | Investigation of source of cortisol excess

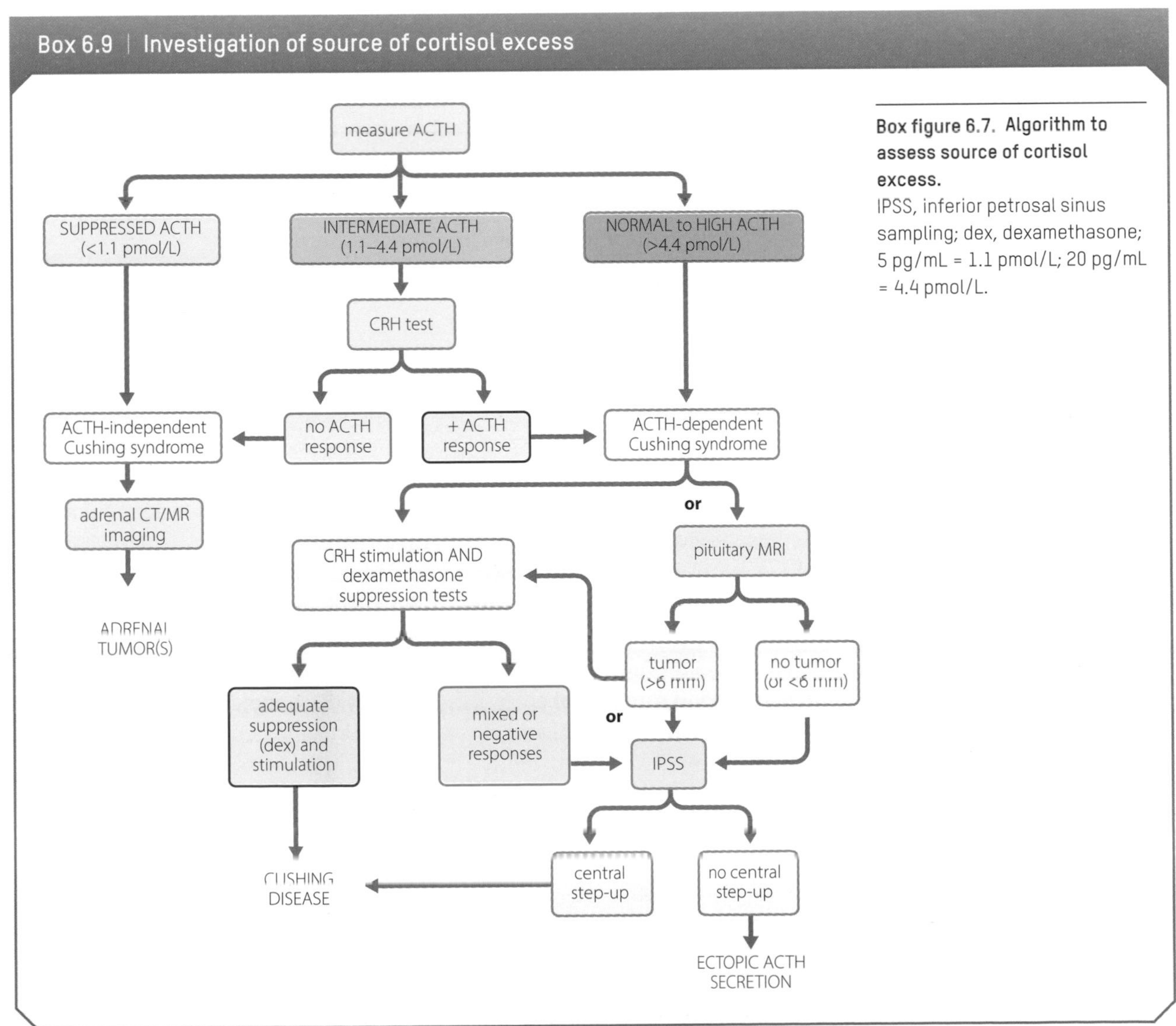

Box figure 6.7. Algorithm to assess source of cortisol excess.
IPSS, inferior petrosal sinus sampling; dex, dexamethasone; 5 pg/mL = 1.1 pmol/L; 20 pg/mL = 4.4 pmol/L.

Determination of cause of cortisol excess

Once abnormality of cortisol secretion has been determined (given the caveats alluded to above) it is necessary to determine whether overproduction is due to pituitary ACTH excess, ectopic ACTH secretion, or primary adrenal disease. This sounds easy but in practice can be challenging.

First, try to ascertain whether there is ACTH-dependent disease (i.e. ACTH excess) or autonomous adrenal oversecretion. Measuring ACTH is a reasonable starting point. If ACTH is low (<1.1 pmol/L) the lesion is likely to be adrenal. If the ACTH is high (>4.4 pmol/L) the likelihood is that the cause is pituitary (an ACTH adenoma) or ectopic ACTH. Intermediate levels tend to be indicative of ACTH-dependent cortisol excess (*Box 6.9*).

If the ACTH is undetectable in the light of hypercortisolism it is reasonable to proceed to adrenal imaging with CT scans. There is no real advantage in MRI scanning. Adrenal adenomas tend to be smaller than carcinomas and have a lower enhancement level (<10 Hounsfield Units). If needed, the washout of contrast can be calculated and should be greater than 50% if there is an adenoma. Carcinomas in contrast have less washout and may demonstrate calcification, necrosis, or hemorrhage. Biochemically, carcinomas also present more commonly with elevated levels of adrenal androgens. If there is a suspicion of adrenal cancer, further imaging with MRI or 18FDG-PET may help (see *Box 6.14*).

A unilateral adenoma in the light of clear biochemical evidence of non-ACTH dependent hypercortisolism is usually enough evidence to warrant laparoscopic or open surgical intervention to achieve a cure. Bilateral disease or suspicion of adrenal cancer will usually require further investigation (see *Section 6.5*).

CASE 6.1 284 292

- Woman of 45 years with PCOS, presents with amenorrhea, weight gain, hirsutes, and hypertension
- Metformin and oral contraceptive pill used for treatment but stopped; currently on bendroflumethiazide and ramipril
- Tests showed high fasting sugar, undetectable ACTH, and failure to suppress cortisol, confirming Cushing syndrome
- Patient admitted for 09.00h and 00.00h blood tests: no diurnal variation in cortisol and undetectable ACTH
- CT scan of abdomen revealed a mass in the left adrenal gland – a full recovery was made after removal

The initial investigations pointed to Cushing syndrome with lack of suppression of cortisol after an overnight dexamethasone test: 1 mg dexamethasone given at 22.00h and cortisol measured at 09.00h the following morning, with cortisol and ACTH having been previously measured at 09.00h pre-dexamethasone. The patient was admitted and blood samples taken at 09.00h and 00.00h for cortisol and ACTH. Cortisol levels were persistently high (in the range of 7–800 nmol/L) and showed no variation with time of day. ACTH levels remained undetectable. The low levels of ACTH suggested an ACTH-independent cause (primary adrenal adenoma) and the patient proceeded immediately to a CT scan of the abdomen which revealed a 3.2 cm mass in the left adrenal gland. Laparoscopic unilateral adrenalectomy was performed and histology revealed a benign functional lipid-rich adrenal adenoma. The patient made an uneventful recovery and was discharged on a low dose of hydrocortisone pending reassessment. Within a few weeks, adequate cortisol reserve in the remaining adrenal gland was confirmed and the patient is now free of medication.

It should be noted that many cases of Cushing syndrome are far more complex and challenging than Case 6.1.

CASE 6.2 284 293

- Man of 31 years with features highly suggestive of Cushing syndrome
- Tests showed no diurnal variation in cortisol, high ACTH, and no cortisol suppression on dexamethasone testing
- High dose dexamethasone testing showed a failure to suppress cortisol by >50%
- Diagnosis was either ectopic ACTH or pituitary Cushing syndrome, but no imaging could locate a tumor
- Patient started on adrenolytic chemotherapy and then treated with prednisolone replacement

Initial investigations demonstrated cortisol excess with failure to suppress cortisol after a low dose dexamethasone suppression test. Unlike Case 6.1, ACTH levels were consistently high, suggesting ACTH-dependent disease (pituitary Cushing's or ectopic ACTH). The patient was admitted for a high dose dexamethasone suppression test (2 mg of dexamethasone 6 hourly for 48 h) with basal and post-dose samples taken for cortisol and ACTH measurements. Again there was failure to suppress cortisol by more than 50% at 48 hours. A pituitary MRI was unhelpful and showed no obvious lesion. CT scanning of the adrenals showed bilateral adrenal hyperplasia. A peripheral CRH test (an intravenous bolus injection of 100 μg CRH) did not stimulate a rise in either cortisol or ACTH. CT scans of the chest were unremarkable.

The differential remained either ectopic ACTH or pituitary Cushing syndrome. The lack of a response to peripheral CRH and the failure to suppress cortisol after a high dose dexamethasone suppression test support a diagnosis of ectopic disease, although subsequent imaging (including octreotide scans and MRI of the thorax) failed to show a source. Pituitary disease could not be discounted and petrosal sinus sampling was planned but refused by the patient. A decision was made (in view of the absence of a clear ectopic source and the patient's age) to proceed to hypophysectomy where no tumor was seen and biopsy histology was negative. Post-operative cortisol levels remained impressively high necessitating the use of adrenolytic chemotherapy and the patient was started on both mitotane and metyrapone (*Box 6.10*) resulting in a rapid drop in cortisol levels. He was treated with prednisolone replacement. The disease remained active and the patient eventually underwent bilateral adrenalectomy followed by hormone replacement therapy with hydrocortisone and fludrocortisone. He remains well, and the search for his presumed ACTH-secreting tumor (probably neuroendocrine in origin) is ongoing.

6.4.3 Treatment of Cushing syndrome

The aim of treatment is to normalize levels of cortisol secretion. Ideally this should be achieved without resultant deficiency of other hormones (i.e. pituitary hormones) obviating the need for long-term hormone replacement. In practice this is often difficult to achieve. Tumors resulting in excess cortisol secretion (i.e. pituitary adenomas or ectopic sources of ACTH) need to be treated effectively. In addition, Cushing's causes a number of other co-morbidities (e.g. osteoporosis, diabetes, hypertension), all of which will need to be treated either in the short term (whilst awaiting a cure for the underlying problem) or in the long term.

Exogenous steroid excess

Unsurprisingly the answer here is to stop the offending steroid, but there are two problems with this approach. Occasionally patients cannot stop steroid treatment and the risks of continuing the treatment are outweighed by the risks of stopping it. Secondly, many patients will have been on steroids for a long time and the

Box 6.10 | Adrenolytic drug therapy in cortisol excess

The treatment of choice for an adrenal adenoma is laparoscopic or open adrenalectomy, and for pituitary Cushing disease it is transsphenoidal hypophysectomy (with or without adjunctive external radiotherapy). Hypercortisolism can be controlled either pre-operatively or (where a cure or remission has not been achieved) post-operatively with adrenal enzyme inhibitors. The final 'cure' for Cushing's is bilateral adrenalectomy which can be either surgical (bilateral adrenalectomy) or chemical (mitotane).

Mitotane

Mitotane (also known as *o,p'*-DDD) is a derivative of the insecticide DDT and inhibits 11β-hydroxylase and cholesterol side chain cleavage enzymes. It also causes necrosis and destruction of adrenocortical cells through binding of its metabolite (acyl chloride) to adrenocortical cell mitochondria. Exogenous glucocorticoid replacement (in the form of hydrocortisone or more commonly prednisolone or dexamethasone) is necessary during mitotane treatment and close monitoring with urinary or serum cortisol is essential. The cells of the zona glomerulosa (i.e. mineralocorticoid producing cells) are relatively spared, so fludrocortisone replacement is not always essential. Adverse effects of mitotane are shown in *Box 6.15*.

Adrenal enzyme inhibitors

A number of pharmacological agents can block steroid synthesis by inhibiting the actions of various enzymes along the steroid synthesis pathway *(Figure 6.3)*.

- Aminoglutethimide (an anticonvulsant) blocks the first step in the cholesterol side chain cleavage pathway (cholesterol to pregnenolone). It is less effective than many other inhibitors but is relatively cheap.
- Ketoconazole (better known as an antifungal) inhibits side chain cleavage and, to a lesser extent, conversion of 11-deoxycortisol to cortisol. It can also modify ACTH secretion by impairing adenylate cyclase activity in pituitary corticotrophs. It is sometimes hepatotoxic (liver function needs to be regularly assessed) and is contraindicated in pregnancy (teratogenicity).
- Metyrapone blocks the final step in cortisol synthesis (11-deoxycortisol to cortisol by 11β-hydroxylase). It can be associated with a concomitant rise in adrenal androgen production (unfortunate for women) and may provoke worsening of hypertension by increasing levels of deoxycorticosterone.

Other adrenolytic drugs have been used with varying efficacy. Mifepristone (better known for its role in chemical termination of pregnancy) is an 'anti-progestogen' which at high doses can compete for binding at the glucocorticoid receptor. Etomidate (an anesthetic which also blocks action of 11β-hydroxylase) is theoretically effective but less commonly used in practice. Various reports have suggested mixed results with bromocriptine (a dopamine agonist), fluconazole (another antifungal) and sodium valproate (an anti-epileptic). The mainstay of chemical adrenal enzyme inhibition, however, remains ketoconazole with or without the addition of metyrapone.

hypothalamic–pituitary access will be shut down; in this situation it is necessary to taper off the steroids slowly and review the situation regularly to assess restoration of adrenal reserve.

Cushing disease

Once cortisol excess secondary to an ACTH-producing pituitary adenoma has been confirmed, transsphenoidal surgery is the treatment of choice. Usually, after successful removal of an adenoma, the post-operative cortisol will be undetectable (the adrenal glands have been subjected to long-term ACTH drive and normal regulatory pathways have shut down – the adrenals have 'gone to sleep'). Restoration of normal adrenal function following hypophysectomy is variable and patients often require a period of medical support (with hydrocortisone). Surgery for Cushing disease is often followed by targeted radiotherapy. Cushing disease is difficult to cure following transsphenoidal surgery (*Figure 2.7*) and the recurrence rate is higher than that for most pituitary tumors (see *Chapter 2*).

Ectopic ACTH/CRH

Surgical removal of the source of ectopic ACTH is the aim of curative therapy in Cushing syndrome caused by unregulated excess ACTH. This is possible in localized neuro-endocrine tumors and pulmonary and other carcinoid tumors that produce ACTH. Some other tumors responsible for the syndrome (e.g. small cell cancers of the lung) will often have metastasized at diagnosis. In these cases, chemotherapy and radiotherapy may occasionally be helpful, and cortisol excess can be controlled with 'chemical adrenalectomy' using drugs designed to inhibit cortisol production (*Box 6.10*).

In ACTH-dependent Cushing syndrome (both ectopic ACTH and pituitary disease) bilateral adrenalectomy may be considered to control cortisol excess when other approaches have failed. In the presence of a pituitary ACTH-secreting adenoma, adrenalectomy may result in the development of Nelson syndrome – the progression of the corticotroph adenoma (*Box 6.11*). This is much rarer with the use of prophylactic pituitary irradiation.

Box 6.11 | Nelson syndrome

In patients with pituitary Cushing disease who are treated by bilateral adrenalectomy, progression of the causative corticotroph adenoma can occur. This results in an enlarging pituitary tumor (with the possibility of developing local effects due to tumor size (see *Chapter 2*). Additionally, the inexorably increasing ACTH levels can cause hyperpigmentation. Nelson syndrome occurs more commonly in the younger patient, and can be ameliorated (although not always completely prevented) by prior irradiation of the pituitary.

ACTH levels may be impressive in Nelson syndrome, ranging from 90 pmol/L to >4500 pmol/L (NR 4.4–18). Expansion of the pituitary adenoma can prove difficult to treat and there is a risk of transformation to pituitary cancer. Surgical hypophysectomy is the treatment of choice; proton beam irradiation, stereotactic [^{60}Co]-gamma knife, or linear accelerator photon knife radiosurgery may be effective (see *Chapter 2*). Medical therapy is relatively ineffective, although isolated case reports have claimed some success with dopamine agonist therapy (bromocriptine or cabergoline) or somatostatin analogs.

Adrenal Cushing syndrome

Unilateral adrenal adenomas causing Cushing syndrome are cured by unilateral adrenalectomy – usually laparoscopically, but occasionally requiring open surgery.

Bilateral adrenal adenomas have two forms:

- micronodular adrenal hyperplasia (also called primary pigmented nodular adrenocortical disease, PPNAD)
- macronodular adrenal hyperplasia.

In these conditions bilateral adrenalectomy is the treatment of choice (although some reports suggest unilateral surgery may be effective in low grade forms of macronodular hyperplasia). Obviously bilateral adrenalectomy will cause lifelong loss of adrenal hormones and thus replacement with glucocorticoid (hydrocortisone) and mineralocorticoid (fludrocortisone) is essential.

When surgical/radiotherapeutic procedures have failed to cure Cushing syndrome, or where the patient is too infirm or simply refuses surgery, adrenolytic drugs can be used. These are either adrenal cytotoxic drugs (mitotane) or inhibitors of key enzymes in the cortisol synthetic pathway (e.g. ketoconazole, metyrapone, mifepristone, and etomidate) (*Box 6.10*).

6.5 Adrenocortical cancer

6.5.1 Epidemiology

Adrenocortical tumors are present in at least 3% of the population over the age of 50, but adrenocortical cancers (ACCs) are rare tumors causing less than 0.2% of all cancer deaths in the USA (incidence 1–2 per 1 million population). Women are affected more than men (ratio about 1:5) and there are two peaks of age distribution, one in childhood and a higher second peak in adulthood (fourth and fifth decades).

6.5.2 Clinical presentation

ACC can present in two ways:

- a result of mass effect
- symptoms and signs of hormone excess produced by the tumor cells.

The majority of functioning tumors (85%) secrete cortisol, although co-secretion of cortisol and androgens is the most frequent manifestation of ACC and this results in rapidly progressing Cushing syndrome with or without virilization.

- Androgen-secreting ACCs in women present with male-pattern hair loss, hirsutism, and oligomenorrhea.
- Estrogen-secreting tumors (5–10% of male patients) present with gynecomastia and testicular atrophy. They are almost always pathognomonic of ACC.
- Aldosterone-producing tumors (rare) present with severe hypertension and hypokalemia. Hypokalemia can also be a feature of cortisol excess because incomplete renal inactivation of cortisol by 11β-HSD2 (*Figure 6.9*) results in cortisol interacting with mineralocorticoid receptors (*Figure 6.14*).

Tumors secreting multiple hormones are almost always malignant.

On occasion, tumors may secrete steroid precursors and have ineffective steroidogenesis, making them appear clinically hormonally inactive. Urinary steroid analysis (by gas chromatography/mass spectroscopy, GC/MS) to identify the types of hormonal excess can be used later as a tumor marker. As many as 75% of ACCs are associated with subclinical hypercortisolism, and this can only be detected by hormone assays.

Clinical features, presenting because of symptoms related to distant metastases (liver, bones, lung, lymph nodes), of a non-functioning ACC include:

- nausea
- vomiting
- back pain caused by the tumor mass
- abdominal fullness
- occasionally, fever, anorexia, and weight loss may be present.

Other features may indicate hereditary forms of ACC. They include: hyperparathyroidism, pancreatic and pituitary tumors (MEN-1); familial susceptibility to breast carcinoma, soft tissue sarcomas, brain tumors, osteosarcomas, leukemia (Li–Fraumeni syndrome); macroglossia, neonatal macrosomia, and omphalocele (Beckwith–Wiedemann syndrome).

6.5.3 Histopathology and staging of adrenocortical tumors

The pathological diagnosis of ACC can be difficult due to lack of a consensus on morphological criteria. Generally, they have a heterogeneous texture with an average size of 10 cm and weighing more than 100 g. They may exhibit vascular, local, or capsular invasion. The Weiss criteria are widely used to diagnose ACC and these identify nine morphological criteria related to tumor structure, tumor cytology, and invasion (*Box 6.12*).

Box 6.12 | Histopathology and staging of adrenocortical tumors

The pathological diagnosis of ACC can be difficult due to lack of a consensus on morphological criteria. Generally, they have a heterogeneous texture with an average size of 10 cm. They may exhibit vascular, local, or capsular invasion. Malignant tumors weigh more than 100 g.

Weiss criteria are widely used to diagnose ACC. These combine nine morphological criteria: three are related to tumor structure (cytoplasm, architecture, necrosis), three are related to cytology (atypia, atypical mitotic figures, mitotic figures count), and three are related to invasion (tumor capsule, sinusoids, veins). Each features scores 0 (absent) or 1 (present). A score of less than or equal to 2 is likely to be an adenoma and a score of 3 or more is more suggestive of ACC. However, a score of 2 or 3 is ambiguous and requires other criteria to define the histopathologic features. Some investigators advocate the use of adjunct pathologic tools to reach accurate diagnosis, including: insulin-like growth factor 2 (IGF-2) over-expression, allelic loss at 17p13, Ki-67, cyclin E expression, telomerase activity, topoisomerase I, and N-cadherin.

Tumor staging has been shown to be one of the most important predictors of disease-free survival and the TNM classification is widely used (*Box table 6.2*).

Box table 6.2. **Staging classification for ACC**

Stage	UICC/WHO 2004	ENSAT 2008
I	T1, N0, M0	T1, N0, M0
II	T2, N0, M0	T2, N0, M0
III	T1–2, N1, M0 T3, N0, M0	T1–2, N1, M0 T3–4, N0–1, M0
IV	T1–4, N0–1, M1 T3, N1, M0 T4, N0–1, M0	T1–4, N0–1, M1

T1, tumor ≤5 cm; T2, tumor >5 cm; T3, tumor infiltration in surrounding tissue; T4, tumor invasion in adjacent organs (ENSAT: also venous tumor thrombus in vena cava / renal vein. N0, no positive lymph nodes; N1, positive lymph node(s). M0, no distant metastases; M1, presence of distant metastases.

6.5.4 Diagnosis of adrenocortical tumors

Hormonal work-up

A thorough hormonal work up for adrenal tumors is essential prior to surgery. Hormonal secretory pattern may point to the malignant potential of the tumors (e.g. estradiol in males, DHEA-S and steroid precursors). It is important to identify autonomous cortisol production (risk of post-operative adrenal crisis) and catecholamine excess (intra-operative hypertensive crisis) prior to surgery, to prevent unnecessary complications. Furthermore, the hormonal work-up will identify tumor markers to use for monitoring after surgery.

Box 6.13 | Hormonal work-up for the diagnosis of adrenocortical cancer

Box table 6.3. **Recommended diagnostic work-up in patients with suspected or proven ACC**

Hormonal work-up	
Glucocorticoid excess (minimum 3 out of 4 tests)	• dexamethasone suppression test (1 mg, 23.00h) • excretion of free urinary cortisol (24 h urine) • basal cortisol (serum) • basal ACTH (plasma)
Sexual steroids and steroid precursors	• DHEA-S (serum) • 17-OH-progesterone (serum) • androstenedione (serum) • testosterone (serum) • 17β-estradiol (serum, only in men and post-menopausal women)
Mineralocorticoid excess	• potassium (serum) • aldosterone:renin ratio (only in patients with arterial hypertension and/or hypokalemia)
Exclusion of a pheochromocytoma	• Catecholamine or metanephrine excretion (24 h urine) • metanephrine and nor-metanephrine (plasma)
Imaging	
	• CT or MRI of abdomen and CT thorax • Bone scintigraphy (when suspecting skeletal metastases) • FDG-PET (optional)
Staging during follow-up	
	• CT or MRI of abdomen and CT thorax every 2–3 months (depending on treatment)

Recommendations of the ACC working group of the European Network for the Study of Adrenal Tumours (ENSAT), May 2005; adapted from www.ensat.org.
FDG-PET, [18F]-2-fluoro-2-deoxy-D-glucose positron electron tomography (see *Box 6.14*).

Many steroid-synthesizing enzymes in ACC lead to the production of steroid precursors found in adrenal enzymatic blocks. Urinary steroid profile analysis (over 24 h) using GC/MS can identify the secretion of steroid precursors by the tumor in almost all the patients with ACC. A suggested scheme for hormonal diagnostic work-up in ACC is shown in *Box 6.13*.

Fine-needle biopsy

This is not used as part of the work-up of diagnosis of adrenal tumors because of the possibility of breaching the tumor capsule which can result in tumor spillage and seeding along the track of the biopsy needle. It may be indicated in cases of heterogeneous masses (>20 Hounsfield Units) with a history of other cancers (lung, breast, kidney), no distant metastases, and after the exclusion of a pheochromocytoma.

Imaging

Diagnostic imaging is an essential step in the diagnostic work-up for adrenal tumors. CT/MRI may help identify size, texture, extent, and the presence of local and distant metastases. Functional imaging also has an important place in the diagnosis of ACC (*Box 6.14*).

Box 6.14 | Imaging in the diagnosis of adrenocortical cancer

Adrenal protocol CT scan is the method of choice especially when investigating an incidentaloma (see *Section 6.5.7*). ACCs tend to have irregular margins; a non-homogeneous texture and calcifications may sometimes be seen. CT scans can also be used to evaluate local invasion or extension and distant metastatic spread of ACC (see *Box figures 6.8* and *6.9*). By measuring the X-ray attenuation in Hounsfield Units (HU) it is possible to distinguish benign from malignant adenomas. Fat-containing tissues tend to have lower HU values. Ten HU (sensitivity 71% and specificity 98%) is accepted as a cut-off to distinguish an adenoma from a potentially malignant lesion. Adrenal lesions of >10 HU or an enhancement washout of <50% and delayed attenuation of >35 HU (on 10–15 min delayed enhanced CT) are suspicious of malignancy.

Box figure 6.8. Right adrenal carcinoma.
(a) Axial CT image shows a large non-homogeneous right adrenal mass (thin arrow), and an enlarged retroperitoneal lymph node (thick arrow).
(b) Enhanced axial CT image obtained more distally shows a minimal non-homogeneously enhancing liver nodule (arrow), and multiple enlarged retroperitoneal lymph nodes (thick arrow)
(c) Enhanced axial CT image obtained at the dome of the liver shows an enhancing liver nodule.
(d) Enhanced coronal reconstructed CT image shows a large non-homogeneous right adrenal mass (white arrows) with displacement of the right kidney downward.

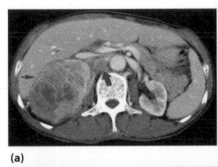

(a)

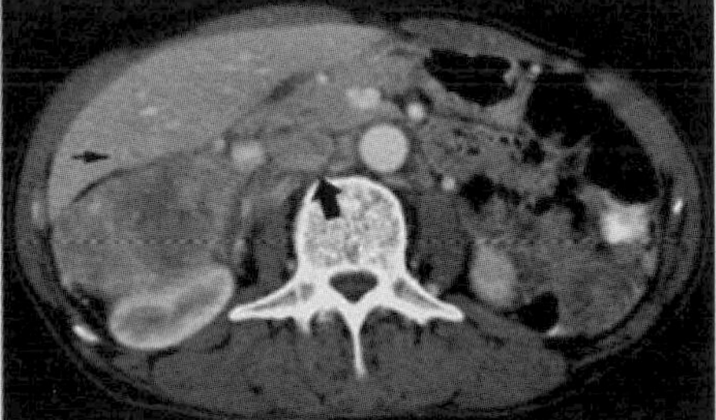

(b)

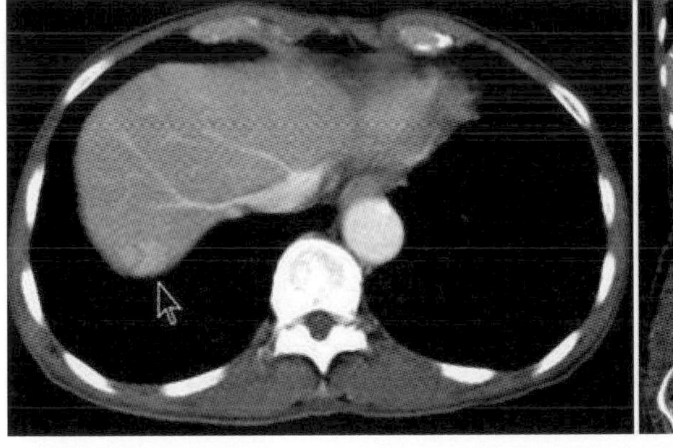

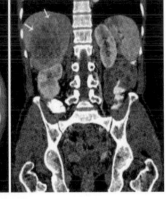

(c)

(d)

Box figure 6.9. Left adrenal carcinoma.
(a) Precontrast CT showing a heterogeneous 8 cm left adrenal mass (★) containing a small amount of calcification (arrow).
(b) The mass shows moderate heterogeneous enhancement after contrast.

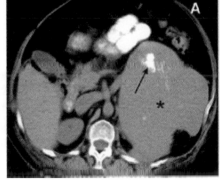

(a)

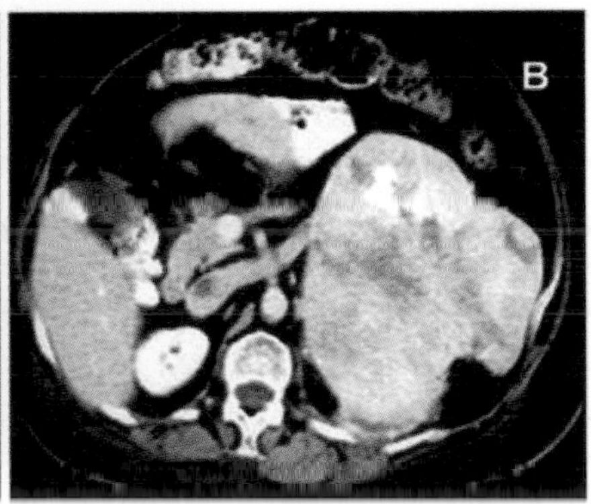

(b)

MRI using the gadolinium enhancement and chemical shift technique is as effective as CT in determining the nature of adrenal lesions. Fat content is used to differentiate a benign from a malignant lesion. MRI can be used if CT is equivocal or contrast administration is contraindicated.

Box 6.14 | continued

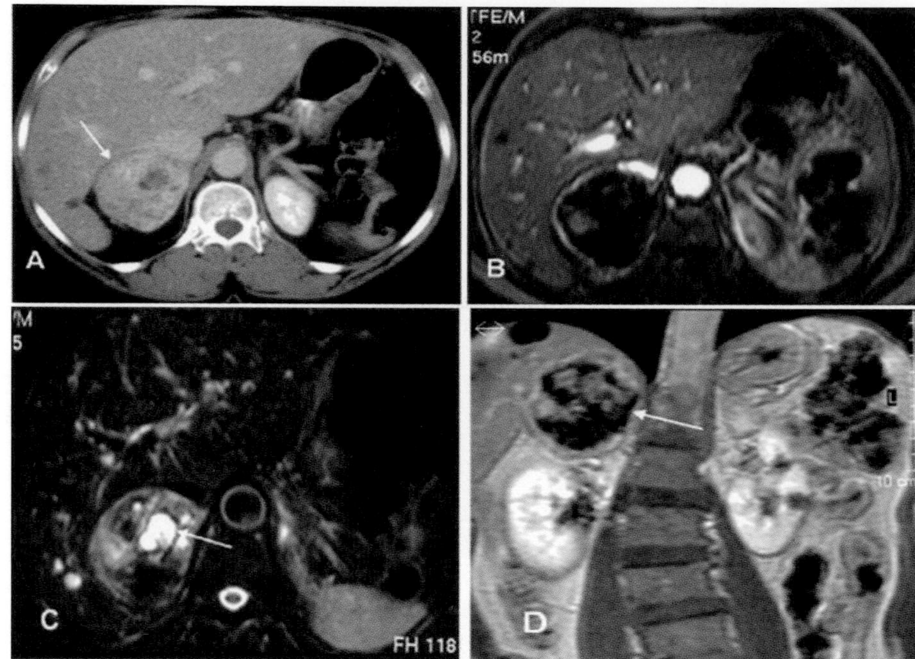

Box figure 6.10. Cushing syndrome due to adrenal carcinoma.
(a) Post-contrast CT shows a heterogeneous right adrenal mass (arrow) with a non-enhancing area.
(b) T1-weighted GRE sequence.
(c) The T2-weighted sequence (with fat suppression) shows that most of the mass is moderately hyperintense, with a very hyperintense area (arrow) corresponding to the non-enhancing area on CT – this represents an area of necrosis.
(d) Coronal image following intravenous administration of Gd-DTPA which shows heterogeneous enhancement (arrow).

Functional imaging (18-fluorodesoxyglucose (18-FDG)) appears to distinguish benign from malignant tumors because malignant cells almost invariably have high uptake of 18-FDG. Another imaging modality that targets the adrenal cortex is [^{11}C]-metomidate (MTO)–PET which binds to 11β-HSD2. Thus it has high sensitivity and specificity in differentiating adrenocortical from non-adrenocortical tissues.

6.5.5 Treatment of ACC and prognosis

Treatment modalities for ACC include surgery, medical therapy, radiotherapy, and radiofrequency ablation, or chemoembolization. Both the choice of treatment and prognosis of the disease are dependent on the staging of ACC and further details of treatment and prognosis are given in *Box 6.15.*

6.5.6 Adrenal incidentalomas

An adrenal incidentaloma is defined as a >1 cm lesion in the adrenal gland found by accident when undertaking another investigation (e.g. abdominal CT scan) for an apparently unrelated reason, e.g. investigation of non-specific abdominal pain. Initial prevalence figures for adrenal incidentalomas were based on autopsy studies and were quoted as being between 9 and 12% (higher in patients with pre-existing hypertension). A review of a major series of CT scans from the Mayo clinic suggested a prevalence rate of 0.4%, but other series have suggested rates of up to 4.4%.

Clearly, before the discovery of an incidentaloma patients should have no suggestive symptoms prior to imaging; however, retrospectively several patients may have rather subtle signs of hormonal excess (e.g. weight gain, bruising, etc.). Pre-existent hypertension, obesity, and type 2 diabetes increase the likelihood of finding an adrenal incidentaloma.

Box 6.15 | Treatment, prognosis, and follow-up of adrenocortical cancer (ACC)

Treatment modalities available to treat ACC include:

- surgery
- medical therapy (mainly mitotane)
- radiotherapy
- tumor-directed radiofrequency ablation or chemoembolization.

Choice of the treatment modality depends on the stage of the disease. A multidisciplinary team approach to the management of ACC is essential. An algorithm for the treatment of ACC is shown (*Box figure 6.11*).

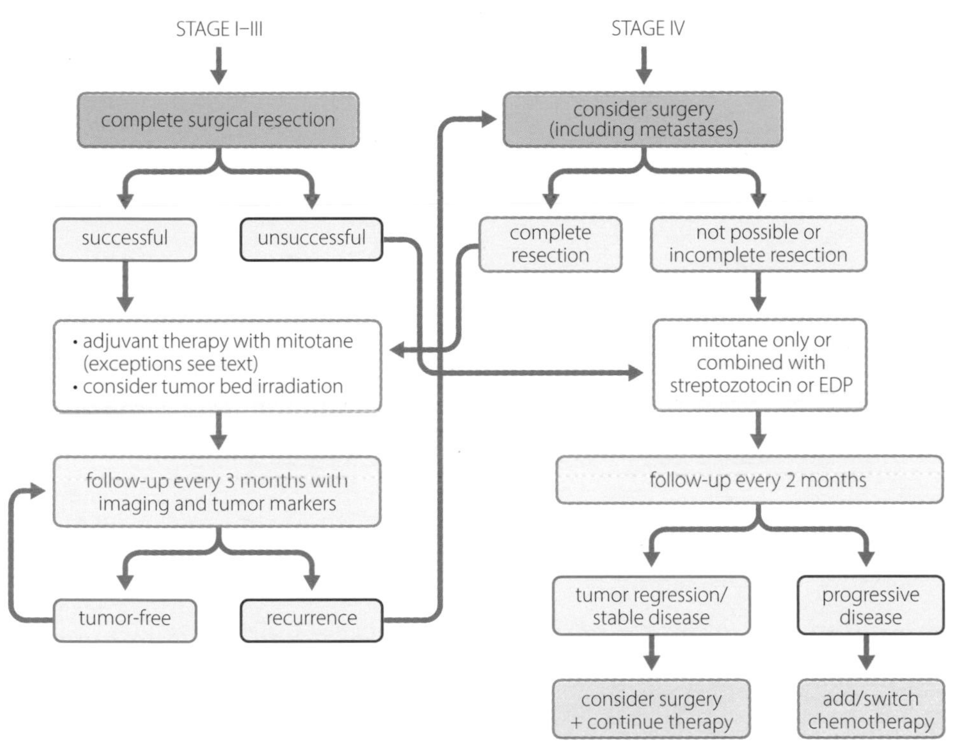

Box figure 6.11. Treatment algorithm for patients with ACC. Reproduced from Fassnacht M and Allolio B (2009) *Best Pract. Clin. Endocrinol. Metab.* **23**: 273–89, with permission.

Surgery

The aim of the surgery is to achieve complete tumor resection to prevent recurrence. It is the major treatment for patients with stage I–III. Only complete tumor removal can lead to long-term remission. Open adrenalectomy is recommended, because laparoscopic removal of the tumor can be associated with a high risk of tumor spillage. Starting glucocorticoid replacement for autonomous cortisol producing tumors will prevent adrenal insufficiency post-operatively. In stage IV patients, tumor debulking can be discussed to improve prognosis and reduce steroid excess. Surgery for metastases can be considered to prevent complications such as fractures (bone metastases) and neurological symptoms (spinal metastases).

Medical therapy – mitotane and emerging therapies

As discussed in *Box 6.10*, mitotane (*o,p'*-DDD) is an adrenolytic compound with specific adrenocortical activity. It has anticortisol effects and inhibits steroid synthesis by acting on enzymes such as 11β-hydroxylase and cholesterol side chain cleavage. It has a major role in the medical therapy for ACC as an adjuvant treatment and in advanced disease.

Mitotane is given orally according to tolerability and blood levels (levels of 14 mg/L have been established as an antitumor threshold). Levels exceeding 20 mg/L have been associated with increased risk of significant toxicity. A detailed adverse effects profile is shown in *Box table 6.4* below.

Box 6.15 | continued

Box table 6.4. **Adverse effects of mitotane**

Adverse effect	Frequency
Gastrointestinal – nausea and vomiting	
Diarrhea	Common
Anorexia	Common
Mucositis	Common
Hepatobiliary	
Increase in hepatic enzymes (especially GGT)	Common
Hepatic microsomal enzyme induction leading to increased glucocorticoids and drug metabolism (barbiturates, phenytoin, warfarin)	Common
Autoimmune hepatitis	Rare
Liver failure	Rare
CNS	
Lethargy and somnolence	Common
Vertigo and ataxia	Common
Confusion	Common
Dizziness	Common
Decreased memory	Common
Psychiatric	
Depression	Common
Endocrine	
Adrenal insufficiency	Common
Primary hypogonadism in males	Common
Gynecomastia	Common
Increase in hormone binding globulins (CBG, SHBG, TBG, vitamin D binding protein)	Common
Abnormal thyroid function test	Common
Skin	
Rash	Common
Hematological	
Prolonged bleeding time	Common
Leukopenia	Common
Thrombocytopenia	Rare
Anemia	Rare
Hematuria and albuminuria	Rare
Cardiovascular	
Hyperlipidemia	Common
Hypertension	Rare
Ophthalmological	
Blurred vision	Rare
Double vision	Rare
Toxic retinopathy	Rare
Cataract	Rare
Macular edema	Rare
Urinary tract	
Hemorrhagic cystitis	Rare

Box 6.15 | continued

Mitotane induces adrenal insufficiency, and the glucocorticoid doses required for replacement need to be twice or three times the doses used to treat adrenal insufficiency due to other causes (such as Addison disease). This is because mitotane induces hepatic microsomal enzymes and increases the levels of cortisol binding globulin, resulting in reduced availability of cortisol. Insufficient glucocorticoid replacement results in the enhancement of the gastrointestinal side-effects of mitotane.

Cortisol excess caused by the tumor cells can increase the disease burden and interferes with the quality of life of patients with ACC. Mitotane treatment alone is not sufficient sometimes to control the cortisol excess, in which case other inhibitors of cortisol synthesis can be used (see *Box 6.10*).

Several newer and somewhat experimental therapies are undergoing active investigation with varying degrees of success. These include:

- blockade of IGF-1 receptor
- figitumumab (anti-IGF-1R monoclonal antibody)
- therapies targeting growth factors and cytokines (TGF-α, FGF-2, TGF-β1, VGEF) involved in regulating the growth and function of the adrenal gland
- anti-angiogenesis such as thalidomide
- tyrosine kinase inhibitors such as sunitinib
- adrenocortical cell proliferation inhibitors (*in vitro*) such as the transcription factor steroidogenic factor-1 (SF-1) inhibitors (alkyloxyphenol class) and inverse agonists (isoquinolinone class).

Chemotherapy and radiotherapy

Several chemotherapy regimes have been used to treat ACC. They are considered in cases of disease progression or failure of mitotane to control the disease (because of drug toxicity or side-effects). Experience is still limited. There are two currently accepted regimes. The first (EDP regime) is the combined use of mitotane, cisplatin, etoposide, and doxorubicin. The second regime is the combined use of streptozotocin and mitotane. Trials are currently underway to assess the best regime in cases of locally advanced and metastatic ACC.

The evidence for use of radiotherapy to treat ACC is limited. Anecdotal reports suggest it is as effective in ACC as in other solid tumors. However, radiotherapy is recommended in the treatment of metastases (brain, bone, etc.). It is recommended in treatment of local recurrence. It can also be administered to patients with incomplete local resection in whom total resection was not possible.

Chemoembolization and radiofrequency ablation

These forms of therapy are used in lesions <5 cm in diameter. They show impressive results in limited disease and in functional tumors. However, the tumor recurs without systemic treatment. Radiofreqeuncy ablation has been used in liver and lung metastases (4–5 cm) as an alternative to surgery. Chemoembolization has been used to treat liver metastases. There are no current guidelines to introduce such therapies or information on whether they exert any survival benefit.

Prognosis

Prognosis is closely related to the staging of ACC (see *Box figure 6.12*). When applying the new ENSAT staging system (see *Box table 6.2*), the 5 year survival rates were 84% for stage I, 63% for stage II, 51% for stage III, and 15% for stage IV.

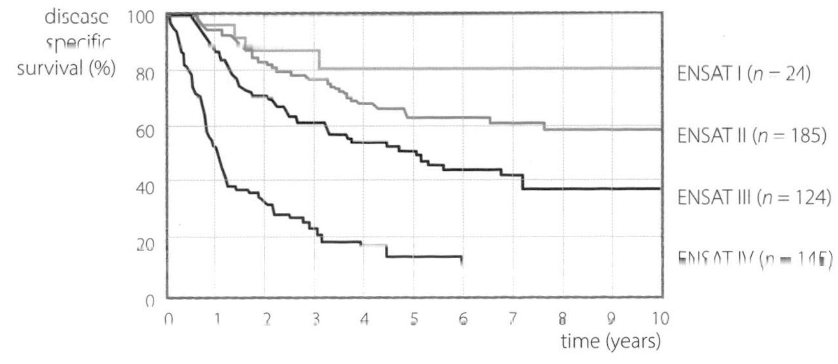

Box figure 6.12 ACC survival rates according to ENSAT (2008) staging criteria.

Box 6.15 | continued

There is limited evidence to support prognostic markers other than staging. Functionality, age, and gender have no major role. Large tumor size (>12 cm) has been associated with worse prognosis after surgical resection. Ki-67 is a promising immunohistochemical proliferation marker to predict prognosis.

Follow-up

Patients who have undergone complete tumor resection should be followed-up every 3 months with endocrine tests (depending on the hormone excess identified in the pre-operative investigations) as well as radiological surveillance. CT scanning is a convenient and sensitive investigation to use for follow-up. MRI and FDG–PET can be useful in patients with equivocal findings or occult recurrence detected on endocrine investigations.

Patients with metastatic disease undergoing medical therapy should be followed-up every 3 months (or less) to assess efficacy and treat complications.

The majority of lesions will turn out to be benign and require no treatment at all (or at most surveillance). It is sometimes difficult to know how aggressively to investigate an incidental finding, but the discovery of a mass lesion in the adrenal gland(s) leads to two immediate questions: is the lesion functional (i.e. hormone producing) and is there a suggestion of malignancy (primary adrenocortical cancer or metastatic lesion)? Clinical evaluation, biochemical screening, and appropriate imaging are usually necessary in the work-up of an incidentaloma. These would include:

- history and examination
- 24 h urinary catecholamine check if there is a suggestion of a pheochromocytoma (see *Section 6.9*)
- overnight or formal dexamethasone suppression testing to exclude cortisol overproduction (see *Section 6.4*)
- aldosterone and renin estimations if there is a suggestion of primary aldosteronism (hypertension/hypokalemia – see *Section 6.7*)
- a lesion of <4 cm diameter with no suspicious features and rapid contrast washout suggests a benign lesion
- a lesion of >4 cm of irregular shape, calcification, high CT attenuation values with delayed contrast washout suggests a malignant lesion.

The risk of any hormonal activity (resulting in subclinical Cushing syndrome, pheochromocytoma, or aldosterone excess) increases with increasing size and any tumor of 3 cm or more should be thoroughly evaluated. It is important to remember, however, that aldosterone-secreting tumors tend to be small (see *Section 6.7*) and if there are suspicious features (hypokalemia, hypertension, metabolic alkalosis) then even smaller lesions should be fully evaluated.

Active adenomas producing catecholamines (pheochromocytoma) or aldosterone (Conn syndrome) should be surgically removed. The management of those patients with subclinical Cushing's is slightly more controversial because it is not completely clear how many will progress to overt Cushing syndrome and what the time frame is. Nevertheless, evidence increasingly suggests that patients undergoing unilateral adrenalectomy in this situation have more easily controlled hypertension, improved glycemic control, a reduction in obesity and more favorable bone mineral density.

Any tumor greater than 6 cm in diameter should be removed (after full endocrinological work-up), and those between 4 and 6 cm removed if there is a suggestion of malignancy on imaging. Thus any hormonally active incidentaloma and any tumor greater than 6 cm (or 4–6 cm if suspicious) should be treated surgically. Follow-up scans beyond 12–24 months are unlikely to be helpful if the incidentaloma remains unchanged. FNA is not indicated unless (in cancer patients) the incidentaloma is the only evidence of a possible metastasis. An investigation algorithm helpful for the evaluation of adrenal incidentalomas is shown in *Figure 6.13.*

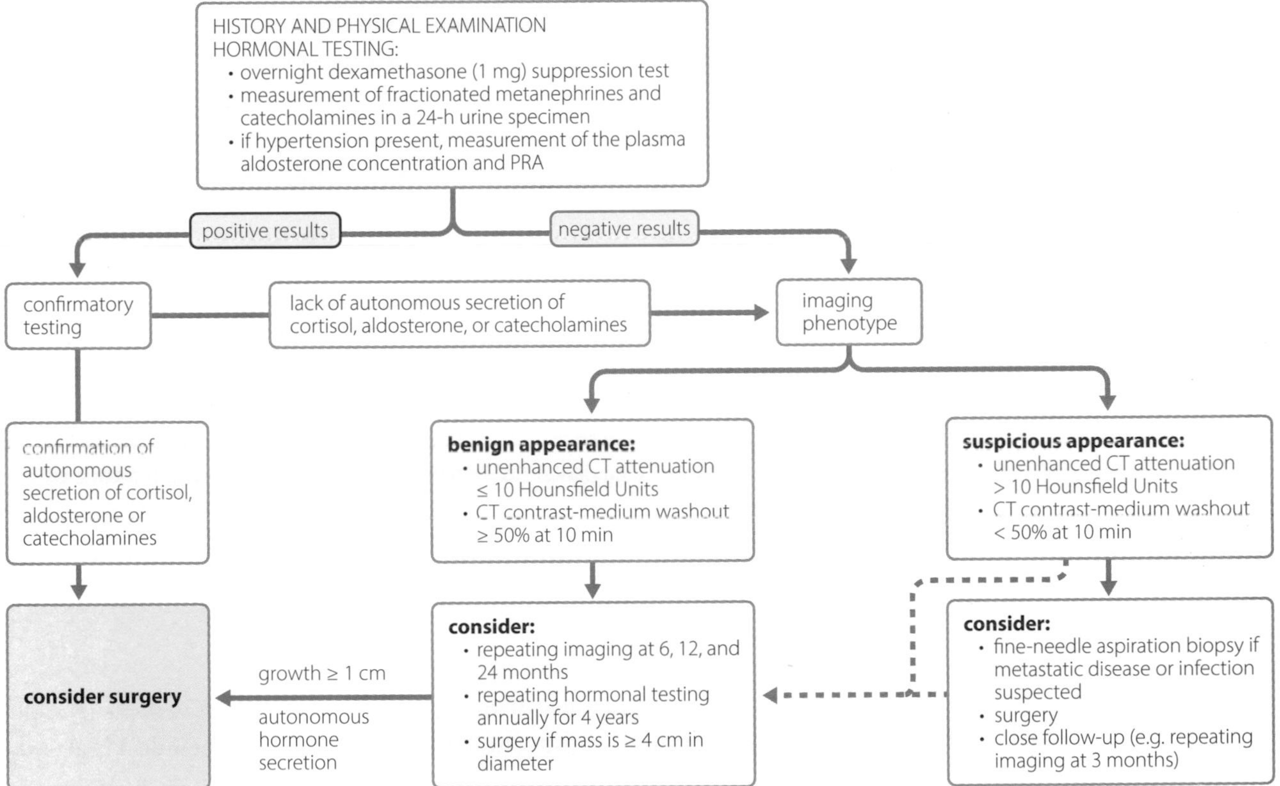

Figure 6.13. Evaluation of adrenal incidentalomas.

The algorithm must be personalized to the clinical situation, including consideration of imaging results, age of the patient, etc. Initial investigations are designed to assess functionality of the lesion which would sway opinion toward a surgical cure. For non-functional lesions intervention is based on imaging findings, including size of the lesion. In some situations, where a lesion is slightly suspicious the dashed line can be followed if the physician considers that serial imaging and hormonal testing are more appropriate than FNA or surgery for certain patients.

6.6 Adrenal insufficiency – Addison disease and other causes

6.6.1 Causes of adrenal insufficiency

Overall, the most common cause of adrenal insufficiency or hypoadrenalism (in approximately 99% of cases) is the result of sudden withdrawal of exogenous glucocorticoids. This occurs because exogenous glucocorticoids suppress CRH and ACTH secretion and the ability of the adrenal cortex to produce glucocorticoids (sometimes referred to as tertiary hypoadrenalism). It takes time for the adrenal glands to 'wake up' and to start producing normally regulated glucocorticoid in

CASE 6.3 306 311

- Female student of 22 years with D&V of 24 h duration; significant fatigue, with weight loss and anorexia (BMI 17) in last few months
- Examination showed hypotension, pigmentation of buccal mucosa, high urea, hyperkalemia, hyponatremia, and low blood sugar – likely cortisol deficiency

A 22 year old medical student was admitted to the medical assessment unit after presenting to the emergency department with diarrhea and vomiting of 24 hours duration. She had recently attended a rock festival. None of her friends had become unwell, she had no history of recent foreign travel and was not feverish. On questioning she gave a history of significant fatigue over the last few months, with weight loss and anorexia. She often felt faint on standing after lectures. Her periods were erratic. Her mother had hypothyroidism and a maternal aunt was on vitamin B_{12} injections.

On examination she was hypotensive at 90/55 mmHg with a postural drop of 20 mmHg. Her buccal mucosa was significantly pigmented, as were her palmar creases, and she had an old appendectomy scar. She was underweight (BMI of 17 kg/m^2). Initial investigations revealed:

- urea of 12 mmol/L (NR 3–7)
- potassium of 5.8 mmol/L (NR 3.5–5.1)
- sodium of 130 mmol/L (NR 135–146)
- glucose of 3.6 mmol/L (NR 3.5–6.1)

It was clear from the baseline investigations that the patient had mild hyperkalemia, hyponatremia, a low blood sugar, and moderately increased urea. This pattern of electrolytes is compatible with cortisol deficiency. As the patient was unwell it was essential to undertake further investigations to confirm cortisol deficiency, but also to initiate treatment on the balance of clinical probability prior to the results coming back.

response to need. Phased withdrawal of the prescribed steroids over variable periods may be required to re-establish normal ACTH secretion and adrenocortical function. In some clinical situations it may even be necessary to continue lifelong steroid support for patients who have been on extremely long-term immunosuppressive doses of steroid.

Other causes of adrenal insufficiency may be primary, secondary, or tertiary (*Box 6.16*). In primary adrenal insufficiency (Addison disease) the adrenal gland has impaired secretory function with intact hypothalamic and pituitary reserve. Thus there is a loss of both cortisol (*Figure 6.12d*) and aldosterone secretion. Secondary adrenal insufficiency results from disruption of ACTH secretion (hypopituitarism) and tertiary from loss of CRH caused by hypothalamic damage or long-term glucocorticoid treatment. Secondary and tertiary causes do not result in loss of aldosterone secretion because aldosterone is not controlled by ACTH. Finally, there are some very rare resistance syndromes of the hypothalamic–pituitary axis which either manifest as resistance to ACTH or to glucocorticoids (*Box 6.17*).

Addison disease is the most common form of spontaneous primary adrenal insufficiency and, whilst tuberculosis may remain the most common cause worldwide (often in combination with HIV infection), in Western populations autoimmune adrenal destruction accounts for 80–90% of all cases, the majority of whom have autoantibodies against 21-hydroxylase. The reported prevalence of

Box 6.16 | Causes of hypoadrenalism

Primary adrenal insufficiency (Addison disease)

- Autoimmune adrenalitis
  - Isolated adrenal failure
  - Autoimmune polyglandular syndrome types I and II
- Infectious causes
  - HIV/AIDS
  - Tuberculosis
  - Fungal infections (e.g. histoplasmosis)
  - Syphilis
- Metastatic disease
  - Usually breast, lung, prostate, or colon cancer
- Adrenal hemorrhage or infarction
- Drugs
  - Adrenolytic drugs (mitotane, metyrapone, ketoconazole, etomidate) (see *Box 6.10*)
  - Rifampicin
  - Phenytoin
  - Barbiturates
- Rare causes
  - Congenital adrenal hypoplasia
  - Adrenoleukodystrophy
  - Familial glucocorticoid resistance or deficiency
  - Defective metabolism of cholesterol

Secondary adrenal insufficiency

- Panhypopituitarism
- Isolated ACTH deficiency
- Chronic opiate usage
- Traumatic brain injury

Tertiary adrenal insufficiency

- Long-term glucocorticoid treatment (approximately 99% of cases of adrenal insufficiency)
- Directly following cure of Cushing syndrome
- Processes leading to hypothalamic impairment
  - Infiltrative diseases (e.g. sarcoidosis)
  - Tumors
  - Irradiation

Box 6.17 | Resistance syndromes in the hypothalamic–pituitary–adrenal axis

Inherited ACTH and glucocorticoid resistance syndromes are rare and they show genetic heterogeneity so that the same clinical phenotypes may result from defects in different genes or more than one gene. The ACTH/melanocortin-2 receptor (MC2R) resistance syndromes include familial glucocorticoid deficiency (FGD) and triple A syndrome (also known as Allgrove syndrome). Patients with FGD usually present in early childhood with symptoms related to cortisol deficiency and high levels of ACTH due to loss of negative feedback. Their renin–angiotensin–aldosterone axis is normal. Clinical features include hypoglycemia, frequent infections, and ACTH-induced hyperpigmentation as in Addison disease. Mutations in both the MC2R and the melanocortin-2 receptor accessory protein (MRAP) have been identified, both of which are necessary to provide a functional MC2R at the cell surface. FGD arising from mutations in the genes coding for MC2R and MRAP has been termed Type 1 and Type 2 FGD, respectively, although these mutations only account for about 50% of all cases of FGD. Triple A syndrome is characterized by adrenal failure, alacrima (absence of tears), achalasia (loss of relaxation in smooth muscle fibers in the GI tract) and progressive neurological symptoms; 90% of such cases will have isolated glucocorticoid deficiency, although about 10% will also develop mineralocorticoid deficiency due to destruction of the adrenal cortex. The syndrome has been linked to defects in the *AAAS* gene and although the function of this gene is not fully understood, it is highly expressed in the adrenal cortex and neural tissue and encodes a protein, ALADIN, which localizes to the nuclear pore.

Whilst resistance to ACTH produces hypocortisolism and raised levels of ACTH, generalized resistance to glucocorticoids increases the activity of the hypothalamic–pitutary axis (due to the loss of negative feedback effects of glucocorticoids) and increases steroid production of the adrenal cortex. As a consequence, patients present with signs of overproduction of mineralocorticoids (hypertension and hypokalemic alkalosis) due to excess cortisol interacting with aldosterone receptors and, in women, hirsutism due to the excess androgens. Although hypercortisolism exists, patients will not present with features of Cushing syndrome because of resistance to this hormone. Several mutations in the gene that codes for the glucocorticoid receptor have been identified, most of which lie in the ligand binding domain. There are, however, a substantial number of patients with unexplained glucocorticoid resistance showing no mutations in the glucocorticoid receptor gene.

autoimmune and idiopathic Addison disease is 100–140 per million in Caucasians, so it is a rare disorder. Other rare causes of this disease are given in *Box 6.16.*

6.6.2 Symptoms and signs of adrenal insufficiency – chronic and acute

Chronic primary adrenal insufficiency may be due to deficiency of glucocorticoid, mineralocorticoid and (in women) androgen action. It frequently manifests as an insidious process with gradual, rather non-specific symptoms along with common signs and laboratory abnormalities (*Box 6.18*).

A number of these symptoms and signs appear non-specific. The most characteristic clinical sign, however, is hyperpigmentation of the skin due to excess ACTH secretion (loss of negative feedback by cortisol). ACTH stimulates melanocytes in the skin by acting on melanocortin-1 receptors (*Box 6.5*) and is, in fact, an equipotent or more potent stimulator of melanogenesis than α-melanocyte stimulating hormone (MSH) itself. Skin darkening may be homogeneous or blotchy and additional darker areas can occur at the palmar creases, sites of friction, flexural areas and genital skin.

Box 6.18 | Symptoms and signs of adrenal insufficiency

Symptoms

- Weakness (fatigue)
- Anorexia
- GI symptoms:
  - nausea
  - vomiting
  - constipation
  - abdominal discomfort
  - diarrhea
- Salt craving
- Postural dizziness
- Myalgia, joint pain

Signs

- Weight loss
- Hyperpigmentation
- Systolic hypotension
- Vitiligo

Laboratory tests

- Hyponatremia
- Hyperkalemia
- Hypercalcemia
- High urea
- Anemia
- Eosinophilia

(a)

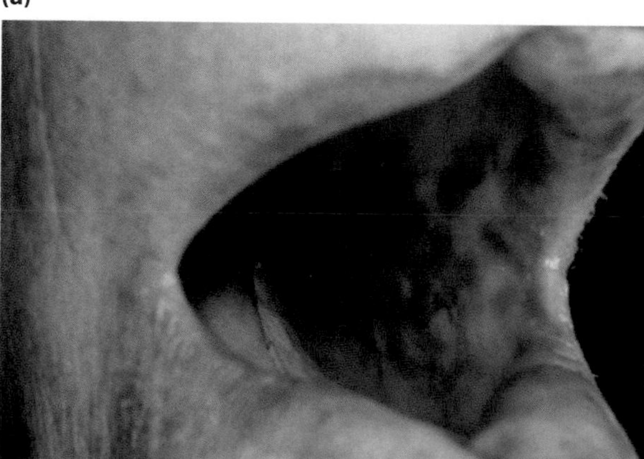

(b)

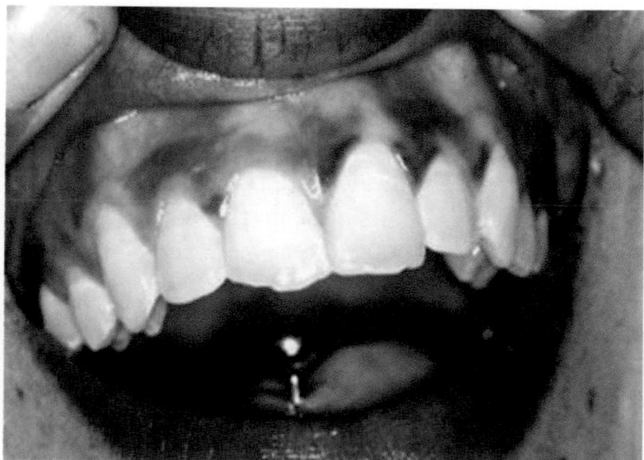

Box figure 6.13. Buccal and gum pigmentation in newly presenting Addison disease.

The buccal, periodontal, and vaginal mucosa may also exhibit areas of increased pigmentation (*Box 6.18*). Thus skin pigmentation is the hallmark of primary adrenal failure and does not occur in secondary or tertiary causes of adrenal insufficiency where ACTH is low.

Due to the potentially rather indolent nature of the condition, it may go undiagnosed for some time and indeed may only become apparent at a time of intercurrent illness or with other stress sufficient to produce an acute adrenal or Addisonian crisis. Situations associated with development of acute adrenal crisis include:

- serious infection or major stress in a previously undiagnosed patient
- persistent vomiting in a diagnosed patient (failure to adequately replace cortisol orally)
- failure to increase dose of replacement glucocorticoid in a patient with known adrenal insufficiency and an intercurrent major illness or surgical procedure
- acute bilateral adrenal infarction or hemorrhage
- pituitary apoplexy (see *Section 2.11.1*).

Acute primary adrenal failure or *adrenal crisis* presents with orthostatic hypotension, confusion, circulatory collapse, fever, and hypoglycemia. The hypotension is due to the excess excretion of Na^+ and water by the kidneys due to the loss of aldosterone that normally promotes Na^+ and water reabsorption in the distal tubule. Blood volume is reduced and hyponatremia and hyperkalemia occur. Hypoglycemia is the result of loss of cortisol which normally raises blood glucose levels.

6.6.3 Diagnosis of adrenal insufficiency

Once adrenal insufficiency is suspected it is necessary to confirm cortisol deficiency and ascertain whether this is due to primary adrenal disease (low cortisol with high ACTH, *Figure 6.12d*) or secondary causes (low cortisol and low ACTH).

The synacthen test

This is generally the most useful diagnostic test. Synacthen is synthetic ACTH(1–24) which has the same biological activity as native ACTH(1–39). The test is generally performed first thing in the morning to obviate the influence of circadian variation in cortisol levels and, in a standard test, a blood sample is taken for cortisol and ACTH just prior to an injection of 250 μg of synthetic ACTH. A normal response, defined as a 30 minute value of cortisol above 500–550 nmol/L, will exclude all patients with primary and the majority with secondary adrenal insufficiency, because a good response of the adrenal gland to synacthen indicates an endogenous source of ACTH maintaining adrenal function.

In the context of adrenal crisis, which has a significant untreated mortality, it is essential not to delay treatment whilst waiting for results of blood tests. If this condition is suspected it is reasonable to take blood samples at baseline for later measurement of cortisol (and, if possible, ACTH, renin, and aldosterone) and then immediately start resuscitation of the patient (see below) with intravenous saline and steroid (either hydrocortisone or dexamethasone). Dexamethasone has the advantage of not cross-reacting in the cortisol assay, allowing a synacthen test to be carried out in a timely fashion once the patient is clinically improved.

Insulin stress test

In those patients with suspected pituitary disease or those who have low basal ACTH and cortisol on the synacthen test, it may be necessary to proceed to an insulin stress test which will determine whether there is secondary adrenal deficiency. The aim of this test is to mimic stress by causing hypoglycemia, thereby activating the hypothalamic–pituitary axis. Insulin is given intravenously at a dose of 0.15 U/kg with the aim of obtaining a nadir sugar of 2 mmol/L or less. Bloods are taken at baseline and then at 15 minute intervals for between 45 and 120 minutes. A 'normal' result is a peak cortisol of greater than 500 nmol/L. The test is contraindicated in patients with known ischemic heart disease or a history of epilepsy.

CRH test

A CRH test can be performed to differentiate between secondary adrenal insufficiency (at the level of the pituitary) or tertiary adrenal insufficiency (at the level of the hypothalamus). After administration of CRH (100 μg, or 1 μg/kg, IV), the normal response is a rise of serum ACTH of 30–40 pg/mL; patients with pituitary failure do not respond, whereas those with hypothalamic disease usually do. In secondary adrenal insufficiency there is no response to CRH, whilst in tertiary insufficiency basal ACTH levels are low but there will be a brisk and exaggerated response to CRH. In practice this is rarely necessary or of clinical value.

6.6.4 Determining the etiology of adrenal insufficiency

Once the diagnosis of primary (as opposed to secondary or tertiary) adrenal insufficiency is confirmed, identification of the cause is the next step. Adrenal CT scans may be helpful. If the adrenal glands are enlarged or calcified this makes an infectious, hemorrhagic, or metastatic cause more likely and an autoimmune cause less likely. Tuberculous adrenal disease (once the commonest cause of adrenal insufficiency) usually coexists with clear evidence of tuberculosis elsewhere; a chest X-ray, urine culture for mycobacterium, and tuberculin skin testing may be useful.

Most primary adrenal disease in the developed world is autoimmune in origin. Assays for a target antigen in autoimmune adrenalitis (21-hydroxylase/P_{450}c21) are available and are positive in the majority of cases. Autoimmune diseases often associate with one another and it is reasonable to look for evidence of other autoimmune endocrinopathies by measuring calcium, phosphate, glucose, and TSH. If calcium is low it is worth measuring parathyroid hormone to look for evidence of hypoparathyroidism (see *Chapter 4*). Women may present with oligomenorrhea or amenorrhea and this may be a result of chronic illness or may point to an associated autoimmune hypogonadism; thus it is worth measuring LH, FSH, and estrogen (*Chapter 7*).

Rare causes of primary adrenal insufficiency include X-linked adrenoleukodystrophy and adrenomyeloneuropathy, and these should be excluded in young males (less than 14 years of age) even in the absence of classic neurological symptoms/signs which may post-date the onset of impairment of adrenal function.

There are several causes of pituitary or hypothalamic dysfunction (*Section 2.11.1*). If secondary or tertiary adrenal dysfunction is suspected, it is sensible to request a pituitary MRI or CT to exclude a mass lesion or evidence of pituitary apoplexy. There are numerous causes of hypopituitarism and a number of causes of isolated ACTH deficiency are discussed in detail in *Section 2.11*.

6.6.5 Treatment of adrenal insufficiency – adrenal crisis and long-term treatment

As mentioned above, adrenal insufficiency is a potentially life-threatening condition and requires rapid treatment, particularly if the patient presents in adrenal crisis.

In this situation the patient requires rapid resuscitation with large volumes of normal saline to correct hypotension and the circulatory volume deficit, followed by glucocorticoid replacement with either parenteral hydrocortisone or dexamethasone (as discussed above). Once stable the patient can be converted to a maintenance dose of oral hydrocortisone (15–30 mg/day in divided doses), usually along with fludrocortisone (100–200 μg/day). Education is crucially important here because the patient needs to take control of their own disease, realize that the treatment is lifelong, and understand the need to increase the dose of steroid replacement at times of stress (intercurrent illness, surgery, etc.). Injectable steroid should be made available (with appropriate training) to patients and relatives for times of acute stress. The need for identification of the condition cannot be overemphasized and patients need to carry written documentation of their condition and chronic treatment and also wear some form of identification (e.g. 'Medic Alert' bracelet or pendant).

Primary adrenal insufficiency differs from secondary/tertiary insufficiency in that it also results in mineralocorticoid deficiency. Destruction of adrenal tissue involves all layers of the adrenal cortex, whereas in secondary or tertiary hypoadrenalism, mineralocorticoid function is preserved because the renin–angiotensin–aldosterone system remains intact (see *Section 6.7*).

Mineralocorticoid replacement (100–200 μg 9-α-fluorohydrocortisone daily) should prevent sodium loss and hyperkalemia with concomitant intravascular fluid depletion. The adequacy of the replacement dose of fludrocortisone is based on its ability to suppress the elevated plasma renin activity associated with adrenal insufficiency.

The adrenal gland is the sole source of post-menopausal androgens in women, and recent evidence suggests a benefit in replacing DHEA-S in this group (in terms of libido and well-being). At present, however, DHEA-S is not available on prescription in either the USA or UK.

CASE 6.3 306 311

- Female student of 22 years with D&V of 24 h duration; significant fatigue, with weight loss and anorexia (BMI 17) in last few months
- Examination showed hypotension, pigmentation of buccal mucosa, high urea, hyperkalemia, hyponatremia, and low blood sugar – likely cortisol deficiency
- Resuscitated with 4 L normal saline over 12 h, plus hydrocortisone = improved within 24 h
- Discharged on maintenance dose of hydrocortisone

After taking blood for cortisol and ACTH, the patient was resuscitated with large volumes of normal saline (4 liters over the initial 12 hours). She was given a stat dose of 100 mg hydrocortisone i.v. followed by a further 100 mg 4 h later. At 7 hours, the cortisol level came back at 50 nmol/L (NR 140–690) and the following day the ACTH was reported at 110 pmol/L (NR <26). After 24 hours of intravenous glucocorticoid therapy and saline resuscitation she improved dramatically. Adrenal CT was unremarkable, and the adrenal antibody screen was positive. She was discharged on a maintenance dose of hydrocortisone: 10 mg in the morning on waking, 5 mg at lunchtime and 5 mg in the early evening along with 100 μg of fludrocortisone. She bought an alert necklace engraved with her medical details and at review was well and happy and about to enter her final year of medical school.

Secondary/tertiary hypoadrenalism also requires hydrocortisone therapy in doses similar to those used in primary adrenal disease. The differences here are that ACTH cannot be used to monitor adequate replacement (there isn't any) and mineralocorticoid replacement is not necessary. Clearly a full pituitary/hypothalamic assessment is required because other hormones may need to be replaced (see *Section 2.11.2*).

6.7 More basic physiology

6.7.1 Aldosterone and its actions

Aldosterone acts on the distal nephron and the distal colon to promote Na^+ reabsorption and K^+ excretion through regulation of specific ion transporters across the apical and basolateral membranes of epithelial cells. In the kidney Na^+ is reabsorbed from the ultrafiltrate at the apical surface of distal convoluted tubule cells through the epithelial Na^+ channel (ENaC). At the basolateral suface it is pumped out of the cells by the Na^+/K^+-ATPase pump. The latter provides the electrochemical driving force for the luminal influx of Na^+ and the basolateral efflux of K^+.

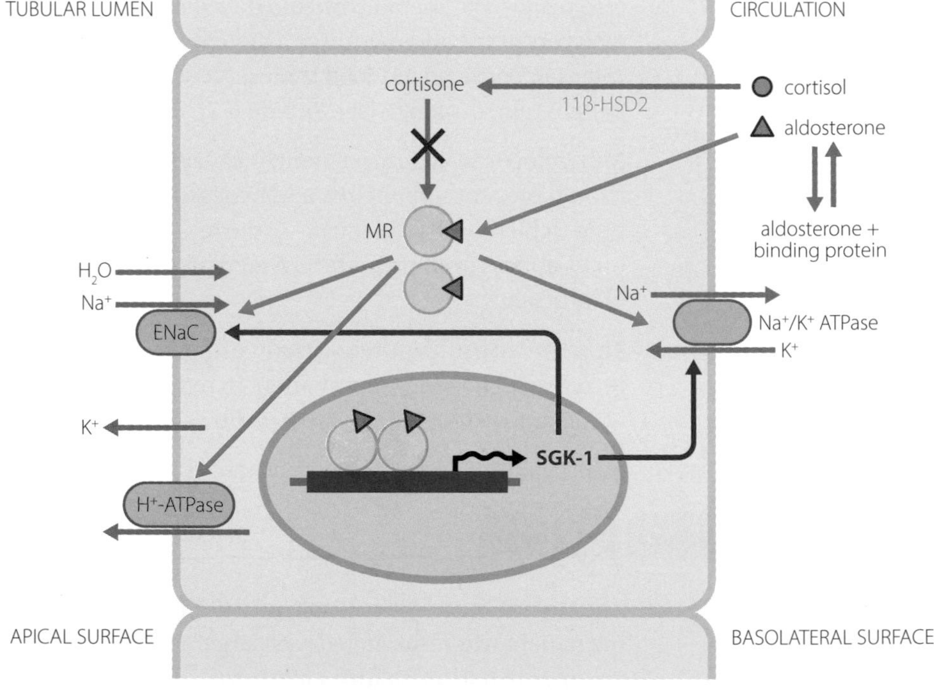

Figure 6.14. Actions of aldosterone on the ascending loop of Henle, distal convoluted tubule and cortical collecting ducts of the kidney controlling the reabsorption of salt (Na^+) and water. Unbound aldosterone diffuses across the cell membrane and interacts with the mineralocorticoid receptor (MR). Once activated, it dimerizes with another activated receptor and the dimer translocates to the nucleus where it induces transcription of serum glucocorticoid-activated kinase (SGK-1). This increases expression of the epithelial Na^+ channel (ENaC) and Na^+/K^+ ATPase transporters increasing Na^+ and water reabsorption. Activated MRs also have rapid non-genomic effects which may directly or indirectly activate the activity or trafficking of these transporters as well as other transporters such as the H^+-ATPase pump in the apical membrane. Cortisol, which diffuses into tubular cells, is rapidly inactivated to cortisone by 11β-hydroxysteroid dehydrogenase (HSD)2. Thus cortisol is prevented from interacting with the MR for which it has equal affinity.

Aldosterone interacts with classical cytoplasmic steroid receptors located in the thick ascending loop of Henle, distal convoluted tubule, and the cortical collecting ducts (*Figure 6.14*). Like other steroid receptors, once activated by ligand binding, they dimerize and translocate to the nucleus where they initiate gene transcription. One of the earliest genomic events induced by aldosterone is the increased expression of serum glucocorticoid-activated kinase (SGK-1) which either directly or indirectly regulates the activity and membrane trafficking of the Na^+/K^+-ATPase and ENaC transporters. Later genomic actions of aldosterone include the increased expression of these membrane transporters. Aldosterone also has very rapid, non-genomic

Box 6.19 | Endocrine hypertension

Hypertension, conventionally defined as a systolic blood pressure >140 mmHg and diastolic pressure >90 mmHg, is the main cause of cardiovascular disease. It is divided into two forms: primary hypertension, otherwise known as essential hypertension (a synonym for idiopathic or no known cause), and secondary hypertension which has a diagnosable cause. Over 95% of cases of hypertension are classified as essential hypertension that requires life-long management. Secondary hypertension occurs as a result of another disease such as renal disease and certain endocrine disorders. The most common causes of endocrine hypertension, which account for <1% of all cases of hypertension, are excessive production of mineralocorticoids, glucocorticoids, or catecholamines.

Primary hyperaldosteronism (PA) is the most common form of endocrine hypertension usually caused by idiopathic bilateral hyperplasia or a unilateral aldosterone-producing adenoma (Conn syndrome). Hypertension is caused by increased sodium retention which increases the ECF volume. The increased tubular reabsorption of Na^+ and hence water leads to hypokalemic acidosis, although plasma sodium increases only slightly and usually remains in the normal range due to the intervention of vasopressin and thirst that control water balance. Patients rarely have symptoms, except hypertension, although hypokalemia may cause muscle weakness.

Excess glucocorticoids induce Cushing syndrome and the excess glucocorticoids may be from endogenous sources (usually a pituitary adenoma) or from exogenous steroidal anti-inflammatory drugs such as prednisone. The exact mechanisms of this endocrine hypertension are unknown but can include:

- glucocorticoid stimulation of hepatic synthesis of angiotensinogen leading to an increased activity of the renin–angiotensin–aldosterone pathway
- increased vascular reactivity leading to increased peripheral resistance and elevation of blood pressure
- inappropriate interaction of cortisol with the aldosterone receptor due to oversaturation of 11β-HSD2 activity which inactivates cortisol in renal tubular cells, converting it to cortisone.

Deficiency of 11β-HSD2, a rare autosomal recessive disorder, is known as apparent mineralocorticoid excess (AME). Similar to patients with primary hyperaldosteronism, affected individuals will have hypertension and hypokalemia with low renin and aldosterone levels, but normal plasma cortisol levels. The ratio of urinary free cortisol:free cortisone, however, is elevated.

Excess circulating catecholamines are caused by chromaffin cell tumors of the adrenal medulla known as pheochromocytomas. These tumors are rare but cause labile hypertension and paroxysmal symptoms such as headache, sweating, and palpitations. The hypertension is caused by the stimulatory effects of epinephrine and nor-epinephrine on increasing heart rate, stroke volume, and vasoconstriction.

Other endocrinopathies may also cause hypertension and these include:

- hyperthyroidism due to the inotropic and chronotropic effects of thyroid hormones on the heart
- excess growth hormone (acromegaly) related to effects of GH and/or insulin like growth factor-1 (IGF-1) on renal function
- insulin resistance and myocardial hypertrophy
- primary hyperparathyroidism due to excess intracellular calcium and non-specific effects of raised parathyroid hormone.

effects on tubular cells such as increasing intracellular Ca^{2+} concentrations and activating protein kinase C isoforms, and these effects also increase the activity of these membrane transporters. In addition, aldosterone also regulates the trafficking and activity of other ion transporters in the distal nephron such as the Na^+/H^+ exchangers (NHE) and the H^+-ATPase pumps in the apical membrane (*Figure 6.14*).

The systemic effect of aldosterone on the kidney is to raise blood pressure as a result of the osmotic movement of water that follows the Na^+ reabsorption. Excessive Na^+ conservation leads to hypertension, thus increasing the risk of stroke and myocardial infarction, both major causes of mortality. Indeed, excess aldosterone (primary aldosteronism (see *Section 5.8*)) is the most common form of endocrine hypertension (*Box 6.19*).

However, it is now well accepted that aldosterone also has physiological and pathophysiological actions on non-epithelial cells resulting in cardiac fibrosis

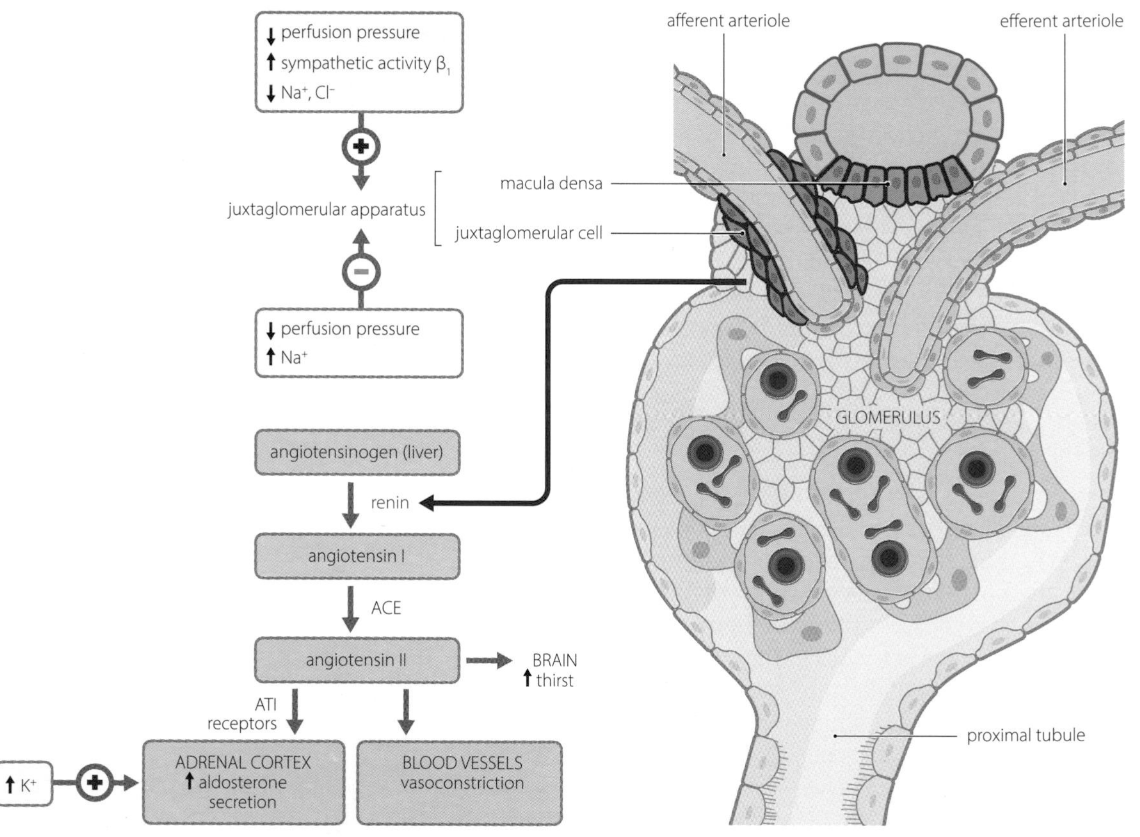

Figure 6.15. Control of aldosterone secretion.

- Juxtaglomerular (JGA) cells are modified smooth muscle cells which secrete renin.
- The macula densa are tubular cells of the thick ascending limb of the loop of Henle which can detect circulating concentrations of sodium.
- In response to the indicated stimuli, renin is secreted and converts angiotensinogen (synthesized in the liver) to angiotensin I.
- Angiotensin-converting enzyme (ACE) converts angiotensin I to angiotensin II and this then acts on AT1 receptors in the adrenal cortex (glomerulosa), blood vessels and brain (via circumventricular organs).
- In addition to angiotensin II, high circulating concentrations of K^+ also stimulate aldosterone secretion.

and inflammatory actions in the heart and vasculature. This led to clinical trials investigating the use of low doses of spironolactone (a mineralocorticoid receptor antagonist) as an adjunctive therapy to diuretics and ACE inhibitors in the treatment of moderate to severe heart failure. The use of mineralocorticoid receptor antagonism is now first line and has reduced morbidity although hyperkalemia may limit the therapeutic utility of spironolactone.

6.7.2 Control of aldosterone secretion

The control of aldosterone synthesis and release is through the renin–angiotensin system (*Figure 6.15*). Smooth muscle cells in the afferent and efferent arterioles of the kidney synthesize, store, and release renin. The release of this enzyme is stimulated by a reduced perfusion pressure in the kidney, increased activity of sympathetic nerves innervating the smooth muscle cells, or a reduction in Na^+ delivery to the macula densa. Once released, renin cleaves angiotensinogen to angiotensin I and this peptide is further converted by angiotensin-converting enzyme (ACE), found in the endothelial cells of the lung and kidney, to the octapeptide, angiotensin II. Angiotensin II then acts on the glomerulosa cells of the adrenal cortex to stimulate the production of aldosterone. High K^+ levels will also directly stimulate the release of aldosterone.

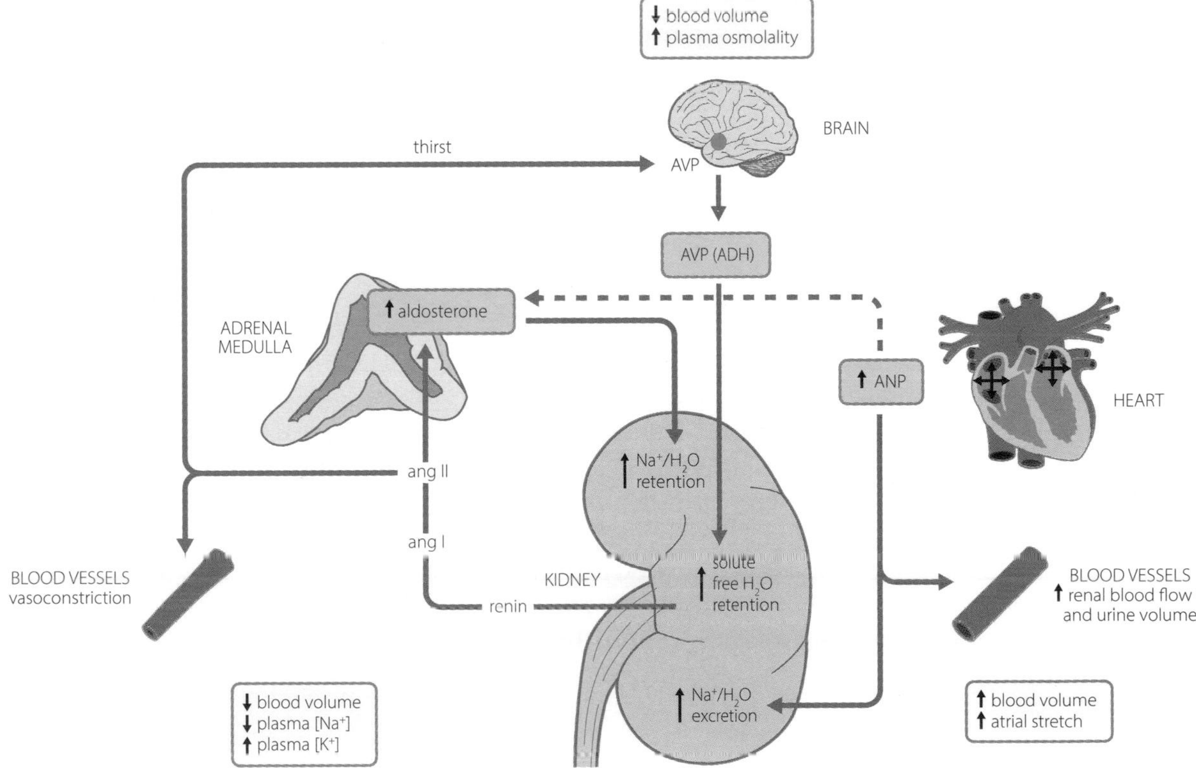

Figure 6.16. Integrated control of salt and water balance.
The renin/angiotensin system stimulates aldosterone secretion, and angiotensin II potentiates the release of AVP and stimulates thirst. Vasopressin secretion is also directly stimulated by hypothalamic osmoreceptors and volume receptors in the cardiovascular system. Atrial natriuretic peptide (ANP) is released in response to atrial stretch and also inhibits the synthesis and release of aldosterone, and inhibits renin production and AVP release.

6.7.3 Integrated endocrine control of salt and water balance

Aldosterone stimulates Na^+ and water retention, helping to maintain salt and water balance and, thus, blood pressure. The two other major hormones involved in this control are atrial natriuretic hormone (ANP) and arginine vasopressin (AVP) (*Figure 6.16*).

ANP antagonizes the overall effects of aldosterone, i.e. it promotes the excretion of sodium and, thus, reduces ECF volume. The 28 amino acid peptide is synthesized and stored in atrial myocytes. An increase in atrial tension caused by an increase in central venous pressure (CVP) stimulates ANP release. ANP inhibits Na^+ reabsorption in the distal convoluted tubules and collecting ducts via a cGMP-dependent mechanism. It also inhibits AVP, aldosterone, and renin secretion, and increases the GFR (and therefore the sodium load delivered to the kidneys). The overall effect is to reduce the ECF volume, although it should be noted that the cardiovascular effects of ANP in man are minimal.

Normally, sodium balance determines the ECF volume and thus blood pressure and the perfusion pressure within the vascular system. An increase in ECF stimulates Na^+ and water excretion through a reduction in aldosterone secretion and ANP release. A decrease causes Na^+ and water retention through aldosterone secretion. Sodium salts are the major determinants of osmolality in the ECF since they are the most abundant solutes. Changes in sodium balance affect serum osmolality.

Regulation of serum osmolality is achieved by the action of AVP decreasing solute-free water clearance by the kidney (i.e. retention of water without electrolytes). Increases in osmolality are detected by osmoreceptors in the hypothalamus and these stimulate AVP secretion from the magnocellular neurosecretory cells in the supraoptic and paraventricular nuclei of the hypothalamus. AVP increases the reabsorption of water in the kidney by inserting water channels (aquaporins) into the membranes of tubular cells in the distal convoluted tubules and collecting ducts. The secretion of AVP is inhibited by a reduction in serum osmolality resulting in reduced water reabsorption and increased excretion.

AVP secretion is also stimulated by a reduced ECF volume. This is achieved through low-pressure volume receptors in the cardiac atria and pulmonary vessels. High-pressure sensors in the aortic arch, carotid sinus, and the afferent arterioles of the kidney inhibit AVP secretion. Thus, whilst AVP controls solute-free water balance, maintaining both osmolality and ECF volume, aldosterone and ANP regulate the ECF volume by controlling Na^+ balance. The relationship between Na^+ balance and ECF volume is complex, particularly under certain pathological conditions.

6.8 Primary aldosteronism

Originally described by Conn over 50 years ago, primary aldosteronism (PA) was a relatively rare curiosity, but more recent studies have suggested that PA is more common. This discovery was established by the widespread measurement of the aldosterone:renin ratio and studies show that the prevalence of suppressed plasma renin activity with elevated or normal aldosterone levels is between 5 and 20% of the population.

CASE 6.4

317 319

- Male of 41 years with uncontrolled hypertension and hyperkalemia
- Beta-blockers, ACE inhibitors, calcium channel blockers, and diuretic all tried unsuccessfully

A 41 year old hedge fund manager was referred by his primary care physician with uncontrolled hypertension and hypokalemia. He was treated with a beta-blocker, an ACE inhibitor, a calcium channel blocker and a diuretic (bendroflumethiazide), but his 24 hour mean ambulatory blood pressure remained at 160/104 mmHg with no obvious nocturnal dipping (i.e. reduction of blood pressure whilst asleep at night). He was a non-smoker with no other personal or family medical history. He was on no other medication and drank only an occasional glass of fine wine in the evening. ECG showed mild left ventricular hypertrophy confirmed by echocardiography. Renal function was normal apart from the persistent hypokalemia (2.9 mmol/L; NR 3.5–5.1). He remained asymptomatic. Investigations for secondary causes of hypertension were carried out.

6.8.1 Clinical features of PA

The clinical features are variable and rather non-specific. The most common features include renal potassium loss usually (though not always) resulting in hypokalemia, hypertension (which may be severe and difficult to control, as in Case 6.4), and metabolic alkalosis (secondary to hypokalemia). Low potassium may result in muscle cramps, weakness, and paresthesia, and occasionally in cardiac dysrhythmias. Aldosterone also has direct effects on the cardiovascular system and can contribute to cardiac hypertrophy and (rarely) fibrosis.

6.8.2 Etiology of PA

Primary hyperaldosteronism may be caused by:

- an aldosterone-producing adenoma (APA, as originally described by Conn)
- bilateral adrenal hyperplasia (BAH)
- glucocorticoid remediable aldosteronism (GRA)
- unilateral adrenal hyperplasia (UAH)
- adrenal carcinoma.

The most common cause of PA is BAH which accounts for about 65% of cases, followed by APA (30%) and primary UAH (3%). Other cases are rare, although the incidence of GRA is increasing with higher indices of suspicion and improved diagnostics.

APAs are generally small tumors (<2 cm) and are more common in men. BAH is more common, and of idiopathic etiology, although there have been suggestions of exaggerated responsiveness to angiotensin II. GRA is an autosomal dominant condition (confusingly also known as familial hyperaldosteronism type I) in which the promoter sequence of the 11β hydroxylase gene is fused to the aldosterone synthase gene making aldosterone synthesis dependent on ACTH, hence 'glucocorticoid remediable' because exogenous glucocorticoids will suppress ACTH activity and reduce blood pressure. UAH is rare and behaves in much the same way as APA, but without an obvious lesion on imaging; the diagnosis is generally based on finding unilaterally high levels of aldosterone on adrenal vein sampling (see below). Adrenal carcinomas are rare causes of hypertension (see *Section 6.5*).

Secondary hyperaldosteronism is the result of increased stimulation of the renin–angiotensin system (RAS) and differs biochemically from primary aldosteronism in that both renin and aldosterone levels are high. Secondary hyperaldosteronism commonly arises from conditions causing an effective reduction in blood volume, e.g. nephrotic syndrome, congestive cardiac failure, and liver failure. Where hypertension is associated with secondary hyperaldosteronism the causes are almost always reno-vascular in nature; the most common being atherosclerosis or fibromuscular hyperplasia of the renal arteries. This leads to decreased perfusion of the kidneys with resultant activation of the RAS. Very rarely, secondary hyperaldosteronism may be caused by renin-secreting tumors of the kidney.

6.8.3 Diagnosis of PA

The importance of diagnosing primary aldosteronism is the growing evidence that aldosterone may have deleterious cardiovascular, renal, and metabolic effects in addition to its direct hypertensive effects (*Box 6.19*). Patients with PA and aldosterone-related hypertension appear to be at higher cardiovascular and renal risk than comparable patients with essential hypertension.

A measurement of renin and aldosterone levels and determination of the aldosterone:renin ratio is useful. Various cut-off levels have been suggested ranging from 200 to 2774 pmol/L/µg/L·h (from 7.2 to 100.1 ng/dL/ng/mL·h). In practice, where renin is measured in ng/dL and PRA (plasma renin activity) in ng/ml·h, a ratio of less than 20 makes primary aldosteronism extremely unlikely and a ratio of >60 makes it almost certain.

It is also important to remember that many patients will be on one or more antihypertensive agents and these may well affect measurements of renin and aldosterone (indeed that is how many of them work). In simple terms, and in an ideal world, all agents should be stopped. This is rarely possible, however, and the most important agents to stop are inhibitors of aldosterone, spironolactone, and epleronone which increase renin levels and beta-blockers which lower renin levels. Both drug types should be stopped at least 4 weeks before testing. ACE inhibitors and angiotensin receptor blockers both suppress aldosterone; if levels remain high on the drugs then the patient is likely to have hyperaldosteronism. Alpha-blockers and calcium channel blockers have rather neutral actions on the RAS.

An abnormal ratio (which remains undiagnostic) can be followed up with further tests designed to result in volume expansion.

- Isotonic saline test: 500 ml of saline are injected over 4 h – a normal result is suppression of aldosterone to below 166 pmol/L and a level greater than 277 pmol/L (10 ng/dL) is considered diagnostic.
- Oral salt loading: patients are given a salt-rich diet (200 mmol/day) for 3 days followed by a 24 h urine collection for measurement of aldosterone and sodium excretion. Levels of aldosterone exceeding 40 nmol/day with a sodium excretion exceeding 200 mmol/day are considered diagnostic.
- Fludrocortisone suppression test: fludrocortisone is given in a dose of 0.1 mg 6 hourly along with oral sodium chloride (200 mmol/day) for 4 days. Failure to suppress upright aldosterone levels to less than 140 pmol/L by day 4 confirms the diagnosis of primary aldosteronism.

Once the biochemical diagnosis is confirmed the etiology is sought. APA is suggested by a younger age, more impressive hypokalemia (<3 mmol/L), and higher aldosterone levels (>700 pmol/L).

Fine cut adrenal spiral CT scanning is the most useful imaging modality to locate a small adenoma. A clear adenoma on imaging with strong biochemical evidence is probably justification for laparoscopic surgery.

In difficult cases adrenal vein sampling may help – samples for aldosterone and cortisol are taken from the left and right adrenal veins and the inferior vena cava. The test is sometimes done under continuous stimulation with ACTH. A cortisol/aldosterone ratio is derived from each sample; if one side is more than four times the contralateral this favors APA, but less than three times suggests BAH.

If there is a suggestion of secondary hyperaldosteronism and the initial tests have confirmed an elevated level of renin, structural abnormalities can be identified by a variety of imaging techniques including CT, angiography, magnetic resonance angiography (MRA), or duplex ultrasonography. A captopril angiogram may also be useful; here the ACE inhibitor (captopril) is given 30 minutes prior to a nuclear medicine renogram. Delayed excretion of the tracer is exaggerated by captopril on the side where there is arterial narrowing.

6.8.4 Management of PA

As suggested above, APA is treated by surgery and is one of the few conditions where hypertension can be effectively 'cured' rather than just treated. Unfortunately, some patients will have co-existing primary hypertension and will need to continue antihypertensive medication.

Where surgery is contraindicated or where there is BAH, medical treatment with aldosterone antagonists (epleronone or spironolactone) is used. Spironolactone (in men) has rather potent anti-androgenic side-effects and its use is often limited by symptoms of gynecomastia, erectile dysfunction, and libido loss. Epleronone is better tolerated because it does not bind the androgen or progesterone receptors. In GRA, hypertension is proportional to ACTH activity, so exogenous low-dose glucocorticoids (e.g. dexamethasone) can control hypertension. In secondary hyperaldosteronism caused by renal artery stenosis, renal angioplasty is the treatment of choice.

CASE 6.4

317 319

- Male of 41 years with uncontrolled hypertension and hyperkalemia
- Beta-blockers, ACE inhibitors, calcium channel blockers, and diuretic all tried unsuccessfully
- CT revealed 3 cm lesion in right adrenal gland a full recovery was made after removal

The patient underwent testing for random aldosterone and renin 3 weeks after stopping his beta-blocker and diuretic. An alpha-blocker (doxazosin) was added to his treatment to maintain acceptable blood pressure. Aldosterone levels were high (750 pmol/L) with undetectable PRA. An adrenal protocol spiral CT revealed a 2.8 cm lesion in the right adrenal gland with a normal left adrenal gland. He underwent unilateral laparoscopic adrenalectomy and had an unremarkable post-operative course. Six months after surgery he remains symptom free and is on no antihypertensive blood pressure medication with a mean blood pressure of 132/72 mmHg.

6.9 Excess adrenal androgens – congenital adrenal hyperplasia

CASE 6.5 320 324

- Woman of 18 years with excess hair growth, acne, and irregular periods
- Normal weight but short for her age

An 18 year old woman was referred by her family doctor with increased hair growth, acne, and irregular periods. Her acne was severe and affected her face, neck, and chest. Her hair growth was prominent on her upper lips, chin, neck, chest, arms, lower abdomen, back, and legs. Cosmetic approaches (shaving and plucking) had become increasingly unsatisfactory. She reported unhappy teenage years when she was bullied because of her appearance. She started menstruating aged 15 but her periods had always been irregular, often not occurring for months; her last period was about 3 months ago.

There was nothing remarkable in her childhood history and she had no significant medical or drug history. She had never been sexually active and at college she preferred to play football. She had Jewish antecedents and denied any significant family history. On examination, she was 9 cm below the height expected from her mid-parental target height but she was normal weight for her height. There was considerable hair growth in the areas mentioned. Her abdomen was soft and non-tender. Her external genitalia were normal.

Congenital adrenal hyperplasia (CAH) describes a group of autosomal recessive disorders in which mutations of the genes coding for steroidogenic enzymes result in complete or partial loss of synthesis of one of more steroids secreted from the adrenal cortex. The clinical features will depend on which particular enzyme is affected, the severity of the defect and the sex of the patient. The more proximal the deficiency in the steroidogenic pathway (*Figure 6.3*) the more widespread the defect, so both the adrenal glands and gonads will be affected (*Boxes 6.20* and *6.21*).

The most common form of CAH is a loss of function mutation in the *CYP21A2* gene, which codes for 21-hydroxylase, and this mutation accounts for 95% of all cases of CAH. The severe or classic form of CAH occurs in 1:15 000 live births worldwide, although the incidence varies according to ethnicity and geographic area. For example, amongst the Yupic Eskimos of Alaska the incidence is 1 in 280 live births and in the French island of La Réunion the incidence is approximately 1 in 2000. CYP21A2 (CYP21B) is important in the synthesis of adrenal glucocorticoids and mineralocorticoids (*Box 6.20*) and patients with the classic form of CAH have a cortisol deficiency with or without an absolute aldosterone deficiency; salt-losing or non-salt-losing reflecting the degree of the aldosterone deficiency. The precursors of these steroids are consequently shunted into androgen synthesis, resulting in androgen excess, which causes virilization of a female fetus and ambiguous genitalia. The adrenal hyperplasia is caused by high production rates of the trophic hormone, ACTH, due to loss of negative feedback of endogenous cortisol.

In the non-classic mild or late onset form patients do not have cortisol deficiency but have manifestations of hyperandrogenism, generally later in childhood or in early adulthood (*Box 6.21*). These patients may present with precocious pubarche (see *Section 7.3*), or as young women with hirsutism (*Box 6.4*), oligo- or amenorrhea,

Box 6.20 | Congenital adrenal hyperplasia

- A group of autosomal recessive disorders.
- All share an enzyme deficiency involved in the synthesis of cortisol, aldosterone, or both.
- Clinical manifestations related to degree of cortisol/aldosterone deficiency.
- In some cases the excess of precursor hormones may have physiological significance.
- Phenotype varies from clinically inapparent disease through a milder late onset form of the disease (non-classical adrenal hyperplasia) to severe disease characterized by adrenal insufficiency in infancy +/- virilization and salt wasting.
- Most common form is 21-hydroxylase deficiency divided into three subtypes – simple virilizing, salt wasting, and non-classical.

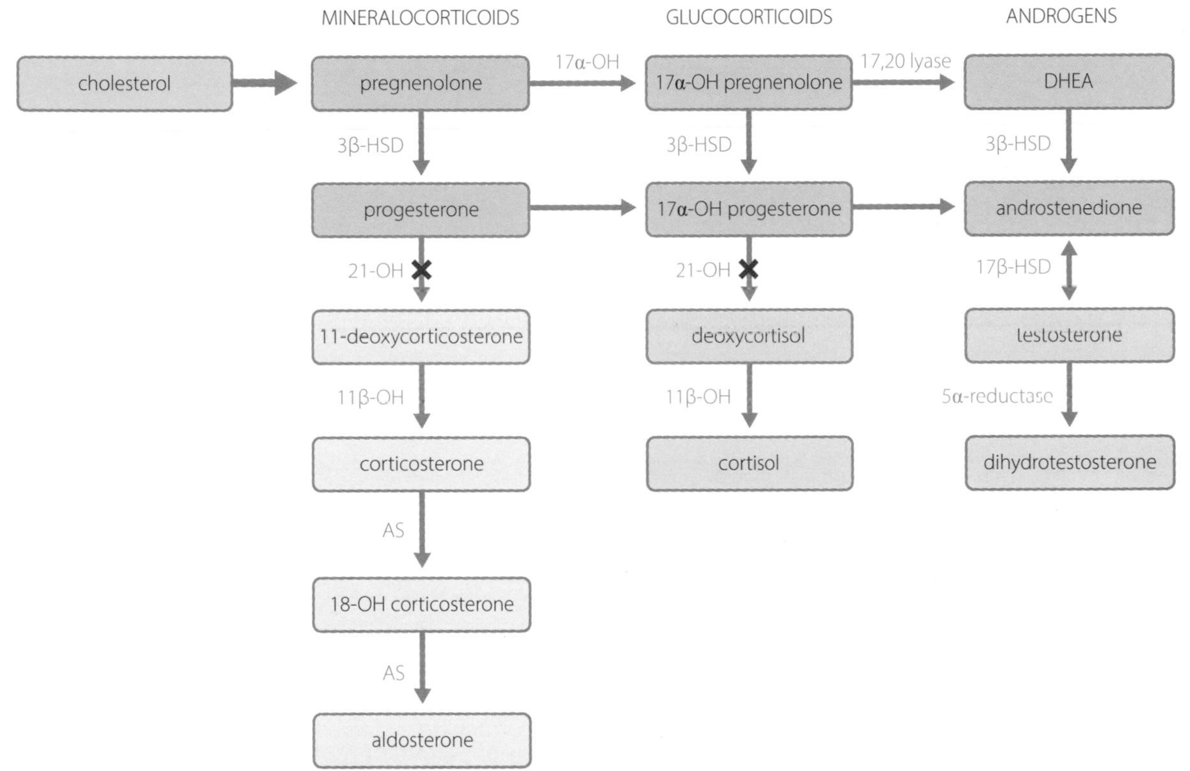

Box figure 6.14. Steroid synthesis in the adrenal cortex showing how a deficiency of 21-hydroxylase (21-OH) shunts precursors into the synthesis of androgens.

The *CYP21A* gene codes for 21-hydroxylase (OH), *CYP11B1* codes for 11β-hydroxylase, *CYP17* codes for 17α-hydroxylase, and *CYP11B2* codes for aldosterone synthase (AS).

- In the first step of adrenal steroidogenesis, cholesterol enters mitochondria via a carrier protein called StAR. ACTH stimulates cholesterol cleavage that results in the formation of pregnenolone, the rate-limiting step of adrenal steroidogenesis.
- Decrease in cortisol production leads to increased ACTH activity leading to excessive synthesis of adrenal products in those pathways unimpaired by the enzyme deficiency, and a build-up of precursor molecules in pathways blocked by the enzyme deficiency.

Box 6.20 | continued

Box table 6.5. A summary of enzyme deficiencies resulting in CAH

% of CAH	Deficient enzyme	Substrate	Product	Androgen	Mineralo-corticoid
	Steroidogenic acute regulatory protein (STAR)	–	Mediates cholesterol transport across mitochondrion	Deficiency [1]	Deficiency [2]
	3β-hydroxysteroid dehydrogenase (3β-HSD)	Pregnenolone, 17α-hydroxypregnenolone, DHEA	Progesterone, 17α-hydroxyprogesterone, androstenedione	Deficiency [1]	Deficiency [2]
	17α-hydroxylase	Pregnenolone Progesterone	17α-hydroxypregnenolone 17α-hydroxyprogesterone	Deficiency [1]	Excess [3]
>90%	21-hydroxylase	Progesterone 17α-hydroxy progesterone	Deoxycorticosterone 11-deoxycortisol	Excess [4]	Deficiency [2]
5%	11β-hydroxylase	Deoxycorticosterone	Corticosterone	Excess [4]	Excess [3]

[1]Males undervirilized at birth.
[2]Associated with salt wasting.
[3]Associated with hypertension.
[4]Females virilized at birth or later.
More details of clinical features associated with specific enzyme deficiencies are given in *Box 6.21*.

polycystic ovaries, and acne. Some women have no apparent clinical symptoms and men with non-classic CAH remain symptom free. The proportion of patients who remain symptom free is unknown and thus the incidence of mild 21-hydroxylase deficiency is unknown.

Measuring the relative concentrations of precursor molecules will generally allow diagnosis of the specific enzyme defect. Thus patients with classic CAH resulting from a mutation of *CYP21A2* will have high concentrations of 17α-hydroxyprogesterone (more than 242 nmol/L; normal range is <3 nmol/L at 3 days in a full-term infant) with salt-losing patients typically having higher levels compared with non-salt-losing patients. In patients with non-classic CAH, 17α-hydroxyprogesterone levels may be normal and the gold standard diagnosis is usually with a CRH stimulation test with measurement of 17α-hydroxyprogesterone at 60 minutes. A stimulated concentration of 17α-hydroxyprogesterone higher than 45 nmol/L is diagnostic of 21-hydroxylase deficiency.

It is now possible to screen for this genetic defect from chorionic villus sampling and very early prenatal treatment with dexamethasone (which readily crosses the placenta and inhibits fetal ACTH secretion) reduces sexual ambiguity. Postnatally, patients can be treated with appropriate steroid replacement, although this has to be monitored and titrated carefully according to the age of the patient, for example, neonates are particularly vulnerable to electrolyte imbalances (salt wasting) and

Box 6.21 | Clinical features of congenital adrenal hyperplasia associated with the specific enzyme deficiencies

21-hydroxylase

- Females virilized at birth.
- Adrenocortical function begins at 7/40 therefore female fetus exposed to androgens at critical time of sex differentiation.
- Degree of virilization divided into 5 Prader stages ranging from clitoromegaly through penile clitoris and scrotum-like labia (complete labial fusion).
- Internal female genitalia develop normally (normal ovaries – no production of AMH).
- Premature pubarche, excess growth in childhood but short final height due to premature epiphyseal closure.
- Problems with gender role behavior.
- Males who are recognized and treated normally undergo normal puberty.
- Some have small testes and oligo-azoospermia.
- Adrenal rest tumors in the testes may lead to subfertility.
- Salt wasting occurs in >75%.
- Adrenal crisis can occur between 1 and 4 weeks postnatally.
- Salt wasting is not related to the degree of virilization.

Non-classic 21-hydroxylase

- Most common recessive disorder.
- Incidence as high as 1:27 with Ashkenazi Jews.
- No virilization at birth.
- Varying degrees of hyperandrogenism postnatally.
- Commonly occurs in association with PCOS.
- May result in subfertility in males.
- Up to 80% may have adrenal incidentalomas.
- Diagnosis based on 17α-hydroxyprogesterone response to synacthen.

11β-hydroxylase

- Virilization and low renin hypertension.
- Virilization similar to 21-OHD.
- Hypertension due to overproduction of DOC causing salt retention.
- Hypertension usually appears in late childhood.
- Hypokalemia is variable.
- Renin and aldosterone are both low.

3β-hydroxysteroid dehydrogenase

- Two forms of 3β-HSD – Type II is expressed in the adrenals and gonads.
- Δ^5 precursors converted to active Δ^4 steroids in the periphery leading to female virilization
- 3β-HSD deficiency in the gonads leads to insufficient Δ^4 gonadal androgens in males.
- Genital ambiguity thus occurs in both sexes – virilization in females and incomplete virilization in males.

17α-hydroxylase, 17,20 lyase deficiency

- 1% of CAH.
- Affects steroid synthesis in adrenals and gonads.
- Low renin hypertension due to excess DOC and corticosterone.
- Females born with normal external genitalia.
- Males undervirilized due to defective gonadal testosterone production.
- Females fail to develop secondary sex characteristics.

Lipoid hyperplasia

- Very rare and very severe.
- Deficient synthesis of all gonadal and adrenal steroids (failure of conversion of cholesterol to pregnenolone).
- Abnormalities of StAR protein are responsible.
- Males are undervirilized.
- Females appear normal but do not progress through puberty.
- Severe salt wasting and hypoadrenalism are present from birth.
- Universally fatal if not rapidly treated.

hypoglycemia (lack of glucocorticoids). Conversely, excess glucocorticoids suppress growth and excess sex steroids derived from androgens may induce premature epiphyseal closure and contribute to infertility in females. The treatment is to remove the ACTH drive to androgen synthesis by giving exogenous glucocorticoid, but not in doses high enough to totally suppress the HPA axis. In classic (severe) cases of CAH, mineralocorticoids are also given to return electrolyte concentrations to normal.

CASE 6.5 320 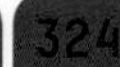

- Woman of 18 years with excess hair growth, acne, and irregular periods
- Normal weight but short for her age
- Synacthen stimulation test confirmed diagnosis of late-onset CAH; treated with low-dose dexamethasone and oral contraceptive

Due to clinical suspicion, the patient was investigated with a basal 17α-hydroxyprogesterone level which was normal. She went on to have a stimulation test with synthetic ACTH (synacthen 250 μg) and 60 minutes after injection of synacthen her 17α-hydroxyprogesterone had risen significantly to 1100 nmol/L. Other biochemical investigations (early morning cortisol, LH, FSH, and androstenedione) were all normal, although her testosterone level was marginally elevated at 4.1 nmol/L.

These tests confirmed a diagnosis of late-onset or non-classic CAH. As alluded to above, this is a variant form of CAH with fewer clinical signs and symptoms. The exact prevalence is unknown because many women probably go undiagnosed. Prenatal virilization and salt wasting at birth is not present; the degree of postnatal virilization is variable and often manifests as acne and hirsutes.

As fertility was not an issue at this time she was treated with a combination of very low dose glucocorticoid (0.25 mg dexamethasone at night) and the oral contraceptive pill. At 6 months of follow-up her hirsutes and acne had markedly improved.

6.10 The adrenal medulla and pheochromocytoma

The adrenal medulla is the location of the majority of the body's chromaffin cells, although sympathetic ganglion cells are also present in the gland. The chromaffin cells, so named for their characteristic brown staining (pheo-) with chromic acid (hence pheochromocytes), are arranged either in clusters or cords, whereas the ganglion cells are found singly or in nests interspersed between the chromaffin cells. Other groups of chromaffin cells (paraganglia) are located on both sides of the aorta.

Epinephrine and lesser amounts of nor-epinephrine are synthesized by and secreted from the chromaffin cells in response to stimulation of pre-ganglionic (cholinergic) sympathetic nerves originating from the thoracic spinal cord from T5 to T11. Thus chromaffin cells are modified post-ganglionic nerve cells, but because they release hormones into the circulation they are considered to be neurosecretory cells. The gland can be considered to be a specialized sympathetic ganglion. The adrenal medulla receives blood either directly from medullary arterioles or from the venules of the cortex (rich in cortisol) that drain centripetally to medullary venules.

The catecholamines are synthesized from tyrosine and the rate-limiting step in their synthesis is the one catalyzed by tyrosine hydroxylase, converting tyrosine to dihydroxyphenylalanine (DOPA). Subsequent decarboxylations and hydroxylations convert DOPA to dopamine, nor-epinephrine and finally to epinephrine (*Figure 6.17*). Cortisol, reaching the adrenal medulla from venules of the cortex, promotes epinephrine synthesis by up-regulating phenylethanolamine *N*-methyltransferase (PNMT), the enzyme that converts nor-epinephrine to epinephrine.

Through an energy-requiring process, catecholamines are stored in secretory granules in association with ATP (4 catecholamine molecules to 1 ATP) and a

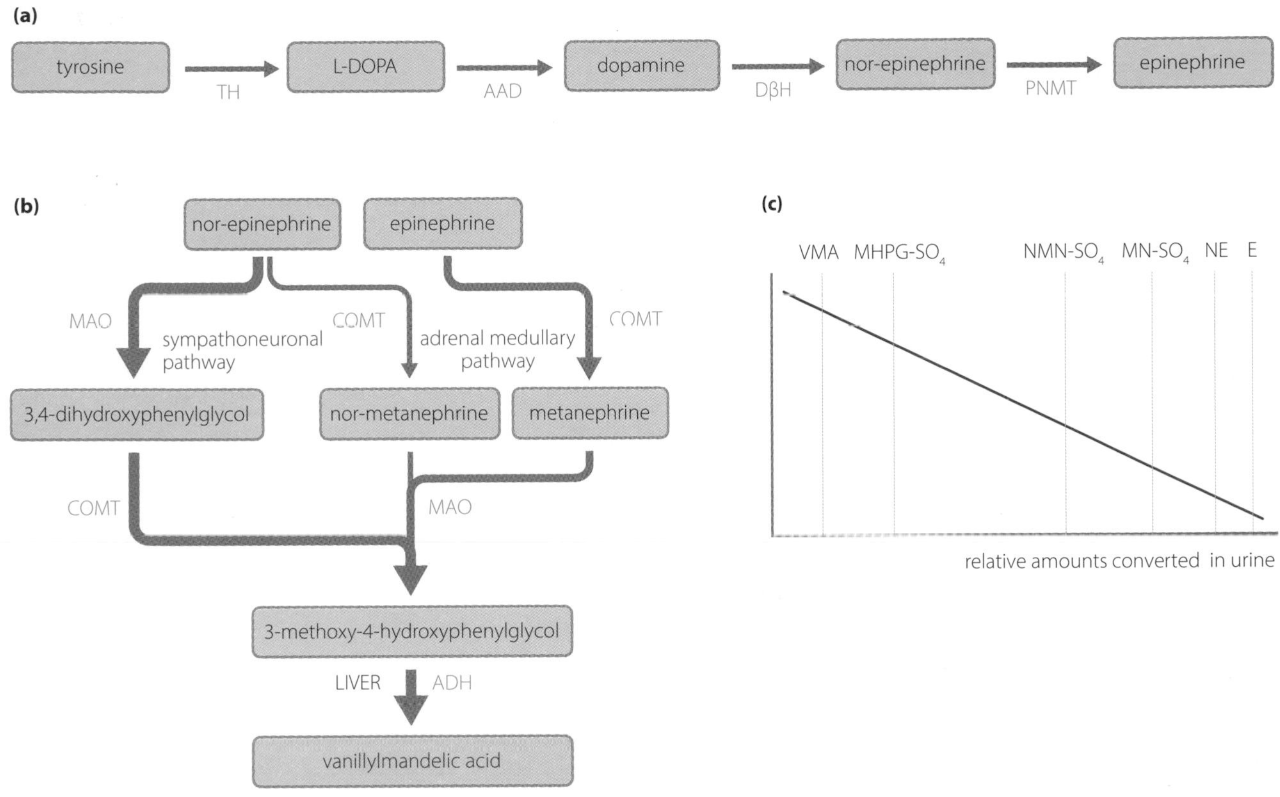

Figure 6.17. Synthesis (a) and metabolism (b) of nor-epinephrine and epinephrine derived from sympathetic neurons and adrenal chromaffin cells. (c) The relative amounts of metabolites secreted in the urine.
(a) Synthesis of epinephrine. TH, tyrosine hydroxylase; AAD, amino acid decarboxylase; DβH, dopamine β-hydroxylase; PNMT, phenylethanolamine-*N*-methyltransferase.
(b) The two major pathways for the metabolism of nor-epinephrine (NE) and epinephrine (E) in sympathetic neurons and adrenal chromaffin cells. *Metabolites*: DHPG, 3,4-dihydroxyphenylglycol; MN, metanephrine, NMN, nor-metanephrine, MHPG, 3-methoxy-4-hydroxyphenylglycol; VMA, vanillylmandelic acid. *Enzymes*: MAO, monoamine oxidase; COMT, catechol *O*-methyl transferase, ADH, alcohol dehydrogenase.
(c) The relative amounts of metabolites secreted in the urine. Sulfate conjugation of catecholamines and catecholamine metabolites, particularly MHPG, occurs mainly in mesenteric organs, whereas production of VMA occurs mainly in the liver.

number of proteins, including adrenomedullin. The output of the adrenal gland is controlled by nerve cells within the posterior hypothalamus which, via the spinal cord, ultimately stimulate the cholinergic pre-ganglionic nerve fibers innervating the adrenal medulla. This induces depolarization of the chromaffin cells and exocytosis of the catecholamine-containing granules following a transient rise in intracellular calcium concentration. The half-life of epinephrine and nor-epinephrine in the circulation is very short (approximately 1–2 min).

6.10.1 Actions of catecholamines

Catecholamines act on their target tissues through typical G-protein linked membrane receptors. These receptors are classified as α or β on the basis of the physiological and pharmacological effects induced by hormone binding. Further sub-classification into α_{1A}, α_{1B}, α_{2A}, α_{2B}, β_1, β_2, β_3 is also made depending on what specific drugs antagonize these receptors.

The physiological effects of the catecholamines are manifold and summarized in *Box 6.22*. They have been characterized as preparing us for 'fight or flight' with overall actions to increase heart rate and stroke volume, increase blood pressure, dilate bronchi, mobilize glucose, and stimulate lipolysis. These actions are mediated by β-adrenergic receptors. Blood flow to the splanchnic bed is reduced by vasoconstriction of arterioles via α-adrenergic receptors and this helps to divert blood flow to skeletal muscles.

Box 6.22 | Major actions of neuronal and/or adrenomedullary catecholamines

Cardiovascular actions

- Heart – increase in heart rate and force of contraction.
- Blood vessels – mainly vasoconstriction; dilatation in cardiac and skeletal muscle.

Metabolic and endocrine actions

- Increased glycogenolysis.
- Increased lipolysis.
- Increased glucagon secretion.
- Decreased insulin secretion.
- Stimulation of renin release.

Miscellaneous

- Dilatation of the pupil.
- Contraction of spleen.
- Ejaculation.
- Inhibition of micturition.

Whilst most catecholamines released from sympathetic nerves are taken back up into the pre-synaptic terminal (termed uptake$_1$), catecholamines released into the circulation are taken up by non-neuronal tissues (uptake$_2$) and rapidly converted to *O*-methylated products (metanephrine and nor-metanephrine) by catechol *O*-methyltransferase (COMT). These are subsequently degraded to 3-methoxy-4-hydroxyphenylglycol (MHPG) and finally to vanillylmandelic acid (VMA) (*Figure 6.17*). All these metabolites, as well as a very small proportion of unmetabolized catecholamines, are excreted in the urine in relative proportions and these may be conjugated with sulfate or glucuronide (*Figure 6.17*). The ratio of different metabolites circulating in the plasma or in the urine is important in the diagnosis of pheochromocytoma.

6.10.2 Pheochromocytomas

CASE 6.6 331

- Man of 26 years with sweating and palpitations and unprovoked panic attacks
- Normal electrolytes, chest X-ray, and thyroid function; hypertensive and tachycardic

A 26 year old man was referred to the endocrine clinic with sweating and palpitations. He had been investigated in primary care with normal electrolytes, chest X-ray, and thyroid function. On close questioning he mentioned that he suffered from regular panic attacks for no discernible reason. His partner commented that he would occasionally 'look like death' with extreme pallor. There was no significant personal history, but his sister (who was resident in Ghana) had recently undergone a total thyroidectomy but he was not sure of the reason behind this. On examination he was hypertensive (186/124 mmHg) with a resting tachycardia (92 beats/minute).

Pheochromocytomas are rare catecholamine-secreting tumors that arise from chromaffin tissue. As ever, the classification of these tumors is complex. Essentially, tumors may be intra-adrenal (where they are called pheochromocytomas) or extra-adrenal (where they are often called paragangliomas). Extra-adrenal paragangliomas may arise from sympathetic nervous system associated chromaffin cells (which produce catecholamines and may cause hypertension) or from parasympathetic tissue (usually head and neck tumors, which do not produce significant amounts of catecholamines and therefore are not usually associated with hypertension). To complicate things further, head and neck paragangliomas are frequently referred to as carotid body tumors or glomus tumors.

Around 85% of pheochromocytomas arise from the adrenal medulla and 15% from extra-adrenal chromaffin tissue; 20–30% are familial in origin, often in association with MEN-2 (see *Section 8.6*), the rest being sporadic. Familial pheochromocytomas are more frequently bilateral. The estimated incidence of pheochromocytoma is around 1–2/million/year and although this is low, it is a diagnosis worth considering in the hypertensive patient. Cure rates are excellent (at least 90%) whereas if left undiagnosed/untreated the condition can lead to malignant hypertension with associated heart failure, myocardial infarction, stroke, or death from metastatic disease.

Clinical features of pheochromocytomas

Around 5–10% of patients may be totally asymptomatic and present with an adrenal incidentaloma (see *Section 6.5.7*). Those patients that present with symptoms will generally have hypertension which may be sustained or intermittent. Postural hypotension is not uncommon but the myriad symptoms described are really rather non-specific (*Box 6.23*) and can make clinical diagnosis difficult. Usually investigations are carried out given a high index of suspicion, or in the work-up of a young patient with uncontrolled hypertension, or where there is a family history or a known mutation associated with pheochromocytoma (see below). In an ideal world a patient with pheochromocytoma would present with hypertension, recurrent headaches, palpitations, and sweating, or with extreme 'panic attacks'. Patients may describe an intermittent sensation akin to realizing they have just stepped into the road in front of a bus. Some 'attacks' may be precipitated by certain agents or situations and these include:

Box 6.23 | Symptoms of pheochromocytoma

Hypertension – sustained, intermittent

Hypotension – postural

- headache
- palpitations or tachycardia
- sweating
- pallor
- flushing
- anxiety
- chest pain
- fatigue
- constipation or diarrhea
- weight loss
- fever
- vomiting
- convulsions

This list is not exhaustive and reflects the difficulty in clinical diagnosis.

- drugs – ACTH, histamine, glucagon, tyramine, phenothiazines, metoclopramide
- ingestion of tyramine-containing foods, e.g. cheese, beer, wine
- exertion
- anxiety
- trauma
- pain
- intubation or anesthesia
- endoscopy
- micturition or catheterization (in extra-adrenal bladder tumors).

Diagnosis of pheochromocytoma

The first part of the diagnosis is clinical suspicion: patients presenting with uncontrolled, paroxysmal hypertension or with a clear precipitant warrant investigation. Secondly, a number of potential patients will have been identified through family screening programs where a proband has a known mutation associated with the development of pheochromocytoma. The genetics of this condition are discussed in *Box 6.24.*

Recent evidence strongly suggests that biochemical measurements of catecholamine metabolites (nor-metanephrine and metanephrine) are diagnostically superior to measurements of catecholamines themselves in the diagnosis of pheochromocytoma (*Table 6.1*). These can be measured in plasma or urine (or both). Numerous drugs (especially many classes of antihypertensive) will affect the measured levels of catecholamines or metanephrines, but it is often not practical to stop all medication in a known hypertensive patient while investigating an underlying cause. In this case the antihypertensives that have the fewest effects are selective alpha-blockers (doxazosin) and calcium channel blockers. Other known stimulants (caffeine, nicotine, alcohol) should be avoided for at least 12 hours before testing.

Once a biochemical diagnosis is strongly suggested it is important to localize the tumor(s). Both structural (CT/MRI) and functional scanning are generally employed.

Table 6.1. **Biochemical tests in the diagnosis of pheochromocytoma**

Biochemical test	Sensitivity (%)		Specificity (%)	
	Children	Adults	Children	Adults
Plasma nor-metanephrine and metanephrine	100	99	94	89
Plasma nor-epinephrine and epinephrine	92	84	91	81
Urinary nor-metanephrine and metanephrine	100	97	95	69
Urinary nor-epinephrine and epinephrine	100	86	83	88
Urinary vanillylmandelic acid	–	64	–	95

Children (based on 45 children studied, 12 pheochromocytomas): adapted from Weise *et al.* (2002) *J. Clin. Endocrinol. Metab.* **87**: 5038–43. Adults: adapted from Zelinka *et al.* (2007) *Stress,* **10**: 195–203 and Lenders *et al.* (2002) *J. Am. Med. Assoc.* **287**: 1427–34.

Box 6.24 | Genetics of pheochromocytoma

Several gene mutations are known to be involved in familial pheochromocytomas/paragangliomas:

- the von Hippel-Lindau (*VHL*) gene leading to VHL syndrome
- the *RET* gene leading to multiple endocrine neoplasia type 2 (MEN2A or 2B)
- the neurofibromatosis type 1 (*NF1*) gene associated with von Recklinghausen disease
- the genes encoding B, C, and D subunits of succinate dehydrogenase – associated with hereditary paraganglioma syndromes (PGL4 < PGL3 and PGL1 respectively)
- the gene encoding succinate dehydrogenase 5 (*SDH5*)

Patients with a family history warrant routine screening for pheochromocytoma even in the absence of symptoms and (given the ever increasing number of apparently spontaneous pheochromocytomas that are associated with germline mutations – around 25–30% of all tumors) an underlying hereditary condition should probably be considered even in the absence of an obvious family history. It is not unreasonable to recommend routine gene screening in all patients with pheochromocytoma.

Box table 6.6. **Hereditary pheochromocytoma: facts and figures**

Gene	*VHL*	*RET*	*NF1*	*SDHD*	*SDHB*
Chromosome	3p25–26	10q11.2	17q11.2	11q23	1p36.13
Exons	3	21	59	8	4
Frequency in 'sporadic' tumors (%)	2–11	1–5	Unknown	3–10	4–7
Predisposition to malignancy (%)	~3	<3	11	<2	66–83
Tumor catecholamine phenotype	NE	E	E	Unknown	Unknown
Adrenal disease	++	++	++	+	+
Extra-adrenal disease	+	–	+	++	++

Abbreviations:
VHL, von Hippel–Lindau syndrome; RET, rearranged in transfection; NF1, neurofibromatosis type 1; SDHD and SDHB, succinate dehydrogenase subunit D and B.
Tumor catecholamine phenotypes are designated as either epinephrine-producing (E) or predominantly nor-epinephrine-producing (NE).

von Hippel–Lindau disease

The incidence of pheochromocytoma in VHL is variable and dependent on the site of the mutation, but overall is 15–20%, i.e. about 15–20% of patients with VHL will develop pheochromocytoma. Presentation is usually in the third decade of life and bilateral disease is common (around 50%).

MEN2A and 2B

The development of pheochromocytomas in patients with MEN2A or 2B is common – around 50% – the diagnosis usually following that of medullary thyroid cancer. In MEN2A the majority of pheochromocytomas are benign, adrenal and unilateral, whereas in MEN2B approximately 35% are bilateral and a significant percentage of patients develop a second contralateral pheochromocytoma. Prognosis is good after surgical resection.

Neurofibromatosis type 1

The incidence of pheochromocytoma in neurofibromatosis type 1 is about 1% with a rather later presentation – usually in the fifth decade.

Succinate dehydrogenase mutations

Mutations of these genes are associated with relatively high rates of extra-adrenal tumors. *SDHB* mutations are more frequently associated with a higher rate of malignancy (B = bad). Mediastinal paragangliomas are rare (accounting for only 2% of all paragangliomas) but are commonly associated with *SDH* gene mutations and have a tendency to present with metastatic disease. It is worth screening all patients with mediastinal paragangliomas assessed for *SDH* gene mutations regardless of age.

CT/MRI has around a 95% success rate in initial tumor localization; the abdomen and pelvis would usually be scanned first and, if negative, mediastinum and neck scans would follow. Whilst these scans would confirm structural lesions, functional scanning is usually necessary for confirmation of the diagnosis and to determine the extent of disease. MIBG is a guanethidine analog which is structurally similar to nor-epinephrine and which can be concentrated by chromaffin tissue of the adrenal medulla. [^{123}I]-MIBG scintigraphy is useful in diagnosis, but the sensitivity of the scan is often somewhat reduced in extra-adrenal and malignant disease. Newer modalities including octreotide scans (with radiolabeled somatostatin analogs) and PET scans are an alternative with promising results (particularly in some case of familial paragangliomas).

Treatment of pheochromocytomas

The aim of treatment is surgical resection of the tumor, generally using a laparoscopic approach. One challenging aspect is the risk of uncontrolled catecholamine release resulting in hypertensive crises and arrhythmias. Pre-operative blockade is with alpha-blockers, usually phenoxybenzamine, which is given in a dose of 10–20 mg twice a day, often with an extra dose (about 1 mg/kg) given the night before surgery. This antagonizes the vasoconstrictor effects of catecholamines. Alternatives to phenoxybenzamine include selective α_1-blockers (e.g. doxazosin or terazosin) and occasionally calcium channel antagonists. Beta-blockers can be added to improve control of tachyarrhythmias and angina but it is essential to adequately block alpha activity initially because otherwise the unopposed vasoconstrictive activity of catecholamines may lead to hypertensive crises.

Some centers advocate the use of Demser (metyrosine or α-methyl-L-tyrosine or α-MPT) both pre- and post-operatively, particularly where adequate control cannot be achieved with combined alpha- and beta-blockade. Demser inhibits tyrosine hydroxylase which catalyzes the first step in catecholamine biosynthesis, thus resulting in decreased levels of catecholamines (*Figure 6.17a*).

Post-operative complications also include hypotension and hypoglycemia (due to the sudden loss of excess catecholamines that regulate glucose) and these can be managed by adequate restoration of circulating volume and by dextrone infusion.

The long-term prognosis for non-malignant pheochromocytoma is good, although up to 50% of patients may remain hypertensive; a large proportion of these patients may have co-existing idiopathic hypertension. Biochemical screening to ascertain cure (at about 14–28 days post-operation) and subsequent screening for evidence of recurrence (up to 20% of patients) is required. Long-term follow-up is particularly important in those patients harboring disease-causing gene mutations.

Malignant pheochromocytomas have an incidence varying from 3 to 30% depending on location and genetic background. The prognosis is much worse, particularly where there are lung or liver metastases. The likelihood of metastatic malignant pheochromocytoma is increased in larger lesions, those that are extra-adrenal, and in patients harboring the SDHB mutation (*Box 6.24*). Surgery to reduce tumor size may give symptomatic relief but there is no compelling evidence yet that it increases overall survival rates. Treatment is with [^{131}I]-MIBG (if there is demonstrable MIBG uptake on a localizing scan) or chemotherapy (cyclophosphamide, vincristine, dacarbazine). If these agents fail or are contraindicated there is some evidence for the use of octreotide if the octreotide scan shows positive uptake. A number of experimental chemotherapeutic regimens form the basis of ongoing trials.

CASE 6.6 326 331

- Man of 26 years with sweating and palpitations and unprovoked panic attacks
- Normal electrolytes, chest X-ray, and thyroid function; hypertensive and tachycardic
- Pheochromocytoma suspected; urinary catecholamines revealed elevated epinephrine and slightly raised nor-epinephrine, with normal dopamine
- MRI imaging showed 4 cm lesion in right adrenal gland – a full recovery was made after removal

The combination of hypertension, tachycardia, pallor, and sweating with well-described 'panic attacks' suggested that a diagnosis of pheochromocytoma was a strong possibility. Urinary catecholamines revealed elevated epinephrine, marginally elevated nor-epinephrine and normal dopamine. Plasma metanephrine and nor-metanephrine levels were raised. MRI imaging revealed a 4 cm lesion in the right adrenal gland which avidly took up radiolabeled MIBG. In view of the family history of thyroidectomy, genetic screening for MEN-2 (see *Chapter 8*) was undertaken but was negative. After appropriate medical stabilization, the patient underwent unilateral adrenalectomy and made an uneventful recovery. Two years post-operatively there was no symptomatic or biochemical suggestion of recurrence and he remains well.

6.11 Further reading

Adler JT, Meyer-Rochow GY, Chen H, *et al.* (2008) Pheochromocytoma: current approaches and future directions. *The Oncologist,* **13:** 779–93.

Bertagna X, Guignat L, Groussin L, and Bertherat J (2009) Cushing's disease. *Best Pract. Res. Clin. Endocrinol. Metab.* **23:** 607–23.

Betterie C and Morlin L (2011) Autoimmune Addison's disease. *Endocrine Devel.* **20:** 161–72.

Buckingham JC (2006) Glucocorticoids: exemplars of multi-tasking. *Br. J. Pharmacol.* **147:** S258–68.

Buckingham JC, John CD, Solito E, *et al.* (2006) Annexin 1, glucocorticoids, and the neuroendocrine-immune interface. *Ann. N.Y. Acad. Sci.* **1088:** 396–409.

Connell JMC and Davies E (2005) The new biology of aldosterone. *J. Endocrinol.* **186:** 1–20.

D'Acquisto F (2009) On the adaptive nature of annexin-A1. *Curr. Opin. Pharmacol.* **9:** 521–8.

Fuller PJ and Young MJ (2005) Mechanisms of mineralocorticoid action. *Hypertension,* **46:** 1227–35.

Fung MM, Viveros OH, and O'Connor DT (2008) Diseases of the adrenal medulla. *Acta Physiol. (Oxf.)* **192:** 325–35.

Hammer F and Stewart PM (2006) Cortisol metabolism in hypertension. *Best Pract. Res. Clin. Endocrinol. Metab.* **20:** 337–53.

Husebye E and Løvås K (2009) Pathogenesis of primary adrenal insufficiency. *Best Pract. Res. Clin. Endocrinol. Metab.* **23:** 147–57.

Merke D and Bornstein SR (2005) Congenital adrenal hyperplasia. *Lancet,* **365:** 2125–36.

Newell-Price J, Bertagna X, Grossman AB, and Nieman LK (2006) Cushing's Syndrome. *Lancet,* **367:** 1605–17.

Nieman LK and Chanco Turner ML (2006) Addison's disease. *Clinics Dermatol.* **24:** 276–80.

Nimkarn S and New MI (2007) Prenatal diagnosis and treatment of congenital adrenal hyperplasia. *Hormone Res.* **67:** 53–60.

Rayner B (2008) Primary aldosteronism and aldosterone-associated hypertension. *J. Clin. Pathol.* **61:** 825–31.

Revollo JR and Cidlowski JA (2009) Mechanisms generating diversity in glucocorticoid receptor signaling. *Annals N.Y. Acad. Sci.* **1179:** 167–78.

Rhen T and Cidlowski JA (2005) Antiinflammatory action of glucocorticoids – new mechanisms for old drugs. *New Engl. J. Med.* **353:** 1711–23.

Tritos NA, Biller BM, and Swearingen B (2011) Management of Cushing disease. *Nature Rev. Endocrinol.* **7:** 279–89.

Useful websites

Addison disease:
www.ncbi.nlm.nih.gov/pubmedhealth/PMH0001416/

www.nhs.uk/conditions/addisons-disease

Cushing syndrome:
http://endocrine.niddk.nih.gov/pubs/cushings/cushings.aspx

6.12 Self-assessment questions

(1) The actions of cortisol include which one of the following?
- (a) Stimulation of macrophage function
- (b) Reduction of blood pressure
- (c) Stimulation of glucose uptake into muscle
- (d) Inhibition of insulin signaling in muscle and adipose tissue
- (e) Reduction of glucose levels

(2) The synthesis of adrenal steroids requires which one of the following?
- (a) The transport of cholesterol from lipid droplets to mitochondria by StAR protein
- (b) The conversion of cholesterol to pregnenolone by 3β-hydroxysteroid dehydrogenase
- (c) The conversion of 17α-progesterone to cortisol and androgens
- (d) The conversion of corticosterone to aldosterone by CYP17
- (e) The synthesis of deoxycortisol to cortisol by CYP21A

(3) Which one of the following is most likely to be associated with decreased ACTH secretion?
- (a) Steroidal anti-inflammatory drugs
- (b) Pheochromocytoma
- (c) Cushing disease
- (d) A synacthen test
- (e) Addison disease

(4) The anti-inflammatory and immunosuppressant actions of glucocorticoids include which one of the following?
 (a) Decreased expression of annexin 1
 (b) Increased activity of cyclo-oxygenase
 (c) Activation of macrophages
 (d) Inhibition of prostaglandin synthesis
 (e) Increased antibody production

(5) In Cushing syndrome, which one of the following statements is true?
 (a) ACTH levels are always low
 (b) Pigmentation never occurs
 (c) Hypokalemia is always present
 (d) Long term alcohol excess may produce a similar clinical phenotype
 (e) Very low basal ACTH levels suggest an adrenal lesion

(6) In primary hyperaldosteronism, which one of the following is true?
 (a) Solitary adenomas are the usual cause
 (b) Aldosterone-producing adenomas are usually more than 5 cm in diameter
 (c) Hypokalemia always occurs
 (d) The aldosterone:renin ratio is useful in the diagnosis
 (e) Treatment is always surgical

(7) Which one of the following statements about congenital adrenal hyperplasia is true? It:
 (a) Is an autosomal dominant disorder
 (b) Is most commonly associated with 21-hydroxylase deficiency
 (c) Is always associated with cortisol deficiency
 (d) Is easily diagnosed in male infants
 (e) Is always associated with salt wasting

(8) A 54 year old woman was referred to the outpatient department with weight loss, increasing pigmentation, and a supine systolic blood pressure of 50 mmHg. Addison disease was suspected. Which one of the following tests might best confirm diagnosis?
 (a) Dexamethasone suppression test
 (b) 24 h urinary cortisol measurement
 (c) Measurement of plasma ACTH levels
 (d) Midnight salivary cortisol measurement
 (e) Synacthen test

(9) A 54 year old man was referred for evaluation of a 2.5 cm lesion found on an abdominal CT scan during investigation of non-specific abdominal discomfort. On closer questioning he admitted to weight gain of 9 kg over the last year, muscular fatigue, and easy bruising. He was hypertensive on treatment with an ACE inhibitor and a loop diuretic. There was no previous significant personal history and no family history of note. Initial investigation revealed an elevated fasting blood sugar (7.2 mmol/L), a cortisol level of 622 nmol/L at 09.00h (NR 110–520) with a simultaneous ACTH level of <1 pmol/L (NR <26).
 (a) What is the most likely diagnosis?
 (b) How would you confirm the diagnosis?
 (c) What is the most appropriate treatment?

(10) A 45 year old man complained of excessive fatigue, abdominal cramps, and light-headedness during the last 6–8 months. He had lost 5 kg in weight during this time and a friend recently commented on his sun-tanned appearance. After an intramuscular injection of 250 μg tetracosactrin (synacthen) his circulating cortisol concentrations rose from 180 to 240 nmol/L at 60 minutes (NR >480) and a random ACTH test showed elevated concentrations of this trophic hormone.

(a) Based on this evidence what diagnosis would you suggest?
(b) Why does this patient have a sun-tanned appearance?
(c) Why were his circulating ACTH concentrations raised?
(d) How might you treat this patient?

CHAPTER 07 The gonads

After working through this chapter you should be able to:

- Outline the genetic control of sex differentiation
- Describe how hormones control the differentiation of the internal reproductive tracts and external genitalia
- Outline the hormonal and physical changes associated with puberty (adrenarche and gonadarche) and the concept of consonance
- Identify the causes, investigation, and treatment of precocious and delayed puberty
- Describe the hormones and their effects in controlling testicular and ovarian function and the actions of sex steroids secreted by the gonads
- Outline the processes of spermatogenesis, oogenesis, and folliculogenesis
- Identify the causes, investigations, and treatments of male and female infertility
- Describe the pathophysiology of PCOS and its treatment
- Distinguish between premature ovarian failure and the menopause

7.1 Introduction – hormones of gonadal control

The gonads, like the thyroid gland and adrenal cortex, are controlled by hormone secretions from the hypothalamic–pituitary axis. The hormone secreted from neurons in the hypothalamus is gonadotropin releasing hormone (GnRH), a decapeptide which stimulates the synthesis and secretion of the two glycoprotein hormones, luteinizing hormone (LH) and follicle stimulating hormone (FSH) from the gonadotrophs of the anterior pituitary gland. GnRH acts on GPCRs, with the major signaling pathway being the inositol pathway which produces inositol triphosphate and diacylglycerol (*Chapter* [illegible]) which activate further downstream intracellular signals. GnRH is secreted in a pulsatile manner and the frequency and amplitude of these pulses is controlled by feedback effects of gonadal steroids, primarily testosterone from the testis and progesterone and estradiol from the ovaries.

LH and FSH have distinct targets on the testis and ovaries and both act on GPCRs to activate adenyl cyclase and the production of cAMP (*Chapter 1*). They are essential for stimulating the production of steroids from the gonads and for regulating spermatogenesis and folliculogenesis. Thus, unlike the thyroid gland and adrenal cortex, whose sole function is to secrete hormones, the gonads not only secrete hormones essential for sexual development and maintenance of the reproductive tracts, but they also produce gametes required for reproduction and continuation of the species.

7.2 Sexual determination and differentiation

CASE 7.1 336 343

- Girl of 16 years presenting with primary amenorrhea
- Tall with BMI of 19 and no axillary or pubic hair
- 46,XY, with high LH, FSH, and testosterone but normal estradiol
- Ultrasound revealed absence of ovaries and uterus

A 16 year old girl presented to the endocrine clinic with primary amenorrhea. She was born of non-consanguineous parents and there was a family history of delayed puberty. Her only past medical history was childhood asthma. She was not on any regular medication.

On examination she had a normal female appearance. She was quite tall at 5′9″ (176 cm) with a BMI of 19 kg/m^2. Axillary and pubic hair were absent. She had underdeveloped breasts recorded at Tanner stage 2 (see *Figure 7.7*). External genitalia were normal and her vaginal canal was 5 cm in length.

Investigations revealed:

- LH 38.4 IU/L (NR luteal 0.8–10.4)
- FSH 12.9 IU/L (NR luteal 2.6–9.5)
- testosterone 17.7 nmol/L (NR 0.5–3.0)
- estradiol 138 pmol/L (NR 70–1100)

Androstenedione, DHEA-S, 17-hydroxyprogesterone, prolactin, and thyroid function tests were normal. Pelvic ultrasound showed absence of both uterus and ovaries. MRI showed no obvious gonadal tissue. Chromosome analysis confirmed a 46,XY karyotype.

7.2.1 Development of the gonads and internal reproductive tracts

Phenotypic sexual development can be viewed as a two step process:

- development of either the testes or ovaries (**sex determination**)
- **sexual differentiation** of the male or female reproductive tract.

Since studies in the early 1940s, it had been considered that the genetically determined development of the testis (presence of the Y chromosome) was required for male development and that ovarian development was simply passive. Subsequently the sex determining region on the Y chromosome, *SRY*, was identified as the gene directing male development. However, more recent genetic studies have shown that complete or partial sex reversal of XX embryos to a male phenotype has been observed in humans with loss or gain of function of genes expressed in early sexual determination of the female phenotype. It has therefore been established that ovarian development is dependent on the active repression of one or more genes in the testicular pathway rather than it depending entirely on a passive 'default' pathway (*Figure 7.1*). However, the male determining region of the Y chromosome

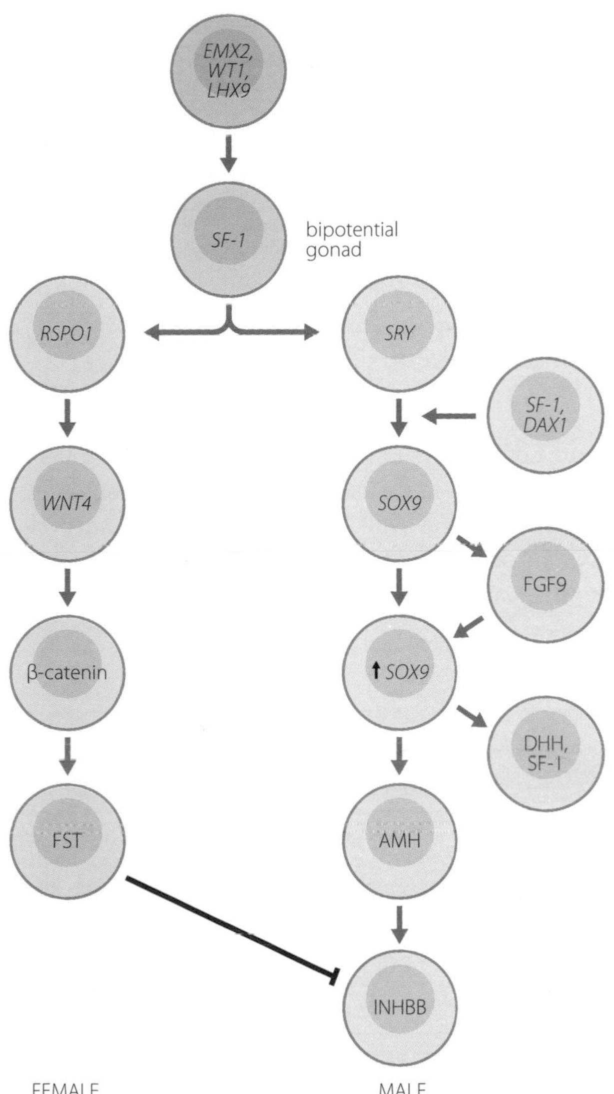

Figure 7.1. Genetic control of sex determination.

Current evidence suggests that the expression of *EMX2, WT1,* and *LHX9* determines the development of the bipotential gonad into which the germ cells migrate. The expression of steroidogenic factor 1 (*SF-1*) then initiates the transient expression of *SRY* in pre-Sertoli cells of an XY gonad. In turn *SRY*, along with *DAX1* and *SF-1*, up-regulates the expression of *SOX9*. *SOX9* also up-regulates *FGF9* that signals back through the FGFR2 to maintain or increase *SOX9* expression, thereby creating a positive feedback loop. When the expression of *SOX9* reaches a critical level the expression of *SRY* is switched off. The target genes of *SOX9* include *AMH* (anti-Müllerian hormone), *DHH, SF-1,* and *prostaglandin D synthase*. The ovarian differentiation pathway involves *RSPO1* increasing signaling of *WNT4* which up-regulates β-catenin and this in turn stimulates the expression of follistatin (FST). β-catenin suppresses *SOX9* expression whilst the testis pathway appears to mainly antagonize the ovarian pathway through decreasing *β-catenin* expression. Loss of function mutations of *RSPO* and *WNT4* can cause sex reversal of an XX genotype to a male phenotype despite absence of the *SRY* gene, whilst overexpression of *WNT4* or *DAX1* induces XY sex reversal, known as dosage sensitive sex reversal. Mutations of the *SRY* gene or an insufficiency of *SOX9* expression also causes XY sex reversal. Thus female sex determination can no longer be considered as the 'default pattern'.

is very powerful in that individuals with 47,XXY (Klinefelter syndrome) or even 49,XXXXY are unequivocally male at birth, whilst the inheritance of only one chromosome X0 (Turner syndrome) still leads to the development of the female phenotype (see *Section 7.4.3*).

Around the 5th week of gestation, primordial germ cells begin to migrate from the yolk sac into the bi-potential germinal ridges which are first recognized as thickenings underlying the coelomic epithelium adjacent to the mesonephros (*Figure 7.2*). The migration is complete by about the 6th week and the germ cells are incorporated into the primary sex cords formed from somatic cells derived from the coelomic epithelium. These sex cords will eventually become the Sertoli cells of the testis. After this point XY germ cells arrest in mitosis and do not divide again until postnatally as spermatogonia, whilst the XX germ cells continue to divide mitotically before entering their first meiotic division and arresting at the diplotene stage. The oogonia remain in this stage until they finally emerge as the oocyte of a dominant follicle that will be ovulated in any one menstrual cycle. Some eggs will remain in this state of suspended animation for about 50 years until the occurrence of the menopause.

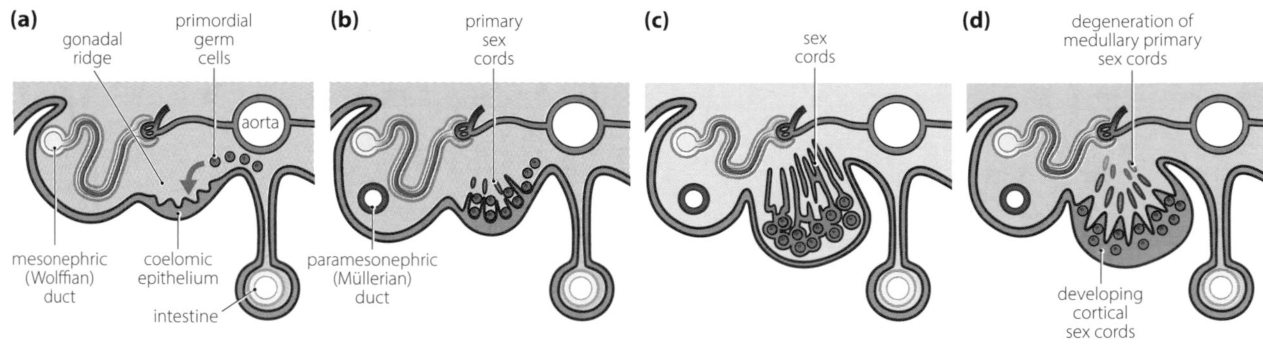

Figure 7.2. Embryogenesis of the gonads.
(a) Between embryonic weeks 4 and 6, primordial germ cells migrate from the yolk sac into the genital ridge.
(b) Cells of the thickened coelomic epithelium then proliferate and invade the gonadal ridge where they form the primary sex cords. The anlage of both the paramesonephric (Müllerian) and mesonephric (Wolffian) ducts have developed.
(c) Differentiation of the testis begins around embryonic week 7, when the somatic cells of the sex cords (the future Sertoli cells) incorporate the primordial germ cells and they begin to secrete AMH. By the 8th fetal week, Leydig cells begin to differentiate from the somatic cells and these secrete testosterone which is essential to the development of the male reproductive tract.
(d) In females the primary sex cords degenerate and the primordial cells retain their connection to the surface epithelial cells (the cortical region). These somatic cells will become the granulosa cells and stromal cells of the ovary.

By week 8, Leydig cells differentiate from interstitial cells in the fetal testis and begin to secrete testosterone. At this time the primary sex cords are degenerating in the female fetus and the cortical sex cords are beginning to form. These will eventually break up into clusters, surround the primitive oogonia, forming primordial follicles and subsequently differentiate into granulosa cells. Interstitial cells in the female will become ovarian stromal cells, some of which will develop into theca cells during folliculogenesis. At week 8 the human fetus has both Wolffian (mesonephric) and

Müllerian (paramesonephric) ducts that are the embryonic precursors of the male and female reproductive tracts, respectively (*Figure 7.2*).

The transcription factor SOX-9 stimulates the production of anti-Müllerian hormone (AMH) in the Sertoli cells which causes the Müllerian ducts to regress and, under the influence of testosterone, the Wolffian ducts develop into the epididymis, the vas deferens, and the seminal vesicles (*Figure 7.3*). Testicular descent during sexual development occurs in two phases. In the first phase it migrates from the kidney and by week 24 it has reached the inguinal ring. The second phase occurs in the last 2 months of fetal life with the testis passing through the inguinal canal to reach the scrotum, i.e. from the abdomen to the scrotum. This movement is dependent on the differential development of one of two ligaments – the gubernaculum and the cranial suspensory ligament (CSL). In male development the gubernaculum grows and the CLS regresses, and evidence suggests that regression of the CLS is induced by testosterone whilst development of the gubernaculum is stimulated by insulin-like hormone 3 (Insl3) which is expressed in fetal Leydig cells. Thus both testosterone and Insl3 are an absolute requirement for migration of the testis and in 97% of newborns the testes are in a scrotal position. In the female fetus the gubernaculum regresses and the CSL holds the ovaries in a position lateral to the kidneys.

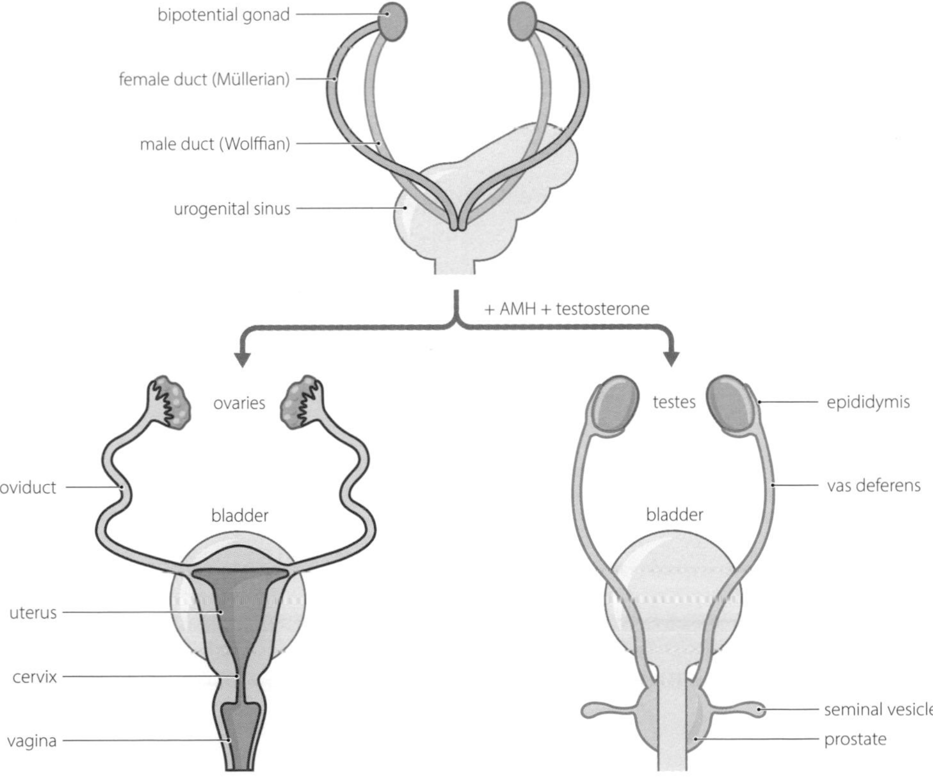

Figure 7.3. Sexual differentiation of the gonads and of the male and female internal reproductive tracts from the Wolffian and Müllerian ducts.
The differentiation of the bipotential gonadal anlage into either an ovary or testis is initially dependent on the expression of specific sets of genes (see *Figure 7.1*) and subsequently the production of testosterone and AMH in male fetuses. These hormones are important in testicular development, Müllerian duct regression and, under the action of testosterone, the development of both the internal and external parts of the reproductive tract (see *Figure 7.6*).

Development of female internal genitalia in an XY fetus is due to the incapacity of the Sertoli cells to secrete bioactive AMH or to defects in the AMH receptor type 2. These result in persistent Müllerian duct syndrome and affected patients present with a male phenotype, usually with bilateral cryptorchidism (undescended testes) and inguinal hernia. Leydig cell function is retained but azoospermia is common due to malformation of the vas deferens or agenesis of the epididymis.

In the absence of AMH, the Müllerian ducts develop to form the fallopian tubes, uterus, cervix, and upper part of the vagina, while the Wolffian ducts begin to degenerate (*Figure 7.3*). This female differentiation begins around the 10th week of gestation. Around the same time the germ cells, now destined to become oogonia, begin to enter their first meiotic division and by about week 15 of gestation they become surrounded by a layer of granulosa cells to form primordial follicles (some 8 weeks after the differentiation of the testes). At birth each ovary contains approximately 2 million primordial follicles, though this declines to around 400 000 by menarche (*Figure 7.4*). There is a vast overprovision of potential follicles and many become atretic well before the menopause. Thus females are born with all the eggs they will ever have, in contrast to the male germ cells or spermatogonia that continue to divide from puberty throughout life.

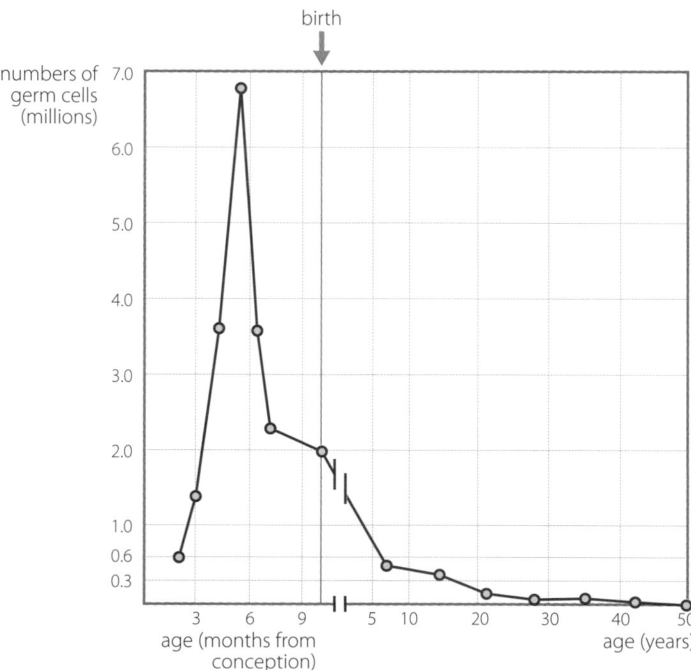

Figure 7.4. Changes in the number of germ cells in the human ovary during fetal development and throughout postnatal life.
Primordial follicles are formed in the fetus between 6 and 9 months after conception. During this period, a marked loss of oocytes occurs due to apoptosis. At birth the ovary contains approximately 2 million oocytes which are half-way through their first meiotic division. Throughout a woman's reproductive life only about 0.02% of the eggs she is born with will ever reach maturity and be ovulated, the rest gradually becoming depleted through atresia. At the menopause, all remaining ovarian follicles will undergo atresia with their oocytes having been in arrested meiosis for over 50 years.

7.2.2 Sexual development of the external genitalia

Like the bipotential gonads, the structures that develop into the external genitalia are initially identical in both sexes and develop from the same precursors: the genital or labioscrotal swelling, the urogenital or urethral fold, the genital tubercle, and the urogenital sinus (*Figure 7.5*).

In the male fetus between weeks 7 and 13 of gestation the labioscrotal swellings migrate and become the scrotum; the urogenital folds enlarge and enclose the penile urethra and corpus spongiosa; the genital tubercle becomes the glans penis and the urogenital sinus forms the prostate gland. Hypospadias arises when the urethra is not completely enclosed by the urogenital or urethral folds. The development of the

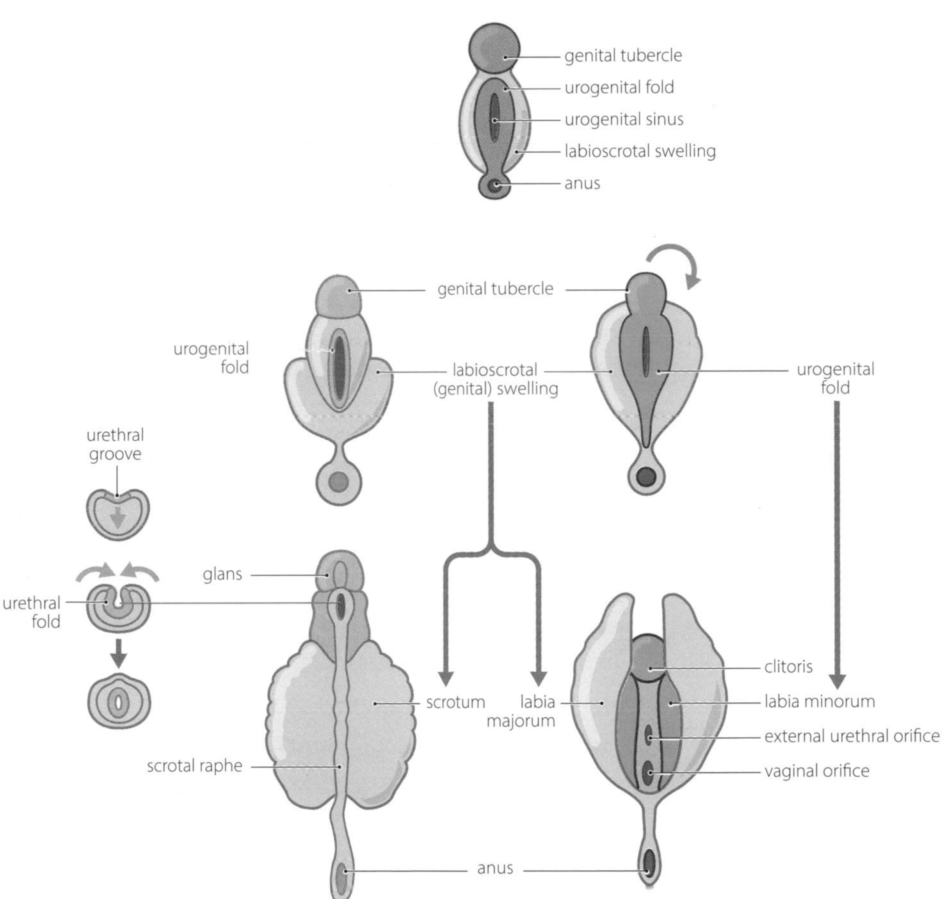

Figure 7.5. Sexual differentiation of the external genitalia.
In males the genital tubercle elongates and forms the shaft and glans of the penis. As the genital tubercle is elongating and growing to form the penis, the urogenital folds, which lie on either side of the urogenital sinus, begin to move towards each other forming a groove, known as the urethral groove. The urogenital folds eventually fuse together on the ventral side of the developing penis, enclosing what will now become the spongy urethra. If the urogenital folds fail to close, hypospadias results. The tip of the penis, which is now called the glans, then begins to form a cord of epithelial cells which meets the penile urethra and, when the cord canalizes, formation of the urethra is complete. The labioscrotal swelling folds to form the scrotum. The line of fusion long the scrotum is called the scrotal raphé.
In females the genital tubercle bends inferiorly to form the clitoris. The urogenital folds, which do not fuse, form the labia minora and the labioscrotal (genital) swelling develop into the labia majora. The vagina and the urethra open into the vestibule of the urogenital sinus.

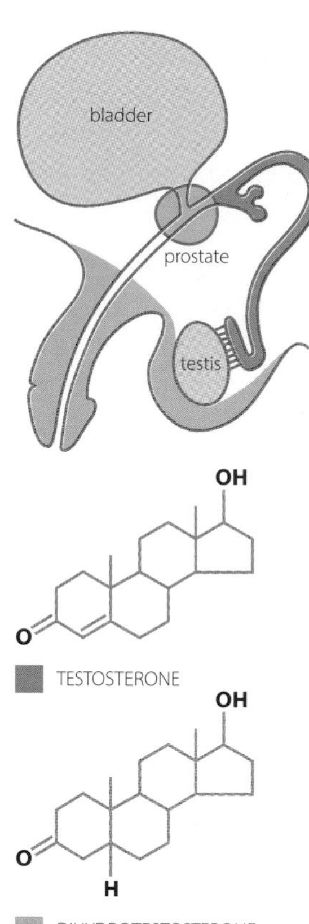

Figure 7.6. Roles of testosterone and dihydrotestosterone in the development of the internal and external male reproductive tract.
Testosterone is required for the development of the vas deferens and the seminal vesicles whilst its metabolite, dihydrotestosterone (formed by the enzyme 5α-reductase), is important in the development of the external genitalia (see *Figure 7.5*) and the prostate gland.

external male phenotype also requires testosterone secreted by the fetal Leydig cells, but unlike differentiation of the internal reproductive tract the testosterone must first be converted to 5α-dihydrotestosterone within the embryonic cells that will form the scrotum, penis, and prostate gland (*Figure 7.6*).

Female differentiation begins later and, in the absence of testosterone, the labioscrotal swellings form the labia majora; the urogenital folds remain unfused and form the labia minora; the genital tubercle forms the clitoris and the urogenital sinus the lower two-thirds of the vagina (*Figure 7.5*). Unlike male differentiation, this development appears to be independent of gonadal steroids. Up until 15 weeks of gestation the size of the external genitalia are roughly similar in males and females and it is not until the 2nd and 3rd trimesters that the growth of the male external genitalia and descent of the testes into the scrotum take place.

7.2.3 Androgen insensitivity syndromes

In view of the essential role of testosterone in the development of the male reproductive tract, it is obvious that defects in androgen signaling, or in the synthesis of androgens, would have marked effects on sexual differentiation. The androgen insensitivity syndrome (AIS) may be either complete (complete AIS, CAIS) or partial (PAIS). It results from a mutation in the androgen receptor gene located on chromosome Xq11–12. Several mutations may occur, inherited in an X-linked recessive fashion, although they can occur spontaneously. Major gene deletions result in CAIS but the more common amino acid substitution can result in any of the phenotypes. The incidence is 1:20 000 to 1:64 000.

The clinical picture of CAIS is quite homogeneous and, whilst the genotype is 46,XY, the main phenotypic characteristics of individuals with CAIS are: female external genitalia, a short, blind-ending vagina, absence of Wolffian duct derived structures (epididymides, vasa deferentia and seminal vesicles), and absence of the prostate gland and pubic and axillary hair, all of which depend on androgens for their development. The testes also fail to descend. Müllerian duct derived structures are usually absent because AMH is produced by the embryonic testes.

If CAIS is not detected in prenatal screening, it can be identified at puberty with complete breast development (androgens secreted by the patient's undescended testes are converted to estrogens), primary amenorrhea (no ovaries), and reduced or absent pubic hair. Removal of the undescended testes is indicated because of a high risk of testicular tumors.

In PAIS, several phenotypes ranging from individuals with a predominantly female appearance (e.g. external female genitalia and pubic hair at puberty, or with mild clitoromegaly, and some fusion of the labia) to those with ambiguous genitalia, or individuals with a predominantly male phenotype (also called Reifenstein syndrome). Patients from this latter group can present with a micropenis, perinea hypospadias, and cryptorchidism. In this group of PAIS individuals, Wolffian duct derived structures can be partially or even fully developed, depending on the biochemical phenotype of the androgen receptor mutation. At puberty, elevated LH, testosterone, and estradiol levels are observed, but in general the degree of feminization is less than that seen in individuals with CAIS. Individuals with mild symptoms of undervirilization and infertility have also been described. There is a 9% risk of seminoma (germ cell tumors of the testis).

Investigations and management

Testosterone levels are usually within the normal range (10–40 nmol/L) or are slightly elevated, while elevated LH levels (>10 IU/L) are also found, indicating androgen resistance at the hypothalamic–pituitary level. The high testosterone levels are also a substrate for aromatase activity, resulting in substantial amounts of estrogens, which are responsible for further feminization in CAIS individuals.

Orchidectomy is usually performed in adolescence, after attaining puberty, to prevent malignancy. In phenotypic females with partial androgen insensitivity, gonadectomy may be performed before puberty to avoid virilization. Estrogen replacement therapy is indicated in aphenotypic women. High dose androgen therapy in males with Reifenstein syndrome may improve virilization.

Several different 46,XY disorders of sex differentiation due to defects in testosterone synthesis have been described. These range from complete or partial forms of Leydig cell hypoplasia (from complete absence to a reduction in testosterone secretion) to defects in the enzymes responsible for the synthesis of testosterone and 5α-dihydrotestosterone (*Figure 7.6*). The degree of impairment will determine a range of phenotypes: a complete female (but absence of an internal female reproductive tract), ambiguous genitalia, and milder defects in male development with male external genitalia but micropenis and/or hypospadias.

CASE 7.1 336 343

- Girl of 16 years presenting with primary amenorrhea
- Tall with BMI of 19 and no axillary or pubic hair
- 46,XY, with high LH, FSH, and testosterone but normal estradiol
- Ultrasound revealed absence of ovaries and uterus
- Following counseling patient was started on estrogen replacement

It was clear that this patient was genetically (karyotypically) male but with feminine features and a female upbringing. The key here is to establish the way forward with the patient and to involve psychological support and counseling from the earliest stage: the role of a multidisciplinary team cannot be overstressed. The patient was appropriately counseled and it was clear that she had a female identity. Estrogen replacement was initiated. Serial imaging was unable to demonstrate any gonadal tissue, so the risk of malignancy and the need for surgical intervention to remove gonadal tissue was reduced. The absence of a uterus clearly made fertility sadly impossible.

7.2.4 Steroid production in the fetal and neonatal gonads

The development of the hypothalamic–pituitary connection through the hypophyseal portal veins is only established between 11 and 12 weeks after conception, some 3 weeks after the onset of testosterone production by the developing Leydig cells. Early sexual differentiation therefore depends on the secretion of human chorionic gonadotrophin (hCG) from the placenta. This hormone has a high affinity for the LH receptor and is secreted in high concentrations in the first trimester of pregnancy and is mainly responsible for the first peak of testosterone secretion which occurs between weeks 12 and 14 of gestation during fetal differentiation of the Leydig cells. The detection of hCG, which is secreted shortly after conception, forms the basis of the pregnancy test.

Gradually, the fetal hypothalamic–pituitary–gonadal axis matures and peripheral blood concentrations of fetal pituitary LH and FSH peak around mid-gestation,

Box 7.1 | Secretion of gonadotropins

The secretory patterns of LH and FSH vary widely throughout life (*Box figure 7.1a*), and the differential release of LH versus FSH, or vice versa, is partly dependent on the secretory patterns of GnRH secretion. The release of GnRH into the hypophyseal portal blood occurs in bursts and the frequency of these pulses (approximately each hour) is controlled by the GnRH 'pulse generator', a term used to describe the highly synchronized firing of the hypothalamic neurons. GnRH acts on the gonadotrophs in the anterior pituitary gland and stimulates the synthesis and pulsatile release of LH and FSH into the circulation.

The frequency and amplitude of the GnRH pulses are regulated by feedback effects of gonadal steroids and other factors affecting the hypothalamic–pituitary–gonadal axis. In turn the pattern of pulsatile GnRH release will determine the magnitude of the LH and FSH responses because GnRH regulates its own receptors on the pituitary gonadotroph. This has important implications in the normal physiology of gonadal function because increasing pulsatile frequency can increase the gonadotropin responses and the frequency and amplitude of the pulses can determine the preferential release of one or other of the gonadotropins. Loss of endogenous GnRH secretion results in the loss of GnRH receptors and the LH response to a bolus injection of GnRH is very low.

In complete contrast, when the gonadotrophs are exposed to a continuous GnRH stimulation, as occurs when patients are given long-acting GnRH agonists or antagonists, the GnRH receptors become down-regulated and internalized and LH and FSH secretions are completely suppressed (*Box figure 7.1b*). Whilst both antagonists and agonists are used clinically to suppress LH and FSH secretions, GnRH agonists will initially stimulate gonadotropin secretion prior to down-regulation of the GnRH receptors; an effect not observed with pure antagonists. Such analogs can be used in the treatment of precocious puberty, IVF cycles (to inhibit endogenous hormone secretions prior to exogenous gonadotropin therapy), endometriosis, and for endocrine-dependent cancers (in this regard antagonists are always used to avoid the initial flare of gonadotropin secretion). Essentially, analogs induce a 'chemical' (and reversible) gonadectomy. Thus patients who have hypothalamic hypogonadotropic hypogonadism (e.g. in Kallmann syndrome) have to be treated with pulsatile GnRH therapy administered intravenously via a programmable infusion pump.

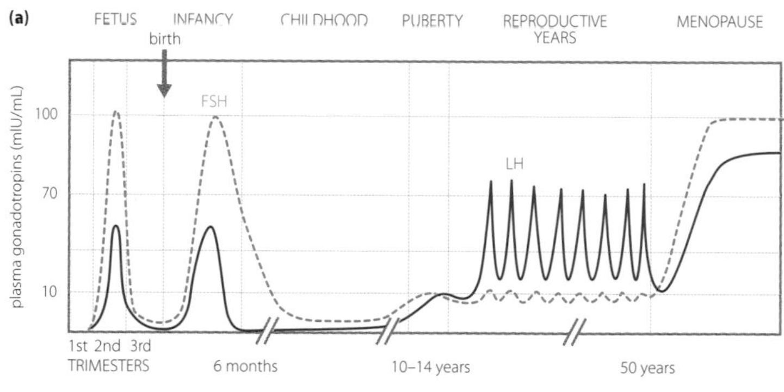

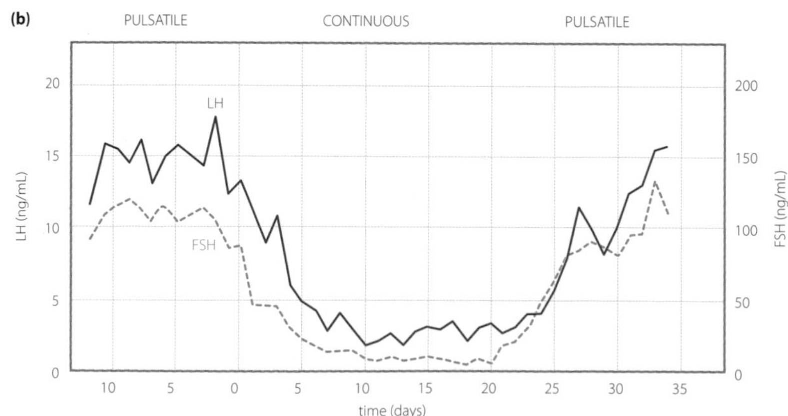

Box figure 7.1. Secretion of gonadotropins.
(a) Secretion over an entire lifetime (female).
(b) Secretion during pulsed and continuous GnRH stimulation.

falling to low levels by the time of birth (*Box 7.1*). This latter reduction is thought to result from the maturation of the negative feedback effects of steroids on the hypothalamic–pituitary axis. Whilst there is an absolute requirement for testosterone in male sexual differentiation and development, the role of fetal estrogens in female development is poorly understood. However, during the latter two-thirds of pregnancy these steroids are required for further virilization (e.g. growth of the penis) and the final shaping of the female genitalia.

A second peak of LH and FSH secretion occurs during the first 3–4 postnatal months, stimulating steroid secretion. This is thought to be due to the loss of negative feedback from the steroids secreted by the feto-placental unit. This postnatal period of relatively high steroid production allows investigation of the hypothalamic–pituitary–gonadal axis, which is not possible again until the onset of puberty. It also provides a therapeutic window in which male children born with micropenis or cryptorchidism can be treated with depot injections of testosterone to increase penis size or encourage testicular descent. After 3–4 months, circulating estrogen and androgen concentrations fall to very low levels and they become unmeasurable in most clinical assays. They do not rise again until the turbulent years of puberty.

7.3 Puberty

CASE 7.2 345 359

- Girl of 16 years with primary amenorrhea and short stature
- Poorly developed secondary sexual characteristics and no axillary or pubic hair
- 45,X0/46,XX – Turner syndrome with mosaicism
- High FSH and LH but low estrogen

A 16 year old girl presented to the endocrinology clinic with primary amenorrhea and short stature. There was no relevant past medical history of mumps, tuberculosis, or any major systemic illness. It was clear from the age of about 8 years that she was shorter than her peers and that there was a significant delay in development of her secondary sexual characteristics. She had three brothers who were doing well.

On examination she was of short stature with a height of 3′11″ (120 cm). She had cubitus valgus (deformity of the elbow), a slightly webbed neck and poorly developed secondary sexual characteristics. She also had a broad chest with widely spaced nipples. There was an absence of axillary and pubic hair. The rest of her systemic examination was unremarkable. A gynecological examination failed to reveal any abnormality.

Baseline investigations which included thyroid function tests, liver function tests, lipid profile, and bone profile were normal. Plasma FSH and LH were elevated while estrogen levels were low, in keeping with hypergonadotropic hypogonadism. A radiograph of the hand revealed short metacarpals. Karyotyping confirmed the diagnosis of Turner syndrome with mosaicism: 45,X0/46,XX. Ultrasound of the abdomen revealed streak gonads with a small atrophic uterus. No renal pathology was seen. Echocardiography was normal.

Normal puberty is a time of widespread endocrine changes during which children attain reproductive capability, develop secondary sexual characteristics, undergo a growth spurt with skeletal changes (e.g. increase in hip width in females), increase their muscle and fat tissue, and experience profound psychological changes. The onset is described as the first appearance of breast development in girls and an

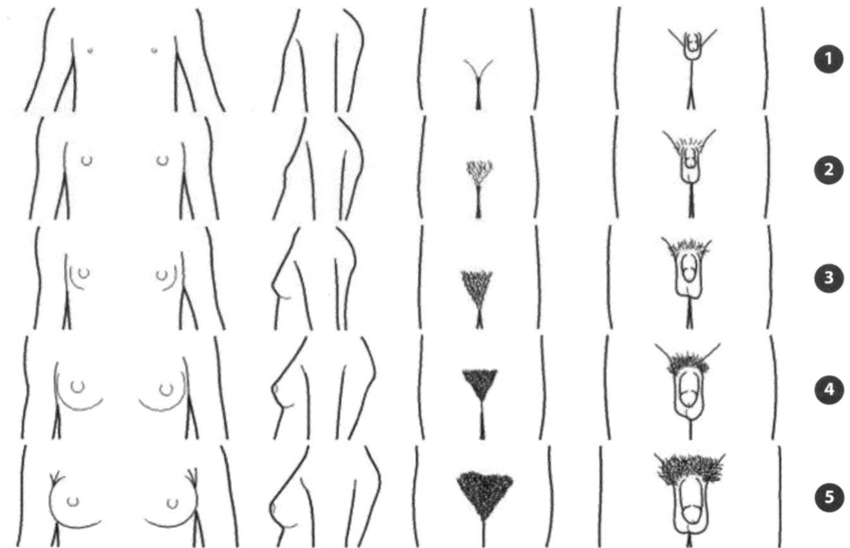

Figure 7.7. Tanner stages of puberty.

STAGES	BREAST DEVELOPMENT (girls)	PUBIC HAIR DEVELOPMENT (both sexes)	GENITAL DEVELOPMENT (boys)
1	no breast tissue	none	prepupertal
2	areolar enlargement, breast bud	few dark hairs along labia or base of penis	testis enlarged to 4mL, scrotum larger, skin coarser
3	enlargement of breast and areola as single mound	curly pigmented hairs across pubes	penis enlarges in length, continued growth of penis and scrotum
4	projection of areola above breast	small adult configuration	growth of penis in length and diameter, pigmentation of scrotum
5	papilla projects out of areola forming part of breast contour	adult configuration with spread onto inner thighs	testis, scrotum, and penis adult size

increase in testicular volume in boys as described by the Tanner definitions (*Figure 7.7*). Both genetic and environmental factors influence the timing of puberty and, though the onset of puberty has been happening earlier during the last century (often attributed to better nutrition), there is evidence that within the last 50 years the onset of puberty in the developing world has been stable.

Early puberty has been linked with adverse outcomes in the adult and these include shorter stature, increased BMI, and increased risk of developing type 2 diabetes mellitus, cardiovascular disease, and premenopausal breast cancer. The current evidence that childhood obesity is associated with earlier puberty is equivocal and as yet the genes that control pubertal onset remain elusive, although genetics are now thought to be the major determinant in the timing of puberty.

7.3.1 Hormonal changes during puberty – adrenarche and gonadarche

The term puberty is derived from the Latin word *pubes* meaning hair, and it not only involves the activation of the hypothalamic–pituitary axis (gonadarche) but also increased secretion of adrenal androgens (adrenarche).

Adrenarche is the prepubertal onset of increased adrenal androgen secretion, especially DHEA, DHEA-S, and androstenedione, and occurs in children at about 6–8 years. The subsequent phenotypic outcome a few years later is pubarche, the development of pubic and axillary hair and also the development of acne (teenage

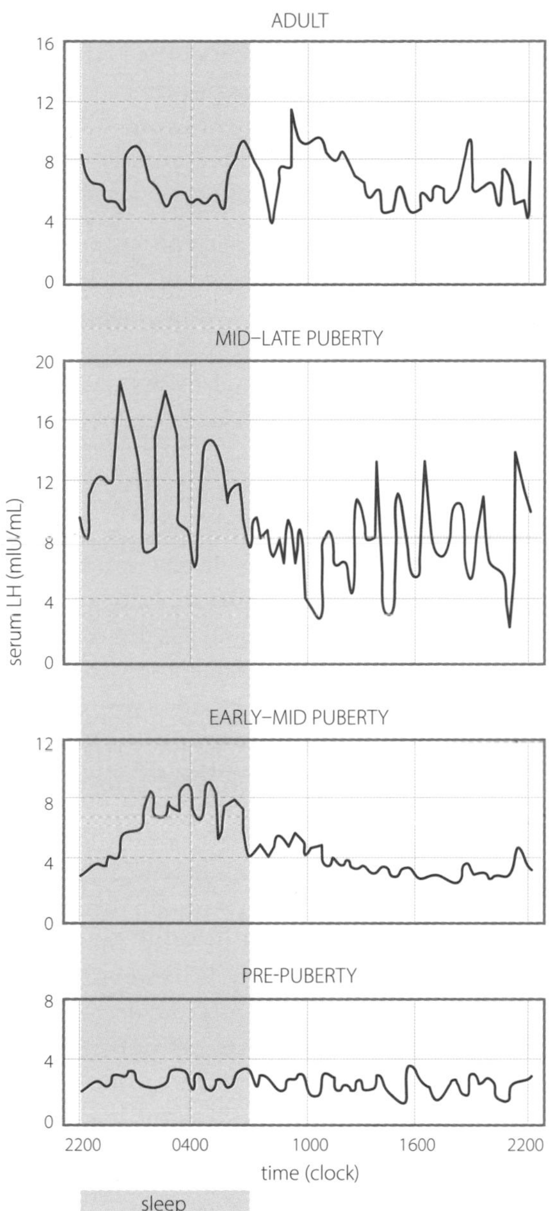

Figure 7.8. Pubertal changes in LH secretion showing increasing activity of the GnRH pulse generator and nocturnal surges of LH secretion.

spots). Serum DHEA and DHEA-S continue to rise, peaking at around 25–30 years, thereafter followed by a slow decline (the andropause). The trigger for adrenarche is unknown, though insulin-like growth factor, prolactin and growth hormone have all been implicated. Any form of excess androgen secretion, whether of adrenal (Case 6.4) or ovarian origin (Case 7.5) will cause hirsutism in females (see *Box 6.4*).

A few years later (typically at about 11 years) gonadarche is initiated and is associated with nocturnal sleep-associated increases in LH pulse amplitude and frequency, driven by an increased pulsatile release of GnRH from neurons in the hypothalamus (*Figure 7.8*). This increased pulsatility begins about a year before breast budding (Tanner stage 2, see *Figure 7.7*) in girls and continues to increase so that by the time Tanner stage 3 is reached, LH and FSH pulse amplitude have increased dramatically. During this time estradiol levels, which stimulate breast development and changes in the reproductive tract, have continued to increase. Moving towards Tanner stage 4, gonadotropin pulses become diurnal and both LH and FSH mature into the adult pattern of hormone release. Menarche occurs near the end of Tanner stage 4 as a result of FSH stimulating folliculogenesis and subsequent estrogen withdrawal. It should be noted that early cycles are anovulatory because estrogen levels are insufficient to induce the pre-ovulatory LH surge.

Similar rises in gonadotropins are seen during puberty in the male. The rising levels of LH stimulate testosterone production from the Leydig cells and the adult generation of Leydig cells begins to differentiate and is complete by 12–13 years of age. Testosterone also induces growth of the penis and other changes in the reproductive tract, whilst FSH stimulates Sertoli cell division and growth. Because Sertoli cells form the bulk of testicular tissue FSH is responsible for testicular enlargement.

7.3.2 Onset of puberty and consonance

The onset of puberty is highly variable amongst individuals but is initiated by an increase in nocturnal pulsatile GnRH secretion (*Figure 7.8*). A fundamental question that remains unanswered is what initiates this rise in pulsatile GnRH secretion? Several theories and factors have been proposed.

- There is an inherent, genetically driven maturation of the 1000–3000 GnRH secreting neurons in the hypothalamus and it has been argued that this could be related to rising levels of adrenal androgens.
- Leptin, a hormone secreted by adipose tissue that signals satiety to the hypothalamus (see *Section 8.3*), might be responsible. This suggestion arose from original observations that a certain percentage of body fat (22%) needed to be achieved before the onset of puberty. This was corroborated by the fact that anorexia nervosa or intense physical exercise (low body fat) post-pubertally was associated with low levels of leptin and decreased gonadotropin levels resulting in amenorrhea and a reversion to pre-pubertal levels of hormones. It was also shown that mutations of the leptin gene or its receptor were associated with low levels of LH and infertility. However, leptin levels begin to rise about 2 years prior to puberty and the current general consensus is that leptin is permissive to puberty and not the 'driver'.
- A few years ago a new neurohormone was discovered, kisspeptin, along with its receptor GPR54. Kisspeptin was found in specific hypothalamic neurons and its receptor expressed on GnRH neuron (*Figure 7.9*). Inactivating mutations of the kisspeptin gene or mutations of GPR54 cause abnormal development of GnRH neurons leading to hypogonadism, failure to enter puberty, and hypothalamic hypogonadism. In contrast, activating mutations of GPR54 induce precocious puberty. But if the kisspeptin system is pivotal in the initiation of puberty, what switches on the kisspeptin system?

Whatever the mechanism that initiates puberty, normal puberty (adrenarche and gonadarche) consists of a smooth ordered progression of processes often termed consonance (*Figure 7.10*). If such consonance occurs either early or late then puberty is considered to be precocious or delayed, but if one aspect of pubertal development occurs before and outside of consonance then it is considered to be precocious pseudopuberty.

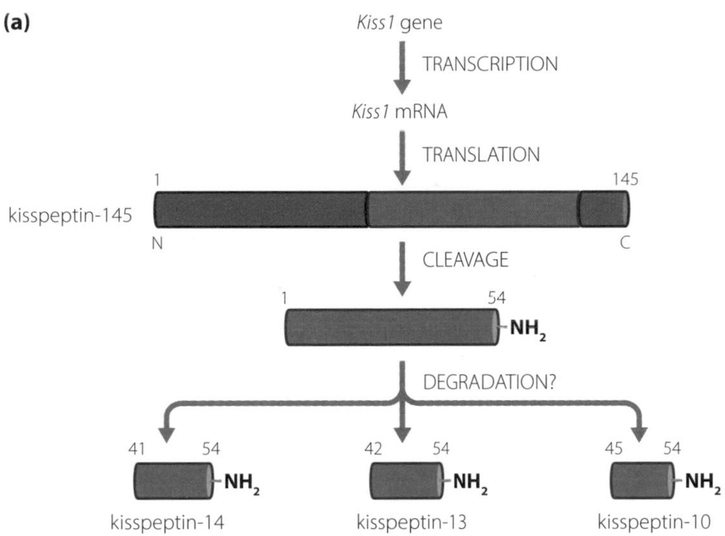

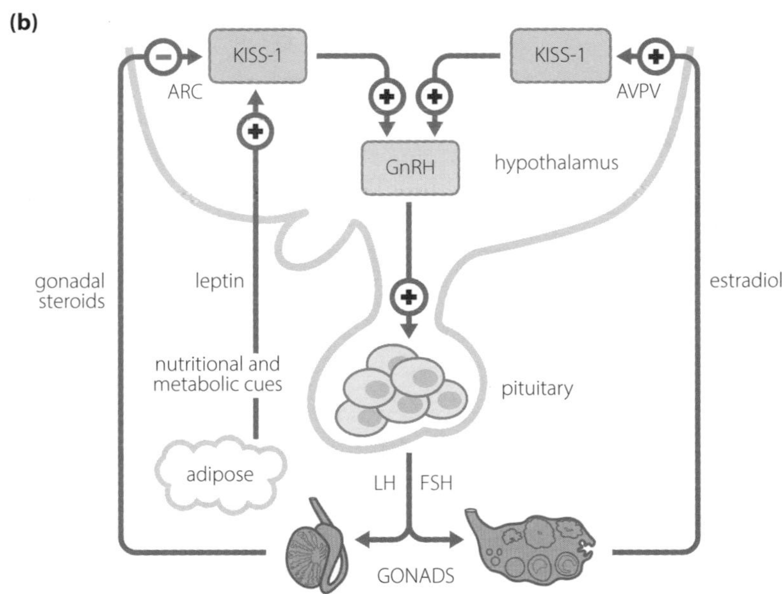

Figure 7.9. The synthesis of kisspeptin and the role of kisspeptin neurons in the hypothalamus in the regulation of GnRH secretion.

(a) Kisspeptin is a 54 amino acid peptide cleaved from a large prohormone derived from the *Kiss1* gene. Other smaller fragments are found in the circulation which may also have biological activity.

(b) Kisspeptin neurons in the hypothalamus stimulate the release of GnRH and hence LH/FSH secretion. Kisspeptin neurons in the arcuate nucleus (ARC) of the hypothalamus are sensitive to the negative feedback effects of gonadal steroids, whilst neurons in the anteroventral periventricular nucleus (AVPV) appear to be more important in mediating the positive feedback effects of estradiol that occurs prior to ovulation. The activity of these kisspeptin neurons also plays an important role in the initiation of puberty which is characterized by an increase in GnRH pulsatility. Patients with activating mutations of the GPCR for kisspeptin (GPR54) show precocious puberty.

Kisspeptin neurons may also mediate metabolic signals to the hypothalamic–pituitary–gonadal axis. In starvation, leptin secretion from adipose tissue is decreased and this is associated with decreased *Kiss1* gene expression (leptin receptors are present on kisspeptin neurons) and loss of pulsatile LH release and gonadal steroid production. This can be reversed by giving exogenous leptin.

ENDOCRINE EVENT	SEXUAL MATURATION
increased GnRH ⟶ increased LH/FSH ⟶ increased steroid production	
estrogen secretion	breast development
testosterone secretion	penile and scrotal development
FSH secretion	testicular enlargement/follicular development
adrenal androgen secretion	pubic and axillary hair
sex steroid and GH secretion	growth acceleration
estrogen withdrawal	menarche (anovulatory)
induction of LH surge	ovulatory menstrual cycles

~3–4 years

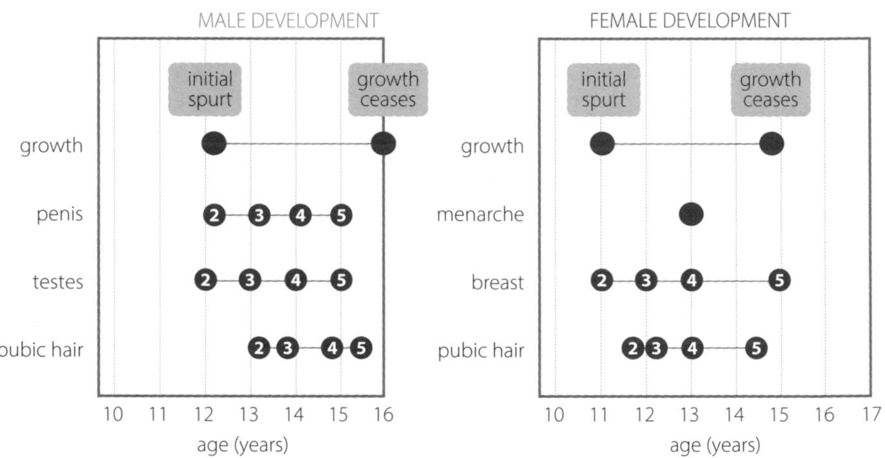

Figure 7.10. Development of secondary sexual characteristics and the progression of consonant puberty.
Numbers indicate Tanner stages (see *Figure 7.7*). Age in years will vary between individuals, body habitus, and ethnicity.

7.3.3 Precocious puberty, precocious pseudopuberty, and delayed puberty

The development of any secondary sexual characteristic prior to the age of 8 years in girls or 9 years in boys is defined as precious puberty or precocious pseudopuberty/precocious sexual development (*Box 7.2*). Precocious puberty can be caused by excess gonadotropin secretion which may either be due to excess hypothalamic GnRH secretion (idiopathic or secondary) or excess gonadotropin secretion from the pituitary itself (e.g. a pituitary tumor).

Examples of precocious pseudopuberty are McCune–Albright syndrome, testotoxicosis, premature adrenarche and premature thelarche. The McCune–Albright syndrome is caused by an activating mutation of the α-subunit of the G protein through which many hormone receptors (including the LH and FSH receptors) and other ligands stimulate cell signaling. This induces hyperactivity of the gonads and other endocrine glands and is an example of a gonadotropin-independent precocious pseudopuberty. Testotoxicosis is very rare and is caused by an activating mutation of the LH receptor. This produces high levels of testosterone that stimulate penile development, linear growth, and pubic hair development but, in the absence of the FSH that stimulates Sertoli cell development and hence growth of the testis, testicular volume is small compared with other aspects of development.

Box 7.2 | Investigating and treating precocious puberty and precocious pseudopuberty

It is not uncommon for girls (and boys) to present with premature adrenarche: development of pubic and axillary hair and sometimes associated body odor. This is non-progressive and a normal variant. Premature thelarche refers to breast development (sometimes occurring before the age of 3 years). It is important to differentiate what is essentially a normal variant from true precocious puberty; this can be achieved by careful clinical examination along with investigations and monitoring of growth charts.

Precocious puberty

Precocious puberty is diagnosed if there is evidence of sustained and **consonant** pubertal maturation in a girl younger than 8 and a boy younger than 9 or 10. It is important to remember that current generations of children start puberty much younger than their ancestors, and that there is a racial difference, with African and African-American girls commonly developing pubic/axillary hair by the age of 7 or 8.

If the diagnosis is likely, the next stage is to determine whether this is 'true' precocious puberty, i.e. driven centrally by increases in gonadotropins (as occurs during normal puberty), or pseudoprecocious puberty as a result of gonadotropin-independent increased sex steroid production.

The frequency of precocious puberty obviously depends on the age that is considered abnormal for the onset of pubertal development. Current data, based on the assumption that development of breasts and pubic hair is abnormal in Caucasian girls of 7 or less and black girls of 6 or less, suggest a rate of around 4% in both ethnic groups. It is probably reasonable to suggest that any girl who shows rapid progression of puberty before the age of 8 or who menstruates before the age of 9 should at least be fully evaluated by an endocrinologist. There are few data on the prevalence of early sexual maturation in boys but the ratio of girls:boys presenting in clinics is probably between 10:1 and 5:1. As with girls, the age at start of sexual maturation (e.g. expressed as the mean age of testicular enlargement) is reducing.

Pathophysiology

The majority of children with true precocious puberty have no underlying CNS structural cause; however, the frequency of abnormal findings on CT/MRI increases with decreasing age of the patient at presentation. One study suggests about 2% of patients presenting with puberty at the age of 6–8 have abnormalities on brain imaging; this increases to 20% for those patients presenting before 6 years.

True precocious puberty is caused by the early development of high amplitude hypothalamic GnRH pulses which in turn result in pulsatile release of LH and FSH from the pituitary. This stimulates sex steroid production from ovarian granulosa cells or testicular Leydig cells (LH) and ovarian/testicular enlargement (with subsequent folliculogenesis in girls and spermatogenesis in males).

In the somewhat rare cases where a CNS cause is associated, these may include:

- CNS tumors (gliomas, astrocytomas, hCG-producing germ cell tumors)
- hamartomas (benign brain tumors) of the hypothalamus
- CNS injury – trauma, radiation, abscess, inflammation, surgery
- congenital abnormalities (arachnoid cysts, hydrocephalus).

Where an intracranial cause is not found, there is no evidence that precocious puberty has any adverse effects on mortality (although there is a theoretical risk of early and prolonged exposure to sex steroids which may result in increased risk of, for example, breast cancer). Eventual short stature is not uncommon, although the growth spurt may occur earlier and often these children are taller than their peers at diagnosis, earlier bone maturation and epiphyseal closure can result in eventual short stature. The assessment of bone age (using X-rays of the wrist) can help with the choice of patients who need treatment; those with a bone age well in advance of their chronological age should result in a lower threshold for treatment.

Presentation and investigation

In girls an obvious sign of estrogen exposure is breast development, which may be unilateral. With advancing puberty, the areola becomes darker and thicker and the nipple more prominent. Pubic hair development may be associated with a lightening of the color of the vaginal mucosa.

In boys, as puberty develops the scrotum becomes thinner and the testes enlarge – a testicular size greater than 4 mL suggests active FSH production. If pubic hair occurs without testicular/penile growth, this suggests premature adrenarche rather than true precocious puberty. Some evidence suggests that (particularly

Box 7.2 | continued

in Caucasian girls) early onset of puberty might be associated with increased BMI.

Laboratory studies include:

- serum testosterone
- serum estradiol measurements are less useful due to variability and assay sensitivity; however, very high levels for age (>100 pg/mL) may suggest ovarian tumors
- DHEA-S levels are high in premature pubarche
- 17α-hydroxyprogesterone measurement is useful to exclude CAH
- LH levels – normally undetectable in pre-puberty (<0.1 IU/L) – a level of 0.9 IU/L is strongly suggestive of central precocious puberty
- FSH levels are less useful (however, undetectable LH/FSH levels with high testosterone or estradiol suggest precocious pseudopuberty, see below)
- the GnRH test, which measures the LH and FSH response to exogenous synthetic GnRH or GnRH analog (e.g. leuprolide in a dose of 20 μg/kg), is useful. A peak LH >6–8 IU/L is diagnostic of precocious puberty. (No response in association with high sex steroids suggests precocious pseudopuberty.)
- thyroid function tests – severe hypothyroidism is rarely associated with precocious puberty.

Imaging

- Head MRI (especially if the child is under 6 years of age – see above).
- Pelvic ultrasound – to exclude ovarian pathology.

Treatment

Treatment is largely based around the use of GnRH analogs (agonists) to reduce LH and FSH levels (*Box 7.1*). Leuprolide is available in a long-acting depot preparation given every 28 days or so. The treatment rarely needs to be continued beyond the age of 11–11.5 when the child can be allowed to resume normal pubertal development. An alternative is histrelin which can be given as an implant releasing about 50–60 μg/day. This also desensitizes the pituitary and results in suppression of LH/FSH.

Several other GnRH agonists are available, and these can be given by daily or twice daily intranasal routes of administration, although this may lead to compliance problems.

It is important to follow up these children with regular auxology, determination that progression through puberty has been arrested, and assessment of bone age. The aim is to see a reduction in the accelerated growth, a reduction in breast/testicular size, and in boys a return of testosterone to the pre-pubertal range.

It is also important to remember that all patients are individuals and in some cases it might be perfectly reasonable to allow puberty to progress. This would certainly be the case in the older age group (>8–9), and in those without evidence of significantly advanced bone age, and where height projections fall within the normal range. Finally, some children may well benefit from psychological support; the impact of early pubertal development at an age where hormonal changes cannot be fully understood can be great, as can the effects of increased libido (particularly in boys).

Precocious pseudopuberty

Precocious pseudopuberty refers to those cases where puberty is not centrally driven, i.e. by early maturation of the hypothalamic–pituitary–gonadal axis, but is independent of GnRH.

Because there is no coordinated central stimulation, levels of FSH and LH are low and there is no response to exogenous GnRH. The syndrome is rarer than true GnRH-dependent precocious puberty (about 1:5) and affects 1 per 5–10 000. There are some ethnic differences depending on the etiology; for example, the incidence of non-classical CAH is far higher in Ashkenazi Jews.

Etiology

The causes of precocious pseudopuberty are many and varied and include:

- exposure to exogenous sex steroids
- congenital adrenal hyperplasia (CAH, see *Section 6.9*)
    - the commonest forms are secondary to deficiency of 21-hydroxylase and 11α-hydroxylase; these lead to a reduction in cortisol levels associated with a rise in ACTH production and an increase in cortisol precursors which are shunted into androgenic forming pathways
- hCG secreting tumors (e.g. choriocarcinomas of the retroperitoneum, pineal, gonads, and mediastinum and hepatomas)
- adrenal tumors; cortical tumors are rare in childhood but may occur and give rise to excess androgen secretion (virilization of girls and early puberty in

Box 7.2 | continued

boys) or very rarely excess estrogen (feminization in males and precocious pseudopuberty in females)

- ovarian tumors (these may be masculinizing or feminizing)
  - benign ovarian cysts (estrogen producing)
  - granulosa cell tumors – produce pseudoprecocious puberty as a result of excess estrogen production
  - sex cord tumors
- Leydig cell tumors or arrhenoblastomas (which are rare ovarian tumors that occasionally occur before adolescence and which are associated with virilization and relatively high levels of androstenedione)
- McCune–Albright syndrome
  - prolonged activation of stimulatory G-proteins in the absence of stimulatory hormones
- testotoxicosis
  - activating mutation resulting in the spontaneous activation of the LH receptor in the absence of ligand binding
- severe hypothyroidism
  - unknown mechanism (arrested rather than advanced growth)

Investigations and treatment

- High levels of sex steroids with suppressed LH/FSH.
- No response of LH/FSH to exogenous GnRH.
- Elevated steroid precursors in CAH:
  - high 17α-hydroxyprogesterone in 21-hydroxylase deficiency
  - high 11-deoxycortisol and deoxycorticosterone in 11β-hydroxylase deficiency
- hCG – elevated in hCG-producing tumors.
- High urinary 17-ketosteroids in adrenal tumors.
- High testosterone in testotoxicosis caused by an activating mutation of the LH receptor. FSH/LH low.
- High TSH – in hypothyroidism.

Imaging studies will include ultrasound scans of the uterus/ovaries to determine the duration of estrogen exposure and the presence of ovarian cysts/tumors and ultrasound of the testes which may demonstrate impalpable (Leydig cell) tumors. A skeletal survey (X-ray) may reveal evidence of polyostotic fibrous dysplasia in McCune–Albright syndrome. Bone age (as above) should be determined in every young patient with evidence of early puberty.

The treatment of precocious pseudopuberty depends on the etiology. As this form of early puberty is independent of normal maturation of the hypothalamic–pituitary–gonadal axis, GnRH analogs (*Box 7.1*) have no place. Ketoconazole (an anti-fungal) reduces androstenedione biosynthesis by inhibition of C17,29 desmolase and 17α-hydroxylase. Anti-androgens (e.g. spironolactone) and aromatase inhibitors (e.g. testolactone) are useful in slowing the effects of precocious pseudopuberty by blocking androgen action or inhibiting estrogen production. Anti-estrogens (such as tamoxifen – more commonly used in the treatment of breast cancer) have shown some promise in the treatment of precocious pseudopuberty associated with McCune–Albright syndrome. CAH is treated with exogenous glucocorticoids in doses adequate to replace steroids and to suppress ACTH (*Chapter 6*).

An identifiable tumor responsible for pseudopuberty clearly requires consideration of surgical intervention.

Premature adrenarche (or indeed congenital adrenal hyperplasia with high levels of adrenal androgens, see *Section 6.9*) can induce precocious development of pubic and/or axillary hair. Premature thelarche (breast development) can occur in the absence of any other pubertal development and this is often cyclical, with growth and regression occurring within a 2 year period. Estrogens in these cases are typically very low or undetectable. If there is no regression of growth this may indicate the onset of precocious puberty. The investigation and treatment of precocious puberty and precocious pseudopuberty are outlined in *Box 7.2*.

Delayed puberty (*Box 7.3*) is defined as no secondary sexual maturation by the age of 13 years in girls and 14 years in boys. About 90% cases are constitutional, affecting both growth and pubertal development; it is about ten times more common in boys than girls and is sometimes associated with chronic illness. In terms of endocrinology there are two causes of delayed puberty: hypogonadotropic

Box 7.3 | Investigating and treating delayed puberty

As its name suggests, delayed puberty refers to the situation where pubertal signs are not present at an age considered to be normal, i.e. 13 for girls and 14 for boys. An alternative definition is testicular size below 3–4 mL in boys and absence of breast development in girls (aged 14 and 13 respectively).

The prevalence of delayed puberty is unknown. Epidemiologically, the onset of puberty is less well defined in males and there seems to have been little change in age of onset over the last few generations. Many more boys than girls will seek medical attention for delayed puberty.

Although the vast majority of patients will have no worrying underlying diagnosis and will be described as having 'constitutional' delay of puberty, some patients will have underlying conditions directly or indirectly responsible for pubertal delay.

Causes of delayed puberty

- Constitutional (often runs in families, usually boys) may present with short stature which will usually be associated with delayed skeletal age/maturation.
- Temporary delay in puberty secondary to underlying chronic illness (diabetes, cystic fibrosis, celiac disease, etc.) or secondary to excessive exercise (e.g. in young gymnasts), anorexia and malnutrition and even excessive stress.
- Hypothalamic–pituitary disorders (hypogonadotropic delayed puberty):
  - congenital gonadotropin deficiency (e.g. Kallmann syndrome, septo-optic dysplasia)
  - genetic associations of congenital gonadotropin deficiency include mutations in several genes including *KAL-1* (Kallmann syndrome), *FGFR-1, Kiss-1, GnRHR, FSH* and LH beta subunit, leptin, leptin receptor, prohormone convertase-I, *PROK-2, PROKR2, DAX-1*
  - acquired gonadotropin deficiency as a result of trauma, surgery, cranial radiotherapy, tumors; iron overload in patients receiving multiple transfusions (e.g. for hemoglobinopathies)
- Gonadal disorders (hypergonadotropic delayed puberty):
  - cryptorchidism and anorchia
  - chromosomal disorders – Klinefelter/Turner syndromes, XY gonadal dysgenesis
  - testicular torsion, mumps, pelvic/abdominal irradiation, testicular/ovarian surgery or torsion, polyglandular autoimmune syndromes.

History and examination

As stated above, far more boys than girls tend to appear in clinic with possible delayed puberty, and this is often due to concern over linear growth. Constitutional delay of growth and puberty (sometimes referred to as CDGP) is the commonest cause. This tends to occur in families and patients should progress through puberty spontaneously (albeit a little later than their peers) and should achieve a normal final height.

Although it is usually clinically fairly obvious, CDGP is essentially a diagnosis of exclusion and it is important to rule out other causes. A detailed history and examination are important. Underlying chronic disease (for example, poorly controlled diabetes, celiac disease, inflammatory bowel disease, cystic fibrosis, severe asthma, renal failure, malignancy) needs to be ruled out. Eating disorders are increasingly common (in both boys and girls) and it is important to rule out anorexia or bulimia.

The history may also highlight previous cranial or pelvic surgery or radiotherapy, or use of chemotherapeutic agents. It is important to consider a history of mumps or testicular pain secondary to torsion, both of which can cause primary gonadal failure.

The pituitary gonadotrophs are very sensitive to iron and repetitive transfusions (e.g. in sickle cell disease or thalassemia) frequently result in gonadotropin deficiency and delayed puberty. Other pituitary hormone deficiencies may be evident, for example, secondary hypothyroidism, growth failure due to GH deficiency, or adrenal dysfunction secondary to ACTH deficiency. Anosmia is a frequent accompaniment to Kallmann syndrome.

It is important to record the heights of both parents and calculate a predicted height from standard nomograms (information as to the age of onset of parental puberty is also useful).

In terms of examination, pubertal staging is key and is assessed according to standards first published by Tanner and Whitehouse in the UK. In males, testicular size should be assessed using an orchidometer (*Box figure 7.2*).

The onset of puberty can confidently be diagnosed if the testes are of 4 mL or greater (or 2.5 cm in linear measurement). Other features (such as deepening of the voice and facial hair growth) are less useful. Linear growth spurts with increases in growth velocity occur in mid-puberty. In girls, breast development is

Box 7.3 | continued

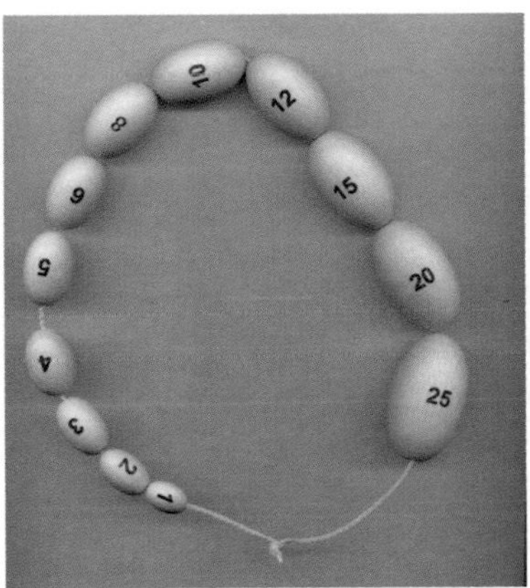

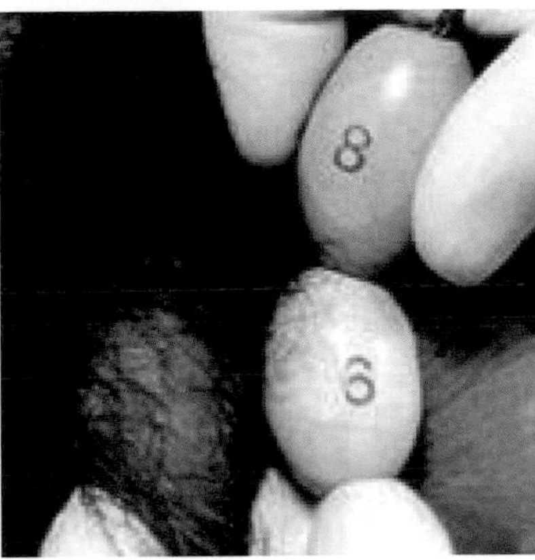

Box figure 7.2. Assessment of testicular size using the orchidometer.

the first sign of puberty but may often be pre-dated by adrenarche, the onset of pubic and axillary hair growth and body odor. Menarche usually occurs at about Tanner Stage 4 of breast development (*Figure 7.7*).

It is useful to plot previous height/weight measures if available. Evidence of underlying chronic disorders should be sought. Other clues on examination might include gynecomastia and gynecoid (female type) habitus in boys with Klinefelter syndrome or typical features of Turner syndrome in girls (see *Section 7.4.3*). Several syndromes that may include pubertal delay (e.g. Prader–Willi, Bardet–Biedl, septo-optic dysplasia) have specific clinical features.

Investigations

An assessment of bone age is useful. An X-ray of the wrists can be compared against an atlas of normal skeletal maturation and a bone age derived (this may be very different from the chronological age). Two atlases are in common use (Greulich and Pyle's *Radiographic Atlas of Skeletal Development of Hand and Wrist* in the USA, and Tanner and Whitehouse's *Assessment of Skeletal Maturity and Prediction of Adult Height (TW2 Method)* in the UK). Children in the USA tend to have a slightly advanced bone age compared with their UK peers, presumably as a result of better nutrition and weather. A typical progression of bone maturation is shown in *Figure 1.22*. Measurements of LH and FSH can sometimes differentiate primary gonadal failure (high gonadotropins) from secondary (low gonadotropins), but it needs to be remembered that pre-pubertal gonadotropin levels are physiologically very low, even in CDGP.

Stimulated gonadotropins, i.e. after injection with GnRH, may be useful, but again will sometimes not differentiate CDGP from true gonadotropin deficiency with no effective gonadotropin response to stimulus in both groups. In these cases it is often necessary to induce puberty with exogenous sex steroids and then re-test the axis at the end of growth and puberty to determine if long-term sex steroid therapy is necessary (see *Treatment* below). In males, administration of human chorionic gonadotropin (hCG, which resembles LH) is sometimes useful: a testosterone response to hCG suggests CDGP, whereas a blunted response suggests that gonadotropin deficiency is more likely. Outside of the hCG test, measurements of testosterone and estradiol are rarely useful.

Chromosomal analysis should be undertaken if there is clinical suspicion of Klinefelter or Turner syndrome; in the latter an abdominal/pelvic ultrasound scan is useful to determine gonadal morphology and renal tract abnormalities which are more common in this condition. If there is a strong suspicion of true gonadotropin deficiency, other pituitary hormones should be measured (either basally or after stimulation) and appropriate imaging (i.e. a hypothalamic–pituitary MRI scan) carried out. Thyroid function tests should probably be measured in all children with possible delayed puberty because hypothyroidism is an easily treatable cause (and sometimes relatively easy to miss clinically).

Treatment

Treatment is aimed at initiating pubertal development and ensuring its association with the normal growth spurt in order to attain predicted adult height. As the majority of cases of delayed puberty are constitutional and temporary, it is often necessary just to watch and wait, to make recurrent height, weight, and Tanner pubertal staging measurements, and to check that relevant hormone levels are increasing as puberty progresses. If there is an underlying

Box 7.3 | continued

chronic disease, treatment is directed towards that. Hormonal manipulation is reserved for cases of true hypogonadotropic hypogonadism (hypothalamic–pituitary disorders with gonadotropin deficiency), primary gonadal failure (for example, Klinefelter or Turner syndrome) and those cases where pubertal delay is resulting in significant psychosocial concern. Basal (and GnRH-stimulated) gonadotropins may be low in both CDGP and true hypogonadotropic hypogonadism and, in cases where there is doubt, it is often reasonable to induce puberty with exogenous sex steroid therapy. The hypothalamic–pituitary–gonadal axis can be re-tested on completion of growth and puberty.

Constitutional delay:

- Monitoring of growth and development.
- If there are significant psychosocial concerns a course of oxandrolone (a synthetic anabolic steroid derived from dihydrotestosterone, helpful in increasing growth velocity) or testosterone (for induction of puberty) might be considered.
- In girls a short course of estradiol treatment may help.

Permanent delay:

- Induction of puberty followed by lifelong sex steroid therapy is needed in patients with chromosomal abnormalities (Klinefelter or Turner syndrome), those with gonadal dysgenesis, gonadotropin deficiency (acquired or congenital), or gonadal failure (mumps, cryptorchidism, torsion, surgery, etc.).

Pubertal induction is with increasing doses of testosterone in males (given usually as intramuscular injections) or increasing doses of estrogen in females (low dose transdermal or oral estradiol without progesterone). In females, once breast development is satisfactory or when uterine breakthrough bleeding occurs, a progestogen should be added to induce regular menstruation. In females with Turner syndrome, growth hormone is licensed and effective in gaining an increase in final adult height.

Once puberty is complete, and if there is evidence of a persistent deficiency of sex steroids (through either gonadotropin deficiency or primary gonadal failure), sex steroid should be continued: testosterone can be given intramuscularly, transdermally, or orally, and estrogen orally or transdermally. Progesterone is always needed in women with an intact uterus: this can be given orally for about 10 days each cycle, or transdermally in a combined preparation, or even locally using the Mirena coil. Anorchic males may require testicular prostheses, and women with inadequate breast development should be offered restorative surgery.

hypogonadism and hypergonadotropic hypogonadism. The former is exemplified in Kallmann syndrome (*Box 7.4*) in which mutations of the *KAL* gene on the short arm of the X chromosome result in failure of development of the olfactory nerves from the nasal cavity to the olfactory bulb. Normally, GnRH neurons, which also arise in the nasal cavity embryologically, migrate along this olfactory tract to the hypothalamus; but in the absence of the product of the *KAL* gene the GnRH neurons remain in the nasal cavity and the result is hypothalamic hypogonadism. Another cause of hypogonadotropic hypogonadism is hypopituitarism, in which a defect in pituitary function suppresses LH and FSH secretion so there is no or reduced stimulus to the gonads.

In contrast, hypergonadotropic hypogonadism results from gonadal dysgenesis, such as seen in Turner syndrome (46,XO) (see *Section 7.4*) and Klinefelter syndrome (47,XXY and its variants) (see *Section 7.5.6*). It may also result from other causes of pre-pubertal gonadal dysfunction that have no clearly defined genetic basis, for example, mumps and other viral infections, or radiation exposure.

7.4 Turner syndrome

Turner syndrome is the most common X chromosome abnormality in women, affecting 1:2500 live female births. It is due to the result of complete (45,X

Box 7.4 | Investigations and treatment in Kallmann syndrome

- 9 am serum testosterone (repetitively low).
- Low LH and FSH, normal inhibin B and AMH.
- Formal testing of the first cranial nerve to investigate anosmia.
- GnRH test (rarely performed): GnRH is injected after a baseline blood test has been taken and LH and FSH are measured 30 minutes after a bolus injection of GnRH. This can distinguish hypothalamic (LH and FSH response) from pituitary (no LH or FSH response) causes of hypogonadism, but may not be helpful because there may be a subnormal LH response in both settings.
- Anterior pituitary testing to assess the rest of the pituitary axis and to ensure the defect is isolated to the hypothalamic–pituitary axis.
- Prolactin estimation to rule out hyperprolactinemia as a cause of hypogonadotropic hypogonadism (either a macroprolactinoma, microprolactinoma or (extremely rarely in this age group) a large non-functioning pituitary adenoma).
- Ferritin level is measured to exclude hemochromatosis.
- Semen analysis to assess sperm production, count, motility, and morphology.
- DEXA scan to assess bone mineral density as the patient is at risk of osteoporosis and delayed bone age.
- MRI to exclude other pituitary pathology (e.g. craniopharyngioma) and reveal any abnormality of the hypothalamus.

Treatment

- Testosterone replacement may be given transdermally, as a topical gel applied daily, or by injections given every few weeks, or with the newer preparations, every few months.
- Treatment with gonadotropins would induce pubertal development (for example, hCG 1500–2000 IU i.m. may be given twice a week). Most patients would also require FSH 75–150 IU i.m. three times a week. Pulsatile gonadorelin using a subcutaneous infusion pump (dose varying from 25 to 500 ng/kg every 90–120 minutes) is titrated to normalize LH, FSH, and testosterone. Serum testosterone and testicular size should be monitored. Once the testes are above 8 mL, semen analysis is undertaken every 3–6 months. It will take at least 2 years to maximize spermatogenesis. Once spermatogenesis is induced it may be maintained by hCG alone.
- In secondary irreversible gonadal failure, treatment with GnRH is a possibility in order to restore fertility.
- To assist fertilization, intracytoplasmic sperm injection (ICSI) may be offered. ICSI fertilization rates are 50–60% and pregnancy rates are around 30% per cycle. Couples will require genetic counseling before undergoing ICSI because there is an increased risk of chromosomal abnormalities.

or XO) or partial absence of one of the two X chromosomes and is generally characterized by short stature and gonadal dysgenesis, although there is a wide variation in the severity of its presentation. The characteristic phenotype includes a webbed neck, micrognathia, low-set ears, high arched palate, widely spaced nipples, and cubitus valgus. Patients may present with any combination of these features (*Figure 7.11*).

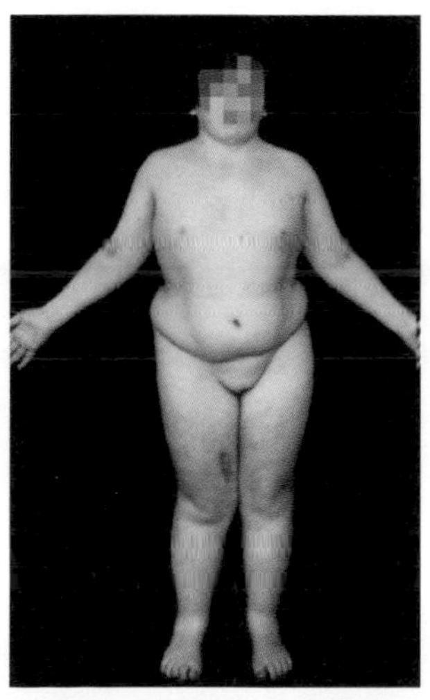

Figure 7.11. A patient with Turner syndrome.

Other associated abnormalities include aortic coarctation and other left-sided congenital heart defects, hypothyroidism, osteoporosis, skeletal abnormalities, lymphedema, celiac disease, congenital renal abnormalities, and ENT abnormalities.

The diagnosis is ultimately made by karyotype analysis and the associated abnormalities will depend on the specific karyotype (*Box 7.5*).

Management

The mainstay of treatment is with sex hormone replacement therapy – a natural estrogen will promote the development of secondary sexual characteristics. Treatment should be started with a low dose estrogen alone and gradually increased.

Box 7.5 | Turner syndrome: correlation of karyotype with phenotype

- 45,X (50%) – most severe phenotype; high incidence of cardiac and renal abnormalities.
- 46,Xi(Xq) (20%) – highest prevalence of thyroiditis, inflammatory bowel disease, and deafness.
- 45,X/46,XX (10%) – least severe phenotype; spontaneous puberty and menses in up to 40%.
- 46,Xr(X) (10%) – spontaneous menses in 33%; congenital abnormalities uncommon; cognitive dysfunction in those with a small ring chromosome.
- 45,X/46,XY (6%) – highest risk of gonadoblastoma, an unusual mixed germ cell–sex cord–stromal tumor that has the potential for malignant transformation.
- Other (4%).

Box 7.6 | Counseling patients with Turner syndrome and premature ovarian failure

All Turner syndrome patients should be counseled about their increased risk of dilatation, dissection, and rupture of the ascending aorta. Because most previous deaths occurred after misdiagnosis, Turner patients should be counseled to make healthcare providers aware of this possible diagnosis when being evaluated for disproportionate symptoms of indigestion and upper abdominal or chest pain; it is possible that many deaths could be avoided with timely diagnosis and surgical repair. Turner syndrome patients need evaluation for horseshoe kidney and for other less frequently diagnosed autoimmune disorders such as diabetes, hypertension, dyslipidemia, and hearing impairment.

Patients with 46,XX gonadal dysgenesis should be evaluated for permutations of the fragile X (*FMRI*) gene. This finding should prompt counseling for themselves and other family members and prohibit use of their similarly affected sisters as oocyte donors. In addition, 46,XX ovarian failure patients should be screened regularly for the development of Hashimoto thyroiditis and at least at baseline for adrenal steroid cell or 21-hydroxylase antibodies. Continued surveillance should be considered for the presence of hypoparathyroidism, adrenal insufficiency, and other autoimmune disorders such as pernicious anemia. All gonadal dysgenesis patients with a Y cell line need extirpation of their gonads including Turner patients with 45,X/46,XY (or those with a Y chromosome fragment) gonadal dysgenesis and the 46,XY gonadal dysgenesis patients.

It is important to remember that rare Turner patients with an apparent single 45,X cell line might have undetected mosaicism for a Y cell line. Screening 45,X single cell line patients and those individuals with an unidentified chromosomal fragment with Y DNA centromeric probes may be prudent to uncover those additional individuals at-risk for gonadal malignancies. Counseling is of utmost importance for these individuals and should cover expectations for all aspects of these young women's lives including alternatives for reproduction. While the use of donor oocytes and IVF has proven safe for 46,XX and 46,XY gonadal dysgenesis patients, an estimated maternal death rate of at least 2% exists for Turner syndrome patients and pregnancy may increase the risk of uterine rupture in future years. While it is often easier to include pregnancy by donor oocyte as an alternative during counseling, until more information is available such discussions should be framed with the above concerns. The patient guidelines of national organizations such as the American Society for Reproductive Medicine (ASRM) and the American College of Obstetricians and Gynecologists (ACOG) should be considered. The use of 'buddy programs' in which these patients are paired with others who have previously confronted the same issues during adolescence, and support groups such as the Turner Syndrome Society, are an excellent complement to this counseling.

After 1–2 years, maintenance treatment with cyclical combined estrogen and progestogen therapy can be substituted.

It is important that patients with Turner syndrome receive counseling (*Box 7.6*) and are regularly followed up, ideally in a dedicated clinic with experience of the condition and with facilities to treat the growth, fertility, and psychological aspects of the condition. Awareness of the potential complications of Turner syndrome is highly important and regular review will include the following:

- baseline renal ultrasound scan
- thyroid autoantibodies
- annual BMI, blood pressure, thyroid function test (increased incidence of primary autoimmune hypothyroidism), lipids, fasting blood glucose, and liver function
- 3–5-yearly echocardiogram; a bicuspid aortic valve is the commonest cardiac abnormality and may be associated with progressive aortic root dilatation
- bone densitometry; there is increased risk of developing osteoporosis and based on the scan results extra bone protection treatment may be necessary
- audiometry and ENT review if necessary – hearing loss may occur as a result of recurrent middle ear infections.

Despite the absence of demonstrable GH deficiency, treatment with recombinant GH may increase final height and may allow a more normal childhood stature (concordant with mid-parental height).

In terms of fertility, 2–5% of patients with Turner syndrome will have spontaneous periods, although only 0.5% have ovulatory cycles and an early menopause is likely. Contraception and genetic counseling are important in this subgroup because there is a 30% risk that their offspring will have a congenital anomaly. For the majority of cases, however, specialist fertility input is required if they wish to conceive by *in vitro* fertilization or gamete intrafallopian transfer (GIFT) using a donor ovum. Pre-pregnancy cardiovascular and renal screening is imperative.

CASE 7.2 345 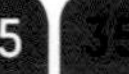

- Girl of 16 years with primary amenorrhea and short stature
- Poorly developed secondary sexual characteristics and no axillary or pubic hair
- 45,XO/46,XX – Turner syndrome with mosaicism
- High FSH and LH but low estrogen
- No cardiac abnormalities – patient opted for treatment with combined oral contraceptive pill

The patient had Turner syndrome and was referred to a multidisciplinary clinic with an interest in the management of 45,XO. She underwent initial screening and echocardiography which showed no cardiac abnormalities. Renal function and structural imaging of the renal tract also revealed no abnormality. The possibility of growth hormone treatment was discussed but was declined by the patient and the family. Treatment with estrogen was discussed and because of her concerns over potential bullying at school the patient herself elected to start treatment with a standard combined oral contraceptive. The possibility of future egg/embryo donation was discussed. The Turner Syndrome Support Society (www.tss.org.uk) in the UK proved helpful, providing sensible advice and offering access to a forum with fellow patients. Three years after diagnosis she remains well, is attending university in her first year of a law degree and has her first boyfriend.

7.5 Testicular function and its control

7.5.1 Anatomy of the testis

The two testes lie outside of the body freely moving in the scrotal sac where they are maintained at a temperature about 2°C lower than core body temperature (see

Figures 7.12 and *7.13*). Each adult testis is oval in shape with a volume of about 25 mL ($4 \times 2 \times 3$ cm) and weighing between 10 and 14 g. They are surrounded by three layers of membranes and extensions of the fibrous tunica albuginea form septa that divide the gland into 200–300 lobes. The functional components of the testis are the seminiferous tubules, of which there are approximately 200 m in each testis (constituting 70–80% of testicular mass), and the interstitial or Leydig cells (which constitute about 4% of the mass). The seminal vesicles drain into the rete testes, the epididymis, and finally the vas deferens (*Figure 7.12*).

CASE 7.3

360 370

- Man of 37 years with reduced libido and failure to conceive
- Sparse pubic hair and small soft testes
- High FSH and LH, and low testosterone; 47,XXY – Klinefelter syndrome

A 37 year old man was seen in the endocrine clinic with history of reduced libido, erectile dysfunction, and premature ejaculation. Despite relatively regular intercourse, he and his partner had failed to conceive over the previous 4 years. His only significant past medical history was that he developed acute scrotal pain lasting 3 days with no associated rash or parotid swelling when he was 30 years of age. He denied use of anabolic steroids. He shaved daily and there was no loss of body hair or muscle mass.

He had a history of type 2 DM (for 3 years) and was on metformin 500 mg twice daily and gliclazide 80 mg once daily. He was a non-smoker and did not drink alcohol. On examination he was 5′10″ (180 cm) tall with a weight of 83.4 kg (BMI 27 kg/m^2).

Facial, chest, and pubic hair was sparse but axillary hair pattern was normal. His testes were small and soft: (right 1 mL and left 1.5 mL in volume). There was no gynecomastia. Systemic examination was unremarkable. Investigations revealed:

- FSH 30.9 IU/L (NR 2.6–9.5)
- LH 20.4 IU/L (NR 3–12)
- testosterone 4.7 nmol/L (NR 14–28)
- prolactin 402 mIU/L (NR 70–360)

Full blood count, urea and electrolytes, liver function test, thyroid function test, and ferritin were normal. An ultrasound confirmed bilateral small atrophic testes. Semen analysis showed no spermatozoa. Chromosome analysis revealed a 47,XXY karyotype.

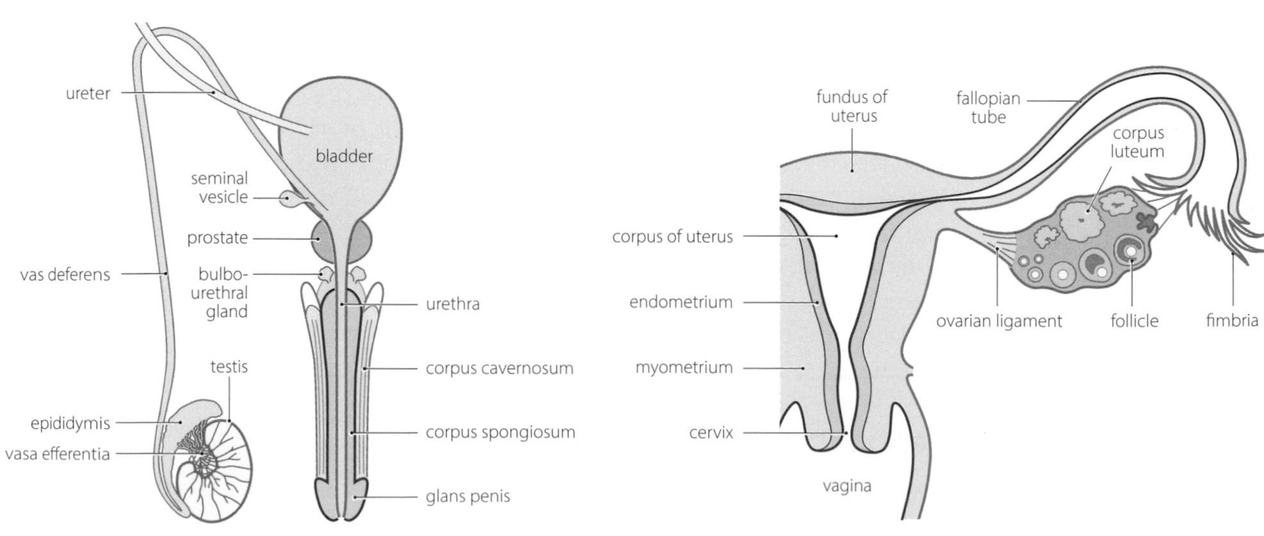

Figure 7.12. Comparative gross anatomy of the male and female reproductive systems.

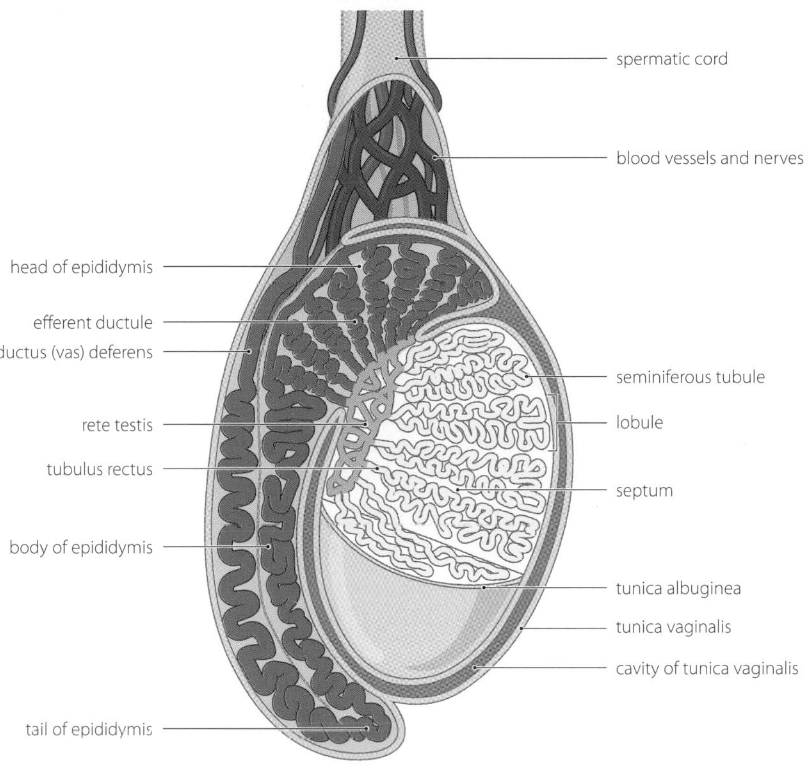

Figure 7.13. Structural organization of the testis.
The testis is enclosed in a tough fibrous capsule, the outer layer being the tunica vaginalis and immediately underneath, the tunica albuginea. It is divided by fibrous septa into about 200–300 lobes. At puberty there are about 700 curled seminiferous tubules, each as long as an arm and as thin as a hair. The seminiferous tubules drain into a network of ducts, the rete testis, and then into the head (caput) of the epididymis which comprises 8–12 efferent ducts. These taper into the body (corpus) of the epididymis, but in the tail (cauda) of the epididymis the diameter of the duct enlarges. The entire epididymal length is 5–6 m and drains into the vas deferens which is about 30–35 cm in length and terminates in the ejaculatory duct near the prostate (see *Figure 7.12*). Each testis is suspended from the body wall by a spermatic cord which penetrates into the pelvic cavity through the inguinal canal. Each spermatic cord contains the vas deferens, a testicular nerve, and three coiled blood vessels – the testicular or spermatic artery and two testicular or spermatic veins. The testicular veins receive tributaries from the epididymis which unite to form a convoluted plexus, called the pampiniform plexus, which constitutes the greater mass of the spermatic cord.

7.5.2 Functions of the testis

There are two functions of the testis: sperm production in the seminiferous tubules and testosterone secretion from the Leydig or interstitial cells that lie between the tubules (*Figure 7.14*). Testosterone is not only essential in maintaining spermatogenesis but is also essential for sexual differentiation and development (see *Section 7.2*) and maintenance of male secondary sex characteristics and other aspect of male physiology.

Both spermatogenesis and testosterone production are regulated by pulsatile secretion of GnRH from hypothalamic neurons (*Box 7.1*) and this hormone stimulates the secretion of LH and FSH. LH stimulates testosterone biosynthesis in the Leydig cells and this requires the activities of four enzymes: P_{450}scc, 3β-hydroxysteroid dehydrogenase (HSD), 17α-hydroxylase (CYP17), and 17β-

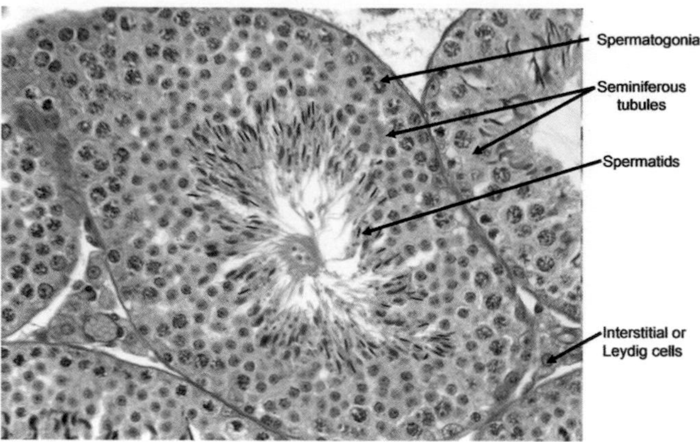

Figure 7.14. Histology of the testis.

HSD (*Figure 7.15*). Testosterone enters the testicular blood capillaries that are immediately adjacent to the Leydig cells and, once in the systemic circulation, 95% becomes complexed with the high affinity sex hormone binding globulin and the low affinity albumin. The adult production of testosterone is estimated to range from

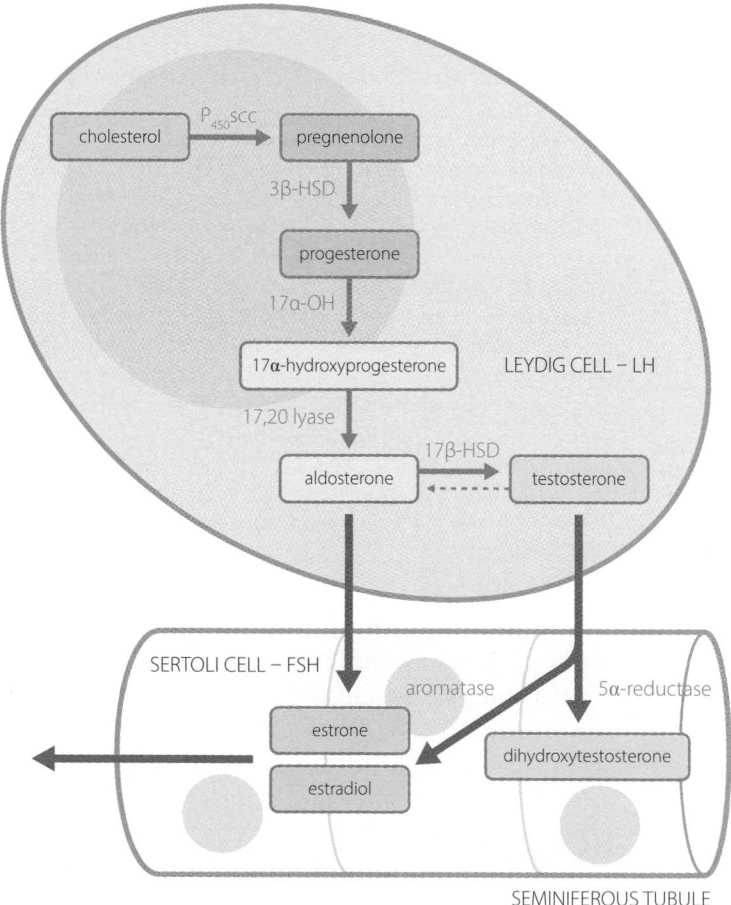

Figure 7.15. Steroid synthesis in the testis.

3β-HSD, 3β-hydroxysteroid dehydrogenase, 17α-OH, 17α-hydoxylase, 17β-HSD, 17β-hydroxysteroid dehydrogenase.

5 to 7.5 mg/day and the levels of total testosterone in normal men range from 14 to 28 nmol/L in most assays. If the testes are removed, testosterone levels decline by 95%, the remainder being derived from peripheral conversion of androstenedione and DHEA produced by the adrenal cortex. Levels of testosterone are controlled by a classic negative feedback effect on the hypothalamus, which regulates the synthesis and pulsatile amplitude and frequency of GnRH release and thus LH and FSH secretion. High levels of testosterone suppress GnRH release and the reverse occurs when testosterone levels decline.

Normal men also produce small amounts of estradiol and estrone from testosterone and androstenedione by the action of the enzyme aromatase. This enzyme is present in Leydig cells, but most estrogens are thought to be derived from aromatase in peripheral tissues such as adipose tissue, skin, kidney, and the brain. Rare cases of aromatase deficiency in men cause delayed bone aging and thus increased height and there is some evidence that estrogens may regulate testicular cell mass in the newborn testis. From experimental observations it is now considered that estradiol is important for male fertility.

The Sertoli cells of the seminiferous tubules, that provide nourishment, growth factors and organization for the developing germ cells, are the target for FSH and the classic view was that FSH stimulates spermatogenesis and LH stimulates testosterone production. However, it now appears that spermatogenesis is qualitatively maintained by testosterone alone and that FSH simply amplifies the basal level of germ cell production by stimulating a factor in Sertoli cells that rescues spermatogonia from programmed cell death. Like LH, FSH secretion is also regulated by feedback effects of gonadal steroids on GnRH release but, in addition, FSH is also controlled by the negative feedback effects of inhibin B (*Figure 7.16*) produced by the Sertoli cells in response to FSH. Inhibin selectively inhibits FSH secretion by an action on the pituitary gland. FSH secretion is also modulated at the level of the pituitary gland through activin produced by the folliculostellate cells. Activin stimulates synthesis of the FSH β subunit, although its action is moderated by the paracrine action of follistatin which binds to activin and prevents it interacting with its receptors (*Figure 7.17*). It should also be noted that while spermatogenesis is dependent on hormonal drive, this process is impaired if the testis is maintained at 'normal' core body temperature, as occurs in cryptorchidism (no testicular descent) or through tight clothing.

Figure 7.16. Hormonal regulation of testicular function.

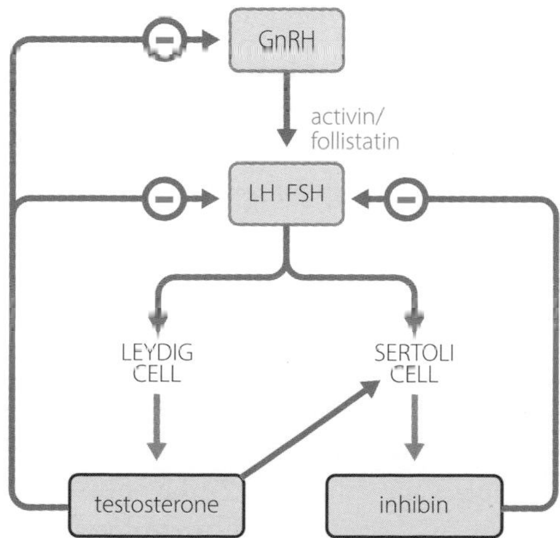

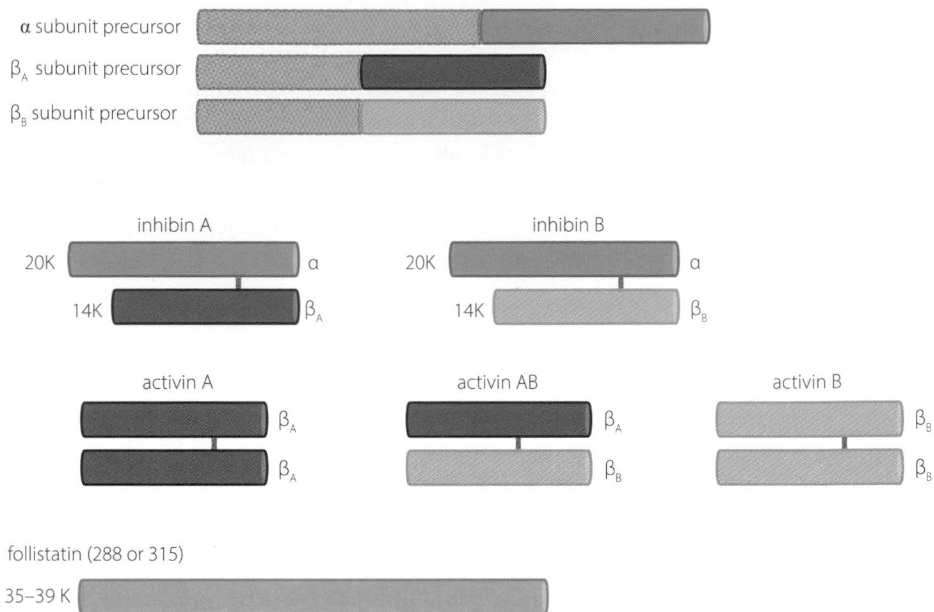

Figure 7.17. Inhibins, activins, and follistatin.
Inhibins and activins are produced by three different subunit precursors. Inhibins inhibit FSH synthesis and release, while activins stimulate FSH synthesis and secretion. Follistatin, coded by a different gene, is an activin-binding protein and inhibits the action of activin.
Activin and follistatin act in the pituitary gland to regulate gonadotropin secretion.
Inhibins are mainly produced in the gonads.

7.5.3 Spermatogenesis

The Sertoli cells and the germ cells (the precursors of spermatocytes) are the major components of the seminiferous tubules. The Sertoli cells span the thickness of the seminiferous tubules which are surrounded by a basement membrane and the germ cells or spermatogonia are always adjacent to this membrane. Near the basement membrane the Sertoli cells are connected to each other by tight junctions (*Figure 7.18a*) and these form the blood-testis barrier that enables the Sertoli cells to maintain an extracellular environment within the tubule that is different from the extracellular environment. This barrier helps to protect maturing sperm from potential toxins and immune assault and leakage of sperm out of the tubule.

Spermatogonia are classified as type A stem cells, or type B which are differentiated spermatogonia. Type A spermatogonia may divide to produce more type A or the first generation of type B. Type B are committed to produce more type B. The last generation of type B spermatogonia divide to produce primary spermatocytes, the last diploid germ cells in the production of spermatozoa. They then move away from the basement membrane, through the tight junctions towards the lumen of the tubule; during the whole process of spermatogenesis the germ cells bind to Sertoli cells through specialized cellular junctions and remain so until they are released into the lumen of the seminiferous tubules. Each spermatocyte undergoes two meiotic divisions, meiosis I giving rise to two secondary spermatocytes and, almost immediately after, meiosis II giving rise to four secondary spermatocytes (*Figure 7.18b*).

At this stage they are simple round cells and they then undergo the long phase of morphogenesis, termed spermiogenesis. The major changes during this phase are formation of a head with an acrosome (essential for fertilization), formation of a tail for motility, and loss of cytoplasm. The spermatocytes are then extruded from the Sertoli cells into the lumen of the seminiferous tubule. The whole process of spermatogenesis takes approximately 74 days and every second about 300–600 sperm/g of testis are produced. Not all sperm survive although a fully functioning

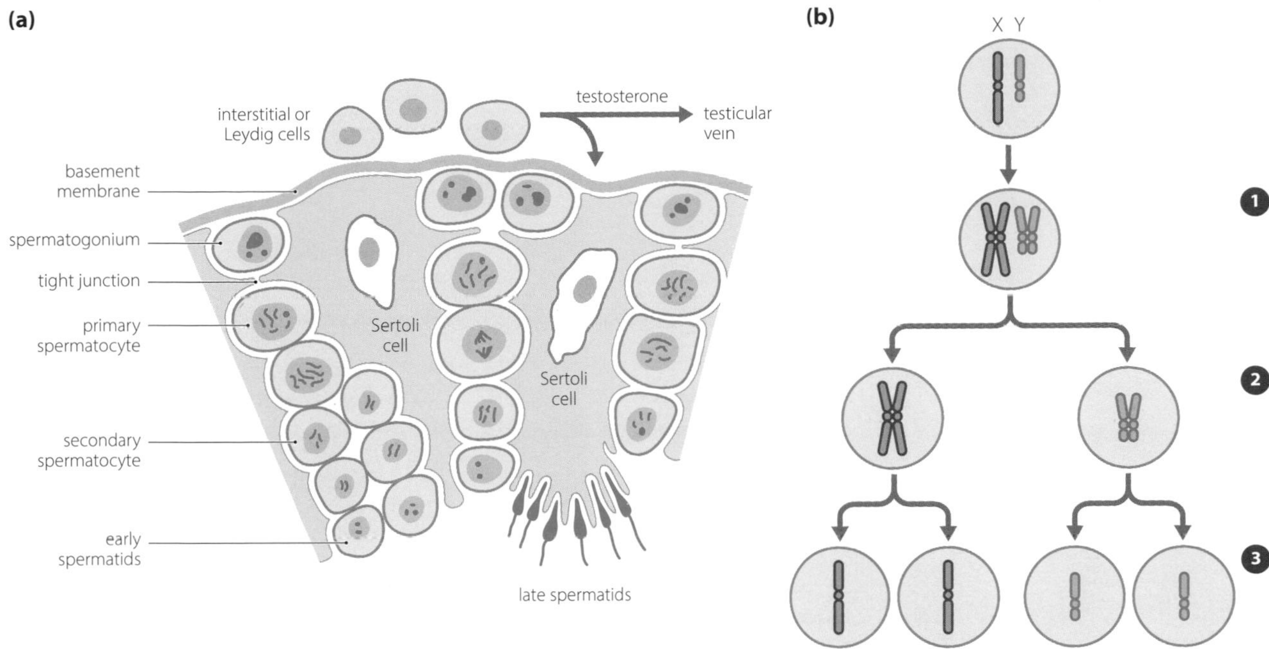

Figure 7.18. Cross-section of a seminiferous tubule (a) and the process of spermatogenesis (b).
(a) The seminiferous tubules form the bulk of the testis. Each tubule is made up of columnar epithelium, the Sertoli cells, which are connected to each other at their bases by tight junctions. These form the blood–testis barrier. The spermatogonia, halfway through their first meiotic division push through the tight junction and, nurtured by the Sertoli cells, they undergo the process of spermatogenesis. (b) Sequential meiotic divisions lead to the production of mature sperm. At the first meiotic division (1) each chromosome makes a duplicate copy and they become sister chromatids. Crossing over rarely occurs in the sex chromosomes, although it is common in autosomal chromosomes. Each pair of chromatids separates to form two new haploid cells ($n = 23$) but each chromosome is made up of two chromatids (2). At the second meiotic division (3), each chromatid separates and becomes a chromosome – 23 per cell.

testis, normally achieved by the age of 16 years, has the capacity to produce over 200 million sperm each day.

From the seminiferous tubules, the sperm are washed towards the rete testis which drains into the vasa efferentia and from there into the epididymis, a highly convoluted tube that finally drains into the vas deferens (*Figure 7.13*). During the 12 day passage from the testis to the vas deferens the sperm become highly motile and mature to reach full fertilizing ability. The sperm also become highly concentrated as a result of fluid absorption in the epididymis.

Sperm can be stored for up to 5 weeks in the tail of the epididymis and vas deferens before they are released at ejaculation. In the absence of ejaculation, sperm dribble into the urethra and are washed away in the urine. In men who have undergone a vasectomy (ligation of the vas deferens) sperm build up behind the ligation and are either removed by phagocytosis in the epididymis or leak through the epididymal wall.

7.5.4 Erection and ejaculation

The ejaculatory response is evoked by a complex series of reflexes and the physiological phases of this response have been defined as erection, emission, and ejaculation (*Figure 7.19*). Failure to achieve penile erection has been termed impotence, but because the word conjures up such images of functional incapacity, the term erectile dysfunction is now preferred.

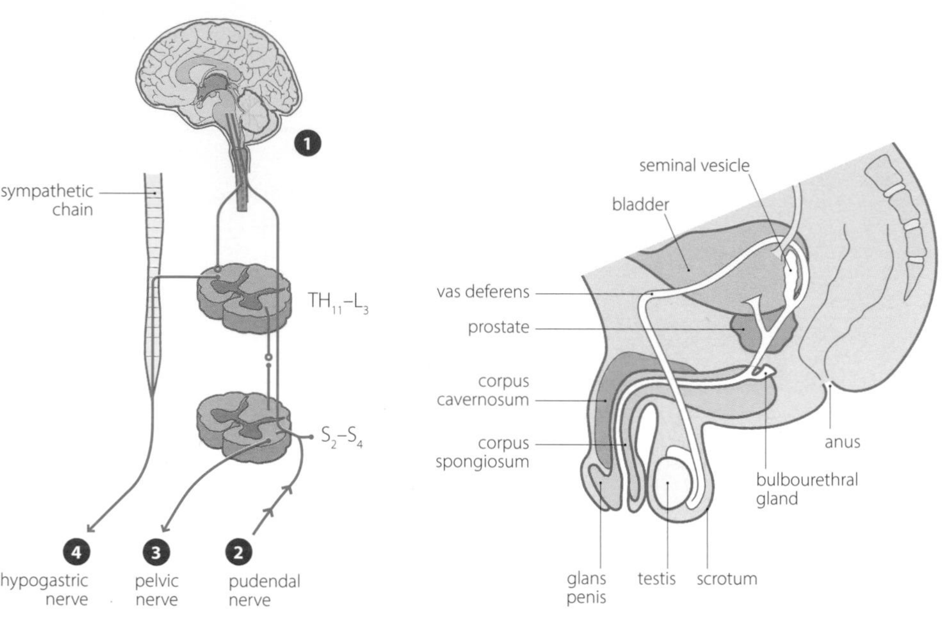

Figure 7.19. Functional anatomy of erection and ejaculation.
Psychogenic stimuli from the brain (1) or from tactile receptors on the penis (2) via the pudendal nerve activate the parasympathetic fibers (3) of the pelvic nerve. This parasympathetic stimulation causes vasodilatation in the corpus cavernosa and, to a lesser extent, in the corpus spongiosum. This involves the neurotransmitters acetylcholine and vasoactive polypeptide and the production of nitric oxide. The sympathetic outflow of the hypogastric nerve (4), which normally maintains myogenic tone in the flaccid penis, is counteracted by the parasympathetic stimulation during arousal.
Nitric oxide in the corpus cavernosum stimulates the production of cyclic guanosine monophosphate (cGMP) which causes vasodilatation. Sildenafil (marketed as Viagra) inhibits the breakdown of cGMP and increases blood flow to the penis. Other drugs that can cause tumescence are prostaglandin E_1 (or a synthetic analog) and α-adrenergic blockers which can reduce sympathetic tone.

- *Erection* is induced by tactile stimulation, particularly of the glans penis, and from visual cues and psychogenic stimuli. These stimuli activate efferent parasympathetic fibers of the pelvic nerve that activate dilatation of penile arteries which involves acetylcholine, vasoactive polypeptide, and nitric oxide. The corpus cavernosa and spongiosum, which are surrounded by a strong fibrous coat, become engorged with blood and venous outflow is compressed. Simultaneously the parasympathetic nerves stimulate the bulbo-urethral glands to produce a mucoid-like substance for lubrication.
- *Emission* involves contractions of the smooth muscle in the walls of the vas deferens and genital ducts and this pushes sperm into the upper part of the urethra. At the same time the seminal vesicles and prostate gland contract and seminal fluid is released into the urethra.
- *Ejaculation* of semen (sperm and seminal fluid) from the posterior urethra involves contractions of the bulbo-cavernous and urethral muscles. The passage of semen from the upper part of the urethra back into the bladder is normally prevented by sympathetic contraction of the urethral sphincter, but if this fails retrograde ejaculation can occur. The volume of semen generally ejaculated is usually between 2 and 6 mL and the sperm concentration is between 20 and 100 million sperm/mL, although these parameters will depend on the frequency

of ejaculation. Men are considered to be subfertile if their sperm count is <20 million sperm/mL.

It is remarkable that only one sperm is required for fertilization and that less than 1 in 1 000 000 sperm ever makes the journey through the 30–40 cm of the male and female reproductive tract to reach its final destination in the fallopian tube. This distance is 100 000 times the length of a sperm, each of which is only a few thousandths of a millimeter long.

Over 50% of cases of erectile dysfunction have a physical basis such as interference of spinal reflexes or blood supply such as occurs, for example, in diabetic complications. To what extent testosterone contributes towards the male sexual response depends on the individual. However, loss of androgens before puberty reduces the normal pubertal sex drive and androgen deficiency in adulthood causes a gradual loss of sex interest and an increasing incidence of erectile dysfunction. The sexual response may also be suppressed by the central nervous system and psychogenic stimuli from the brain such as performance anxiety and depression can cause erectile dysfunction, loss of sex drive, premature ejaculation, ejaculatory failure, and loss of orgasm. These problems are often amenable to behavioral therapy, although oral sildenafil (Viagra, a phosphodiesterase type 5 (PDE5) inhibitor), which inhibits the breakdown of cGMP and thus potentiates the effects of nitric oxide on vasodilatation (*Figure 7.19*), is now widely used to treat a variety of causes of sexual dysfunction. Newer and possibly more effective PDE5 inhibitors include tadalafil and vardenafil.

Prostagalandin E-1 (PGE_1) is a vasodilator produced by the seminal tubes and so another medical option is alprostadil, a PGE_1, which can be given as an intraurethral suppository (MUSE) or in an intracavernous injectable form (Caverject). This may be given alone or in conjunction with papaverine or phentolamine (an α-adrenergic blocker). In some patients vacuum constriction devices may be useful in inducing erection, and in more extreme cases surgical intervention (implantation of a penile prosthesis or penile arterial reconstruction) might be considered.

The role of testosterone is not clear; many endocrinologists believe that testosterone is there to increase libido rather than performance, although it is often worth restoring testosterone levels into the normal range should they be low.

7.5.5 Causes of male infertility

Male factors are considered to contribute to infertility in 25–50% of infertile couples and the cause can be genetic, hormonal, physical, or psychological. The most common chromosomal defect which causes gonadal dysgenesis (primary testicular failure) and infertility is Klinefelter syndrome (47,XXY) and its variants (see *Section 7.5.6*) which have an estimated frequency of 1:500 to 1:1000 live births. Patients with Klinefelter syndrome typically present with small testes, infertility, low testosterone levels, erectile dysfunction and low bone mineral metabolism, although sperm can be found in a significant percentage of patients, so they are not necessarily sterile. Other causes of primary testicular failure include cryptorchidism (which may be genetically linked), orchitis (inflammation of the testes, typically caused by mumps), trauma, and chemotherapy. In fact, congenital or acquired testicular failure accounts for about 50% of cases of male infertility and typically these patients will have low testosterone levels and high LH and FSH levels, resulting from the loss of negative feedback on testosterone; in other words, hypergonadotropic hypogonadism. In contrast, hypogonadotropic hypogonadism results from any cause of hypopituitarism or pituitary failure, but the incidence of infertility related to this endocrine disorder probably only represents about 2% of all cases of infertility.

Duct obstruction probably accounts for about 15% of all cases of male infertility, and other causes include systemic illness, drugs and toxins, ejaculatory dysfunction, sperm antibodies and sperm abnormalities. Varicocele, an abnormal dilatation of the spermatic veins in the pampiniform plexus of the spermatic cord (see *Figure 7.13*) caused by incompetent valves, has often been quoted as the most common form of male infertility. Whether this is a cause or simply an association with infertility continues to be debated.

Finally, mutations of genes controlling sex development (see below) and steroid synthesis in a male phenotype, as well as microdeletions in the Y chromosome which cause defects in spermatogenesis, can all cause infertility, though such cases are rare. There are many causes of infertility and the clinical evaluation of the infertile male and possible treatment options are outlined in *Box 7.7*.

Box 7.7 | Clinical evaluation and treatments of male infertility

Evaluation

Medical history and physical examination.

Laboratory tests

- Semen analysis.
- Hormone concentrations: testosterone, LH/FSH, prolactin, and estradiol/estrone.

Imaging

- MRI of pituitary and hypothalamus (if indicated).
- Ultrasound/MRI of the testes (if indicated).

Treatments

General

- Lifestyle changes such as stopping smoking, reducing alcohol intake, and the wearing of cool and loose underwear may sometimes lead to an improvement in sperm quality and number.
- Some studies have suggested potential benefits of antioxidants, e.g. folic acid, vitamin E.

Medical

- Males with hypogonadotropic hypogonadism can be treated with exogenous gonadotropins to enhance both spermatogenesis and testosterone production.
- Specific urogenital infections should be appropriately managed.

Surgical

- Surgical intervention in cases of structural abnormalities of the testes, vas deferens and associated structures may be attempted.
- Surgical sperm retrieval can be attempted with or without prior gonadotropin priming followed by ICSI during an IVF cycle (see Case 7.3).

7.5.6 Klinefelter syndrome

Klinefelter syndrome was first described in 1942 as a clinical condition characterized by small testes, azoospermia, gynecomastia, and an elevated serum FSH (*Box 7.8*). The chromosomal basis of the disorder was first described in 1959. Subsequently, the diagnosis of Klinefelter syndrome has required the demonstration of the 47,XXY karyotype or one of its rarer variants.

The prevalence of Klinefelter syndrome appears to be approximately 1 in 660 males, and recent data suggest a rising incidence over the last few decades. It is the most frequent form of primary testicular dysfunction affecting spermatogenesis as well as hormone production and is found in about 12% of men presenting with azoospermia.

Box 7.8 | Klinefelter syndrome (47,XXY or mosaicism)

Clinical features

- Reduced libido and erectile dysfunction.
- Gynecomastia.
- Reduced facial hair.
- Obesity.
- Infertility.
- Mild to moderate mental retardation.

Risks

- Type 2 DM.
- Osteoporosis.
- Thromboembolism.
- Malignancies – extragonadal germ cell tumors.

Investigations

- Karyotyping: 47,XXY in 80%; higher grade chromosomal aneuploidies or mosaicism in the remainder.
- Testosterone: low; elevated FSH and LH.
- Elevated SHBG and estradiol.
- Semen analysis – azoospermia/oligospermia.

Management

- Androgen replacement therapy – lifelong.
- Surgical reduction – gynecomastia.
- Fertility.
- ICSI has resulted in successful pregnancies.
- TESE – microsurgical testicular sperm extraction.
- IVF.
- Cryopreservation for future pregnancies.
- Genetic counseling.
- Psychological support.

A non-mosaic 47,XXY karyotype is found in 80–90% of Klinefelter patients. A mosaic is seen in another 5–10% of patients; 47,XXY/46,XY mosaicism is most common. The 48,XXXY, 48,XXYY, and 49,XXXXY karyotypes constitute 4–5% of all Klinefelter syndrome karyotypes, and structurally abnormal extra X chromosomes are found in less than 1% of patients. Karyotype analysis can be supported by molecular genetic methods which are used to quantify the number of X chromosomes, for example, by quantitative PCR analysis of the androgen receptor gene located on the X chromosome.

Clinical manifestations

Patients with Klinefelter syndrome are usually inconspicuous until puberty, although the velocity of height gain can be increased in the pre-pubertal years. Men with Klinefelter syndrome tend to be tall (mean adult height is about the 80th percentile for the population) and to have relatively long legs compared to their overall height (*Figure 7.20*). In most patients, early stages of puberty proceed normally. Post-pubertally the syndrome is characterized by small testes with a firm consistency remaining in the range of 1–4 mL. Most patients with Klinefelter syndrome are infertile because of azoospermia. The degree of virilization varies widely. In early puberty, LH and FSH increase while serum levels of testosterone plateau at or just below the lower limit of the normal range. After the age of 25 years, about 80% of patients have reduced serum testosterone levels and complain of decreasing libido and potency. On average, serum estradiol levels are at the upper end of, or exceed, the normal range. LH and especially FSH levels may be exceedingly high; serum levels of inhibin B are very low or undetectable.

During puberty bilateral painless gynecomastia of varying degrees develops in about half of the patients. The intelligence of Klinefelter patients is variable; some of the young patients attract attention because of learning difficulties and school problems. In

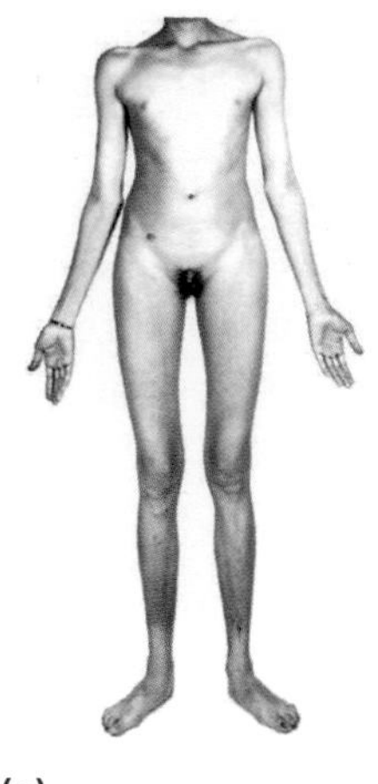

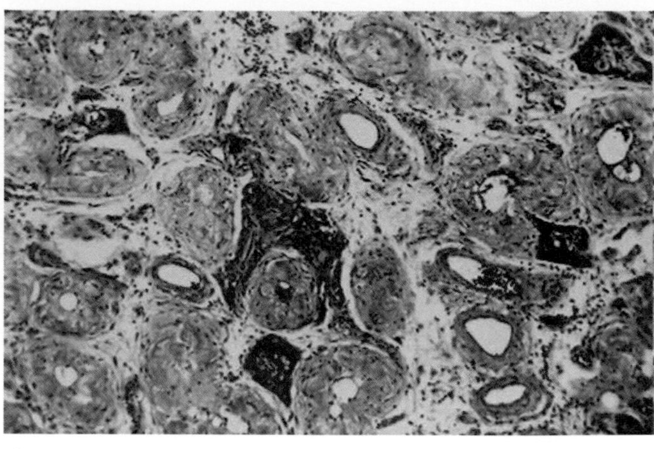

(a) (b)

Figure 7.20. A patient with Klinefelter syndrome (a) and histological appearance of the testis (b) showing gonadal dysgenesis.

general, they fail to reach the level of achievement or professional expectations of their families. Compared with their classmates certain abnormal physical and psychological characteristics of the patients become obvious and they may become socially alienated. Higher-grade aneuploidy of the sex chromosomes (48,XXXY, 48,XXYY, and 49,XXXXY) is associated with mild mental retardation. Klinefelter patients with chromosome mosaics (47,XXY/46,XY) may show very few clinical symptoms.

Management

Regarding infertility treatment, it should be noted that in rare cases sperm can be found in the ejaculate and, exceptionally, spontaneous paternity has been described. Preliminary data suggest that in about 20–50% of patients with Klinefelter syndrome it may be possible to retrieve sperm by testicular sperm extraction (TESE). Several pregnancies have been achieved with testicular sperm used for intracytoplasmic sperm injection (ICSI). When testosterone levels are reduced, substitution with testosterone is indicated. To avoid symptoms of androgen deficiency, hormone

CASE 7.3

360 370

- Man of 37 years with reduced libido and failure to conceive
- Sparse pubic hair and small soft testes
- High FSH and LH, and low testosterone; 47,XXY – Klinefelter syndrome
- Started on testosterone replacement and fertility addressed by IUI with donor sperm

The patient was diagnosed with Klinefelter syndrome on the basis of karyotype. He had no gynecomastia (a common problem in Klinefelter patients which may require surgical intervention for psychological reasons) but he was concerned about the size of his testes. He was commenced on testosterone replacement with Testogel 50 mg daily. A baseline bone mineral density scan showed no evidence of osteoporosis or osteopenia. Fertility was discussed; although he was ambivalent, his partner was extremely keen to start a family. Semen analysis on two occasions revealed azoospermia. In the light of hypergonadotropic hypogonadism it was not possible to attempt to induce sperm production with gonadotropins. Sperm donation was discussed and, after a wedge biopsy of the testes revealed no usable sperm (small numbers of sperm from biopsies can be used effectively in an IVF cycle with ICSI), the couple agreed to sperm donation. His partner was inseminated by donor sperm in an intrauterine insemination (IUI) IVF cycle which was successful. He continues on testosterone replacement, is reasonably happy and well-adjusted.

replacement therapy should be initiated as early as needed. Studies have repeatedly shown that early testosterone replacement not only relieves biological symptoms such as anemia, osteoporosis, muscular weakness, and impotence, but also leads to better social adjustment and integration. Testosterone replacement must be considered a lifelong therapy in Klinefelter patients to assure quality of life. Usually gynecomastia is not influenced by hormone therapy. If it disturbs the patient, a plastic surgeon experienced in cosmetic breast surgery could perform a mastectomy.

7.6 Ovarian function and its control

CASE 7.4

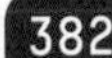
382

- Woman of 29 years complaining of amenorrhea
- BMI of 19 but extensive regular exercise
- FSH and LH both low and estrogen undetectable

A 29 year old medical student attended the endocrine clinic complaining of amenorrhea after stopping the oral contraceptive 14 months previously. She had previously achieved a first class degree in biomedical science and admitted to being a 'workaholic'. She exercised regularly and was currently training for a marathon and was running at least 70 miles a week alongside regular gym workouts. Apart from the amenorrhea she was asymptomatic and there was no previous personal or family history. She was on no medication (including over-the-counter remedies), did not smoke or use recreational drugs or alcohol. There was no galactorrhea. On examination she weighed 49 kg with a BMI of 19 kg/m^2. She was of normal height with no syndromic features. Examination was otherwise unremarkable. Initial investigations revealed:

- FSH 0.7 IU/L (NR luteal 2.6–9.5)
- LH 1.2 IU/L (NR luteal 0.8–10.4)
- prolactin 220 mIU/L (NR 100–550)
- estrogen was undetectable

A transvaginal ultrasound scan revealed a normal uterus and ovaries but a thin endometrial lining (3 mm). She had been having unprotected intercourse with her partner for 12 months and was now keen for a pregnancy. There was no history of pelvic surgery, irradiation, or infection.

7.6.1 Anatomy of the ovary

Each ovary nestles in a small depression of the posterior wall of the broad ligament on each side of the peritoneal cavity and just above the pelvic brim. They are connected to the fimbriated ends of the fallopian tubes (see *Figure 7.12*). The ovaries are dull white in color, oval in shape (3 × 2 × 1 cm) and weigh about 5.8 g. They are enclosed in a tough fibrous capsule, the tunica albuginea, and consist of an outer cortex and an inner medulla. The cortex contains all the follicles and remains of ruptured follicles embedded in vascular fibrous tissue (*Figure 7.21*). The inner medulla is where the blood vessels, lymphatic system, and nerves enter the ovary. The appearance of the ovary varies with the age of the woman. Before puberty the glands are smooth and rather solid in consistency and contain many primordial follicles. Between puberty and the menopause their surfaces become more corrugated in appearance due to the activity of the gland during each ovarian cycle. After the menopause they shrink and are covered with scar tissue, the result of monthly follicular rupture.

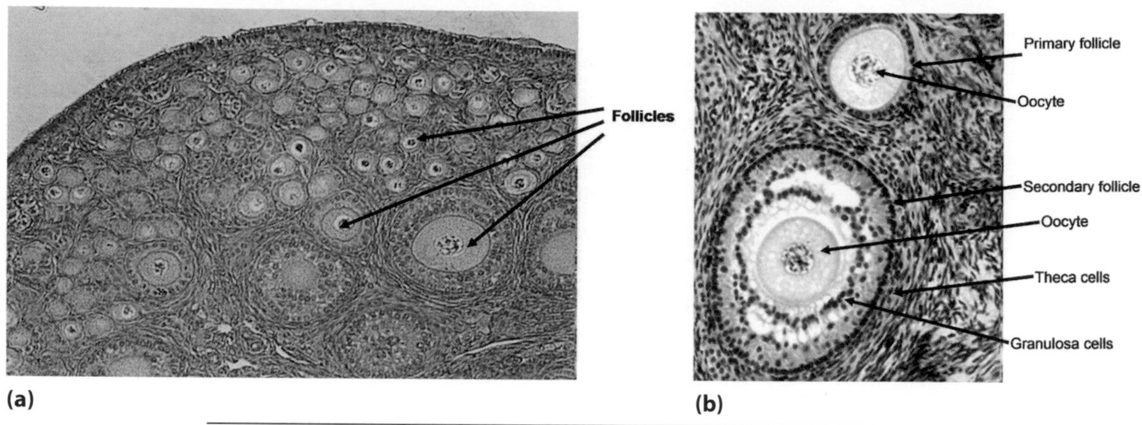

Figure 7.21. Histology of the ovary.
(a) Cortex of the human ovary showing follicles at various stages of development. (b) Higher power image showing a primary and a secondary follicle.

7.6.2 Functions of the ovary

Like the testis, the ovaries have two main functions – to produce and ovulate a mature oocyte during each menstrual cycle and to secrete hormones, notably estrogens and progesterone. These steroids are important for preparation of the reproductive tract for fertilization and subsequent establishment of pregnancy, maintaining pregnancy during the first trimester, in the development of secondary sexual characteristics, and maintaining other aspects of female physiology.

Ovarian function in the adult is controlled by the GnRH pulse generator (see *Box 7.1*) which regulates the synthesis and secretion of LH and FSH. In turn the gonadotropins regulate the latter stages of folliculogenesis, ovulation, maintenance of the corpus luteum, and steroid synthesis in the ovary. Unlike the testis, where only LH is responsible for testosterone secretion, the ovary requires both LH and FSH for steroid synthesis and the gonadotropins act on different cell types of the maturing follicle (*Figure 7.22*). The early stages of folliculogenesis are independent of gonadotropins, but the formation of antral follicles and steroid synthesis requires gonadotropins (see *Figure 7.25b*). At this stage of follicular development, the oocyte is surrounded by many layers of granulosa cells and, separated by the basal lamina, theca cells form the outer layers of the follicle. G-protein coupled LH receptors are present on theca cells and LH stimulates the synthesis of progesterone and androstenedione from cholesterol in these cells. The androstenedione then diffuses into the granulosa cell layer where it is converted to estrone and estradiol by the enzyme aromatase. Granulosa cells in these maturing follicles have G-protein linked FSH receptors and FSH regulates the expression of aromatase. Thus estrogen synthesis in developing ovarian follicles requires two cell types and two gonadotropins (*Figure 7.22*).

Estradiol and progesterone (the dominant hormone secreted by the corpus luteum) exert negative feedback effects on the GnRH pulse generator and hence LH and FSH secretion (*Figure 7.23*). However, just prior to ovulation in each menstrual cycle, there is a switch from negative to positive feedback of estradiol stimulating a surge of LH secretion and a small FSH surge, and this switch is responsible for the release of a mature ovum (see *Section 7.6.4*). Whilst these feedback effects were

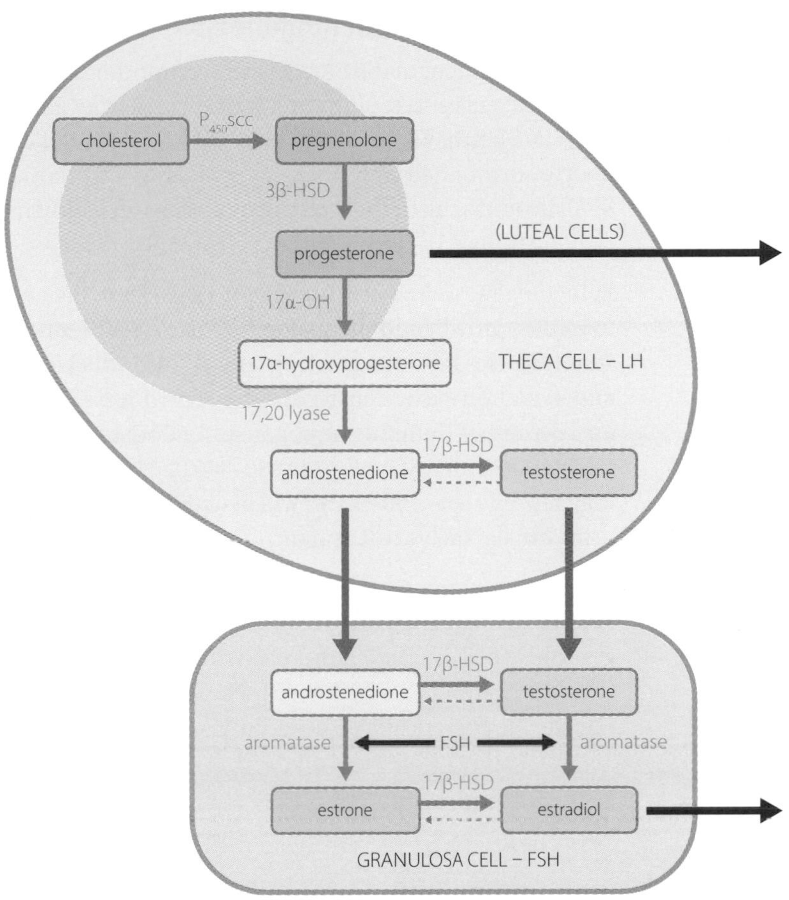

Figure 7.22. Steroid synthesis in the ovary and control by gonadotropins.
Luteinizing hormone (LH) acts on theca cells to produce androgens which diffuse though the basal lamina into the granulosa cell layer where follicle stimulating hormone (FSH) stimulates the synthesis of estrogens from androgens. Just prior to ovulation, the granulosa cells acquire receptors for LH that respond to the pre-ovulatory surge of LH to induce rupture of the follicle. HSD, hydroxysteroid dehydrogenase; 17α-OH (hydroxylase) and 17,20 lyase CYP17.

thought to be mediated by effects on the GnRH secreting neurons, there is now good evidence that both positive and negative feedback effects of ovarian steroids (and negative feedback effects of testosterone in the male) are mediated via groups of hypothalamic neurons that synthesize kisspeptin which acts on its GPR54 receptors on GnRH neurons (see *Figure 7.9*). This system is also thought to be involved in the initiation of puberty (*Section 7.3.2*).

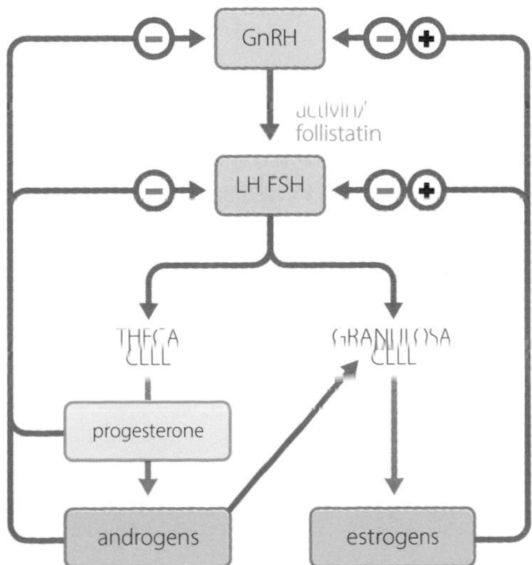

Figure 7.23. Hormonal regulation of ovarian function.

7.6.3 Oogenesis and folliculogenesis

The development of the oocyte and surrounding follicular cells is a highly complex array of events and requires autocrine, paracrine, and endocrine factors and cross talk between the oocyte itself and the follicular cells. Primordial follicles (an oocyte surrounded by a single layer of flattened granulosa cells) are laid down in fetal life and at birth the ovary contains its full endowment of follicles – there is no replenishment.

Folliculogenesis involves two major steps. First, the activation of primordial follicles to initiate growth and then, after puberty, cyclic recruitment of a limited number of small follicles from the growing cohort from which one is selected for dominance and ovulation each menstrual cycle. Activation of primordial follicles begins *in utero* and continues until the menopause. A neonate girl born with 1 million primordial follicles at birth will have only 300–400 000 by puberty (see *Figure 7.4*) and of these follicles only 300–400 (0.1%) will ovulate; by the menopause only about 1000 primordial follicles will remain.

The trigger for the recruitment and initiation of growth-arrested primordial follicles to form primary follicles (an oocyte surrounded by a single layer of cuboidal granulosa cells) is, as yet, unknown but several growth factors have been implicated (*Figures 7.24* and *7.25 b*). These include KIT and KIT ligand signaling between the oocyte, the pre-granulosa cells, bone morphogenic peptides (BMPs), fibroblast

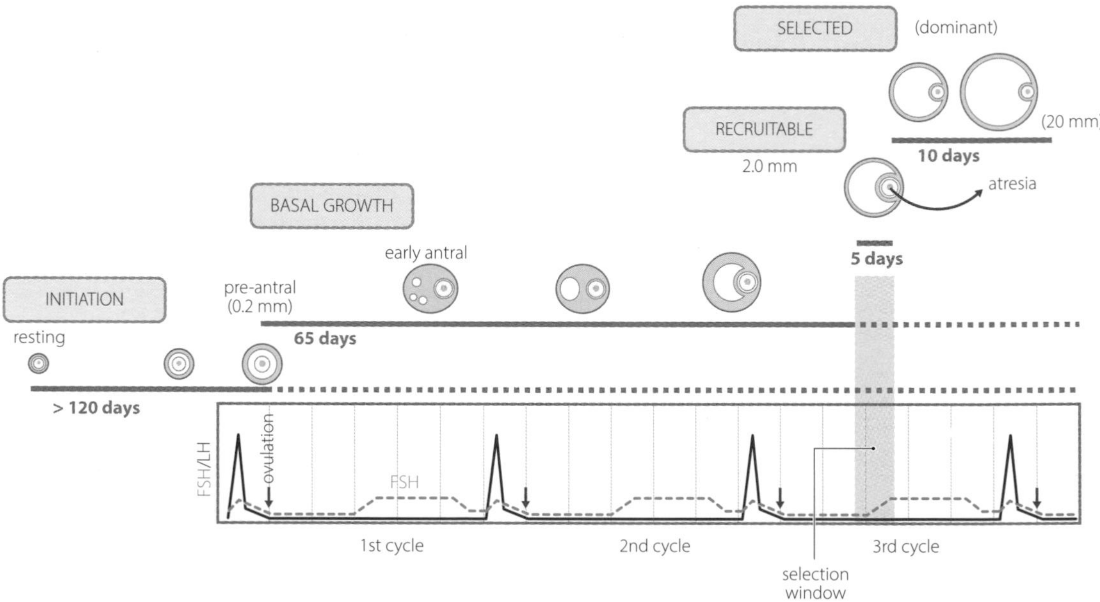

Figure 7.24. The process of folliculogenesis.
During a woman's reproductive years there is a continual initiation of growth of primordial follicles into pre-antral follicles. This stage of follicular growth, which takes several months, is considered to be independent of gonadotropin stimulation, although paracrine effects of local growth factors produced by the oocyte and granulosa cells are important in this initiation. Follicles that reach the pre-antral stage (~0.2 mm) become responsive to gonadotropins, particularly to the intercycle rise in FSH secretion and this stimulates further development of follicles into antral follicles. Over the course of about three menstrual cycles follicular growth continues and if they reach a size of about 2.0 mm they can be recruited and selected to become the dominant follicle. It is thought that the dominant follicle emerges as the one that is most responsive to the intercycle rise of FSH secretion, whilst the rest undergo atresia. The factors that govern continued atresia throughout follicular growth remain poorly understood.

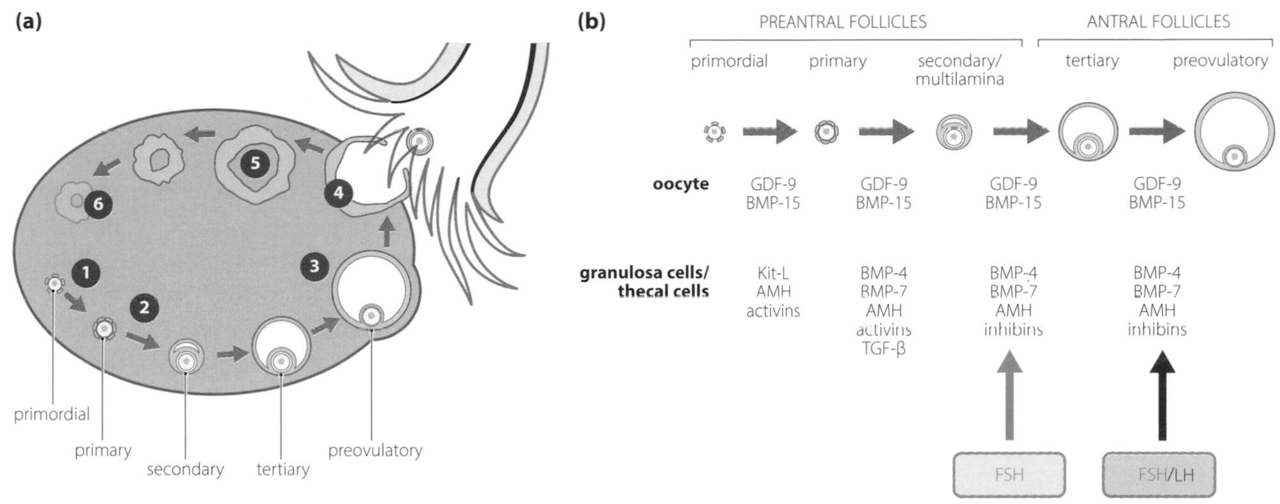

Figure 7.25. The control of folliculogenesis.
(a) Primordial follicle (an oocyte surrounded by a single flattened layer of granulosa cells) begins to grow (1) and becomes a primary oocyte (2) where the single layer of granulosa cells have become cuboidal in shape. The granulosa cells divide and form several layers (creating a secondary follicle) and stromal cells condense round the basal lamina forming layers of theca cells. Growth continues over several menstrual cycles and eventually a dominant follicle emerges which is then ovulated (4). The empty follicle forms the corpus luteum (5) which then undergoes luteolysis toward the end of the menstrual cycle (6).
(b) Growth factors produced by the oocyte and granulosa/theca cells are listed. These control the initiation of follicular growth and then the formation of antral follicles and finally the emergence of the dominant pre-ovulatory follicle. The pre-antral stages of follicular development are considered to be gonadotropin independent.
Kit-L, Kit ligand; BMP, bone morphogenic peptide; AMH, anti-Müllerian hormone; TGF, transforming growth factor; LH, luteinizing hormone; FSH, follicle stimulating hormone.

growth factors (FGFs), and GDF-9 secreted by the oocyte. Further development into secondary follicles which have two, progressing to several, layers of granulosa cells (pre-antral follicles), also require further growth factors such as BMPs, GDF-9, activin, and transforming growth factor (TGF)-β. A negative regulator of all stages of folliculogenesis is AMH which is produced exclusively by the granulosa cells. This progression from primary follicle to the pre-antral phase involves oocyte enlargement, proliferation of the granulosa cells, formation of the basal lamina, and the formation of theca cells from somatic cells which occurs early in secondary follicle development. Essentially, the granulosa cells are the 'nurse' cells of the oocyte and the theca cells supply the granulosa cells with estrogen precursors and the other nutrients and oxygen required for the development of the oocyte. The theca cells are well vascularized but there is no blood supply inside the basal lamina to the granulosa cells or oocyte.

The development of primordial to pre-antral follicles extends over a period of several months and appears to be independent of gonadotropin stimulation (*Figures 7.24* and *7.25*). Females with inactivating mutations of the FSH receptor show a block in folliculogenesis at the pre-antral stage. Thus whilst early folliculogenesis is independent of gonadotropins, transition to the antral stage of development is dependent on FSH, not only to prevent granulosa cell apoptosis and follicular atresia, but for granulosa cell proliferation, estradiol synthesis, and LH receptor expression.

During antral folliculogenesis multiple small, fluid-filled spaces eventually coalesce to form a single antral cavity which separates two functionally distinct granulosa cell populations. The mural cells that line the wall of the follicle are critical for estrogen synthesis and ovulation, whereas the cumulus granulosa cells that surround the oocyte promote its growth and developmental competence. These processes not only involve LH and FSH, but continued intraovarian paracrine secretions which involve BMPs, TGF-β, activin, and inhibins. AMH continues to exert an inhibitory effect on folliculogenesis, probably by inhibiting aromatase and thus estradiol synthesis in the follicles. Circulating levels of AMH correlate with the number of antral follicles and its measurement in the circulation had been used as a marker for ovarian reserve. Levels of AMH decline markedly in the menopausal period. Interestingly, women with polycystic ovary syndrome (see *Section 7.6.7*), which is associated with impaired folliculogenesis, have very high levels of AMH in the follicular fluid filling the antrum of the follicle.

Over two to three menstrual cycles, pre-antral follicles (0.2 mm) grow to about 2.0 mm diameter antral follicles. During this growth period there is continued atresia of many of these follicles, as also occurs in the pre-antral phase of folliculogenesis. When a cohort of developing follicles reaches about 2.0 mm in diameter one follicle is selected to become the 'dominant' follicle which will grow from about 2.0 to 20 mm in 10 days and then be ovulated (*Figure 7.24*). The mechanism(s) responsible for this selection are not known but probably involve up-regulation of FSH receptors by activin A and TGF-β, increased FSH-induced aromatase expression, and possibly other factors including insulin-like growth factor-I (IGF-I).

Ovulation of the dominant follicle requires the expression of LH receptors on the mural granulosa cells (prior to this LH receptors are only expressed on the theca cells). The pre-ovulatory surge triggers a cascade of events including activation of the progesterone receptor and the expression of prostaglandin synthase 2 and epidermal growth factors. These lead to resumption of the first meiotic division of the oocyte and cumulus expansion. Eventually the ovarian surface epithelium ruptures and the oocyte surrounded by cumulus cells (the cumulus–oocyte complex) is extruded and captured by fimbria of the fallopian tube.

7.6.4 The menstrual cycle and its disorders

The ovary shows cyclical activity, unlike the testis that is maintained in a more or less constant state of activity. Hormone secretions vary according the phase of the menstrual cycle and gonadal steroids have both negative and positive feedback effects on the control of gonadotropin secretion in relation to the phase. The average length of a menstrual cycle is 28 days and although considerable variation is seen, in 95% of women each cycle lasts between 25 and 34 days. Most of the variation is due to differences in the length of the first (follicular) phase of the cycle, whilst the second luteal phase is more likely to be about 14 days in length (*Figure 7.26*).

By convention the menstrual cycle begins on the first day of menstruation which is initiated by luteolysis – breakdown of the corpus luteum formed after ovulation in the preceding cycle. Luteolysis results in falling levels of luteal estrogen, progesterone, and inhibin A (*Figure 7.17*) and, as a consequence of relaxed negative feedback, the secretion of LH and FSH rises. This intercycle rise in gonadotropins stimulates growth of cohorts of antral follicles and increases their production of androgens, estrogens and inhibin B. From the cohort of the largest antral follicles one will be selected during this rise in FSH and becomes the dominant follicle which

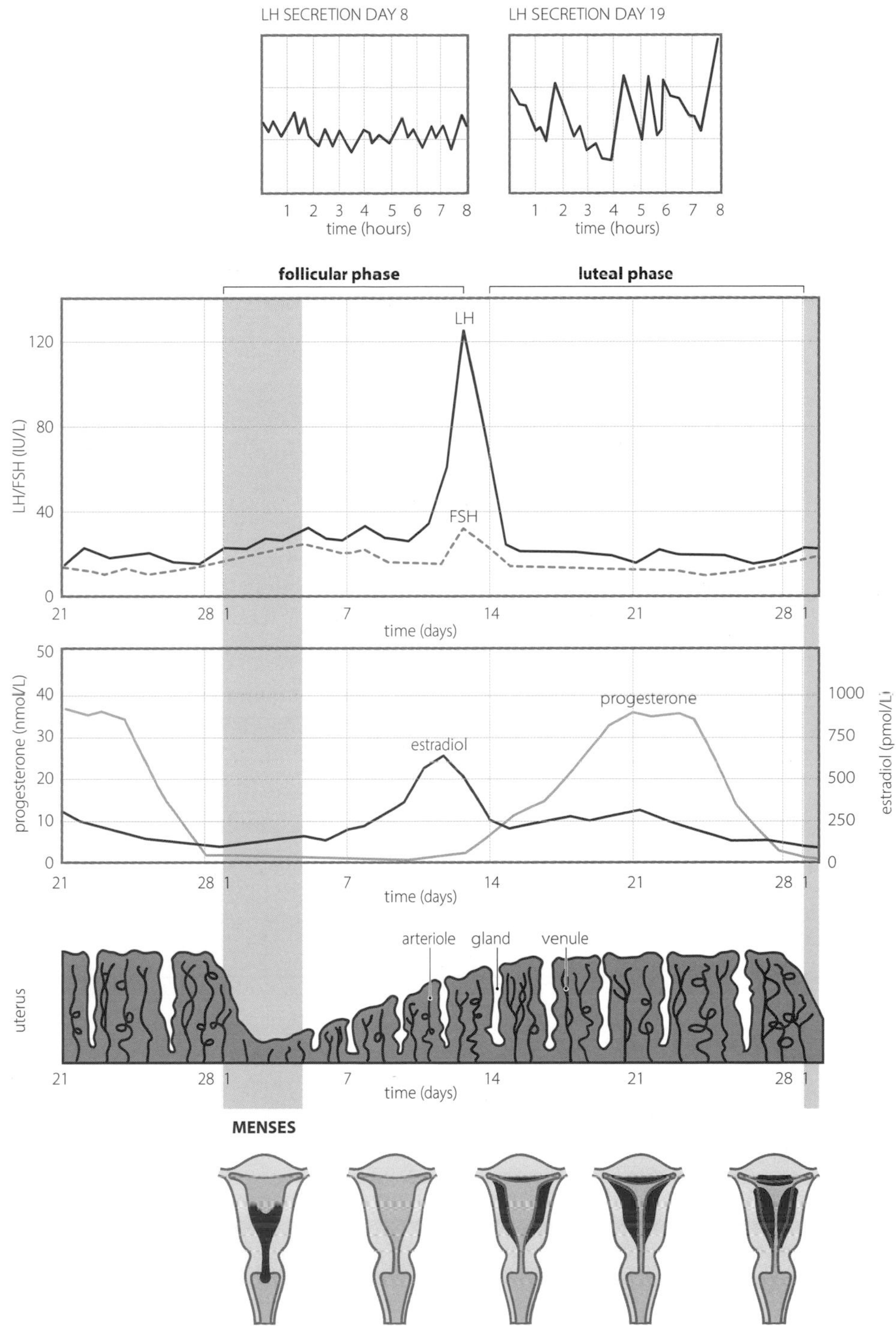

Figure 7.26. The human menstrual cycle.

Average serum concentrations of the gonadotropins (LH and FSH) and the gonadal steroids (estradiol and progesterone) during the follicular and luteal phase of a typical 28-day menstrual cycle. Positive feedback effects of peak estradiol mid-cycle induce the pre-ovulatory LH surge. Also shown are the changes in the uterine endometrium with the development of the spiral arteries and growth of the secretory glands.

The first half of the uterine cycle is known as the proliferative phase and the second half the secretory phase. The breakdown of the endometrium following the decline of ovarian steroids is manifest by menstruation. The pulsatile pattern of GnRH (top) indicates changes in frequency and amplitude of GnRH pulses at different phases of the menstrual cycle. This may be important in determining differential synthesis and secretion of LH or FSH.

will be ovulated at the end of the follicular phase of the cycle. The remainder undergo atresia. The selection of a dominant follicle leads to a further rise in estrogen and androgen synthesis and, when levels of estradiol reach a critical concentration for 24–48 hours, there is a switch from negative to positive feedback effects and estradiol triggers a surge of LH and smaller rise in FSH secretion. This is thought to be due to estradiol increasing the frequency and amplitude of GnRH pulses and increasing GnRH receptors on the anterior pituitary gland.

Ovulation requires that the dominant follicle rises to the surface of the ovary and LH receptors are expressed on the granulosa cells (normally they are only expressed on theca cells). Ovulation occurs 9–12 hours after the pre-ovulatory LH surge and the granulosa cells and theca cells of the empty follicle are remodeled and form the corpus luteum. This is the luteal phase of the cycle and is characterized by rising concentrations of progesterone and 17α-hydroxyprogesterone which peak about 8 days after the LH surge. The luteinized cells also make large amounts of estrogen and inhibin A (*Figure 7.17*) and these secretions exert negative feedback effects on the hypothalamus and pituitary gland and antral development is arrested. If conception does not occur luteolysis begins approximately 10–12 days after ovulation. This involves the collapse of the lutein cells, ischemia, and progressive cell death, but the factors stimulating luteolysis in humans are unknown.

The shifting balance of hormones during the ovarian cycle affects the activity of the female reproductive tract. Estrogens maintain ciliated movement and secretions from the epithelium of the fallopian tube, making the environment suitable for sperm and oocyte transport. Progesterone may inhibit the actions of estrogen. These steroids have more dramatic effects on the uterus. During the follicular phase of the cycle estrogens stimulate myometrial activity and stromal cells of the endometrium proliferate (the proliferative phase of the cycle). The glands enlarge, the endometrium becomes richly supplied with blood vessels, and the epithelial cells secrete a fluid of watery constitution that contains proteolytic enzymes. In the luteal phase there is further growth of the endometrium and the glands secrete a thick fluid rich in nutrients to nourish a fertilized egg and encourage implantation of the conceptus. If fertilization occurs, the hCG secreted by the developing placenta maintains the corpus luteum and hence progesterone secretion. In the absence of fertilization, the steroid support of the endometrium is lost, the spiral arteries that have grown up into the endometrium contract and cells, starved of their normal blood supply, break away and menstrual loss ensues.

In the cervix estrogens relax the smooth muscle and stimulate the epithelium to secrete a mucus that will allow penetration of sperm. Progesterone inhibits mucus secretion and depresses sperm penetration. Thus sperm penetration is low in the early follicular and luteal phase of the cycle and reaches a maximum around ovulation. Finally, estrogen and progesterone also induce cyclical changes in vaginal secretions, varying the metabolic substrates available for bacterial flora: this results in different proportions of volatile alphatic acids generated by bacteria and give distinctive odors to vaginal secretions.

There are several markers to indicate ovulation has occurred.

- Detection of the LH surge in the urine. This is both sensitive and robust.
- Measurement of progesterone levels in the luteal phase (usually at day 21). High levels indicate the formation of a corpus luteum and thus previous ovulation.

- Body temperature. The increase in progesterone after ovulation results in a small rise in body temperature but while this can be used to indicate whether ovulation has occurred, obtaining reliable temperature measurements is difficult.

Total blood loss during each menstruation varies from cycle to cycle and in different women at different stages of their reproductive life. Average blood loss is about 50–60 mL although this can vary from 10 to 80 mL. Excessive blood loss (menorrhagia) can lead to iron deficiency anemia. Finally it should be noted that menstruation can occur in the absence of ovulation because in anovulatory cycles menstrual bleeding results from estrogen withdrawal after the non-ovulatory follicles have degenerated.

Rates of fertility peak around the age of 20 and, thereafter, show a more or less linear decline until the menopause, while the rates of childlessness increase exponentially from around 25 up to the age of 45. This has meant that the rising social trend to delay pregnancy until later in reproductive life has led to an increased demand for assisted conception techniques, although a successful outcome from these methods also decreases with age. With regard to fertility control, there are three socially accepted methods: contraception, induced pregnancy termination, and sterilization. An outline of these methods is beyond the scope of this book, but further details of steroidal contraceptives are given in *Box 7.9*.

Box 7.9 | Steroidal contraception

The first female 'pill' was introduced in the early 1960s and since then a range of steroidal contraceptives has been developed, including:

- combined estrogen and progestogen oral contraceptive (COC)
- oral progestogen only pill (POP)
- progestogen only contraception delivered either by injection (every 2–3 months) or implants (every 5 years)
- progestogen-releasing intrauterine device.

Synthetic steroids are used in these preparations because their half-lives in the body are longer and their effects more sustained. Such synthetic steroids include 17β-ethinyl estradiol and mestranol, and the progestogens such as levonorgestrel (norgestrel), etonorgestrel and drosperidone.

All methods of steroidal contraception (except the intrauterine device) have some effects on suppressing ovulation, although the COC is most effective in this respect. Ovulation is suppressed by inhibiting the formation of pre-ovulatory follicles and the pre-ovulatory LH surge (negative feedback effects of the steroids). All preparations alter cervical mucus, reducing sperm penetrability and reducing the receptivity of the endometrium to implantation of a blastocyst. With progestogen only preparations menstruation is usually irregular, although with the COC menstrual bleeding is regular. COCs are available as biphasic or triphasic preparations. In biphasic preparations estrogen and progestogen are given in the first half of the cycle with the progestogen dose stepped up at mid-cycle followed by seven steroid-free days. With triphasic preparations the first 5–6 days have low estrogen and progestogen, a further 5–6 days with slightly higher doses of progestogen, followed by 10 days with low estrogen and doubled progestogen in an attempt to mimic the hormonal changes of a natural cycle. In the developed world, oral contraceptives are the most commonly used methods of contraception, although their use progressively declines between the age of 30 and 50 years.

There has been a continued search for a male 'pill' with the ultimate goal of achieving 100% oligospermia, which is reversible. Long-acting testosterone injections with a progestogen implant or a daily testosterone gel with a depot injection of progestogen every 3 months result in severe oligospermia in 80–90% of men, but to date a uniformly effective regime remains elusive. Interestingly, there appear to be ethnic differences in the response to testosterone in suppressing gonadotropin secretions, and hence spermatogenesis.

Table 7.1. **Common causes of primary and secondary amenorrhea**

	Approximate frequency (%)
PRIMARY AMENORRHEA	
Breast development	30
Müllerian agenesis	10
Androgen insensitivity	9
Vaginal septum	2
Imperforate hymen	1
Constitutional delay	8
No breast development: high FSH	40
46,XX	15
46,XY	5
Abnormal	20
No breast development: low FSH	30
Constitutional delay	10
Prolactinomas	5
Kallmann syndrome	2
Other CNS	3
Stress, weight loss, anorexia	3
PCOS	3
Congenital adrenal hyperplasia	3
Other	1
SECONDARY AMENORRHEA	
Low or normal FSH	66
Weight loss/anorexia	
Non-specific hypothalamic	
Chronic anovulation including PCOS	
Hypothyroidism	
Cushing syndrome	
Pituitary tumor, empty sella, Sheehan syndrome	
Gonadal failure: high FSH	12
46,XX	
Abnormal karyotype	
High prolactin	13
Anatomic	7
Asherman syndrome	
Hyperandrogenic states	2
Ovarian tumor	
Non-classic CAH	
Undiagnosed	

The World Health Organization (WHO) classification of the causes of amenorrhea

Group I – no evidence of endogenous estrogen production, e.g. no breast development, normal or low FSH levels, normal prolactin levels, no evidence of a hypothalamic lesion.

Group II – evidence of estrogen production, e.g. breast development, normal levels of FSH and prolactin.

Group III – elevated serum FSH indicating gonadal failure.

7.6.5 Amenorrhea

Primary amenorrhea is defined as the failure to start menstruating by the age of 16 years, whilst secondary amenorrhea, which occurs after menarche, is defined by the absence of periods for 6 months. Primary amenorrhea is far less frequent than secondary amenorrhea (*Table 7.1*). It is usually caused by genetic defects, the most common being ovarian dysgenesis which occurs in Turner syndrome (see *Section 7.4.3*) although other genetic causes and indeed unknown causes of gonadal dysgenesis have been observed. It should be noted that gonadal dysgenesis specifically refers to impaired ovarian development, but is often applied to situations of primary amenorrhea or where there is a failure of development rather than dysgenesis.

Other, but rare, causes of primary amenorrhea include:

- failure of Müllerian duct development (there is no female reproductive tract) although ovaries are present and breast development will occur due to estrogens secreted by the ovaries
- CAIS in which an XY fetus develops into a female phenotype but without a female reproductive tract: breast development occurs due to peripheral conversion of androgens to estrogens from the undescended testes (see *Section 7.2.3*)
- anatomical vaginal abnormalities such as vaginal septum and imperforate hymen.

The prevalence of secondary amenorrhea (*Table 7.1*) that is not due to pregnancy, lactation, or menopause is approximately 3–4% and, although the list of potential causes is long, the majority of cases are accounted for by four conditions:

- hypothalamic amenorrhea
- hyperprolactinemia
- polycystic ovary syndrome
- ovarian failure.

Hypothalamic amenorrhea caused by loss of GnRH secretion is characterized by low levels of FSH and low estrogens. It is thus termed hypogonadotropic hypogonadism

Box 7.10 | Suggested flow diagram aiding the evaluation of women with amenorrhea

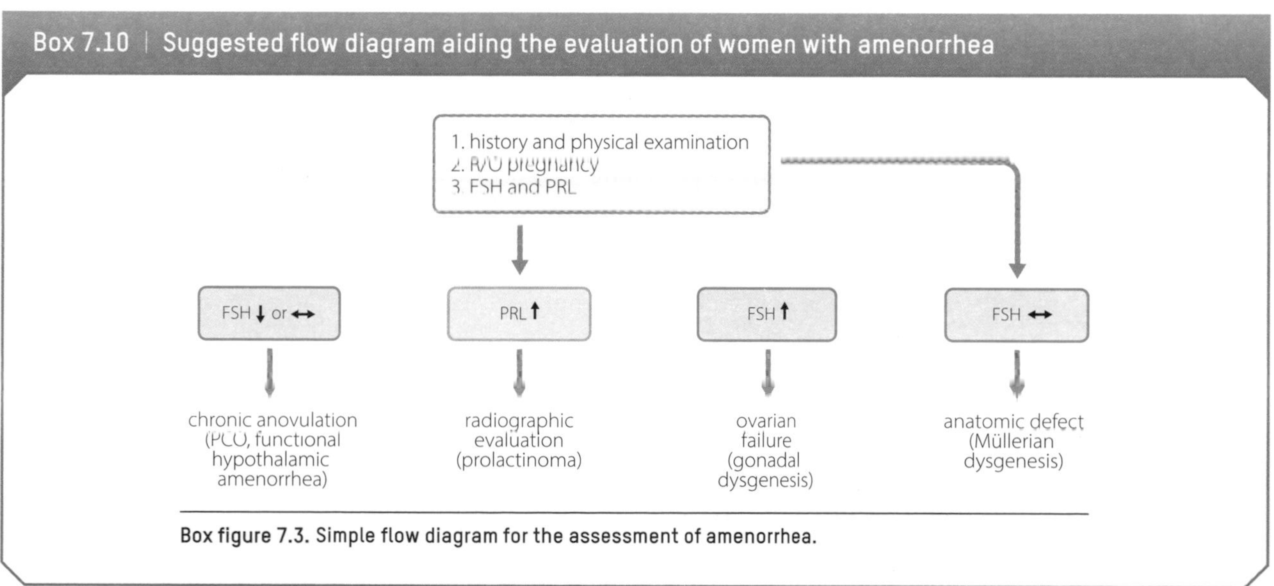

Box figure 7.3. Simple flow diagram for the assessment of amenorrhea.

and can be the cause of either primary or secondary amenorrhea. For example, weight loss/anorexia nervosa is associated with reduced pulsatile GnRH, as is intense exercise training and loss of body fat. Girls with untreated Kallmann syndrome (loss of GnRH neurons, see *Section 7.3.3*) will also have primary amenorrhea. Hypopituitarism causing loss of gonadotropin drive to the ovary is another cause of amenorrhea.

Cushing syndrome, hypothyroidism, chronic anovulation, and prolactinomas (prolactin secreting tumors of the anterior pituitary gland) suppress the endocrine functions of the hypothalamic–pituitary–gonadal axis and these endocrine states also result in amenorrhea. A suggested flow diagram aiding evaluation of women with amenorrhea is given in *Box 7.10.*

CASE 7.4 371 382

- Woman of 29 years complaining of amenorrhea
- BMI of 19 but extensive regular exercise
- FSH and LH both low and estrogen undetectable
- HRT with transdermal estrogen and oral progestogens (10/30) produced a regular withdrawal bleed

The patient had secondary 'post pill' amenorrhea with apparently low levels of gonadotropins and estrogen suggesting a central cause (hypogonadotropic hypogonadism). There was no history of traumatic brain injury or surgery/radiotherapy to the hypothalamic–pituitary area. An assessment of anterior pituitary function by measuring basal anterior pituitary hormones and cortisol at 09.00h was normal, with the exception of low LH, FSH, and estradiol. A pituitary MRI scan was completely normal. On the basis of the biochemistry, a diagnosis of hypogonadotropic hypogonadism was made. It was felt that the combination of significant stress and high level exercise with a low BMI were contributory factors. A DEXA scan was carried out to assess bone density and this was normal with no evidence of osteopenia or osteoporosis.

She was treated with three cycles of clomifene (50 mg for 5 days) and showed no gonadotropin increase or biochemical evidence of ovulation on any cycle and remained amenorrheic. She was started on HRT in the form of transdermal estrogen and oral progestogens for 10 days each calendar month. On this she started a regular withdrawal bleed.

After graduating as a doctor she decided to take a career break . Six months later she had gained weight and achieved a BMI of 23 kg/m^2. She continued to exercise but had reduced this to one gym session a week and was running no more than 30 miles a week. HRT was stopped and she resumed normal menses. Eight months later she conceived naturally. She has now returned to medicine and is working in endocrinology.

7.6.6 Polycystic ovary syndrome

Polycystic ovary syndrome (PCOS) is a heterogeneous disorder characterized by hyperandrogenism (both ovary and adrenal), ovulatory dysfunction and hyperinsulinemia and it is the commonest endocrine disorder in women of reproductive age. The spectrum of clinical features that patients with this disorder may present with is very variable. They range from women with anovulatory cycles or amenorrhea without the clinical features of androgen excess, to women with hirsutism who have regular ovulatory cycles. Some women with polycystic ovaries and androgen excess experience a mixture of ovulatory and anovulatory cycles, or may change from predominantly anovulatory to mainly ovulatory cycles depending on body weight. PCOS is also characterized by significant metabolic abnormalities including insulin resistance, hyperinsulinemia, and obesity.

CASE 7.5 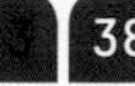 388

- Woman of 23 years with secondary amenorrhea, weight gain, and excess body hair
- BMI of 34, raised prolactin and LH, and reduced SHBG – FSH and testosterone normal
- Pelvic ultrasound revealed bilateral polycystic ovaries

A 23 year old woman attended the endocrine clinic complaining of secondary amenorrhea (of 14 months duration) associated with weight gain of approximately 10 kg over the last year. She had been particularly concerned by the worsening of her acne and the growth of hair around the chin, upper lip, between the breasts and above the umbilicus. She had had menarche at the age of 11 and had no significant previous history. She was on no medication and was using condoms for contraception. Her mother had recently been diagnosed with type 2 diabetes, as had a maternal aunt. Her older sister had problems with weight management and was being investigated for primary subfertility.

On examination she was overweight at 91 kg with a BMI of 34 kg/m^2. She was hirsute and there was a patch of velvety dark skin in both axillae and at the base of the posterior neck. Initial investigations revealed:

- prolactin 606 mIU/L (NR 100–550 mIU/L)
- LH 13.2 IU/L (NR luteal 0.8–10.4)
- FSH 3.7 IU/L (NR luteal 2.6–9.5)
- SHBG 21 nmol/L (NR 28–150)
- testosterone 3 nmol/L (NR 0.5–3.0)

A transvaginal pelvic ultrasound scan revealed bilateral polycystic ovaries with more than 10 small follicles around the periphery of each ovary.

The wide range of symptoms of women presenting with polycystic ovaries makes diagnosis and treatment of PCOS problematic. After excluding other causes of androgen excess, the diagnosis of PCOS is further supported by the presence of polycystic ovaries on ultrasound scanning of the pelvis (ideally a transvaginal rather than a transabdominal scan). The estimated prevalence of PCOS ranges from 5 to 10% on clinical criteria and 95% of women presenting to outpatients with hirsutism have PCOS. However, polycystic ovaries on ultrasound are noted in up to 25–30% of reproductive aged women. Thus the vast majority of women with polycystic ovaries do not have the syndrome.

Rotterdam criteria

In order to diagnose PCOS (rather than simply structural polycystic ovaries) a consensus statement following a meeting of the European Society of Human Reproduction and Embryology (ESHRE) in Rotterdam suggested that two of the following criteria were necessary:

- oligo- /amenorrhea
- hyperandrogenism (clinical or biochemical)
- polycystic ovaries on ultrasound (*Box 7.11, Figure 7.27*).

It is important to remember that other diagnoses that may present as oligo- / amenorrhea with hyperandrogenism should be excluded. The key diagnoses to exclude include congenital adrenal hyperplasia (non-classical), Cushing syndrome/ disease and androgen secreting ovarian/adrenal tumors.

Etiology and pathophysiology

The etiology of this heterogeneous condition remains unknown but may be multi-faceted. Like autoimmune disorders, there is good evidence for a genetic component

Box 7.11 | ASRM/ESHRE consensus recommendations for the ultrasound diagnosis of polycystic ovaries

The ultrasound exam assumes that if there is a follicle >10 mm in diameter the scan should be repeated during a period of ovarian quiescence in order to calculate the ovarian volume.

American Society of Reproductive Medicine and the European Society of Human Reproduction and Embryology.

Polycystic ovaries can be diagnosed either by:

- the presence of 12 or more follicles measuring 2–9 mm in diameter

or

- increased ovarian volume (>10 cm^3)

The presence of a single polycystic ovary is sufficient to make the diagnosis of 'polycystic ovaries'.

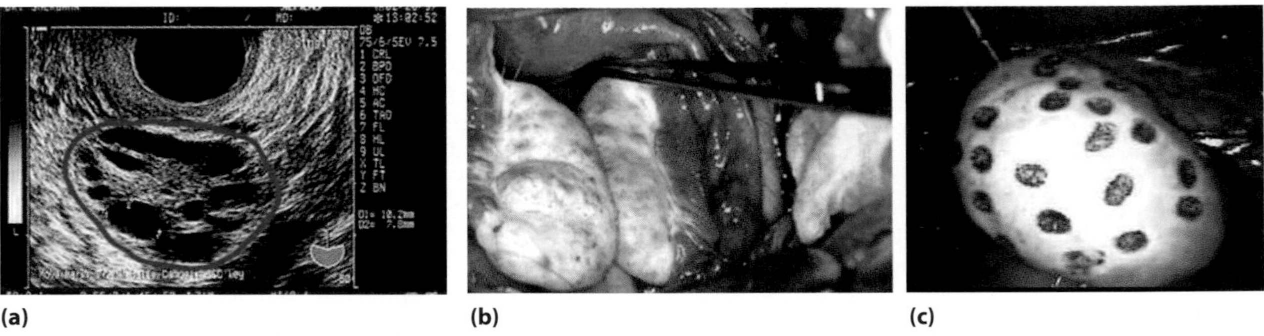

(a) (b) (c)

Figure 7.27. Images of polycystic ovaries.
(a) Ultrasound appearance of a polycystic ovary.
(b) Intraoperative appearance of polycystic ovaries – large ovaries with multiple cysts (representing follicles containing eggs which have failed to mature).
(c) Appearance of ovary after ovarian diathermy (see text).

that can predispose women and this may be linked to environmental factors. However, to date, no candidate genes have been convincingly demonstrated.

PCOS is linked to an increase in the number of developing follicles from the earliest stages of development, i.e. from primary right through to antral follicles, and this has been linked with hyperandrogenism. Why the amount of androgens secreted and number of theca cells increases in PCOS is unknown, but experimental studies suggest follicles exposed to high androgens, not only in adulthood but also pre-pubertally and even prenatally, can affect the normal process of folliculogenesis.

PCOS is also characterized by significant metabolic abnormalities, which include insulin resistance and an increased central adiposity (see *Box 7.12*). These two factors are related but in women with PCOS the insulin resistance relative to central adiposity is much higher than in women without PCOS. The insulin resistance leads to glucose intolerance and can eventually lead to type 2 diabetes mellitus, the prevalence of which is seven times higher in women with PCOS. Pregnancy in itself increases insulin resistance and if gestational diabetes occurs it is possible that a patient may have existing PCOS. If a history suggests this might be the case the patient's ovaries should be scanned after pregnancy along with certain biochemical tests (*Box 7.13*).

Insulin resistance is associated with hyperinsulinemia and this stimulates LH receptors in theca cells and may further increase androgen production. This is

Box 7.12 | Evaluation of PCOS

The following components should be checked during a focused history taking and physical examination.

History

- Onset and duration of oligomenorrhea.
- Hirsutism – onset, extent, severity, and duration.
- History of weight gain.
- Family history for PCOS, diabetes, CVD, endometrial cancer, etc.
- Infertility (also screen for male and tubal factors) and history of previous miscarriages.
- Smoking and substance abuse.

Physical

- Blood pressure.
- BMI (weight in kg divided by height in m^2): 25–30 = overweight, >30 = obese.
- Waist circumference to determine body fat distribution.
- Presence of stigmata of hyperandrogenism/insulin resistance: acne, hirsutism, androgenic alopecia, skin tags, acanthosis nigricans.

exacerbated by the increased central adiposity which contributes to a reduction in SHBG, thus increasing the circulating concentrations of free (biologically active) androgens.

It is not known why no dominant follicle is selected, leading to anovulation and the formation of cysts from the un-ovulated follicle(s). One theory is that the abnormal hormonal environment leads to the premature development of LH receptors on the granulosa cells, stimulating their terminal differentiation and preventing pre-ovulatory growth and an increased production of estradiol required for ovulation. An increased production of AMH has also been implicated in the failure of selection of a dominant follicle and anovulation in PCOS.

Box 7.13 | Suggested laboratory and radiologic examination of women with PCOS

Laboratory

- Documentation of biochemical hyperandrogenemia.
- Total testosterone and SHBG or bioavailable/free testosterone.
- LH concentration – raised in 50–70% of anovulatory patients with reversal of FSH/LH ratio.
- Exclusion of other causes of hyperandrogenism.
- Thyroid-stimulating hormone levels (thyroid dysfunction).
- Prolactin (hyperprolactinemia).
- 17α-hydroxyprogesterone levels to rule out late onset CAH.
- A synacthen test may be needed to rule out non-classical CAH due to 21-hydroxylase deficiency.
- Consider screening for Cushing syndrome and other rare disorders such as acromegaly.
- DHEA-S and androstenedione.
- Evaluation for metabolic abnormalities.
- Annual fasting glucose.
- Fasting lipid profile.

Ultrasound examination

- Determination of polycystic ovaries.
- Identify endometrial abnormalities.

Optional tests to consider

- Gonadotropin measurements to determine cause of amenorrhea.
- Fasting insulin levels in younger women and those with severe stigmata of insulin resistance and hyperandrogenism.
- A 24-hour urine test for urinary free cortisol with late onset of PCOS symptoms or stigmata of Cushing syndrome.

It is now clear that significant abnormalities in the earliest stages of folliculogenesis are very important to the etiology of anovulation in PCOS. However, the broad range of clinical features associated with this disorder has made it difficult to determine the precise sequence of events that can lead to anovulatory infertility, but because it is the most common endocrinopathy in women the stimulus for further research is strong.

Evaluation of women with PCOS

History and physical examination is important in evaluation of women with PCOS (*Box 7.12*), along with laboratory and radiologic examination (*Box 7.13*). It is also important to exclude other causes of androgen excess, insulin resistance, amenorrhea, and other symptoms and signs associated with PCOS. Disorders to consider in the differential diagnosis of PCOS are given in *Box 7.14*.

Box 7.14 | Differential diagnosis of PCOS

Disorders to consider in the differential diagnosis of PCOS:

- Androgen secreting tumor.
- Exogenous androgens.
- Cushing syndrome.
- Non-classical congenital adrenal hyperplasia.
- Acromegaly.
- Genetic defects in insulin action (Donohue syndrome, Rabson–Mendenhall syndrome, lipodystrophy).
- HAIR-AN syndrome (an acronym for an unusual multisystem disorder in women that consists of hyperandrogenism (HA), insulin resistance (IR) and acanthosis nigricans (AN).
- Primary hypothalamic amenorrhea.
- Primary ovarian failure.
- Thyroid disease.
- Prolactin disorders.

Management

The treatment goal depends on the patient's choice and the predominant symptom to be addressed. Main issues in the management of the polycystic ovarian syndrome are:

- menstrual irregularities
- infertility
- hirsutism and acne
- insulin resistance.

Treatment strategies include the following:

Weight loss. Studies have shown that a combination of weight loss and exercise may stimulate ovulation and improve insulin sensitivity leading to significant reduction of hyperandrogenemia.

Metformin. Women with PCOS have markedly decreased insulin sensitivity and there is therefore an increased rate of both impaired glucose intolerance and frank diabetes. There is also an increased incidence of insulin resistance and increased BMI in women with PCOS. Metformin significantly improves the frequency of menstruation, increases insulin sensitivity and reduces serum testosterone and insulin. There is evidence that metformin used alone or combined with clomifene (an anti-estrogen) is effective in improving ovulation rates in women with PCOS.

Ovarian androgen suppression. Estrogen such as ethinyl estradiol or a combined oral contraceptive pill (without an androgenic progesterone) suppress ovarian androgen production in patients in whom the androgen is of ovarian origin. In addition, the combined oral contraceptive:

- provides a regular period
- increases the SHBG and so reduces free testosterone
- increases insulin resistance and may provoke diabetes.

Treatment with progestogens. Where menstrual irregularity is a problem and when estrogen treatment is contraindicated, or not desired by the patient, an alternative method of producing a cycle and minimizing the risk of endometrial hyperplasia is to use cyclical progestogens (given on the first 7–10 calendar days of each month. Or, where periods are not desired and where contraception is important, a levonorgestrel-releasing intrauterine system (e.g. the Mirena coil) may be used. In either situation, estrogen can be added (given as a patch, orally, or as a gel).

Anti-androgens. These competitively inhibit androgens at peripheral receptors and may also reduce androgen synthesis. Cyproterone acetate is often used in a combined preparation (2 mg cyproterone and 35 μg ethinyl estradiol) known as Dianette which is useful in women who also wish to receive oral contraception. An alternative is to add cyproterone to the oral contraceptive pill in a dose of 25–50 mg for the first 10 days of each cycle. Other androgen antagonists include the following.

- *Spironolactone* – occupies androgen binding sites on target tissues and has direct anti-androgenic properties. Some women develop polymenorrhea. Effective contraception is a prerequisite of treatment with spironolactone, because the anti-androgenic properties may lead to failure of embryonic male morphogenesis.
- *Flutamide* – a non-steroidal androgen antagonist which competes with testosterone and DHT for binding at the androgen receptor.
- *Finasteride* – occasionally used in hospital practice; it is a synthetic anti-androgen acting through inhibition of type 2, 5α-reductase, the enzyme responsible for the conversion of testosterone to the more active DHT metabolite.

GnRH analogs. Two to three months of treatment may be required to achieve maximum effect, usually combined with estrogen–progestin replacement or an oral contraceptive pill and an androgen blocker.

Cosmetic treatment of hirsutism. Physical methods of hair removal will usually have been tried by the patient, including waxing, shaving, bleaching, plucking, depilation, and electrolysis. There is evidence for the effectiveness of treatment with the ruby laser in hirsutism. Women who are overweight or obese should be advised on losing weight as this can help. Specific local treatments include 11.5% eflornithine cream. Eflornithine is an irreversible ornithine decarboxylase, marketed as a treatment option to reduce the frequency of the woman's usual method of hair removal (it is not being marketed as a replacement).

Ovulation induction. Clomiphene citrate induces ovulation in 65–80% of patients and is associated with a pregnancy rate of 50–60% following up to six cycles of

CASE 7.5 383 388

- Woman of 23 years with secondary amenorrhea, weight gain, and excess body hair
- BMI of 34, raised prolactin and LH, and reduced SHBG – FSH and testosterone normal
- Pelvic ultrasound revealed bilateral polycystic ovaries
- PCOS confirmed after CAH and Cushing's excluded
- Treated with oral contraceptive, an anti-androgen, and a low GI diet

The patient was diagnosed with PCOS on the bases of biochemical abnormalities (hyperandrogenism with elevated LH:FSH ratio and slightly elevated testosterone), ultrasound appearance of polycystic ovaries, and her phenotype (including menstrual irregularity). Further complementary tests included a normal 17α-hydroxyprogesterone level (excluding CAH), an undetectable cortisol level after a 1 mg dose of dexamethasone taken the night before (excluding Cushing syndrome/disease, see *Section 6.4*) and an elevated androstenedione level.

She was reviewed in a multidisciplinary gynecology/endocrinology clinic. The diagnosis was explained and the importance of lifestyle changes reiterated. Myths around the diagnosis were dispelled and she was informed that with adequate treatment and weight loss there was no reason to suspect any degree of difficulty in conception. She was seen in clinic by a dietician who recommended a low glycemic index diet. She was not hypertensive and there were no familial risk factors or history of breast cancer or thrombosis. She was started on the oral contraceptive pill Yasmin – this was chosen for its weight neutrality and the relative anti-androgenic properties of the progestogen (drosperidone).

Because she was so concerned about the acne and hirsutes, a further anti-androgen (cyproterone acetate) was added for the first 10 days of each pill packet. In view of the probable acanthosis nigricans (the dark velvety patches in each axilla), a fasting insulin was requested and this confirmed hyperinsulinemia (insulin level 38 mIU/L; NR <20). In view of this she was also started on metformin for insulin sensitization, initially at 850 mg once daily but increased to 850 mg twice daily after a week.

Some 6 months later she had lost 10 kg in weight, was happy on the oral contraceptive pill (she had a regular withdrawal bleed) and had joined the gym where she worked out at least twice a week. Unfortunately, although her acne had significantly improved, there had been no effect on her hirsutes and so she had decided to seek cosmetic laser treatment. Two years after diagnosis she remained fit and well and had achieved a BMI of 25. She stopped the oral contraceptive and within 2 months achieved a completely normal and regular ovulatory menstrual cycle.

treatment. Multiple pregnancies occur in about 6% of patients and the rate of miscarriage may be slightly increased.

7.7 Premature ovarian failure and the menopause

7.7.1 Premature ovarian failure

This term is used to describe women under the age of 40 who present with amenorrhea, estrogen deficiency, and elevated gonadotropins (hypergonadotropic hypogonadism) as a result of primary ovarian failure. The term premature ovarian failure (POF) is preferred to premature menopause, but it is still rather a misnomer because about 50% of women diagnosed with POF show varying and unpredictable degrees of ovarian function and some may ovulate and even conceive. It is now

CASE 7.6

389 394

- Woman of 33 years with 9m history of amenorrhea
- High LH and FSH with low estrogen; anti-TPO antibodies strongly positive
- Ultrasound revealed normal ovaries and a thin endometrium

A 33 year old woman was referred to the gynecology clinic with a 9 month history of amenorrhea. On questioning her periods had been somewhat erratic with a cycle of 3–4/30–50 days since stopping the oral contraceptive some 3 years previously. She had been trying for a pregnancy for 2 years but had not sought medical help. She had been more tired than usual over the last few months and had been suffering occasional hot flushes/flashes. She worked as an accountant and did not feel as mentally sharp as usual. Her libido had lessened, and this was further compromised by some mild dyspareunia and vaginal dryness. There was no previous medical history or family history. She was on no drugs (including over-the-counter medicines). Initial investigations from the clinic revealed:

- LH 22 IU/L (NR luteal 0.8–10.4)
- FSH 84 IU/L (NR luteal 2.6–9.5)
- estrogen <60 pmol/L (NR 70–1100)
- prolactin 330 mIU/L (NR 100–550)

Thyroid function tests were normal but anti-TPO antibodies were strongly positive. A transvaginal pelvic ultrasound scan revealed apparently normal ovaries and a thin endometrium (1–2 mm thickness).

considered more appropriate to use the term primary ovarian insufficiency (POI), although it is not yet clear whether this term will come into widespread use and replace POF; consequently we have used POF in this chapter.

Diagnosis is confirmed by demonstrating a high FSH (>30 IU/L) with low estrogen; occasionally, normal women may have an FSH level of 30 IU/L mid-cycle, but the LH level will be significantly higher – in POF the FSH level exceeds that of LH as seen in Case 7.6.

In the UK and USA the average age of the menopause is around 50–52 years, although up to 1% of women will have a spontaneous menstrual bleed after the age of 60 and a similar percentage will cease periods by 40. There are, however, no accurate estimates of the prevalence of POF. They range from 0.3% to 5–10%. Other sources state that the incidence is 1:10 000 in women at the age of 20, 1:1000 at the age of 30 and 1:100 by the age of 40. That said, POF probably accounts for between 15 and 20% of all cases of secondary amenorrhea.

POF is idiopathic in the majority of cases, but where the cause is known it may be familial or sporadic. POF occurs through two major mechanisms: follicle dysfunction (no normal folliculogenesis) or follicle depletion which may be caused by an inadequate pool of primordial follicles being established *in utero* (ovarian dysgenesis), an accelerated loss of follicles, autoimmune/toxic destruction of follicles, or infections (*Box 7.15*).

POF is a heterogeneous disorder and in its severest form patients present with absent pubertal development, primary amenorrhea and depletion of primordial follicles as seen in Turner syndrome. Cases of POF that are post-pubertal are characterized by secondary amenorrhea associated with defective folliculogenesis. The heterogeneity of POF is reflected by the variety of possible causes (*Box 7.15*).

Box 7.15 | Causes of premature ovarian failure

Gonadal dysgenesis

- Turner syndrome (see *Section 7.4.3*, Case 7.2).
- 46,XX gonadal dysgenesis (generally unknown etiology).
- 46,XY gonadal dysgenesis (Swyer syndrome – either deletion of *SRY* [20%] or apparently normal *SRY* genetic material with presumed downstream loss of function – risk of gonadal malignancy).
- Perrault syndrome (gonadal dysgenesis, deafness, short stature – gene defect unknown).

Genetic causes

- Familial ovarian failure – the causative gene defect is rarely identified but many (10–25%) patients will have an affected close family member. Inheritance patterns are unclear.
- Enzyme defects resulting in impaired ovarian estrogen production (sometimes associated with hypokalemic hypertension).
- *FRAXA* mutations (Fragile X syndrome). The *FRAXA* site is in exon 1 of the *FMR1* gene at Xq27.3 and mutations are characterized by more than 60 trinucleotide (CCG) repeats resulting in methylation of the promoter and gene silencing. This results in mental retardation in males and is associated with POF in females.
- FSH/LH receptor mutations – loss of function of the FSH receptor results in hypoplastic ovaries and loss of LH function results in estrogen deficiency. Both defects are extremely rare and are not routinely screened for.
- Galactosemia – possibly due to the toxic effects of galactose or metabolites on the ovary. The presentation is of failure to thrive, hepatomegaly, hypoglycemia and acidosis in infancy. A rare cause and the diagnosis is usually known at presentation of POF.
- BPES – drooping eyelids (blepharophimosis, ptosis,epicanthus inversus) associated with POF in 50% of affected females. Very rare.

Autoimmune disease

- APECED (autoimmune polyendocrinopathy type 1, caused by mutations in the *AIRE* gene) is associated with POF in about 60% of affected females (although, interestingly, testicular function is usually spared in males). APS type 2 (Schmidt syndrome) is the combination of Addison disease, hypothyroidism, type 1 DM and ovarian failure. The association of hypothyroidism and POF is common and probably represents an APS-2 variant.
- Isolated autoimmune ovarian failure may occur outside the classical APS. Evidence suggests that antibodies against 3β-hydroxysteroid dehydrogenase may be causative, but the pathogenetic mechanisms remain unclear.
- Associated with other autoimmune conditions.

Iatrogenic

- Chemotherapy can result in POF – particularly with alkylating agents and cyclophosphamide for hematological malignancies.
- Radiotherapy – again often as a result of total body irradiation in treatment protocols for hematological malignancies.
- Surgery – clearly oophorectomy, but some evidence suggests that the lifespan of functional ovaries after hysterectomy and after ovarian procedures for PCOS (e.g. laser, drilling) is reduced.

Infections

- Viral oophoritis.
- Mumps, CMV, HIV, shigella.

It should be remembered that the vast majority of cases (up to 50%) are idiopathic and no cause is found. Of the remaining, the majority will be Turner syndrome or associated with polyendocrinopathy. *FRAXA* mutations (Fragile X) probably account for no more than 1% of cases.

Clinical presentation and investigation

Presentation is almost invariably with amenorrhea which may be primary, particularly in patients with chromosomal abnormalities. Indeed, patients presenting with primary amenorrhea should always undergo karyotype testing which will confirm the diagnosis of Turner syndrome in those where clinical suspicion is high, and will also diagnose rarer cases of XX/XY gonadal dysgenesis; the presence of Y chromosomal material makes it important to consider removal

Box 7.16 | Symptoms associated with premature ovarian failure and the menopause

Vascular instability

- Hot flashes/flushes and night sweats.
- Migraine.
- Rapid heartbeat.
- Increased risk of atherosclerosis? (contentious issue)

Urogenital (vaginal) atrophy

- Thinning of membranes of vulva, vagina, and cervix. Shrinking and loss of elasticity in genital areas.
- Itching, dryness, and bleeding.
- Increased urinary frequency and urgency.
- Urinary incontinence.
- Increased susceptibility to infection.

Skeletal

- Back pain, joint and muscle pain.
- Osteopenia and risk of osteoporosis developing.

Skin and soft tissue

- Decreased elasticity of the skin, increased dryness and thinning.
- Breast tenderness and atrophy.

Psychological

- Depression/anxiety and mood disturbances.
- Irritability, memory loss, and problems with concentration.
- Sleep disturbances and fatigue.

Sexual

- Painful intercourse due to vaginal dryness and atrophy.
- Decreased libido and difficulty reaching orgasm.

There are mixed conclusions about medical conditions associated with the menopause and at what stage during the peri-menopausal or post-menopausal period they occur. Different cohort studies give different outcomes of reported symptoms and their frequencies.

of gonadal tissue which can undergo malignant transformation. There may be an obvious history of radiotherapy, chemotherapy, or pelvic surgery, and 10% of patients will give a positive family history. It is important to look for evidence of other autoimmune conditions in the history and examination. Occasionally there may be clinical evidence of autoimmunity, for example, the presence of vitiligo or signs of rheumatoid arthritis.

Of women who develop secondary amenorrhea, 75% report hot flushes/flashes, night sweats, mood changes, fatigue or dyspareunia and these symptoms may precede the onset of menstrual disturbances (see *Box 7.16*). The diagnosis is confirmed by serum FSH >30–40 IU/L on at least two occasions at least 1 month apart. Serum estradiol levels are usually undetectable or at the low end of the normal range. It is important to remember that the condition may have a fluctuating course with high FSH levels later returning to normal with possible (usually temporary) restitution of ovulatory function including menstruation.

Perhaps surprisingly, determination of the presence of ovarian antibodies is rarely useful in clinical practice. However, despite absence of biochemical or clinical evidence of hypothyroidism, measurement of thyroid antibodies is useful; if positive it is important to screen for development of hypothyroidism and associated autoimmune disease during follow-up (*Box 7.17*). A baseline DEXA scan to assess bone mineral density (see *Section 4.7* and *Box 4.9*) can be useful in follow-up to check on efficacy of treatment.

Treatment of POF

It is fundamentally important to remember how devastating the diagnosis of POF can be, particularly in young women. Counseling (see below) is as important as

Box 7.17 | Annual assessment of women with POF

Assess adequacy of sex hormone replacement therapy:

- tolerance and compliance
- side-effects and complications
- persistent symptoms of sex hormone deficiency.

Address fertility issues.

Screen for other autoimmune disease (in autoimmune POF):

- clinical evaluation
- TSH and fasting blood glucose
- synacthen test if clinically indicated.

Screen for complications:

- osteoporosis
- cardiovascular disease.

pharmacological intervention and the treatment of these patients should really be in a multidisciplinary setting where psychological as well as physical worries can be adequately addressed.

It is clear that the mainstay of treatment is HRT. Beneficial effects of this on general well-being, quality of life, bone health, and uterine health are clear; long-term beneficial effects on cardiovascular health are likely and the risk of breast cancer in those with no close family history of breast cancer is probably no greater than that of normally menstruating women.

Numerous HRT preparations are available with various routes of administration. Younger women may elect to go on the oral contraceptive pill. This has the benefit of an apparently lower level of stigma, and it is also a contraceptive (remember that HRT is **non**-contraceptive and up to 3% of women with POF will have occasional spontaneous ovulations which may result in conception – these are sometimes unwanted and psychologically devastating). The disadvantage of the oral contraceptive pill is that it uses synthetic estrogen at a higher effective dose with a slightly increased risk of cardiovascular (thromboembolic) side-effects (especially deep vein thrombosis) particularly in women who smoke.

There are numerous forms of HRT and modes of delivery and the final choice is often made after trying more than one preparation (*Box 7.18*). Continuous combined oral preparations (containing estrogen and progesterone) are useful; these are easy to take and give patients the choice of having periods or not. In those with risk factors for thromboembolic disease or with impairment of liver function or with hypertension, transdermal estrogen (patches or gels) may be used; in this case the progestogen (which has to be given in women with an intact uterus in order to prevent endometrial hyperplasia and potential malignant transformation) can be given orally (for the first 7–12 days of each calendar month) or locally in the form of a hormone-secreting contraceptive coil (e.g. the Mirena device). Those women who have significant vaginal dryness resulting in dyspareunia may benefit from added local estrogen given as pessaries or vaginal creams. Although women with preserved adrenal function should be capable of producing sufficient quantities of androgens, it is clear that some women benefit from added exogenous testosterone replacement as part of the HRT protocol. Specific preparations for women (clearly in lower doses than those used in male testosterone replacement regimens) are now available. This is particularly important in those women with autoimmune polyglandular syndrome (APS, see

Box 7.18 | HRT and SERMS

Hormone replacement therapy

The saga of HRT goes back to the 1930s when estrogens were prescribed to women to alleviate the vasomotor symptoms (hot flushes/flashes) of the menopause. In the late 1960s and early 1970s the benefits of HRT in protecting against heart disease and osteoporosis and remaining 'feminine forever' had reached the popular press. Its use was advocated not only for 1–2 years to overcome the initial menopausal symptoms, but for 5–10 years or longer to prevent these health and aging problems. In the mid-1970s unopposed estrogen therapy was linked to an increase in the incidence of endometrial cancer, so progestogens were added to stop endometrial hyperplasia in women who had not had a hysterectomy. Despite this setback and the knowledge that HRT was linked to an increased risk of venous thromboembolic events, there was a significant increase in the use of HRT throughout the 1980s and 1990s.

Between 2002 and 2003 the results of two large studies regarding HRT were published: the Women's Health Initiative (WHI) and the Million Women Study. The outcome was evidence of an increased risk of breast cancer, myocardial infarction, cerebrovascular disease and thromboembolic disease with long-term use of HRT. Conversely, benefits included relief of menopausal symptoms and prevention of osteoporosis and colorectal cancer. Whilst there was criticism of the study designs and evidence continues to be accepted and disputed, media coverage resulted in a significant drop in HRT usage and a re-evaluation of prescribing practices in the clinic. It is now generally accepted that HRT should only be used for 1–2 years to overcome menopausal symptoms and with the lowest possible dose of estrogen. Long-term use for prevention of osteoporosis or cardiovascular disease is no longer recommended. However, women experiencing premature menopause/ovarian failure are advised to start long-term therapy until they reach the normal menopausal age (see *Section 7.7.1*).

Estrogens can be given orally, through transdermal patches or gels, nasal sprays, vaginal rings and implants, though availability differs in different countries and different practices. Most women start with oral therapy, either conjugated equine estrogens or synthetic estrogens such as 17β-estradiol. Women with a uterus should have combined estrogen plus a progestogen (e.g. medroxyprogesterone), given:

- cyclically (estrogens for 25 days with a progestogen added for the last 10–14 days) in which case women will still bleed at the same time a period would be expected
- continuous combined estrogen and progestogen without any withdrawal bleed; this regime may cause irregular bleeding in pre-menopausal women because estrogen production from the ovary may still be fluctuating.

Another steroid preparation is tibolone which has weak estrogenic, progestogenic, and androgenic activities. Its use is increasing, although data on its outcomes such as breast cancer and cardiovascular disease are currently lacking.

Selective estrogen receptor modulators

Estrogen deficiency manifests itself in many tissues and organs, but in post-menopausal women estrogen therapy has both benefical and adverse outcomes. One way of overcoming the adverse effects of estrogen therapy is by developing a SERM that combines with the estrogen receptor and has specific estrogenic and anti-estrogenic effects in selective target tissues.

One of the earliest SERMs to be developed was tamoxifen and this has been used for some time in the treatment of estrogen-dependent breast cancer. It acts as an estrogen antagonist in the breast as well as the brain and vagina, but has an agonist activity on the cardiovascular system and bone, and also on the uterus. Antagonist activity on the vagina and agonist activity on the uterus preclude the use of tamoxifen as an alternative to estrogen replacement therapy. Raloxifen is similar to tamoxifen but it has antagonist actions in the uterus and so does not stimulate endometrial hyperplasia; it has been used to treat osteoporosis associated with the menopause, but bisphosphonates (see *Section 4.7* and *Box 4.5*) are currently the first-line treatment for osteoporosis.

SERMs act by combining with estrogen receptors and altering their confirmation such that the transcription activating factors (AF-1 and AF-2) on the receptors may either attract co-activators or co-repressors or may antagonize their activity (see *Section 1.5.3*). Thus, for example, a SERM can induce a different conformational change in the estrogen receptor than that of estradiol, such that the activity of the AF-2 region is suppressed whilst the AF-1 region can still attract co-regulators of gene transcription. In addition, different tissues express different activities at the AF-1 and AF-2 regions of the receptor and in the expression of co-regulators. In these ways SERMs can have antagonistic and agonistic activities in different estrogen target tissues. Of course, the ideal SERM to replace estrogen deficiency in post-menopausal women would have anti-estrogenic effects on breast and uterus but estrogenic effects on bone, brain, vagina, and the cardiovascular system.

Box 7.15) who have also lost adrenal function. Some evidence suggests that these women may also benefit from administration of oral DHEA-S; while this is not available on prescription in the USA or UK it is readily available on the internet.

Fertility

A minority of females with POF and a normal karyotype will recover spontaneously (albeit often temporarily) and a rate of spontaneous pregnancy after a diagnosis of POF of about 5% is often quoted. Treatment with HRT seems to have a neutral effect on spontaneous ovulation rates, but pregnancy outcomes are probably better in those women on HRT at conception. Because there is likely to be an autoimmune component in many cases of idiopathic POF, glucocorticoid therapy has understandably been used, but efficacy is variable and well controlled trials are lacking.

Oocyte donation and *in vitro* fertilization offer these women their best chance of fertility. Results are promising, with a pregnancy rate of around 35% per patient. The problem is sourcing a donor and women are generally encouraged to find a family member to act as ovum donor (this has the added benefit of shared genetic material in the donated ovum). It is important to remember that both the recipient and donor will need to go through a relatively complex and invasive procedure. Embryo donation (from unrelated patient cycles using non-reimplanted fertilized frozen embryos) is another effective treatment, but plagued with ethical and social dilemmas.

Ovulation induction therapy has been tried but the results have been poor. Recent improvements in methods of oocyte cryopreservation using rapid freezing in liquid nitrogen (vitrification) have allowed women with a high chance of POF (e.g. before chemo/radiotherapy) to store oocytes collected after superovulation. However, this is experimental; quoted success rates are 20–30% per patient and depend on the age and egg quality at time of collection.

CASE 7.6

389 394

- Woman of 33 years with 9m history of amenorrhea
- High LH and FSH with low estrogen; anti-TPO antibodies strongly positive
- Ultrasound revealed normal ovaries and a thin endometrium
- Diagnosis of POF confirmed and patient started on HRT
- Fertility addressed by IVF using donor eggs from her sister

The patient was seen in the reproductive medicine clinic by both endocrine and gynecology consultants. A repeat blood test revealed a persistently high FSH (now at 96 IU/L). The diagnosis of POF was discussed, along with the need for hormone replacement. A DEXA (bone mineral density) scan showed no evidence of osteopenia or osteoporosis. The patient elected to start treatment with combined oral HRT and was keen to discuss fertility options. It was reiterated that occasional cycles may be ovulatory despite the diagnosis, that HRT is not contraceptive, and that a small number of patients may return to a normal ovulatory cyclical menstrual pattern (although this is rare).

At a further review in the fertility clinic, this time with her partner, the possibility of egg/embryo donation during an IVF cycle was suggested. The patient was keen to use her younger sister as a donor and, after relevant socio-legal formalities had been completed, the patient underwent successful IVF with donor eggs from her sister inseminated by her partner's sperm. The family now have a fit and healthy 18 month old daughter. The patient has restarted HRT and is considering a further egg donation next year.

Prognosis

The mortality of women with POF may be increased by twofold. Estrogen deficiency leads to an increased risk of cardiovascular and cerebrovascular disease and osteoporosis. Up to 65% of women with POF and a normal karyotype have a low bone mineral density on DEXA scanning, with a Z score of -1 or lower, despite at least intermittent HRT. This may be due to a combination of factors including an initial delay in initiating HRT, poor compliance with HRT, and estrogen 'under dosing'. The assessment of women with POF is detailed in *Box 7.17.*

7.7.2 The menopause

Unlike POF, in which one can see varying and unpredictable ovarian function in approximately 50% of cases, the menopause results from the permanent depletion of potentially functional primordial follicles and the complete cessation of menses and fertility. The mean age of the menopause is around 50 years but if it occurs before the age of 40 years it is termed POF (see *Section 7.7.1*).

During the time leading up to the menopause, irregular menstrual cycles begin to appear and these are associated with declining numbers of ovarian follicles and a reduced responsiveness to gonadotropins. With decreasing numbers of pre-antral and early antral follicles, the secretion of inhibin B declines and FSH consequently rises. This temporarily salvages small follicles and enough antral follicles survive to maintain estrogen and inhibin A levels. In the latter part of the time leading up to the menopause (the climacteric), when follicles become severely depleted, estrogen and inhibin A levels fall and then LH rises. Thus FSH levels are typically measured to indicate approaching menopause. Paradoxically, androgen levels may rise after the menopause because the high levels of LH stimulate androgen production from ovarian interstitial cells and this adds to the circulating pool of adrenal androgens. This can cause hirsutism in post-menopausal women.

The physical and emotional changes which occur in the peri-menopausal period are driven by these ovarian changes, although experiences of menopausal symptoms vary widely and have been found to relate to social class, ethnicity, and culture (*Box 7.16*). The estrogen withdrawal is responsible for hot flushes/flashes, night sweats, changes in blood lipid profile and a reduction in the size of breasts and uterus. A rise in the pH of vaginal fluids coupled with a reduction in lubrication causes dyspareunia.

The longer-term effects of the menopause include an increased risk of coronary thrombosis and osteoporosis. The former is associated with changes in the circulating lipid profile and perhaps the redistribution of fat with an increase in visceral fat (see *Section 8.3*). The latter is due to increased bone resorption as a result of the loss of estrogen-inhibition on osteoclast differentiation. These symptoms of the menopause can be prevented by estrogen treatment, but results of recent trials have both reduced and changed prescribing practices for HRT (*Box 7.18*).

7.8 Further reading

Arnhold IJP, Costa EMF, Domenice S, and Mendonca BB (2009) 46,XY disorders of sex development. *Clinical Endocrinol.* **70:** 173–87.

Bolyakov A, Fine RG, Kiper J, and Paduch DA (2008) New concepts in Klinefelter syndrome. *Urology,* **18:** 621–7.

Davenport ML (2010) Approach to the patient with Turner syndrome. *J. Clin. Endocrinol. & Metab.* **95:** 1487–95.

DiVall SA and Radovick S (2009) Endocrinology of female puberty. *Endocrinol. Diabetes & Obesity,* **16:** 1–4.

Lamb DJ and Matzuk MM (2008) The biology of infertility: research advances and clinical challenges. *Nature Medicine,* **14:** 1197–213.

Lee PA and Lewis K (2009) Endocrinology of male puberty. *Endocrinol. Diabetes & Obesity,* **16:** 5–9.

Nelson LM (2009) Primary ovarian insufficiency. *New Engl. J. Med.* **360:** 606–14.

Oktem O and Oktay K (2008) The ovary: anatomy and function throughout human life. *NY Acad. Sci.* **1127:** 1–9.

Pangas SA and Richards JS (2010) The ovary: basic biology and clinical implications. *US Nat. Libr. Med.* **120:** 963–72.

Roberts H (2007) Managing the menopause. *Br. Med. J.* **334:** 736–41.

Shalet SM (2009) Normal testicular function and spermatogenesis. *Pediatr. Blood & Cancer,* **53:** 285–8.

Wikstrom AM and Dunkel L (2011) Klinefelter syndrome. *Best Pract. & Res. Clin. Endocrinol. & Metab.* **25:** 239–50.

Useful websites

Infertility:

www.nlm.nih.gov/medlineplus/infertility.html

Menopause:

www.menopause.org/ – North American Menopause Society

www.thebms.org.uk/ – The British Menopause Society for UK health professionals

PCOS:

www.verity-pcos.org.uk/ – a charity for PCOS patients

7.9 Self-assessment questions

(1) Which one of the following cell types is directly controlled by follicle stimulating hormone?
- (a) Leydig cells
- (b) Theca cells
- (c) Spermatogonia
- (d) Oocytes
- (e) Sertoli cells

(2) How long, approximately, does it take for a pre-antral follicle to grow into a dominant (ovulatory) follicle?
- (a) Two years
- (b) Twenty months
- (c) One menstrual cycle
- (d) Two to four menstrual cycles
- (e) Over 120 days

(3) Which one of the following tests indicates that ovulation has occurred?
   (a) Increased estrogen levels during the luteal phase of the menstrual cycle
   (b) A rise in FSH secretion during the follicular phase of the menstrual cycle
   (c) A sudden drop in LH secretion at the onset of menstruation
   (d) A rise in progesterone levels during the luteal phase of the menstrual cycle
   (e) An intercycle rise of FSH secretion

(4) Regarding sexual development of the male reproductive tract, which one of the following structures is dependent on dihydrotestosterone?
   (a) Seminal vesicles
   (b) Prostate gland
   (c) Testis
   (d) Vas deferens
   (e) Urethra

(5) What one of the following is the first physical sign of normal puberty in a girl?
   (a) Development of pubic hair
   (b) Development of axillary hair
   (c) Breast development
   (d) Menarche
   (e) Growth acceleration

(6) Pubertal delay is associated with which one of the following?
   (a) Thelarche
   (b) McCune–Albright syndrome
   (c) Testotoxicosis
   (d) Cushing disease
   (e) Turner syndrome

(7) A 28 year old Asian woman was referred to the Endocrine Clinic because of infrequent periods and evidence of anovulatory cycles. Ultrasound of her pelvis revealed polycystic ovaries. Which one of the following is associated with polycystic ovary syndrome?
   (a) Decreased androgen levels
   (b) Raised FSH levels
   (c) Insulin resistance
   (d) Anorexia nervosa
   (e) Increased estrogen secretion

(8) A 32 year old landscape architect was referred to the infertility clinic after his wife failed to become pregnant even though her tests had revealed normal ovulatory menstrual cycles. He was tall with small (<4 mL) testes and gynecomastia which had developed at puberty. What would be the most likely diagnosis of this case?
   (a) Turner syndrome
   (b) Prolactinoma
   (c) Klinefelter syndrome
   (d) Kallmann syndrome
   (e) Varicocele

(9) A 28 month old boy was brought to the doctor by his mother because over the last 6 months she had noticed growth of coarse pubic hairs. His growth had also increased from the 50th to 85th percentile with a corresponding increase in weight. His past medical history was normal though his father had a history of premature pubertal development and early cessation of growth. The boy's penile and pubic hair development were at Tanner stage 3 with a small but definite testicular enlargement, although this was smaller than expected in relation to penile growth. There was no indication of a testicular adenoma or carcinoma.

Blood tests showed raised levels of testosterone and a slightly elevated androstenedione concentration. Other hormones measured, including LH, FSH, progesterone, DHEA-S, and hCG, were all in the normal range for a 28 month old boy.

(a) What findings would suggest that the raised levels of testosterone are from the testis?

(b) What shows that this precocious sexual development is not caused by true central precocious puberty?

(c) Why is testicular enlargement delayed in relation to penile growth?

(d) What is the most likely diagnosis of this patient?

(10) A 32 year old high school teacher, who had been married for five years, had been trying to conceive for the last year but without success. In the last few years her periods had become irregular and within the last 6 months she had become amenorrheic. She had noted her skin was becoming 'spotty' and there was increased hair growth above her upper lip and on her chin. Otherwise she was fit and healthy and played tennis three times a week and cycled to work. Biochemical tests showed:

LH 13.2 IU/L (NR luteal 0.8–10.4)
FSH 2.9 IU/L (NR luteal 2.6–9.5)
SHBG 19 nmol/L (NR 28–150)
Prolactin 530 mIU/L (NR 100–550)
Testosterone 3.3 nmol/L (NR 0.5–3.0)
17α-hydroxyprogesterone 23 nmol/L (NR follicular 6–30)

(a) Based on these results what would be the most likely cause of the teacher's amenorrhea?

(b) How would this diagnosis be confirmed and the disease defined?

(c) What is the significance of measuring prolactin and 17-hydroxyprogesterone?

CHAPTER 08

Endocrinology beyond the 'classical' endocrine glands

After working through this chapter you should be able to:

- Understand the importance of the suprachiasmatic nuclei in controlling circadian rhythms
- Describe the synthesis and functions of melatonin secreted by the pineal gland
- Outline the endocrinology of adipose tissue and identify the pathophysiological consequences of obesity
- Understand the endocrine functions of the gastrointestinal tract and the consequences of tumors of the gastrointestinal tract including carcinoid tumors and tumors of the pancreas
- Define the differences between type 1 and type 2 multiple endocrine neoplasias, including their etiology, clinical outcomes, and treatment
- Identify endocrine functions of the cardiovascular system, kidney, and bone

8.1 Introduction

There are many organs and tissues in the body which produce hormones that are not considered to be classic endocrine glands because they have other essential functions apart from an endocrine function. However, they play an important role in synthesizing and secreting hormones that regulate diverse functions. These organs and tissues include:

- adipose tissue
- the gastrointestinal (GI) tract
- the cardiovascular system
- the kidney
- bone.

However, the chapter starts with a conventional endocrine gland, the pineal gland. This plays an important role in orchestrating our bodily rhythms, synchronizing various biological clocks and helping our rhythms to be entrained to the light–dark cycle. The main focus of this chapter is on the endocrine functions of adipose tissue and the consequences of obesity, and hormones produced by the GI tract and the clinical consequences of gastroenteropancreatic neuroendocrine tumors (GEP-NETs), which also include carcinoid tumors. From GEP-NETs the chapter moves onto multiple endocrine neoplasia (MEN) which can affect tumors of two or more different endocrine glands including the thyroid and parathyroid glands, and enteropancreatic tumors. It concludes with a brief review of the hormones released by the cardiovascular system, kidney, and bone and, although many of these have been discussed in previous chapters, the purpose of this chapter is to bring together an understanding of endocrinology outside the conventional endocrine glands described in the earlier chapters.

8.2 The pineal gland and biological rhythms

Biological rhythms are a fundamental feature of life and many of these are driven by the suprachiasmatic nucleus (SCN) which receives a direct input from the retina in order to synchronize these rhythms to the light–dark cycle (*Box 8.1*). Oscillations in gene expression of the SCN result in rhythmic physiology at all levels of the body (*Box 8.2*). It is therefore not surprising that disruption of circadian rhythms (as occurs, for example, when rhythms are not synchronized with the light–dark cycle), can affect normal physiological and biochemical function and lead to disease. Epidemiological studies in, for example, shift workers, long-distance flight crews, and patients with sleep disorders have shown that they have a higher prevalence of cancer, psychological disorders, metabolic syndrome, diabetes, and cardiovascular diseases. This is supported by evidence from mice knock-out models of so-called 'clock' genes which indicate a variety of resulting pathologies (*Box 8.3*). Apart from the SCN, the pineal gland is also thought to be important in orchestrating biological rhythms.

The pineal gland was described by Descartes as the 'seat of the soul,' though for much of the twentieth century it has been dismissed as a 'vestige.' It transmits signals to the brain by secreting its unique hormone, melatonin, whose chemical structure (5-methoxy-*N*-acetyltryptamine) was identified in 1958 (*Figure 8.1*). In 1975, it was

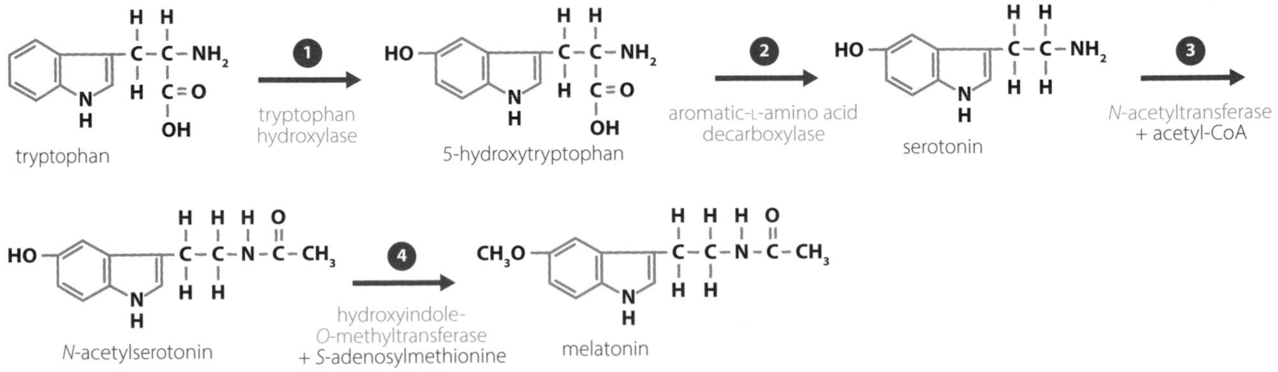

tryptophan → (1) tryptophan hydroxylase → 5-hydroxytryptophan → (2) aromatic-L-amino acid decarboxylase → serotonin → (3) *N*-acetyltransferase + acetyl-CoA → *N*-acetylserotonin → (4) hydroxyindole-*O*-methyltransferase + *S*-adenosylmethionine → melatonin

Figure 8.1. Synthesis of melatonin.

Box 8.1 | Circadian rhythms and their control: the suprachiasmatic nucleus

Many functions of the body show rhythmicity, such as body temperature, sleep–wake cycles, feeding behaviors, endocrine functions and metabolic changes; often these have a circadian (about a day) rhythm. These are driven by the 'master' clock in the suprachiasmatic nucleus (SCN) of the anterior hypothalamus and this clock oscillates with an approximate 24 hour period even in the absence of external cues. This clock, however, is entrained by the light–dark cycle because the SCN receives a direct input from the retina via the retinohypothalamic tract (*Box figure 8.1*). Outputs from the SCN are directed to other parts of the hypothalamus that control endocrine secretions of the pituitary gland, such as ACTH secretion, as well as to other areas of the hypothalamus and medulla that regulate autonomic functions. In turn, the SCN receives inputs from forebrain areas and the locus ceruleus which may modulate the influence of the SCN. Other circadian oscillators that are present in the brain and other organs are referred to as 'peripheral' oscillators and are considered to be orchestrated by the SCN.

The SCN also regulates the secretion of melatonin from the pineal gland. Projections of the SCN, via the paraventricular nucleus (PVN), medial forebrain bundle, and spinal cord, synapse with sympathetic neurons in the superior cervical ganglion (SCG). These neurons project directly to the pineal gland and stimulate the pinealocytes to synthesize melatonin. These sympathetic neurons are most active during night time so that melatonin is secreted during the dark phase of the cycle. However, in the absence of a dark phase circadian melatonin secretion will still occur because it is driven by the inherent oscillations of the SCN. Melatonin is thought to be important in synchronizing various circadian rhythms.

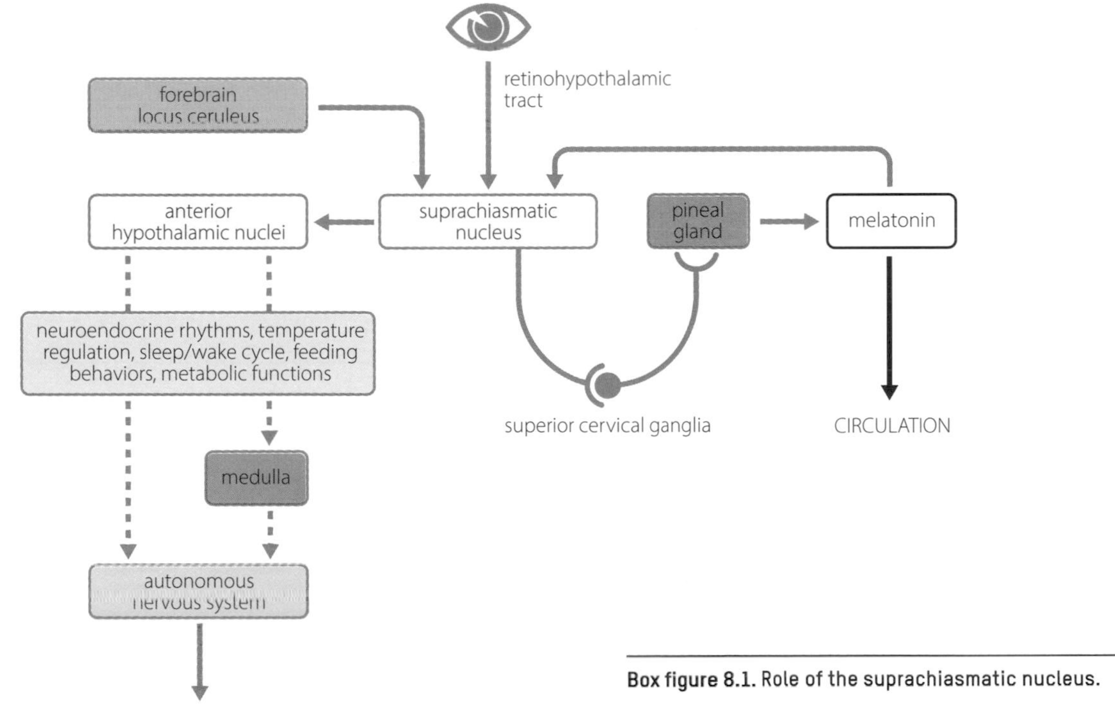

Box figure 8.1. Role of the suprachiasmatic nucleus.

discovered that melatonin secretion in humans, like in other mammals, exhibits a circadian rhythm which is driven by the 'master clock' in the SCN (*Box 8.1*). The nocturnal plasma concentration of melatonin is at least 10 times higher than the daytime concentration (*Figure 8.2*).

The pineal gland is a small central brain structure weighing 100–150 mg in humans and comprises two cell types: pinealocytes and glial-like interstitial cells. The pineal

Box 8.2 | The genetics of the circadian pacemaker: the clock genes

The mechanisms that regulate the oscillatory behavior of the SCN have been identified and involve the transcription of genes and their translational protein products which then feedback to regulate another set of genes and protein products over a 24 hour period. The elements of this feedback loop involve transcription factors. The forward loop comprises the *CLOCK* (circadian locomotor output cycle kaput) and *BMAL1* (brain muscle arnt-like 1) genes and their translational transcription factors and the negative feedback loop involves the period (*PER*) and cryptochrome (*CRY*) genes and their transcriptional protein products (*Box figure 8.2*). During the light period the expression of CLOCK and BMAL1 are high and these two proteins form heterodimers to regulate gene transcription; at the same time they stimulate the expression of *PER* and *CRY* genes by binding to the E-box elements in the promoter region of these genes. When the expression of PER and CRY reaches a critical level (during the dark phase) these two proteins form heterodimers and suppress the transcriptional activity of the *CLOCK/BMAL1* genes. This autoregulatory loop is also post-transcriptionally regulated by casein kinases (CK1ε and CK1δ) which target the PER proteins for degradation.

There is an additional arm to this control system in that *REV-ERB*-α and -β and retinoic acid related-orphan receptor (*ROR*) genes, which are also transcriptionally controlled by CLOCK/BMAL1, create a short feedback loop controlling *BMAL1* expression. REV-ERB negatively regulates the gene expression of *BMAL1* whilst ROR positively regulates the expression of *BMAL1* both through the presence of ROR binding elements (RORE). REV-ERB and ROR are not involved in rhythm generation but are important in controlling the phase and amplitude of circadian gene expression. Melatonin can regulate the expression of REV-ERB and ROR.

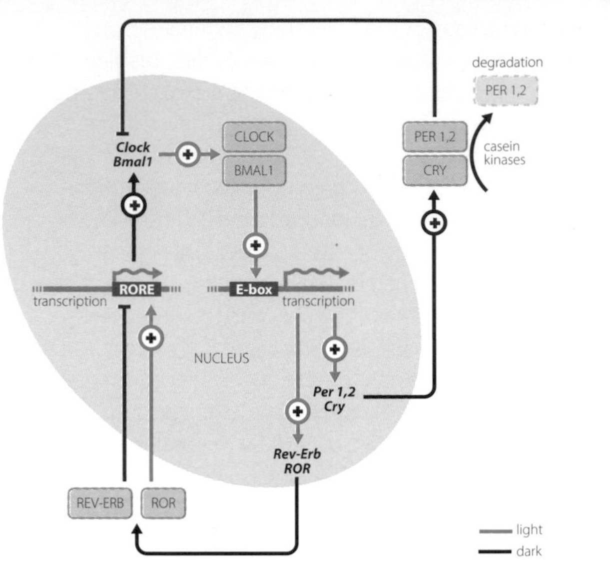

Box figure 8.2. The genes and transcription factors involved in circadian control.

gland receives information via a polysynaptic pathway that has been stimulated by light (*Box 8.1*). This stimulates the production of melatonin as a result of the innervation of the pineal gland by nor-adrenergic sympathetic nerve terminals. The pineal gland contains other compounds beside melatonin, including other biogenic amines, peptides, and GABA.

8.2.1 Melatonin

Melatonin is synthesized within the pinealocytes from tryptophan (*Figure 8.1*). The rate-limiting step in the synthesis is catalyzed by the enzyme *N*-acetyltransferase (NAT). The levels of melatonin and NAT are highest in the dark period of each day. Melatonin is directly released into the blood or CSF. The final step in the production of melatonin is catalyzed by hydroxyindole-*O*-methyltransferase (HIOMT).

Current evidence supports two roles for melatonin in humans: initiating and maintaining sleep and control of other 24 hour rhythms. The majority of excreted melatonin is inactivated by the liver and only 2–3% of the circulating melatonin is excreted into the urine and saliva. Measurement of urinary and salivary melatonin has been used to roughly estimate plasma concentrations (*Figure 8.2*).

Box 8.3 | Biological rhythms, gene expression, and health

Genetic studies indicate that about 10% of genes expressed in any tissue are under circadian regulation and these genes control the cell cycle, proliferation, and metabolism. It is not entirely understood how the central control of circadian rhythms by the SCN is transferred to the periphery, but there is evidence that similar clock genes are present in peripheral tissues and their expression also oscillates as they do in the SCN.

Knock-out mice models have been used to investigate the role of the clock genes illustrated in *Box 8.2* and some of the characteristics of mice with specific deletions of clock transcription factors are summarized below to illustrate the importance of the genes and rhythms in maintenance of health.

Transcription factor	Selected characteristics of mice knock-outs
CLOCK	Obesity, metabolic syndrome, hyperphagia
BMAL1	Hypoglycemia, impaired glucose tolerance, reduced fertility
CRY	Salt sensitive hypertension, lowered incidence of cancer
PER	Increased cellular proliferation, increased incidence of cancer
REV-ERB	Elevated serum VLDL triglycerides, impaired Purkinje cell development
ROR	Low plasma triglycerides, reduced susceptibility to autoimmune and inflammatory disorders, cerebellar atrophy

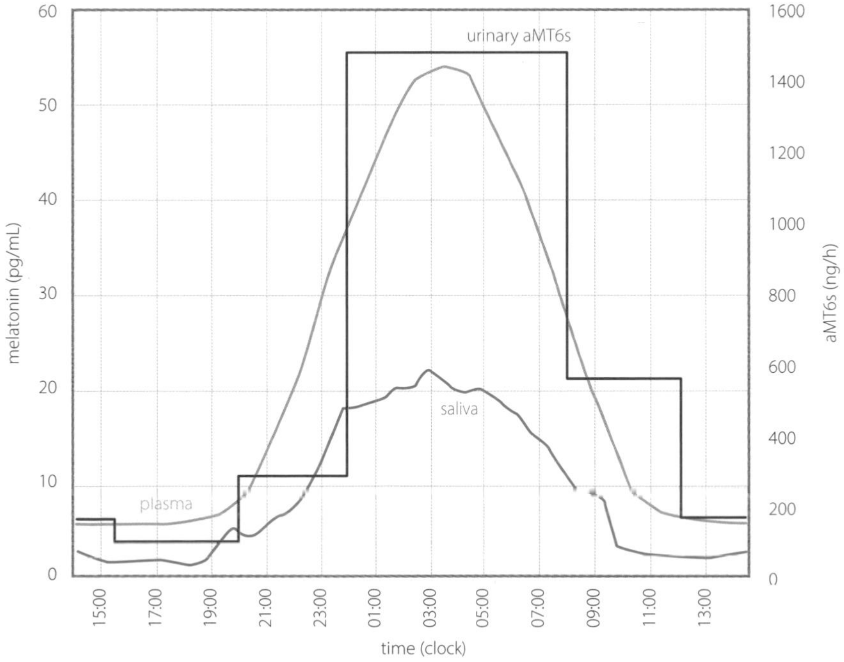

Figure 8.2. Average concentrations of melatonin in plasma (green) and saliva (blue), and a metabolite of melatonin, 6-sulfatoxymelatonin (aMT6s), in urine (red).

Melatonin use in humans

Melatonin has been used to treat sleep disorders, because it is useful in resetting circadian rhythms. Its ability to phase-shift the circadian rhythm underlies its common use to treat or prevent jet lag associated with eastbound travel. Other proposed benefits of treatment with melatonin include slowing or reversing aging, enhancing the immune system, suppressing cancer growth, and helping with depression and seasonal affective disorders.

Pathology of the pineal gland

Pineal gland tumors are rare, comprising <1% of all primary brain tumors. They are more common in children aged 1–12 years. Germ cell tumors, pineal parenchymal tumors, and gliomas account for most of the neoplasms of the pineal gland. These tumors cause neurological symptoms and signs by invasion and/or compression of nearby structures as well as obstruction to CSF flow. Some patients may present with cranial nerve palsies or hypothalamic dysfunction. Distant metastasis is rare, but some patients may present with leptomeningeal spread. MRI is the imaging modality of choice. Treatment is with surgery/radiotherapy depending on the location of the tumor, spread, invasion of adjacent structures and the presence of leptomeningeal spread.

8.3 Basic science – the endocrinology of fat

CASE 8.1 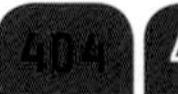 412

- Man of 46 years with BMI of 45.5 and waist of 118 cm
- High fasting blood sugar, high HbA1c, high cholesterol and triglycerides
- Previous diets and attempts at exercise had failed – now motivated to avoid losing job

A 46 year old man was referred to the obesity clinic by his primary care physician who had been looking after him for several years. The physician was concerned that, despite years of advice and apparent efforts of the patient to diet and exercise, his weight was increasing inexorably. The patient freely admitted to having a terrible diet – he worked as a long-distance truck driver and generally ate in roadside cafes or on the ferry. He drank fizzy drinks almost constantly while on the road. He had been increasingly breathless over the last few months. His exercise tolerance was also limited by bilateral knee pain and stiffness in the right hip. He was quite markedly fatigued, and occasionally found himself on the verge of nodding off whilst driving.

On examination he had a BMI of 45.5 kg/m^2 and waist circumference was 118 cm/48 inches. Investigations revealed:

- normal thyroid function
- undetectable cortisol after an overnight dexamethasone suppression test
- fasting blood sugar 8.1 mmol/L (NR 3.5–6.1)
- HbA1c 8.6% or 70 mmol/mol (NR 4.6–5.6% or 20–47 mmol/mol)
- total cholesterol 6 mmol/L (ideal range up to 4.5 mmol/L)
- triglycerides 3.4 mmol/L (upper target is <1.1 mmol/L)

He admitted frustration with previous (albeit rather half-hearted) attempts at weight loss. He now appeared well-motivated, in part helped by the threats of his wife who accompanied him to the appointment. He was concerned about the possibility of getting diabetes which might, he thought, affect his profession as a driver, and was worried about his somnolence at the wheel. He described the weight gain accompanied by joint pain which led to limitation of exercise as a 'vicious circle.'

Adipose tissue was classically thought of as a tissue mass that could store excess fatty acids in the form of triglycerides and provide insulation and padding to the body. It is now known that adipose tissue produces numerous hormones, growth factors, enzymes, cytokines, and complement factors which play a role in varied biological functions including vascular function, lipid metabolism, immune function, fat mass regulation, and regulation of adipocyte differentiation. These secretions may act locally in a paracrine/autocrine manner or be released into the general circulation. They are collectively known as adipokines or adipocytokines. The major secretory products of adipose tissue currently identified are:

- leptin
- adiponectin
- resistin and visfatin
- retinol binding protein-4
- tumor necrosis factor-α (TNF-α)
- various interleukins, plasminogen activator inhibitor-1, growth factors, several chemokines and complement factors.

Adipose tissue is also capable of taking up androgens of gonadal and adrenal origin and converting them to active estrogens. Thus in post-menopausal women, fat and other tissues are important sources of estrogens derived from adrenal androgens. In addition, the amount of body fat is an important contributory component to the onset of puberty and maintenance of fertility in women (see *Sections 7.3* and *7.6*) and this may also be related to the ability of fat to convert androgens to estrogens.

8.3.1 Development of adipose tissue and obesity

Mesenchymal stem cells (MSCs), derived from the mesoderm, are multipotent stem cells that can differentiate into a variety of cell types, including osteoblasts, chondrocytes, skeletal muscle cells, and adipocytes. Two types of adipocytes arise from MSC by a process known as adipogenesis – these are white adipocytes forming white adipose tissue (WAT) and brown adipocytes forming brown adipose tissue (BAT). Once these MSCs have become committed to the adipocyte lineage they are considered to be pre-adipocytes which are devoid of lipid but may proliferate to increase the number of pre-adipocytes, or differentiate into mature lipid-containing adipocytes.

White fat cells contain a single large lipid droplet, whilst brown fat cells contain multiple small lipid droplets throughout the cytoplasm, with the brown color attributed to the large number of mitochondria present in these cells. BAT is specialized for non-shivering thermogenesis whereby the energy derived from fatty acid oxidation is used for the generation of heat as a result of mitochondrial uncoupling. BAT is most prevalent in infants to defend them against cold, although it persists in adulthood with the WAT/BAT ratio being dependent on genetic background, sex, age, nutritional status, and environmental conditions.

Little is known about the development of adipose tissue in humans, although studies from large mammals show that subcutaneous fat deposits develop in specific layers before the internal visceral (intra-abdominal) and epicardial (surrounding heart) fat tissues develop. An excess of visceral fat – central obesity – can be associated with hypertension, insulin resistance and dyslipidemia, giving rise to what is termed the metabolic syndrome.

Obesity is due to an energy intake which exceeds energy expenditure. It has become a worldwide health issue and the World Health Organization has estimated that within a few years about 2.3 billion adults worldwide will be overweight and more than 700 million obese. The cost on health is huge and it is clear that it increases the risk of type 2 DM, cardiovascular disease, stroke, cancer, obstructive sleep apnea, and neurodegenerative diseases.

The control of food intake is complex and involves both hormonal and neural signals from adipose tissue and the GI tract and these are integrated in the brain stem, hypothalamus, and higher cortical areas (*Box 8.4*). Interestingly, the majority of these signals relay satiety messages (anorexigenic) to the brain, but in humans these can be overcome by psychological and emotional factors as well as daily biological rhythms which, if disturbed, can lead to metabolic disturbances. In addition, modern lifestyles have comparatively low levels of energy expenditure and highly palatable high energy foods are readily available. However, our increasing understanding of hormones released by adipose tissue and the GI tract may provide therapeutic targets for the treatment of obesity.

8.3.2 Hormones from adipose tissue

These are summarized in *Figure 8.3.*

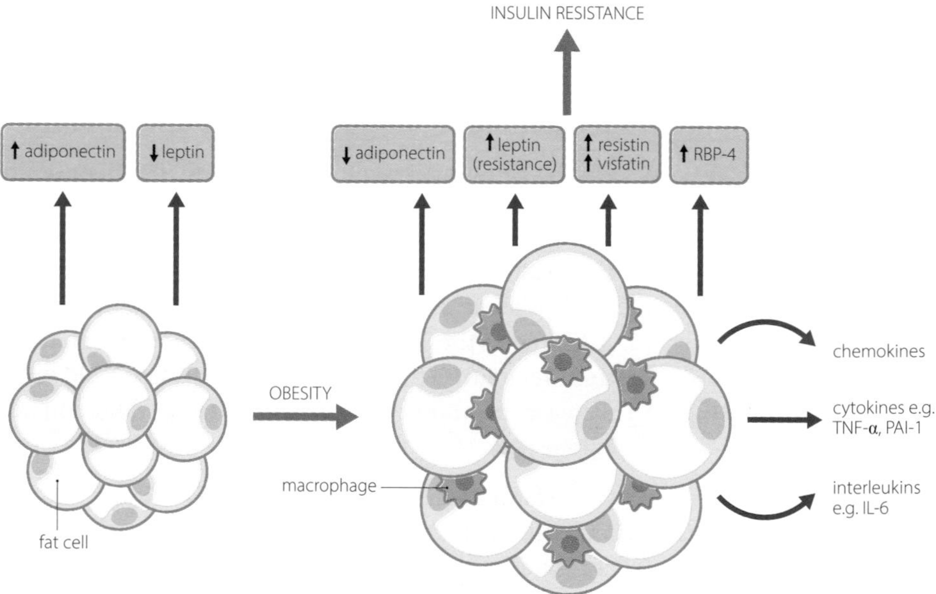

Figure 8.3. Adipose tissue: its secretions and pathology in obesity.

Leptin

Leptin (from the Greek *leptos*, for thin) was the first hormone that was discovered as a secretory product from adipocytes. It was identified through studies on the genetically obese *ob/ob* mouse which is deficient in leptin and the *db/db* mouse which was found to lack functional leptin receptors. Treatment of *ob/ob* mice with leptin was shown to reduce food intake and the percentage of body fat, increase energy expenditure, and restore euglycemia and reproductive functions. In humans, leptin administration did not have similar effects and it became clear that this adipokine was not going to be the cure for human obesity. This is because most obese humans are resistant to leptin, with the exception of a few very rare cases of humans with congenital leptin deficiency who do respond to leptin treatment.

Leptin, known as the prototypical adipokine, is a 167 amino acid peptide with a structure similar to cytokines. It is mainly expressed in adipose tissue but also in

Box 8.4 | Control of food intake

Food intake, body weight, and energy expenditure are coordinated by a complex network of neural and endocrine signals which are integrated in the brain stem and the arcuate nucleus of the hypothalamus. Pivotal to this integration are two neuronal systems in the arcuate nucleus:

- the neuropeptide Y (NPY) and agouti-related peptide (AgRP) neurons which are orexigenic and stimulate food intake
- the pro-opimelanocortin (POMC) and cocaine- and amphetamine-regulated transcript (CART) neurons that signal satiety and are thus anorexigenic.

These central regulators receive inputs from the brain stem (another central integrating center) and from higher brain centers which are important in the psychological and emotional regulation of food intake. Neurons from the arcuate also project to the paraventricular nucleus of the hypothalamus activating anorexigenic pathways involving corticotropin releasing hormone, thyrotropin releasing hormone and oxytocin; these have roles in altering energy expenditure (basal metabolic rate) and sympathetic regulation. Other nuclei in the hypothalamus are also implicated in regulating food intake including the lateral hypothalamic area and the prefornical area which contain neurons releasing the orexigenic hormones, orexins, and melanocyte concentrating hormones.

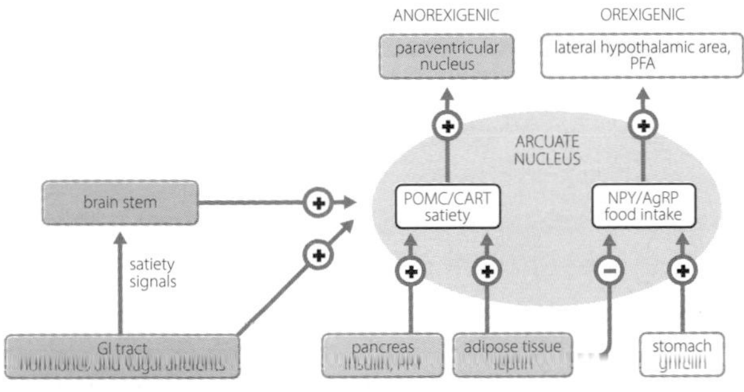

Box figure 8.3. Signaling system in brain stem and arcuate nucleus to control food intake.

Satiety signals from the gastroenteropancreatic tract

Hormones secreted by the GI tract and pancreas are important for short-term information about meal ingestion and they have all been shown to suppress appetite in humans. They include insulin and pancreatic polypeptide (PP), cleavage products of proglucagon (*see Section 5.3, Figure 5.13*), including glucagon-like peptide-1 and oxyntomodulin, and cholecystokinin.

These hormones may reach the brain through the median eminence or area postrema which are outside the blood–brain barrier. Alternatively, they may activate vagal afferents that terminate in the dorsal vagal complex of the brain stem. This area consists of the dorsal motor nucleus of vagus, the area postrema, and the nucleus tractus solitarius. The dorsal vagal complex also receives vagal afferents which detect gut distension – another important signal in the control of food intake.

Leptin

This hormone, secreted mainly by adipose tissue, maintains long-term control of adiposity and influences long-term energy homeostasis. It can inhibit the activity of the orexigenic NPY/AgRP neuronal system whilst stimulating the activity of the anorexigenic POMC/CART neurons. Insulin is also considered to be involved in long-term energy homeostasis. Increases in body adiposity increase both insulin and leptin secretion which pass into the brain in proportion to their circulating concentrations. They both stimulate POMC/CART neurons.

Ghrelin

This is the only known orexigenic hormone, stimulating food intake. It is mainly secreted by oxyntic cells of the stomach but also from other areas of the GI tract. It is the endogenous ligand for the GHRH receptor in the pituitary gland. Experimental studies suggest that ghrelin primarily acts on the NPY/AgRP neuronal system in the hypothalamus to stimulate appetite, although there is evidence it may also act via the brain stem.

NPY/AgRP and POMC/CART

Most neurons in the arcuate nucleus co-express either the orexigenic or anorexigenic peptides. NPY is the most potent orexigen known and NPY neurons may also project to the lateral hypothalamic area and the prefornical area to stimulate the release of orexins (hypocretins) and melanocyte concentrating hormones. POMC is the precursor to several hormones/neurohormones including ACTH and α-MSH. MSH produced by POMC/CART neurons stimulates melanocortin-4 receptors (MC4R) which in turn releases anorexigenic peptides.

Much of the evidence regarding the endocrine control of food intake and the neural circuits involved in this control has been obtained from studies in rodents. That said, naturally occurring mutations in genes coding for hormones and their receptors have greatly added to our understanding of appetite regulation and obesity in humans (*Box 8.5*).

Box 8.5 | Genetics of obesity

Twin and adoption studies during the late 1980s and early 1990s provided evidence that genetics plays an important role in obesity. Parental obesity provides the strongest risk factor and this may reflect both environmental factors as well as genetic mechanisms although twin studies, including twins reared apart, suggest that genetic effects can account for >50% variance in BMI.

These genetic effects can be categorized into two groups:

- rare monogenetic disorders where a mutation of a single dominant or recessive autosomal gene (Mendelian inheritance) gives rise to a one-to-one genotype/phenotype relationship
- polygenetic disorders where traits are due to DNA variation in multiple genes and the phenotype can be variable.

Monogenetic disorders involving hyperphagia and obesity

Prader–Willi syndrome resulting from a deletion of chromosome 15 is a complex genetic disorder, which is present from birth. Its main characteristics are:

- excessive appetite leading to morbid obesity and diabetes during childhood
- low muscle tone
- emotional instability
- immature physical development
- learning disabilities (sometimes very mild).

Prader–Willi patients rarely survive beyond 25–30 years, with eventual death related to diabetes and cardiac failure.

Other monogenetic disorders include:

- Mutations of the leptin (*LEP*) gene in adipose tissue or the leptin receptor (*LEPR*) gene expressed in the arcuate nucleus (*Box 8.4*) lead to abnormal eating behavior and the development of early-onset morbid obesity and impaired fertility. Leptin deficiency has been successfully treated with leptin resulting in a reduction in fat mass.
- Mutations of the *POMC* gene, which produce anorexigenic peptides in the hypothalamus, lead to extreme obesity and adrenal insufficiency as a result of ACTH deficiency.
- Mutations of the *MC4R* gene are associated with early onset obesity. This results from the inability of leptin to signal anorexigenic signals via MSH to other anorexigenic nuclei in the hypothalamus (*Box 8.4*).

Polygenetic disorders

Several polygenetic disorders have been identified including variants in the *MC4R* gene, *CCK, LEP, ghrelin, FTO* (fat mass and obesity-associated gene), *GAD* (glutamic acid decarboxylase), *BNDF* (brain derived neurotrophic factor) and *TASRs* (taste receptors). Such variants can alter the central control of appetite, taste, and ingestive behavior and may all contribute to abnormal food intake and obesity.

other tissues including the ovaries, placenta, mammary epithelium, lymphoid tissue, and bone marrow. It is secreted in a pulsatile manner with highest levels secreted between midnight and early morning; the patterns of secretion appear to be related to food intake. Women tend to have higher levels of leptin than men and this has been attributed to the fact that women accumulate more subcutaneous fat and that leptin expression is higher in subcutaneous fat compared with visceral fat.

Circulating leptin levels reflect both energy stores and acute energy balance. Thus serum levels of leptin show a positive correlation with total body fat mass which is associated with an increased release of leptin from enlarged adipocytes - in obese people these are usually 2–4 times larger than those of lean subjects because of the increased size of lipid storage. Acutely, food restriction results in the suppression of circulating levels of leptin. The mechanisms that control leptin secretion, however, are not well defined.

Several alternatively spliced isoforms of the leptin receptor (ObR, but also known as LEP-R, LR, etc.) have been identified and all have similar extracellular domains but distinct intracellular domains due to alternate RNA splicing. Short isoforms are thought to play a role in transporting leptin across the blood–brain barrier, whilst the long isoform, ObRb/ObR-L, is responsible for leptin signaling. This long receptor is abundantly expressed in areas of the hypothalamus concerned with the regulation of food intake and is also expressed in lower concentrations in several peripheral tissues, including adipose tissue, the gonads, placenta, adrenal medulla, liver, pancreatic beta cells, lung, blood mononuclear cells, chondrocytes, heart, and skeletal muscle. These leptin receptors are classical cytokine receptors and signal through the JAK2/STAT3 pathway (see *Section 1.5*), although leptin can also activate the PI3-kinase and MEK/ERK1/2 signaling pathways as well as AMPK signaling (see *Section 1.5* and *Box 5.8*) in the brain and skeletal muscle.

Functions of leptin

- The major function of leptin is maintenance of energy homeostasis by adjusting appetite and food intake. Leptin, along with insulin and gut hormones, interacts with several neuronal pathways in and outside of the hypothalamus to regulate energy intake via orexigenic and anorexigenic neuropeptides (*Box 8.4*). Leptin is basically an anorexigenic hormone and inhibits eating, but the resistance to leptin in obese individuals suggests that leptin's primary role is a hormone of starvation, controlling the energy deficient state by reduced anorexigenic signals to the brain.
- Leptin has marked effects on metabolism. Leptin deficiency results in insulin resistance and diabetes and individuals with congenital leptin deficiency are profoundly obese and exhibit hyperinsulinemia and dyslipidemia; these can be improved by exogenous leptin. Leptin improves insulin resistance by activating insulin-sensitive tissues including liver and fat.
- Leptin has a modulatory role in neuroendocrine function. In the hypothalamic–pituitary–gonadal axis leptin appears to be important in maintaining pulsatile GnRH/LH secretion and may play a role in the onset of puberty. Its actions are not directly targeted on the GnRH neurons, but probably involve the kisspeptin neuronal system (see *Section 7.3*). Similarly, the hypothalamic–pituitary control of thyroid function may be affected by changes in leptin secretion and some evidence (mainly from rodent studies) points to effects of leptin on the hypothalamic–pituitary control of the adrenal cortex and growth hormone secretion.
- Leptin has a permissive role in immune function promoting T helper cell differentiation and cytokine production. Individuals with congenital leptin deficiency show increased incidence of infection, decreased proliferation of CD4+ T cells, and activation of the TNF-α system.

Adiponectin

Adiponectin, also called adipocyte complement-related peptide, is a 244 amino acid protein which is structurally related to the complement 1q family and has a C-terminal globular domain that is structurally similar to TNF-α. Adiponectin is secreted exclusively from adipocytes, not as a single molecule but in the form of multimers which can range from low molecular weight trimers to high molecular weight dodecamers. The high molecular weight multimers are considered to be the most biologically active, particularly in relation to metabolic function.

Serum levels of adiponectin circulate at a concentration 1000 times higher than leptin and are negatively correlated with body fat, decreasing with obesity and increasing in response to weight loss. The precise role of adiponectin is poorly defined, although experimental evidence from animal models suggests that it has anti-inflammatory properties and a role in protecting against insulin resistance, glucose intolerance and dyslipidemia. Patients with type 2 DM have reduced serum levels of adiponectin. These metabolic effects are mediated by two identified adiponectin receptors, AdipoR1 and AdipoR2, which can activate AMPK (see *Box 5.8*) and increase expression of PPARα and hence PPARα-regulated genes. Obesity can blunt AMPK signaling, but there is little evidence that adiponectin is involved in the regulation of food intake, although adiponectin receptors have been located in the hypothalamus.

Interestingly, PPARγ ligands, the thiazolidinediones which are used in the treatment of type 2 DM, increase circulating levels of adiponectin and it is now thought that part of the insulin-sensitizing effect of these 'glitazones' may be mediated by increased adiponectin secretion.

Resistin

Resistin is a 108 amino acid peptide (including the signal sequence) which is strikingly similar in structure to adiponectin. In humans resistin is secreted from monocytes and macrophages in adipose tissue, although the major source appears to be from mononuclear cells in the circulation. There is controversial evidence about the role of resistin in human physiology and pathophysiology and no receptor has yet been identified. In rodents, resistin is secreted primarily from adipocytes and it had originally been postulated as a risk factor for insulin resistance.

A more likely role for resistin, however, is in inflammation and autoimmunity, i.e. it is a pro-inflammatory hormone. Its expression is stimulated by pro-inflammatory cytokines such as IL-1, IL-6, and TNF-α and there appears to be a positive feedback mechanism in that resistin can up-regulate the expression of these cytokines not only from peripheral blood mononuclear cells but also from macrophages and mononuclear cells in adipose tissue (see below). Visfatin is another adipokine which has similar pro-inflammatory properties to resistin and is also released from peripheral blood lymphocytes as well as adipose tissue. Insulin-mimicking/-sensitizing effects of visfatin have been described, but in humans a metabolic function of this adipokine has not been conclusively established.

Retinol binding protein (RBP-4)

RBP-4 is another adipokine that could be linked to insulin resistance. Whilst the liver is the main source of this specific carrier for retinol (vitamin A), adipose tissue has the second highest expression levels with visceral fat having a higher expression compared with subcutaneous fat. Serum concentrations of RBP-4 correlate with the amount of visceral fat and the raised levels of this adipokine in obesity are correlated with many aspects of the metabolic syndrome including insulin resistance and inflammation.

8.3.3 Obesity, adipose tissue macrophages, and inflammatory cytokines

Obesity is linked with a low grade chronic inflammatory response characterized by altered production of adipokines, increased production of pro-inflammatory cytokines, and over-expression of adipocyte-derived chemokines. In obesity there is hypertrophy of the adipocytes and a recruitment of macrophages into adipose tissue which produce the pro-inflammatory cytokines, notably TNF-α and IL-6. Thus there is a correlative and causative relationship between visceral obesity, insulin resistance, type 2 DM, and inflammation.

TNF-α was originally known as cachectin because its pro-inflammatory effects were accompanied by cachexia, weight loss, and insulin resistance. It is known to disturb insulin signaling and can induce insulin resistance. IL-6 is also over-expressed in adipose tissue of obesity and plasma levels are increased in type 2 DM and positively correlated with body mass and plasma free fatty acid concentrations.

It is only within the last decade that the role of adipose tissue has changed from simply being an inert storage organ to a dynamic endocrine organ and part of the innate immune system. It is clear that there is an important inter-relationship between metabolic signaling and immune signaling and the finding that adipose tissue is infiltrated by macrophages has helped in understanding the link between obesity, inflammation, and insulin resistance. Much research has focused on leptin and adiponectin which shows beneficial effects on insulin action and lipid metabolism whilst resistin and RBP-4 have been linked to the development of insulin resistance. There are, however, many discrepancies between findings in rodent models and humans and the molecular mechanisms through which these adipokines exert their effects. At the same time there are still many outstanding questions to be answered, such as what is the signal that attracts monocytes into adipose tissue, is adipose tissue inflammation a cause or the consequence of insulin resistance, and does the changing endocrine and immune function of adipose tissue in obesity contribute to dyslipidemia, atherogenesis, and other symptoms related to the metabolic syndrome?

BMI is a relatively useful marker of obesity and is calculated from the weight (divided by the square of the height in meters (units: kg/m^2). Classifications of obesity have been agreed by the World Health Organization dependent on BMI, as follows:

Classification	BMI (kg/m^2)	
	Principal cut-off points	Additional cut-off points
Underweight	**<18.50**	**<18.50**
Severe thinness	<16.00	<16.00
Moderate thinness	16.00–16.99	16.00–16.99
Mild thinness	17.00–18.49	17.00–18.49
Normal range	**18.50–24.99**	**18.50–22.99**
		23.00–24.99
Overweight	**≥25.00**	**≥25.00**
Pre-obese	25.00–29.99	25.00–27.49
		27.50–29.99
Obese	**≥30.00**	**≥30.00**
Obese class I	30.00–34.99	30.00–32.49
		32.50–34.99
Obese class II	35.00–39.99	35.00–37.49
		37.50–39.99
Obese class III	≥40.00	≥40.00

In some cases BMI is not a useful marker of obesity, for example in the extremely fit endurance/strength athletes such as rowers who will often have a BMI in the obese range which is unhelpful. Waist circumference is probably a better measure of visceral adiposity and it is this that is a risk factor for cardiovascular and other diseases.

While there is clear and growing evidence for a number of genetic causes of obesity in early childhood (generally associated with hyperphagia and impaired appetite control), an underlying causative disorder of obesity is rarely found in adulthood.

The approach to the management of the obese patient is summarized in *Box 8.6*.

CASE 8.1 404 412

- Man of 46 years with BMI of 45.5 and waist of 118 cm
- High fasting blood sugar, high HbA1c, high cholesterol and triglycerides
- Previous diets and attempts at exercise had failed – now motivated to avoid losing job
- Morbidly obese according to WHO classification and with type 2 DM and possible sleep apnea
- Started on metformin and atorvastatin, then had gastric bypass surgery

The patient was clearly morbidly obese (see *Figure 8.4*) and had developed many of the complications associated with obesity, including type 2 DM, joint pain probably secondary to osteoarthritis, possible sleep apnea, and an adverse lipid profile.

He had no evidence of thyroid dysfunction and a dexamethasone suppression test had ruled out hypercortisolemia. The pattern of weight gain in Cushing syndrome is somewhat different and, in the absence of other clinical features suggesting this diagnosis, it is rarely necessary to proceed to a formal dexamethasone suppression test (see *Section 6.4*).

After a long discussion with the patient it was clear that he was fed up with trying diets and his exercise capacity was so limited as to make an exercise program effectively unworkable. In view of the diagnosis of diabetes and the adverse lipid profile he was started on metformin 850 mg twice daily and atorvastatin 40 mg daily. He was referred for dietary advice, specifically from a nutritionist working in the Diabetes Center, and was given training in glucose monitoring. He was fortunate enough to have been seen in a multidisciplinary obesity clinic and had the opportunity over the next weeks to meet with psychologists and surgeons. It was quickly decided that the best way forward would be to go for early bariatric surgical intervention and he underwent a Roux-en-Y gastric bypass (*Figure 8.5*). He was closely followed up by the obesity service.

Eighteen months after surgery he was off metformin, his cholesterol profile was normal and he had lost 42 kg in weight. He was exercising regularly (without pain), sleeping well at night and was able to drive without falling asleep.

8.4 The endocrinology of the gut and gastroenteropancreatic tumors

The first hormone to be discovered, in 1902, was the gut hormone secretin and the discovery of this 'internal secretion' gave rise to the term hormone from the Greek meaning 'to excite or arouse'. This marked the birth of endocrinology. Gastrin was discovered shortly after and then cholecystokinin (CCK). These three classical gut hormones were considered to control digestive processes. We now know that the gastroenteropancreatic tract is, in fact, the largest hormone producing gland in the body, both in terms of the number of endocrine cells and the number of different hormones it produces. In contrast to other endocrine organs, however, the endocrine

Box 8.6 | Management of obesity

Numerous guidelines aim to unify the approach to the evaluation and treatment of obesity. The rationale for treatment is simple: weight loss results in a significant decrease in the potential for developing weight-related co-morbidity (both physical and psycho-social) and leads to a palpable improvement in quality and quantity of life.

Morbidity associated with obesity

Cardiovascular risk:

- type 2 diabetes mellitus
- hyperlipidemia
- venous thrombosis (PE, DVT, superficial thrombophlebitis)

Respiratory risk:

- obstructive sleep apnea
- alveolar hypoventilation

Gastrointestinal conditions:

- gastro-esophageal reflux
- fatty liver, and non-alcoholic steatohepatitis (which may progress to cirrhosis)
- gallstones
- hernias

Genito-urinary conditions:

- stress incontinence
- PCOS
- subfertility
- hirsutes

Cancer:

- colon, breast, uterus, prostate

Osteoarthritis and degenerative joint disease

Infection, including cellulitis and poor wound healing

Depression

Investigation

Laboratory studies should include:

- lipids: fasting total cholesterol, HDL-C, and triglycerides; this may reveal the typical dyslipidemia associated with the metabolic syndrome – low HDL-C, high LDL-C, and high triglycerides.
- liver function tests: elevated transaminases (ALT, AST, γ-GT) may result from fatty infiltration of the liver and may be a feature of non-alcoholic steatohepatitis.
- thyroid function tests: to exclude hypothyroidism.
- urinary free cortisol or dexamethasone suppression test: if there is a clinical suspicion of Cushing syndrome.
- fasting glucose and insulin: to assess the presence of impaired glucose tolerance or frank diabetes and assess any degree of associated hyperinsulinemia suggesting insulin resistance.

Management

The goal of treatment is to prevent complications (see above) and improve quality of life. Effectiveness requires motivation from the patient and the team involved in the treatment. Patients who already have co-morbidities (e.g. type 2 DM) require aggressive management at an early stage. The presence of components of the metabolic syndrome also suggest active and aggressive treatment should start at a lower BMI. In terms of the metabolic syndrome, BMI is probably a less useful measure than waist circumference. The latter is recorded using a non-expandable tape at the umbilicus with the patient standing.

The metabolic syndrome is defined as:

central obesity with a raised waist circumference of >94 cm / 37 inches (male) and >80 cm / 31.5 inches (female) **AND** any two of the following:

Triglycerides:

- 1.7 mmol/L OR
- treatment for hypertriglycidemia

HDL cholesterol: <1.03 mmol/L in males or 1.29 mmol/L in females

Raised blood pressure:

- systolic BP >130 or diastolic BP >85 mmHg OR
- treatment of previously diagnosed hypertension

Raised fasting plasma glucose:

- >5.6 mmol/L OR
- type 2 DM

General issues

In simple terms, any effective treatment needs to either reduce intake or increase energy expenditure (or be a combination of the two). Sitting inactively in front of the TV uses up about 1100 kcal/day (in processes like maintenance of heartbeat, body temperature and tissue repair). Training as an Olympic rower uses about 10 times this amount of energy.

Box 8.6 | continued

A reasonable target for weight loss would be about 1–1.5 kg (2–3 lb) a week although evidence suggests that programs need to be tailored to the individual. Sadly the majority of programs do not work. Weight losses achieved hardly ever exceed 10% (5% is probably a more realistic norm) and around 60% of weight lost is regained in the first year after diet – weight usually returns to pre-diet levels within 4–5 years.

An intake of 200 kcal/day (usually known as starvation) is associated with adverse changes in electrolytes, vitamin and micronutrient deficiency, and ketosis and so is not recommended. A very low calorie diet usually means limiting intake to around 800 kcal/day and this can result in weight loss of up to 20 kg (44 lb) in 3 months, but it can rarely be maintained, and should probably only be recommended prior to more effective long-term treatment such as bariatric surgery (see below). Low calorie diets usually aim for an intake of between 800–1200 kcal/day and may lead to a weight loss of about 0.5 kg (1 lb) per week. Again, they are rarely sustainable. Normal calorie diets simply aim to reduce the current intake by 500–1000 kcal/day.

Diets may be based on portion control (i.e. reduced meal sizes – dividing total intake into three balanced meals possibly including meal replacement shakes and bars). Alcohol and candy (empty calories) should be avoided. This type of diet has the advantage of maintaining the normal balance of carbohydrate, fat, and protein. Other diets are low carbohydrate (e.g. the Atkins diet) or low fat (e.g. the Ornish diet). Both low fat and low carbohydrate diets probably achieve roughly the same amount of weight loss, but may have differing effects on cardiovascular risk. Either way they are rarely sustained and results are generally disappointing.

Exercise

The ultimate aim is to achieve around 30–45 minutes of aerobic exercise daily. Exercise clearly helps to build muscle mass and to reduce waist circumference – a surrogate marker of visceral fat. Other cardiometabolic risk factors are generally ameliorated by regular effective exercise, especially if combined with a sensible calorie limited diet.

Medication

Very few medications are available for the management of obesity (particularly in the UK and Europe). Along with the basic principles of weight management, drugs should potentially fall into three classes:

- those that limit intake (i.e. centrally acting appetite suppressors)
- those that increase energy expenditure
- those that impair dietary absorption.

In the UK the only licensed medication is orlistat (Xenical) which has been reported to achieve an 8–10% weight loss sustained over 2 years. This drug works by inhibiting pancreatic lipase and so reducing triglyceride absorption.

In the USA several nor-adrenergic drugs retain FDA approval for short-term use, including diethylpropion, phentermine, benzphetamine and phendimetrazine which all suppress appetite. These drugs are not used in the UK and the latter two are likely to be withdrawn from the US market.

Sibutramine, a centrally acting reuptake inhibitor of serotonin, dopamine, and nor-epinephrine was used reasonably extensively until recently when it was withdrawn from the UK and later (2010) the US market due to significant cardiovascular side-effects (MI, stroke, and death).

Other drugs appear to show some potential promise and are occasionally used 'off-license'. These include the anti-epileptic, topiramate which has been reported to achieve a 15–20% weight loss, albeit limited by side-effects including confusion, memory loss, and drowsiness. SSRIs (e.g. fluoxetine) often result in anorexia as a side-effect and this has occasionally been exploited in the medical management of obesity. Caffeine and ephedrine can both increase energy expenditure but are generally not recommended due to the potential for causing palpitations and hypertension.

A huge amount of interest was generated by the availability of a selective antagonist of the cannabinoid type 1 receptor (CB-1). Endogenous cannabinoids induce appetite and have many other potentially adverse effects on components of the metabolic syndrome. The selective antagonist, rimonabant, initially appeared to be a highly effective agent but sadly its lifespan was short because the high incidence of psychiatric side-effects (including suicide) led to its withdrawal.

Newer potential medical interventions include a new dual PPAR agonist (see *Section 5.6* and *Box 5.9*), GFT505, which appears to have useful positive effects on insulin sensitivity, hypertriglyceridemia, and HDL levels. An improved understanding of the complex relationship between the gut and the hypothalamus and a start to

Box 8.6 | continued

the unraveling of the relationship between orexigenic and anorexigenic signals has led to a number of potential new agents, including α-MSH analogs, ghrelin antagonists, β-3-adrenergic agonists, and PYY analogs. Exenatide, the GLP-1 agonist (see *Section 5.6* and *Box 5.2*), has resulted in weight loss in type 2 diabetic patients but is not licensed outside of this diagnosis.

In short, there really is not much available for the medical treatment of obesity. CB-1 antagonists were an exciting addition but have been withdrawn as a result of adverse effects. Metformin shows some promise in obese PCOS patients (and certainly increases insulin sensitivity and reduces incidence of diabetes) but is not licensed for obesity treatment. Hopefully, as the complex endocrine relationships between appetite and hedonistic reward centers in the brain and nutrient sensing mechanisms in the gut continue to be elucidated, new drugs will be designed to block or stimulate these pathways.

Surgery

A surgeon once said "What would you prefer – a gastric bypass or a coronary artery bypass?". It has become clear that really the only effective, sustained (and relatively rapid) treatment modality for morbid obesity is bariatric surgery. Ideally, the decision to proceed to surgery should be made with the patient in a multidisciplinary setting with input from physicians, surgeons, psychologists, nutritionists, and specialist obesity nurses. Currently the majority of recommendations reserve surgery for those with a BMI of 40 kg/m^2 or 35 kg/m^2 with significant obesity-related co-morbidity. Bariatric surgery has been repeatedly demonstrated to have beneficial effects on all the obesity-related co-morbidities highlighted above. Surgical methods and outcomes have improved rapidly and laparoscopic techniques are increasingly being used (especially in the UK and Europe) with reduced surgical morbidity and complications.

An ever growing number of surgical procedures are available and generally these are divided into those procedures that work by restriction (i.e. reducing the effective volume of the stomach so patients are sated after a reduced intake) or by malabsorption (where the effective reabsorptive capacity of the small intestine is reduced). Some procedures combine both restriction and malabsorption. It is becoming clear, however, that in addition to restriction, bariatric procedures also have enormously important effects on neurohormonally regulated energy balance.

Bariatric procedures

Restrictive:

- vertical-banded gastroplasty
- laparoscopically adjusted gastric band (see *Figure 8.5*)
- sleeve gastrectomy

Malabsorption:

- jejuno–ileal bypass
- biliopancreatic diversion (with or without duodenal switch)

Both:

- Roux-en-Y gastric bypass (see *Figure 8.5*)

Roux-en-Y procedures are becoming increasingly common. They are very effective with an estimated excess weight loss of about 65% (excess weight loss refers to the difference between the BMI at decision to operate and a BMI of 25 kg/m^2). Laparoscopic gastric banding is slightly less effective but has the advantage of being a simpler procedure with less peri-operative morbidity, and is also adjustable and reversible.

Overall surgical mortality is around 0.5%. Bypass procedures may result in micronutrient deficiency (especially calcium, vitamin B_{12}, and iron). Operations designed to induce malabsorption may be complicated by diarrhea, development of gallstones, malabsorption of fat soluble vitamins (A, D, E, and K), magnesium and, occasionally, potassium deficiency. Despite these complications, the majority of patients undergoing bariatric surgery demonstrate an improved quality of life and evidence is accruing on the reversal of obesity related complications and adverse cardio-metabolic risk.

secreting cells of the GI tract are diffusely distributed in the mucosa and scattered amongst numerous other cell types that secrete their products (acid, mucus, etc.) into the lumen of the gut or take up nutrients from the gut.

Endocrine cells of the gastroenteropancreatic (GEP) tract are derived from cells of the neural ectoderm (neural crest) and such cells were embryologicaly identified by

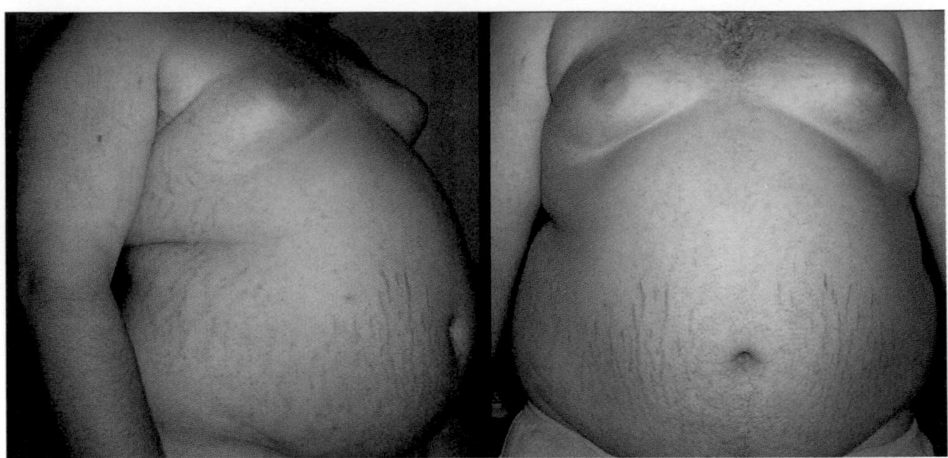

Figure 8.4. A patient with severe obesity (obese class III according to WHO guidelines – see *Section 8.3.3*).

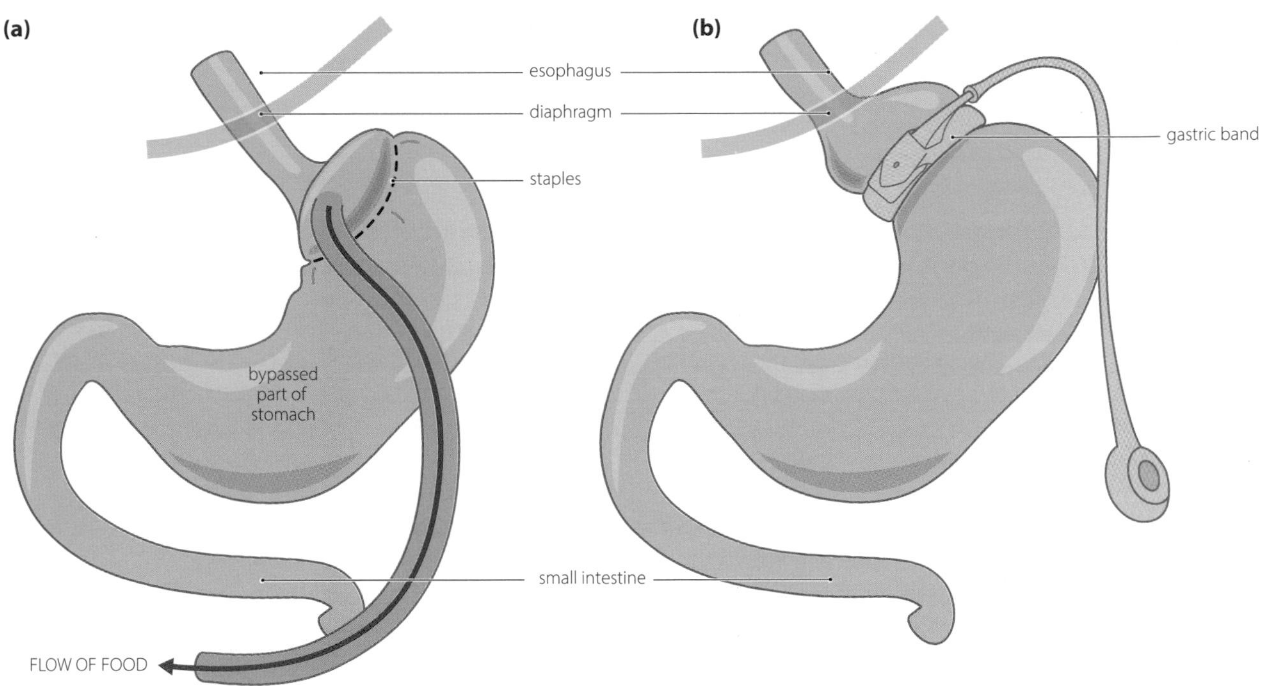

Figure 8.5. Gastric bypass.
(a) Roux-en-Y gastric bypass showing the jejuno-ileal bypass and a small pouch formed from the stomach.
(b) Laparoscopic gastric banding where a soft silicone ring is placed at the entrance to the stomach and this is connected to an injection port placed subcutaneously; injection of saline into the port tightens the band.

their ability to **u**ptake **a**mine **p**recursors and **d**ecarboxylate them – the term APUD cells was introduced for cells that secrete hormones in the GI tract and pancreatic islets. Due to their embryonic origin they are classified as neuroendocrine cells. Some APUD cells are further classified as enterochromaffin cells or Kulchitsky cells, which like the chromaffin cells of the adrenal medulla stain with potassium chromate. They are found throughout the GI tract and secrete serotonin (5-HT) which activates secretory and peristaltic reflexes, stimulates gastrin secretion in the stomach, and activates vagal afferents which are important in the generation of nausea. Another population of chromaffin cells is found only in the stomach and these are termed enterochromaffin-like (ECL) cells because they look like chromaffin cells, but instead of releasing serotonin they release histamine which stimulates the production of gastric acid.

Most neuroendocrine cells of the gut, otherwise termed enteroendocrine cells, extend into the lumen of the GI tract with their luminal surface covered with microvilli. These are termed 'open cells' which can be stimulated by substances in the GI lumen, whilst the 'closed' enteroendocrine cells do not make direct contact with the gut lumen. Both open and closed cells can be stimulated by peptides released from other enteroendocrine cells or by transmitters released from intrinsic or extrinsic neurons.

More than 30 peptide hormone genes are expressed throughout the digestive tract and these may act locally in a paracrine or autocrine function or be released into the general circulation. Many of the hormones are expressed in other tissues and in the brain many of the gut hormones act as neurotransmitters or neuromodulators, hence the term brain–gut peptides. Many neurotransmitters and neuropeptides are also produced in the gut and affect GI function. The plethora of gut hormones that have been discovered and widely expressed outside the GI tract makes the hormones multifunctional regulators. They not only control digestion but also act as acute metabolic hormones, as neurotransmitters and important controllers of food intake and adiposity (*Box 8.4*). *Table 8.1* shows the families of homologous hormones secreted by the enteroendocrine cells of the GI tract and other important gut hormones that have been identified as controlling functions of the GI tract and food intake (*Box 8.4*).

8.4.1 Carcinoid tumors and carcinoid syndrome

CASE 8.2 417 425

- Man of 62 years with hot flushes, severe diarrhea, and weight loss
- Firm hepatomegaly and palpable liver edge

A 63 year old man was seen in the endocrine clinic following concern from his primary care physician. Normally a fit, uncomplaining man, he had been plagued with unusual symptoms for 4 months which included episodes of hot flushes/flashes (up to ten times daily). He had also developed severe diarrhea which necessitated using a large quantity of loperamide purchased over-the-counter; he had lost a significant amount of weight. He had also developed an audible wheeze which kept his wife awake at night. Examination was largely unhelpful but he did have firm hepatomegaly with a liver edge easily palpable 6 cm below the costal margin. He was normotensive. His primary care physician had already determined that he was biochemically euthyroid with normal renal function.

Carcinoid tumors are derived from primitive neuroendocrine cells in the gut. They are usually slow growing and relatively asymptomatic. They are the most common of the neuroendocrine tumors with an incidence of approximately 3 per 100 000 in the UK and USA. It is useful to classify them according to the site of origin in the

Table 8.1. Overview of the major families of hormones secreted by enteroendocrine cells* of the gut and their primary actions on the GI tract

Hormone families	Site of secretion in gut	Stimulus for secretion	Actions on intestinal target cells
Secretin family			
Secretin	Duodenal S cells	Gastric acid	Bicarbonate secretion from pancreatic ducts
Glucagon	Pancreatic α cells	↓blood glucose, ↑alanine/arginine	
Glucagon-like peptides: GLP-1/GLP-2 Oxyntomodulin	L cells of ileum and colon	Glucose and FFAs in ileum, colon	Incretin/trophic effect on gut
Gastric inhibitory polypeptide	K cells of small intestine	Glucose, TGs and amino acids in small intestine	Incretin
Gastrin family			
Gastrin	G cells of stomach	Vagal stimulation, peptides and amino acids in stomach	Acid secretion (HCl) in stomach
Cholecystokinin	I cells of duodenum, jejunum	Long chain fatty acids/ monoglycerides in small intestine	Pancreatic enzyme secretion, gallbladder contraction
PP-fold family			
Pancreatic polypeptide	F or PP cells of pancreas	Food ingestion	Pancreatic enzyme secretion
Peptide tyrosine-tyrosine	L cells of ileum and colon	Food ingestion	Inhibition of pancreatic exocrine secretions
Neuropeptide YL cells small intestine	Glucose, hormones		
Others			
Motilin	Endocrine M cells of duodenum, jejunum	pH of duodenum, fasting?	Gastric motility
Ghrelin	P/D1 cells of stomach, other parts of GI tract	Food ingestion	
Somatostatin	D cells of GI tract	Hormones, acid	Inhibition of GI hormones
Serotonin	Enterochromaffin cells	Vagal stimulation	Gastrin secretion
Histamine	Enterochromaffin-like cells	Stomach	Gastric acid secretion
Vasointestinal peptide	GI tract	Neural	Smooth muscle relaxation

* Other gastroenteropancreatic peptide families include:

- the insulin family including insulin and IGF-1 and -2
- the EGF family including EGF and TGF-α
- the tachykinin family including substance P, neurokinin A and B.

embryonic gut. Foregut tumors (about 20%) occur in the lung, thymus, stomach, and first part of the duodenum; midgut tumors (about 65%) arise in the small intestine, appendix, and proximal colon, and hindgut tumors (about 10–15%) occur in the distal colon. Carcinoid tumors have also been described in the kidney, pancreas, liver, testes, and ovary.

The terminology of neuroendocrine tumors is complex and confusing. It is probably reasonable to use the term carcinoid tumors for those that derive from the embryonic gut. However, carcinoid should not be used to describe pancreatic neuroendocrine tumors (NETs) or islet cell derived tumors. In spite of this attempt at clarity, it would not be real endocrinology if things were that easy, so the World Health Organization has tended to group GI carcinoid tumors together with pancreatic/islet cell neuroendocrine tumors as gastroenteropancreatic neuroendocrine tumors (GEP-NETs).

Neuroendocrine tumors can occur sporadically but are often a manifestation of an autosomal dominant familial multiple endocrine neoplasia (MEN – see *Section 8.5*). The commonest predisposition for NETs is in association with MEN-1, MEN-2, Carney complex, and von Hippel–Lindau disease. Endocrine tumors of the pancreas (and of the pituitary and parathyroids) can also be associated with neurofibromatosis type 1 and with tuberous sclerosis.

The cellular origin of GI neuroendocrine tumors is not entirely clear, but it is likely that they derive from epithelial precursor cells. Various neuroendocrine cells occur through the gut in specific sites and with specific secretory products (see *Table 8.2* below).

Table 8.2. **Gastrointestinal neuroendocrine cells**

Cell type	Location	Secretory product
G cell	Gastric antrum and duodenum	Gastrin
ECL cell	Gastric fundus and body	Histamine
D cell	Stomach, duodenum, jejunum, colon, and rectum	Somatostatin
EC cell	Stomach, duodenum, jejunum, ileum, colon, and rectum	Serotonin, motilin, and substance P
CCK cell	Duodenum and jejunum	Cholecystokinin
GIP cell	Duodenum and jejunum	Gastric inhibitory polypeptide
M cell	Duodenum and jejunum	Motilin
S cell	Duodenum and jejunum	Secretin
PP cell	Duodenum	Pancreatic polypeptide
L cell	Jejunum, ileum, colon, and rectum	Polypeptide YY
N cell	Jejunum and ileum	Neurotensin

CCK = cholecystokinin; D = somatostatin-producing; EC = enterochromaffin; ECL = enterochromaffin-like; G = gastrin; GIP = gastric inhibitory polypeptide; L = enteroendocrine; M = motilin; N = neurotensin; PP = pancreatic polypeptide; S = secretin.

Apart from the cellular origin and secretory products, carcinoid tumors can be classified according to their potential prognosis:

- well differentiated and benign – excellent prognosis
- well differentiated carcinomas with malignant potential but excellent prognosis
- poorly differentiated carcinomas (usually small cell) which are malignant and with poor prognosis.

Carcinoid syndrome

Carcinoid syndrome (sometimes termed malignant carcinoid syndrome) describes a group of symptoms that include bronchoconstriction (wheezing), flushing, abdominal pain, and diarrhea. The syndrome occurs as a result of tumor-derived biologically active vasoactive amines (5-HT and bradykinin) entering the circulation (*Table 8.3*). Normally, if these substances are secreted by gut-derived neuroendocrine tumors they would pass to the liver where they would be degraded and rendered inactive. In the case of disease which has metastasized to the liver, however, this biological inactivation does not occur and active amines enter the systemic circulation. A similar situation occurs with carcinoid tumors in, for example, the lung and ovary where venous drainage is directly into the systemic circulation. Apart from the worrying symptoms, continued exposure to high levels of serotonin (acting through the cardiac 5HT2B receptors) probably contributes to the development of carcinoid heart disease, which is characterized by cardiac valvular fibrosis.

Clinical features of gastrointestinal carcinoids

Due to the rather indolent nature of carcinoid tumors, many remain asymptomatic for years and several are diagnosed fortuitously, e.g. following appendectomy (acute appendicitis may in fact be caused by appendiceal carcinoid). Other clinical features really depend on the site of the tumor and the cell type involved (*Table 8.3*). Small intestinal carcinoids may produce rather non-specific intermittent abdominal discomfort which may be due to obstruction, mesenteric involvement (fibrosis), or volvulus. Midgut derived carcinoid may well present with flushing/flashing – usually of the head and neck. These episodes may be accompanied by sweating, diarrhea, salivation, palpitations, and pruritis (itching). Episodes may be triggered by stress, exercise, anesthesia, or certain foods (cheese is often cited). Diarrhea without flushing/flashing can occur in some patients, as can wheezing secondary to bronchiolar spasm resulting in, essentially, an asthmatic attack. Very rarely, ectopic ACTH or GRH secretion may result in the clinical features and symptoms of Cushing disease (especially from bronchial carcinoids) or acromegaly. As mentioned above, cardiac symptoms may occur as a result of valvular fibrosis (usually on the right side of the heart). Site-specific clinical features of GI carcinoids are somewhat variable and depend on the hormone over-produced or symptoms caused by the size of the tumor itself. Consequently symptoms may include:

- nausea
- vomiting
- abdominal pain
- acid reflux
- hemorrhage from recurrent peptic ulceration

- diarrhea
- jaundice
- pancreatitis
- appendicitis.

Diagnosis of carcinoid

The mainstay of biochemical diagnosis is measurement of urinary 5-HIAA (5-hydroxy indole acetic acid), a metabolite of serotonin. This has relatively high specificity but is of low sensitivity. The test requires a 24 hour urine collection and can be affected by ingestion of various foodstuffs which are rich in serotonin (bananas, tomatoes, walnuts, eggplants). Perhaps even more useful than this is measurement of chromogranin A – a soluble protein fraction of chromaffin granules. If clinical suspicion is supported by biochemical evidence, it is obviously important to attempt tumor localization. This can be complex and difficult, but the variety of imaging modalities available helps.

Most GI carcinoids will express somatostatin receptors – usually type 2 and type 5. Nuclear medicine scintigraphic studies using indium-labeled somatostatin receptor (SSTR) analogs have a high sensitivity (up to 90%). However, very small tumors, or those that do not express the relevant receptor, may be missed. Iodine labeled MIBG (as used in the detection of pheochromocytomas (see *Section 6.10*) can also sometimes be used because carcinoids can concentrate this using the same pathways as for nor-epinephrine.

PET scanning with a radiolabeled serotonin precursor ([^{11}C]-5-hydroxytryptophan) seems a very effective imaging modality; some studies claim a 100% detection rate. Many units will employ endoscopic ultrasonography to detect small tumors.

Prognosis

The overall prognosis is variable and depends on the size and site of the tumor and the extent of disease. Histologically, high levels of the proliferation marker Ki67 and of the tumor suppressor p53 are considered adverse prognostic factors. The coexistence of carcinoid syndrome (suggesting hepatic metastases), carcinoid heart disease, and high concentrations of chromogranin A and 5-HIAA are also adverse prognostic indicators.

In general, tumors arising in the appendix and rectum (and to a certain extent the colon) have a better survival rate than those in the small bowel and stomach. Small intestinal tumors have a higher rate of metastases, although metastatic disease per se is not necessarily an indicator of short-term survival. Tumors presenting as carcinoid syndrome and those with associated carcinoid cardiac disease have a worse prognosis.

8.4.2 Other GEP-NETs: tumors of the pancreas/islets

Section 8.4.1 covered GI neuroendocrine tumors historically known as carcinoid tumors. The current classification of GEP-NETs makes little differentiation between those tumors historically grouped together as carcinoid tumors and the pancreatic (islet cell) neuroendocrine tumors. This section concentrates on hormone secreting tumors of the pancreas/islet cells, although some of these tumors have been previously mentioned in *Chapter 5*.

Table 8.3. **Gastroenteropancreatic neuroendocrine tumors (GEP-NETs)***

	Incidence (per million)	Hormone / peptide	Clinical	Association with MEN-1 (%)
FOREGUT Carcinoid: bronchus, thymus, stomach, proximal duodenum, pancreas	2–5	5-HT, histamine, ACTH, CRH, GH, gastrin, 5-HIAA	Flushing/flashing Syndromes of hormone excess (if biologically active)	10
MIDGUT Carcinoid: distal duodenum, jejunum, ileum, right colon	4–10	5-HT, tachykinins, prostaglandins, bradykinins, 5-HIAA (80%)	Flushing/flashing, wheeze, diarrhea, obstruction	
HINDGUT Carcinoid: Transverse colon to rectum	1–3	Somatostatin, PYY, neurotensin, 5-HT and others	No symptoms (incidental finding) or local symptoms (discomfort, obstruction)	
Insulinoma	1–2	Insulin and proinsulin	Hypoglycemia	10
Gastrinoma	1–2	Gastrin	Zollinger–Ellison syndrome (peptic ulcer, pain, diarrhea)	25
Vipoma	0.1	VIP	WDHA – watery diarrhea, hypokalemic alkalosis, achlorhydria (low or absent gastric acid secretion)	10
Glucagonoma	Up to 0.1	Glucagon	Diabetes	15
Somatostatinoma	Rare	Somatostatin	Gallstones, diarrhea, occasionally diabetes	10
Non-functioning	1–2	Pancreatic polypeptide	Mass effects	25
GRHoma/ACTHoma	Very rare	GHRH/ACTH	Acromegaly/Cushing disease	

*These include those arising from the GI tract historically termed carcinoid tumors and classified according to their site of origin along with pancreatic and gut neuroendocrine tumors (*Box 8.7*).

Table 8.2 classifies GEP-NETs (including carcinoid) of the intestinal tract in relation to their cellular origin and the hormones produced. An alternative approach to trying to understand the complexity of GEP-NETs is to expand this classification to include carcinoid tumors in relation to their location in the GI tract, and hormone producing pancreatic NETs (*Table 8.3*) which include insulinoma, gastrinoma, VIPoma, glucagonoma, somatostatinoma, ghrelinoma, and PPoma (see *Box 8.7*).

Treatment of GEP-NETs

The treatment of GEP-NETs really requires the intervention of a multidisciplinary team including endocrinologists, endocrine surgeons, oncologists, and nuclear medicine physicians. Many of these tumors are slow growing and relatively indolent and treatment is largely targeted at symptomatic relief. The mainstay of treatment remains surgery, either to achieve cure or to debulk the tumor (+/– metastases; *Figure 8.6*) prior to commencement of adjuvant therapies.

Box 8.7 | Pancreatic and gut neuroendocrine tumors

Insulinomas

- Up to 60% of islet cell tumors.
- Generally small (<2 cm in diameter) – larger tumors more frequently associated with malignancy.
- 10% malignant, 10% multiple, up to 10% associated with MEN 1 (see *Section 8.6*).
- Associated with episodes of unexplained hypoglycemia.
- Diagnosed by documenting symptomatic hypoglycemia during a prolonged (48–72 h) fast in association with inappropriately elevated levels of insulin and/or C-peptide.
- Often associated with high levels of chromogranin B.

Gastrinoma

- Gastrin, produced predominantly in the G cells located in the gastric antrum and duodenal bulb, is the principal gut hormone stimulating gastric acid secretion.
- Zollinger–Ellison syndrome is due to the excessive release of gastrin by neuroendocrine tumors of the GI tract and pancreas.
- 85–90% of gastrinomas are located in the pancreatic islets while 10–15% arise from gastrin-producing cells in the duodenum; 60% of patients have metastatic disease at the time of diagnosis.
- Clinical manifestations include severe refractory peptic ulceration complicated by hemorrhage, perforation, and stricture. Malabsorption and diarrhea are also seen.
- Diagnosis is based on finding an inappropriately elevated fasting plasma gastrin in the presence of gastric acid hypersecretion.
- Treatment of choice is complete surgical tumor removal. Medical treatment is by H_2 blockers and PPIs. Check vitamin B_{12} annually.

VIPomas

- VIPomas secrete vasoactive intestinal polypeptide (VIP).
- Also known as pancreatic cholera, Verner–Morrison syndrome, or the WDHA (watery diarrhea, hypokalemia and achlorhydria/acidosis) syndrome and these are the classical symptoms.
- >60% are malignant and metastasize to the lymph nodes, liver, kidneys, and bone.
- Initial treatment is fluid and electrolyte replacement. Somatostatin analogs produce effective symptomatic relief from diarrhea. Definitive treatment requires surgical resection of the tumor.

Glucagonomas

- They arise from the α cells of the pancreas and produce glucagonoma syndrome through secretion of glucagon and other peptides derived from the pre-proglucagon gene.
- A hallmark of this syndrome is necrolytic migratory erythema which is a characteristic rash that occurs in >70% of cases and usually manifests as a well-demarcated area of erythema in the groin before migrating to limbs, buttocks, and perineum.
- Mucous membrane involvement is common with stomatitis, glossitis, vaginitis, and urethritis.
- Gluconeogenesis causes amino acid deficiencies leading to protein catabolism and thereby causing weight loss in >60% of patients.
- Up to 20% of glucagonoma patients will have associated MEN-1.
- Diagnosis is confirmed on finding raised plasma glucagon levels and may also show elevated pancreatic polypeptide. Impaired glucose tolerance may be present.
- Surgery is the only curative therapeutic option. Somatostatin analogs are the treatment of choice with excellent response rates in treating necrolytic migratory erythema.

Somatostatinomas

- They are very rare tumors that arise in the pancreas and the duodenum.
- Classic triad includes diabetes mellitus, steatorrhea, and cholelithiasis.
- Small duodenal somatostatinomas may occur in association with neurofibromatosis type I or, less commonly, von Hippel–Lindau syndrome and therefore may be associated with pheochromocytoma.
- Pancreatic tumors occur sporadically or associated with MEN-1.
- Plasma somatostatin levels will be raised.
- Surgery is considered as the first-line treatment.

Box 8.7 | continued

Ghrelinoma

- Ghrelin, a motilin-related peptide, is a 28 amino acid growth hormone-releasing factor produced by the stomach and which increases during periods of fasting or anorexia.
- Plays an important role in appetite regulation, insulin sensitivity and causes inhibition of pro-inflammatory response in endothelial cells.
- It is characterized by grossly elevated level of ghrelin.
- Ghrelin is also elevated in breast, thyroid, pituitary, and other neuroendocrine tumors.

PPoma

- Pancreatic polypeptides are synthesized by F cells found in islets of Langerhans but also throughout the exocrine pancreas.
- They are found in different locations throughout the GI tract and nervous system.
- They are secreted in response to vagal nerve stimulation.
- PPs are elevated in gastrointestinal endocrine tumors and hence can be used as a tumor marker.
- Stimulated by nutrients, neurotransmitters, gastric distension, insulin-induced hypoglycemia, and vagal nerve stimulation.
- Inhibited by hyperglycemia, bombesin, and somatostatin.

Somatostatin analogs are important in symptom control and may result in at least a slowing of tumor progression (*Box 8.8*). Somatostatin is usually given as a long-acting analog (octreotide-LAR or lanreotide autogel) with durations of action of about 28 days. Newer somatostatin-based therapies employ engineered cyclo-hexapeptides (e.g. Pasireotide/SOM230) which can bind to multiple somatostatin receptor subtypes. Because the majority of NETs express both somatostatin and dopamine receptors, combined or chimeric compounds, such as BIM-23244, are showing great promise.

Interferon-α has been used for about three decades in the treatment of GEP-NETs. Although it is not as effective as somatostatin in controlling tumor growth, it can

Box 8.8 | Somatostatin analogs in the treatment of GEP-NETs

Somatostatin is a natural peptide hormone secreted in various parts of the body including the digestive tract and anterior pituitary gland. In the digestive tract it inhibits the release of numerous endocrine hormones including insulin, glucagon, and gastrin; in the pituitary it inhibits growth hormone secretion. Five somatostatin G-protein linked receptors have been identified (SSTR1–5) all of which bind the natural hormones, somatostatin 14 and 28, with high affinity. The half-life of somatostatin in the circulation is only 1–3 minutes.

Around 80% of GEP-NETs express SSTRs 1–5 and long-acting somatostatin analogs, more resistant to peptidases, were developed to treat hormone-related symptoms of functioning GEP-NETs and acromegaly (see *Section 2.4*). These analogs include the cyclic octapeptides, octreotide, vapreotide, and lanreotide, with half-lives of 1.5–2 hours. Subsequently, depot formulations were developed and these last about 2–4 weeks and eliminate the need for daily injections. These analogs are particularly useful for treating the symptoms of carcinoids and VIPomas, although after 9–12 months of use drug resistance often develops and patients may show a resurgence of their symptoms.

To enable non-invasive imaging of SSTR-positive neuroendocrine and other tumors, octreotide can be labeled with indium-111 (Octreoscan). Furthermore, high resolution and sensitivity can be obtained with gallium-68 labeled octreotide used in positron emission tomography. Aggressive neuroendocrine tumors can also be treated with yttrium-90 or lutetium-177 labeled octreotide (known as peptide receptor radionuclide therapy).

be symptomatically effective and reduce uncomfortable symptoms of diarrhea and flushing/flashing. There does not appear to be any super-additive effect of combining somatostatin analog therapy with interferon-α. Chemotherapeutic regimens have been trialed over several years using a variety of chemotherapeutic agents (e.g. cyclophosphamide, 5-fluorouracil, streptozoticin, etoposide, cisplatin). Varying levels of success have been claimed but, because of the markedly heterogenous nature of the condition, it is difficult to compare studies. A newer chemotherapeutic agent, temezolomide, is an alkylating agent which has been shown to be effective in some studies.

Peptide receptor therapy is based on the fact that NETs express high levels of somatostatin receptors. Consequently a radionuclide bound to somatostatin should be able to bind these receptors and be internalized into the cell resulting in cellular destruction; yttrium and lutetium are commonly used radionuclides. In a similar vein, iodine (^{131}I) labeled MIBG may be used – a treatment similar to that used for pheochromocytoma (see *Section 6.10*).

Newer therapies include:

- tyrosine kinase inhibitors (e.g. imatinib)
- EGFR inhibitors (e.g. gefitinib)
- mTOR inhibitors; mTOR is the mammalian target of rapamycin and a major regulator of cell growth – temsirolimus and everolimus are mTOR inhibitors that have shown some promise in the treatment of NET
- MK0646 is a monoclonal antibody which binds IGF-I and can limit its signaling through the type 1 IGF receptor.

CASE 8.2

417 425

- Man of 62 years with hot flushes, severe diarrhea, and weight loss
- Firm hepatomegaly and palpable liver edge
- 5-HIAA and chromogranin A levels elevated
- Octreotide scan showed uptake in right colon and liver
- Treated with somatostatin analog and then surgery to remove colonic lesion

The patient underwent investigation with a 24 hour urine collection for estimation of 5-HIAA on two occasions and measurement of gut hormones. His urinary 5-HIAA was markedly elevated at 596 μmol/day (NR 10.4–31.2) and chromogranin A levels were also elevated (chromogranin A, also known as parathyroid secretory protein A, is one of the granin family of neurosecretory proteins which is increased in pheochromocytomas and carcinoid tumors). An abdominal CT scan revealed a lesion in the area of the cecum in addition to multiple hepatic metastatic deposits. An octreotide scan confirmed the uptake of tracer in the right colon and liver. He was treated symptomatically with a long-acting somatostatin analog which improved the flushing/flashing and diarrhea. He underwent surgery to remove the colonic carcinoid and to attempt to debulk the hepatic metastases.

Application was made for post-surgical treatment with lutetium dotatate (a somatostatin-based radiopeptide), but his condition sadly deteriorated rapidly and he was readmitted with cachexia complicated by pneumonia. Unfortunately he died before further therapy could be offered.

8.5 Multiple endocrine neoplasia

CASE 8.3 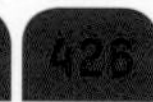 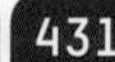

- Woman of 32 years with swelling in region of thyroid
- Euthyroid with firm 3 cm nodule in right lobe; moderately hypertensive
- Ultrasound revealed hypoechogenic lesion; histology confirmed medullary cell carcinoma
- Total thyroidectomy carried out in view of histology

A 32 year old woman presented with a swelling in the region of the thyroid. She was otherwise well but did complain of occasional panic attacks associated with palpitations. She was on no medication. She had been adopted and knew little of her birth family. On examination she was clinically euthyroid, with a firm 3 cm nodule in the right lobe of the thyroid. She was moderately hypertensive at 140/88 and this had previously been assumed to be secondary to the oral contraceptive pill which she had stopped 1 month previously. Initial investigations confirmed euthyroidism:

- calcium 2.48 mmol/L (NR 2.2–2.58)
- phosphate 0.8 mmol/L (NR 0.8–1.5)
- other basic biochemistry was normal

She underwent a thyroid ultrasound and guided fine needle aspiration. Ultrasound revealed a hypoechogenic lesion with intranodular calcification. Histology of the biopsy confirmed medullary cell carcinoma of the thyroid. In view of the histology a decision was made to proceed to surgery (total thyroidectomy with level 6 neck clearance). Surgery was complicated by a hypertensive crisis which was eventually controlled by the anesthetist. Histology confirmed medullary cell cancer with no extra-thyroid spread.

MEN is characterized by primary tumors in at least two endocrine glands. It is a rare autosomal dominant disorder caused by mutations in identified genes which may arise sporadically or may be inherited (familial). The familial form is more common (~90% cases) and is identified in a MEN patient who has one first-degree relative showing at least one of the characteristic endocrine tumors. There are two types of MEN:

- MEN-1 is due to a mutation of the *MEN* gene
- MEN-2, as well as familial thyroid carcinoma, is caused by mutations of the *RET* (rearranged during transfection) gene which codes for the RET receptor.

8.5.1 MEN-1

The MEN-1 locus has been mapped to 11q13 and the gene product is a nuclear protein called menin. The function of this gene is yet to be fully determined, although it is considered to be important in gene transcription, cell proliferation, apoptosis, and genome stability. Over a thousand mutations of the *MEN-1* gene have been reported but there is no correlation between these mutations and the clinical phenotype. Gene screening, however, is useful when patients have a suggestive family history of MEN even though they may present initially with symptoms of a single (sporadic) hormone secreting 'functional' tumor/adenoma such as hyperparathyroidism or gastrinoma.

MEN-1 is relatively rare, with a prevalence of around 1 case per 30 000 and is characterized by hyperplasia/neoplasm of the parathyroids, pituitary, and pancreatic

Table 8.4. Tumors associated with MEN-1 and their penetrance

Localization	Penetrance	Other common non-endocrine manifestations
Parathyroid	**90%**	
Enteropancreatic		
Gastrinoma	40–60%	
Insulinoma	20%–30%	Facial angiofibromas
Non-functioning/other	10–20%	Collagenomas
Pituitary		Lipomas
Prolactinoma	15%	Leiomyomas
Other	20%	
Adrenal		
Non-functioning cortex	20%	
Pheochromocytoma	<1%	
Foregut (carcinoids)		
Gastric	5%	
Thymic	2%	
Bronchial	2%	

islets (the '3Ps'). Extra-pancreatic tumors can occur (e.g. duodenal gastrinomas); in addition carcinoid tumors, adrenal adenomas, and lipomas are encountered more frequently than expected.

Hyperparathyroidism (*Section 4.5*) is usually the first manifestation of the condition and occurs in about 90% of cases (*Table 8.4*). Most patients will have presented by the age of 45–50 and up to 2% of all cases of hyperparathyroidism are associated with MEN-1. It differs from sporadic hyperparathyroidism in the following ways:

- sex ratio equal (female preponderance in sporadic)
- earlier age of onset (two decades or so earlier than sporadic)
- multiple gland hyperplasia (85% of sporadic are single gland adenomas)
- high rate of post-operative recurrence.

Like sporadic forms of hyperparathyroidism, diagnosis is made by elevated serum concentrations of PTH and hypercalcemia. Surgery for hyperparathyroidism in MEN-1 is the preferred option and this may involve subtotal parathyroidectomy (three parathyroid glands and half of the fourth one) or total parathyroidectomy with an autologous parathyroid graft of the 'most normal-appearing' tissue into the non-dominant forearm. There is no general consensus which is the preferred option, although late recurrence of hyperparathyroidism may occur with subtotal parathyroidectomy and may affect up to 50% cases by 8–12 years after surgery.

Recently, calcium-sensing receptor agonists that stimulate the calcium receptor on chief cells of the parathyroid glands have been shown to decrease PTH release. They may also decrease parathyroid tumor growth and thus become an important therapy in the treatment of MEN-1.

The second most common manifestation of MEN-1 is of pancreatic islet cell and GI tumors (*Table 8.4*) which occur in around 35% of MEN-1 patients and may be either benign or malignant. The most common is gastrinoma and some suggest that up to 60% of MEN-1 patients will have either asymptomatic elevation of gastrin levels or symptomatic Zollinger–Ellison syndrome due to gastrinoma(s). The tumors in Zollinger–Ellison syndrome are often small and multifocal and surgical cure is difficult; they often occur in the duodenum and lymph node involvement is common, but not necessarily fatal. Indeed the risk of death from malignant gastrinoma is lower in MEN-I than sporadic Zollinger–Ellison syndrome. The condition should be suspected in patients with recurrent or multiple peptic ulcers. Diagnosis is based on:

- elevated serum gastrin levels
- a brisk gastrin response (>120 pg/mL or >60%) to a test dose of secretin (gastrin-secreting G cells are normally inhibited by secretin but, for reasons that are not understood, secretin causes a brisk and exaggerated release of gastrin from gastrinoma cells)
- elevated chromogranin A (chromogranin A is a non-specific marker for neuroendocrine tumors and does not differentiate a gastrinoma from other gastroenteropancreatic tumors, but may help to differentiate hypergastrinemia due to gastrinoma from other causes of high gastrin, e.g. proton pump inhibitor use or pernicious anemia).

After gastrinoma, insulinomas (see *Section 5.9*) are the most common islet cell tumors occurring in MEN-1 and these tend to be multifocal and may occur in association with other islet cell tumors. Patients will present with symptoms of fasting hypoglycemia which can be relieved with glucose intake. Diagnosis is made with a prolonged fast and serial levels of glucose and insulin during the period of hypoglycemia. Other tumors may secrete vasoactive intestinal peptide (VIPomas), glucagon (glucagonomas), pancreatic polypeptide or be non-functioning (*Box 8.7*).

Non-functioning pancreatic endocrine tumors may produce hormones that have no apparent clinical effect; this may be due to abnormal hormone processing or secretion. Nevertheless these tumors may be malignant and may result in hepatic metastatic disease, the risks being higher with increasing tumor size.

The third type of tumor associated with MEN-1 is adenoma of the anterior pituitary gland (*Section 2.1*). They occur in about 20% of patients with MEN-1, the most common form being benign non-functioning macroadenomas (≥1 cm) which usually present with hypopituitarism and bi-temporal hemianopia, the latter due to compression of the optic chiasm. Only 10–15% of pituitary tumors associated with MEN-1 are functioning, the most common being prolactinomas, although GH and ACTH secreting tumors are not uncommon. The pituitary tumors in MEN patients tend to be rather larger and more aggressive than sporadic tumors. Diagnosis and treatment is the same as for other pituitary tumors (see *Chapter 2*).

Other GEP-NETs may be associated with MEN-1 (see *Section 8.3* and *Box 8.7*); carcinoid tumors are seen in approximately 5% of patients. Non-functioning tumors of the adrenal gland and non-endocrine tumors (including tumors of adipose tissue and the skin giving rise to lipomas, facial angiofibromas, and collagenomas) may also occur.

MEN-1 is a familial disease and therefore an accurate family history should be taken in all suspected patients, e.g. those presenting with Zollinger–Ellison syndrome and/or hyperparathyroidism. Gene screening is useful in those cases where there is a suggestive family history even though the patient currently has what appears to be isolated hyperparathyroidism or sporadic Zollinger–Ellison syndrome. However, since mutations of *MEN-1* do not correlate with specific tumors there is currently no rationale in guiding therapeutic intervention in patients diagnosed with *MEN-1* mutations. Patients diagnosed with a mutation should therefore be closely monitored for evidence of tumors associated with this rare genetic disorder and treated accordingly.

8.5.2 MEN-2

MEN-2 results from mutations in the *RET* proto-oncogene which is located on chromosome 10q11 and codes for isoforms of the RET receptor (*Figure 8.7*). The RET receptor is expressed in the parafollicular C-cells of the thyroid gland, adrenal medullary cells, parathyroid cells, and enteric autonomic ganglion cells, all of which are derived from neural crest cells. The signal transduction pathways for the RET receptor are complex, but they are important in regulating cell survival, differentiation, proliferation, migration, and chemotaxis in target cells. Because mutations of this receptor related to MEN-2 are usually activating mutations leading to ligand-independent activation of the receptor, it is therefore not surprising that MEN-2 is associated with tumors of the thyroid gland, adrenal medulla, and parathyroid gland.

Like MEN-1, MEN-2 is also a rare disorder with an estimated prevalence of about 1 case per 20 000 and exists in two distinct clinical subtypes: MEN-2A or MEN-2B, with

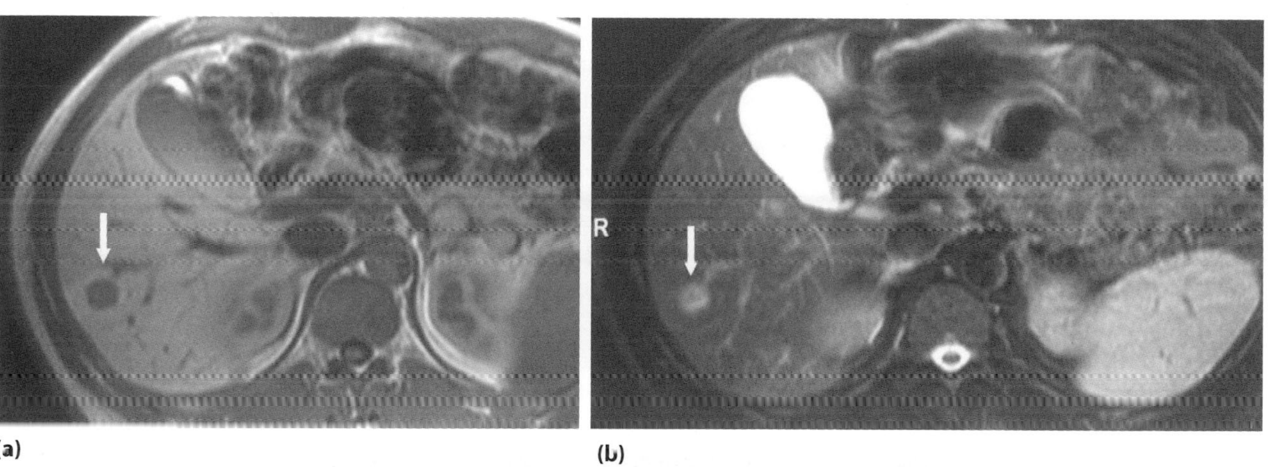

(a) (b)

Figure 8.6. CT/MRI imaging for detection of large tumors and metastases.
(a) T1-weighted MRI of a hepatic metastasis (white arrow) in a patient with a metastatic NET. The lesion is hypodense compared to the surrounding liver parenchyma.
(b) The lesion appears hyperintense on T2-weighted images.

Table 8.5. **Tumors associated with MEN-2A, MEN-2B and FMTC and their penetrance**

Tumor	Penetrance	Other non-endocrine manifestations
MEN-2A		
Medullary thyroid carcinoma	100%	
Pheochromocytoma	50%	Multigland parathyroid tumors
Hyperparathyroidism	30%	
MEN-2B		
Medullary thyroid carcinoma	100%	Marfanoid habitus, mucosal neuromas, intestinal ganglioneuromas
Pheochromocytoma	50%	
FMTC		
Medullary thyroid carcinoma	100%	None

MEN-2A accounting for about 80% cases of MEN-2. Medullary thyroid carcinoma (MTC) of the calcitonin-secreting C-cells, as opposed to differentiated thyroid carcinomas of follicular cells, occurs in **all** MEN-2 patients and in patients with familial MTC (FMTC) (*Table 8.5*). It is usually the first manifestation of MEN-2 and most patients have raised levels of calcitonin (>10 ng/mL) which can provide a good plasma marker for MEN-2 and FMTC.

Pheochromocytomas, which develop in the background of adrenomedullary hyperplasia of the chromaffin cells, affect about 50% of MEN-2 cases. Mostly these are benign and tend to be bilateral and give rise to clinical features typical of excess catecholamines (see *Section 6.10*). It should be noted, however, that most cases of both MTC and pheochromocytomas are sporadic and only about 10% of all cases are related to MEN-2.

Hyperparathyroidism (see *Section 4.5*) occurs in 20–30% of MEN-2A patients but not in MEN-2B patients. Instead, MEN-2B patients suffer from multiple mucosal neuromas and/or diffuse ganglioneuromatosis of the GI tract and show developmental abnormalities such as a Marfanoid phenotype, decreased upper/lower body ratio and skeletal deformations. Morbidity and mortality are greater for MEN-2B than for MEN-2A.

Unlike MEN-1 there is a distinct genotype/phenotype with MEN-2. The majority (>90%) of MEN-2A patients have mutations in the extracellular domain of the RET receptor whilst most MEN-2B patients have mutations in the intracellular, tyrosine kinase domain (*Figure 8.7*). Because there is 100% penetrance of MTC with MEN-2, early diagnosis is imperative so that patients may undergo a prophylactic thyroidectomy. MTC is the most common endocrine-related cause of death in patients with MEN-2 and FMTC. Diagnosis can be made by evaluating the calcitonin response to pentagastrin or calcium but the test is not always reliable and may not allow for early detection of a tumor. Commercial *RET* mutation tests are now available and these can identify 97% of patients with MEN-2 or FMTC.

CASE 8.3

426 431

- Woman of 32 years with swelling in region of thyroid
- Euthyroid with firm 3 cm nodule in right lobe; moderately hypertensive
- Ultrasound revealed hypoechogenic lesion; histology confirmed medullary cell carcinoma
- Total thyroidectomy carried out in view of histology
- Post-operative investigations revealed raised epinephrine, nor-epinephrine and calcitonin
- *RET* gene sequencing showed a Cys634Arg mutation, and CT/MRI scanning confirmed an adrenal lesion
- Histology after unilateral adrenalectomy confirmed pheochromocytoma
- 2 years after adrenalectomy she is well on just thyroid hormone replacement

As a result of the peri-operative hypertensive crisis and the confirmed medullary cell cancer, further investigations were undertaken. Two separate 24 hour urine collections assayed for catecholamines revealed:

- epinephrine 550 µg/mL/24h (NR 0–15)
- nor-epinephrine 1400 µg/mL/24h (NR 0–100)
- calcitonin (on a pre-operative sample) 29 pmol/L (NR 0.8–7.6)

Sequencing of the *RET* gene revealed a Cys634Arg mutation. Abdominal CT and MRI scan confirmed a 5 cm lesion in the left adrenal, and nuclear medicine scanning with MIBG confirmed avid uptake in this area but no uptake elsewhere. After alpha and beta blockade she underwent unilateral laparoscopic adrenalectomy and histology confirmed pheochromocytoma.

One month after surgery, she had had no further hypertensive episodes and no more panic attacks. Urinary catecholamines and metanephrines were normal and calcitonin levels reduced to 1.8 pmol/L. As her family were unknown, counseling and screening of family members could not be undertaken. She underwent regular follow-up and at 2 years post-operation she remains entirely well on thyroid hormone replacement and no other medications.

At presentation there was no evidence of concomitant parathyroid pathology, and subsequent regular investigations revealed no signs of symptomatic or biochemical hypercalcemia. The initial histology of the pheochromocytoma showed no evidence of malignant change and subsequent urinary catecholamine testing and repeat imaging with MRI and MIBG scans revealed no suggestion of missed lesions or recurrence. The final diagnosis was MEN-2A syndrome with no evidence of parathyroid involvement. Whether this was a sporadic or familial case remains unknown in the absence of family screening.

CASE 8.4

431 436

- Man of 59 years with severe breathlessness and swelling of his ankles
- BNP levels very elevated, tachycardic with audible 3rd heart sound
- Chest X-ray showed cardiomegaly and pulmonary edema

A 59 year old man was referred to hospital by his primary care physician. He had experienced increasing breathlessness over the last year or so, to the extent that he now had to stop twice when climbing one flight of stairs and could walk a maximum of 50 yards on the flat. He slept propped up with 3–4 pillows and often woke at night 'gasping for air'. He had also experienced increasing swelling of his ankles, now progressing as far as mid shin. He was on no medication and reported no significant past medical history. His primary care physician had measured levels of B-type natriuretic peptide (BNP) and reported it as markedly elevated at 1600 pg/mL (NR <167 pg/mL). On examination he was breathless at rest, there were coarse crackles in both lung bases, he was tachycardic at 105 beats/min with a clearly audible third heart sound. A chest X-ray showed cardiomegaly and clear evidence of pulmonary edema.

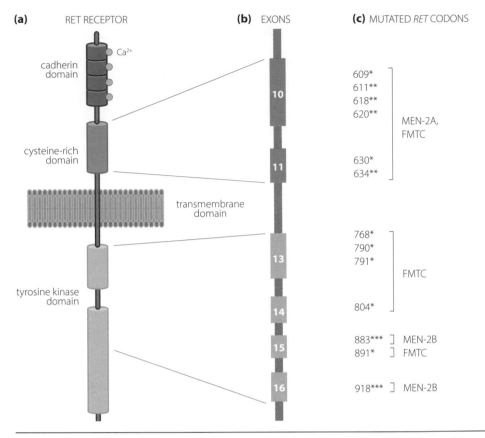

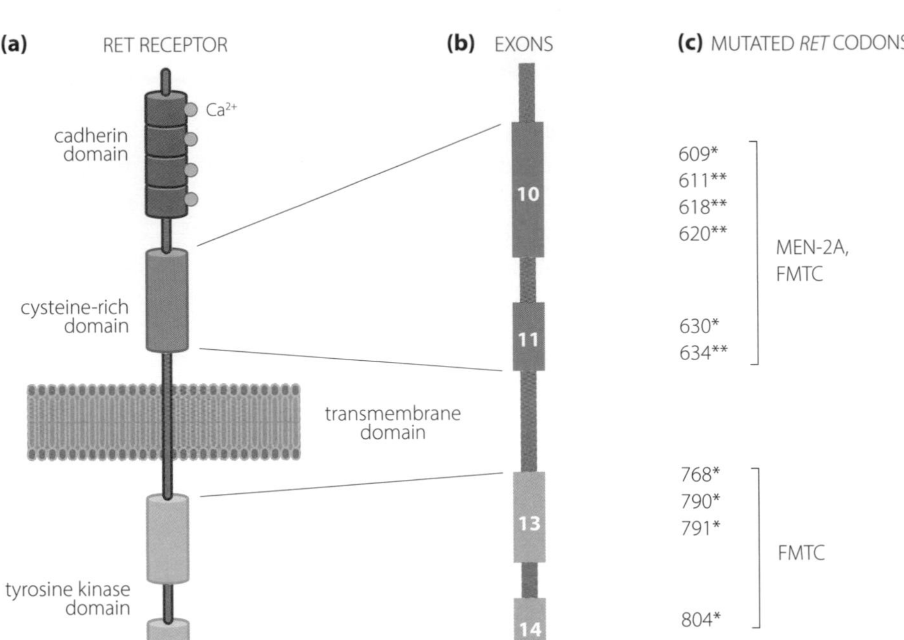

Figure 8.7. Structure of the RET receptor and the most common mutations in the *RET* gene associated with MEN-2A, -2B, and/or FMTC.
(a) RET receptor showing the different domains of the receptor protein.
(b) *RET* mRNA showing the exons which code for extracellular cysteine-rich domain and the intracellular tyrosine kinase domain in which most germline mutations have been identified.
(c) The location of the most common mutated codons that have been identified to date and the genotype–phenotye correlations of MEN-2A and MEN-2B and FMTC. Mutations in the extracellular domain of the receptor lead to ligand-independent activation of the RET receptor and are mostly identified in MEN-2A and FMTC. They account for the majority (93–98%) of MEN-2A cases and the majority (80–96%) of patients with FMTC only. Whilst rare cases of MEN-2A and FMTC have been linked to mis-sense mutations in exons 13, 14, and 15, most MEN-2B cases are associated with activating mutations of this domain leading to constitutive activation of the receptor and uncontrolled cell proliferation.
Hirschsprung disease (a congenital disorder of the development of the colon) is associated with germline mutations at 609, 611, 618, 620 and loss of function mutations all over the gene.
* low risk, **high risk and ***highest risk of developing FMTC which has 100% penetrance in both MEN-2A and -2B and will determine the timing of total thyroidectomy and lymph node dissection.

8.6 Hormones secreted by the cardiovascular system, kidney, and bone

8.6.1 Hormones of the cardiovascular system

Natriuretic peptides

The natriuretic peptide family comprises atrial natriuretic peptide (ANP), B-type natriuretic peptide (BNP), C-type natriuretic peptide (CNP), *Dendroaspis* natriuretic peptide (DNP), and urodilatin (*Figure 8.8*). The natriuretic peptides are a family of

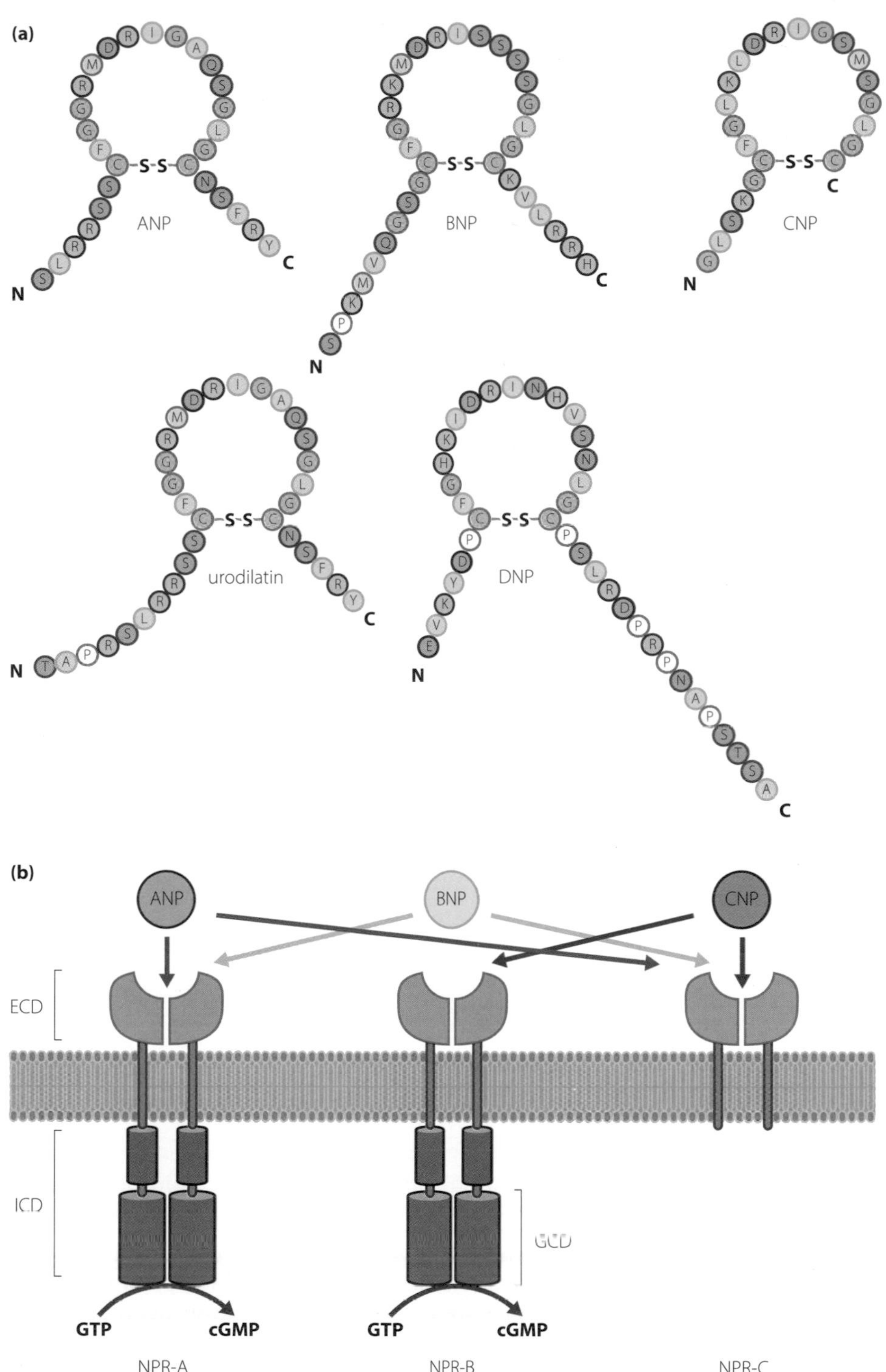

Figure 8.8. The structures of the natriuretic peptide family and their major receptors.
(a) Schematic of the structure of atrial natriuretic hormone (ANP), B-type natriuretic hormone (BNP), C-type natriuretic hormone (CNP), urodilatin and *Dendroaspis* natriuretic peptide (DNP), showing the C and N terminals.
(b) The three different types of natriuretic peptide receptors (NPRs) showing ligand specificity to these receptors, the extra- and intracellular domains (ECD/ICD) and the region of the receptor which contains the guanylyl cyclase domain (GCD). Note that the NPR-C, which is responsible for the clearance of natriuretic peptides, is a truncated receptor. Binding of natriuretic peptides induces dimerization of two receptors prior to activation of guanylyl cyclase.

widely distributed polypeptides that exert a range of effects throughout the body, although their most established function is in relation to blood volume and blood pressure homeostasis.

Three types of receptors for natriuretic peptides have been identified. Two are single transmembrane receptors with guanylyl cyclase activity on the intracellular domain of the receptor. They are termed natriuretic peptide receptor-A (NPR-A) and -B (NPR-B) and their activation and dimerization catalyzes the synthesis of cGMP, which mediates most of the known effects of natriuretic peptides. ANP and BNP activate NPR-A whilst CNP activates NPR-B. The third receptor, natriuretic peptide-C (NPR-C) clears natriuretic peptides from the circulation through receptor-mediated internalization and degradation, although a signaling function for this receptor has also been suggested (*Figure 8.8*).

ANP. The natural response to expansion of extracellular volume following a sodium load is enhanced urinary sodium excretion. This occurs in part secondarily to a suppression of the renin–angiotensin–aldosterone system (see *Section 6.7*) with a modest increase in glomerular filtration rate. ANP also has a role in this regulatory process; it is released by the atria (and also by the ventricles in chronic heart failure) in response to atrial cell stretch secondary to volume expansion. Its actions are mediated through the NPR-A (a specific cell membrane receptor). Binding of ANP (*Figure 8.8*) activates guanylyl cyclase-A leading to an increase in the intracellular concentrations of cyclic GMP.

ANP acts as a diuretic and vasodilator, enhancing sodium excretion through a variety of actions including:

- increase of GFR without increase in renal blood flow (i.e. afferent dilatation and efferent constriction)
- reduction of sodium reabsorption in the collecting ducts of the kidney and in the proximal tubule
- inhibition of renal renin secretion
- inhibition of aldosterone release by the adrenal
- inhibition of ADH-induced water reabsorption in the collecting tubules.

ANP is derived from the C-terminal end of a pro-protein, pro-ANP. Classical ANP is a 28 amino acid peptide including amino acids 99 to 126 of pro-ANP. Other fragments derived from pro-ANP have also been identified in the circulation with varying effects on lowering blood pressure and altering sodium excretion. Urodilatin, a rather interesting and relatively novel peptide form of ANP, has been identified in human urine. The peptide encompasses amino acids 95–126 of pro-ANP and appears to be produced entirely within the kidney rather than the heart. The action of urodilatin is to promote natriuresis and diuresis through a reversible deactivation of renal Na^+/K^+-ATPase (*Figure 6.14*) and thus it has been considered as the kidney's atrial natriuretic hormone.

BNP. This was previously called brain natriuretic peptide, although it is found in both atria and ventricles of the heart as well as in the brain. The predominant form of BNP is a 32 amino acid peptide which is a cleavage product of the C-terminal end of pro-BNP 108. The remaining N-terminal pro-BNP 76 fragment can also be readily measured in the circulation. Plasma concentrations of BNP are normally around 20%

of those of ANP, and whilst the levels of both peptides are raised in cardiovascular disease the magnitude of the BNP increase is usually greater than the increase in ANP, and in heart failure levels can exceed those of ANP. This makes BNP a clinically useful diagnostic marker for several pathophysiological conditions including heart failure and pulmonary hypertension (Case 8.4).

CNP. This is structurally similar to ANP and BNP, but acts on NPR-B and not NPR-A. CNP derives from vascular endothelium and also from the heart. Its role(s) is not yet as well defined but it would appear to have local (paracrine) actions on sodium excretion and regulation of local blood flow. Thus CNP represents the paracrine element of the natriuretic peptide axis which complements the endocrine actions of ANP and BNP.

DNP. This has been isolated from the venom of the green mamba snake (*Dendroaspis angusticeps*) and, whilst DNP-like immunoreactivity has been detected in human plasma and the heart, the gene for DNP has yet to be identified. DNP is a potent natriuretic and diuretic peptide which, like ANP and BNP, increases urinary and plasma cGMP. However, it is more potent than ANP and BNP and more resistant to degradation. Thus DNP has provided new therapeutic drug leads.

Physiology and therapeutic aspects of ANP and BNP

ANP is released in response to increases in volume load and has the potential to be an important co-regulator of natriuresis and reduction in volume-induced hypertension. It is not totally clear whether the blood pressure lowering effects of ANP are more important than its impact on sodium regulation; it is possible that the hypotensive effects limit the effectiveness of natriuresis by reducing the sodium load going to the collecting tubules of the kidney. It is also possible that locally (renally) produced urodilatin is a more effective natriuretic peptide than ANP.

The efficacy of ANP as a therapeutic agent is not yet proven. Rather than exogenous administration of ANP (or BNP), it may be more effective to prevent the breakdown of endogenous ANP/BNP by inhibiting the endo-peptidases responsible for its destruction. Initial studies have been promising, suggesting that inhibition of peptidases responsible for the catabolism of ANP or of its second messenger, cyclic GMP, may produce an effective diuresis without significant hypotensive effects, despite induction of systemic vasodilatation. At the moment, however, these drugs are largely theoretical and have no significantly proven advantages over widely used (and cheap) standard diuretics.

Whilst the functions of ANP and BNP have been established, other hormones that may regulate electrolyte and water balance have recently been identified. These include peptides that belong to the guanylin peptide family and endogenous cardiotonic steroids (*Box 8.9*).

Case 8.4 illustrates the rather close relationship between physiology and pathology and between endocrinology and cardiology. The algorithm for treatment of heart failure is based on a sound understanding of the principles of salt/water homoeostasis, regulation of vascular tone and the fundamentally important interplay of hormones and cardiovascular efficacy.

Endothelin

Endothelin is a potent vasoconstrictor which circulates as a 21 amino acid peptide. It is derived from cleavage of a pre-prohormone (big ET-1) resulting in a prohormone

Box 8.9 | The guanylin peptide family and endogenous cardiotonic steroids in the regulation of electrolyte and water balance

The guanylin family of peptides includes guanylin and uroguanylin and other more recently discovered peptides such as lymphoguanylin. Guanylin and uroguanylin are small peptides (consisting of 15 and 16 amino acids respectively) and they are mainly produced in the intestine and kidneys though other sites of production have also been identified. Like the natriuretic family of peptides, they act on cell surface receptors with intrinsic guanylate cyclase activity and thus signal via cyclic GMP.

Guanylin and uroguanylin are secreted from enterocytes in response to a salty meal and are released both into the lumen of the gut and into the circulation. In the gut they inhibit the absorption of sodium and induce chloride, bicarbonate, and water secretion. Simultaneously they increase electrolyte excretion by inducing natriuresis, kaliuresis, and diuresis, thereby serving a direct link between the gut and kidney in regulating electrolyte balance. Guanylin peptides can synergize with low levels of ANP and can also complement other well-known hormonal systems that are involved in regulating water and electrolyte homeostasis such as the renin–angiontensin system, vasopressin, ANP, BNP, and CNP.

Two cardiotonic steroids have recently been identified in humans: endogenous cardenolide (endogenous ouabain) and bufadienolide (marinobufagenin). They act in a complex manner with other systems that regulate renal salt handling and contribute to salt-sensitive hypertension. Endogenous ouabain appears to be produced exclusively in the adrenal gland and is under the control of angiotensin II, ACTH, and epinephrine. It has a direct effect on ion transport and vascular tone and is also a growth factor, stimulating proliferation and differentiation of cardiac and smooth muscle. Marinobufagenin can also affect ion transport and vasoconstriction via effects on Na^+/K^+-ATPase, but precisely how these cardiotonic steroids act according to sodium status, blood pressure, and salt-sensitive hypertension is currently not known.

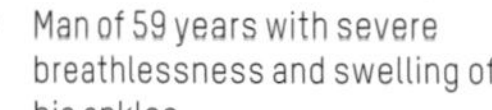

CASE 8.4

431 436

- Man of 59 years with severe breathlessness and swelling of his ankles
- BNP levels very elevated, tachycardic with audible 3rd heart sound
- Chest X-ray showed cardiomegaly and pulmonary edema
- Heart failure treated with furosemide initially, then ACE inhibitor added
- Echocardiogram showed poor left ventricular function so beta-blocker started and then an aldosterone antagonist added

The patient was admitted to hospital. The combination of physical signs, X-ray appearances, and the markedly elevated level of BNP were all in keeping with heart failure. Initial therapy in this case was with a loop diuretic in order to deal with fluid overload; furosemide was commenced at a dose of 40 mg a day and then increased to 80 mg daily in order to achieve a weight loss of 1 kg a day. Clinical examination supported by echocardiography excluded valvular disease as a contributory factor to his heart failure, so an ACE inhibitor was added. Blockade of the renin–angiotensin–aldosterone system at various levels is important in the treatment of heart failure and there is clear evidence from numerous trials that ACE inhibitors have an important role in patient survival even in asymptomatic left ventricular dysfunction.

At review, 4 weeks later, the patient was still experiencing breathlessness on relatively minimal exertion. A repeat echocardiogram showed poor left ventricular function with a left ventricular ejection fraction of 35%. He was started on a beta-blocker (1.25 mg bisoprolol, titrated up at 2 weekly intervals to an eventual dose of 10 mg). The aldosterone antagonist, spironolactone, was added once the bisoprolol had been titrated up to 10 mg. At a further review some 10 weeks later the patient was markedly improved symptomatically and was able to walk up to a mile on the flat. He did complain of lack of libido and rather painful gynecomastia, so the spironolactone was switched to an alternative aldosterone antagonist, eplerenone, which has fewer anti-androgenic side-effects in men.

(pro-ET) which is subsequently the target of several converting enzymes (ETE). Three isoforms have been described to date:

- ET-1: the most potent vasoconstrictor and major isoform which is synthesized in the vasculature
- ET-2: similar vasoconstrictive properties to ET-1 and found in the kidney and intestine
- ET-3: minimal vasoconstrictive activity, found in the CNS.

Endothelin binds to two receptors (ET-A and ET-B) which are present on various cardiovascular cell types including endothelial cells, cardiac myocytes, and vascular smooth muscle cells. The actions of endothelins vary depending on the site and type of receptor to which they bind; in smooth muscle binding to both ET-A and ET-B produces vasoconstriction, whereas binding to ET-B receptors on endothelial cells produces vasodilatation as a result of generation of nitric oxide (*Box 8.10*). In humans, ET-1 is the most important and its major effect is vasoconstriction, although ET-1 may also have a role in inflammation (through increases in cytokine release and vascular permeability).

In the normal human heart endothelin is expressed in the myocardium and has positive inotropic effects (inotropism refers to the power of contraction of the heart and chronotropism to its rate of contraction). ET-A receptors predominate on the cardiac myocytes and ET-B receptors on the fibroblasts.

In experiments, ET-1 production can be increased by hypoxia, ischemia, inflammation, and certain neurohormones (AVP, angiotensin II, and nor-adrenaline), all of which are increased in myocardial failure. Elevated levels of ET-1 in turn can increase levels of these neurohormones and add to renal vasoconstriction and sodium retention through effects on the renin–angiotensin system and renal function. In addition, the activities of ET-1 and the natriuretic hormones ANP and BNP are strictly interrelated. ET-1 stimulates synthesis of ANP and BNP, whilst these peptides inhibit the synthesis of ET-1. In pathological conditions, the predominance of one of these systems can often be identified.

Levels of ET-1 are raised in heart failure and this is probably a result of increased production from myocardial cells (and possibly the lung) rather than reduced excretion. The levels of ET-1 correlate well with the degree of heart failure present, and measurements of both ET-1 and big ET-1 are useful prognostically as markers of long-term survival. In view of this it seems reasonable to look at the efficacy of ET-1 inhibition in heart failure (and indeed in more acute myocardial injury); ET receptor antagonists, either specific for ET-A or inhibiting both ET-A and ET-B, have been used in clinical trials but the results to date are disappointing.

8.6.2 Hormones of the kidney

Chapter 4 described the role of the kidney in synthesizing the active form of vitamin D and in regulating calcium homeostasis. *Chapter 6* addressed the production of renin by the kidney and its role in controlling sodium and water excretion via the renin–angiotensin–aldosterone system. Apart from the production of various prostaglandins and pre-kallikreins, the other major hormone secreted by the kidneys is erythropoietin (also known as EPO, hematopoietin or hemopoietin). EPO is synthesized by specialized peritubular capillary lining cells of the renal cortex,

Box 8.10 | The role of endothelins in vascular homeostasis

Endothelin-1 (ET-1) is synthesized from Prepro-ET-1 (*Box figure 8.4*). This is first cleaved to give Pro- or 'Big' ET-1 which is further cleaved by endothelin-converting enzyme (ECE) to produce the active hormone in endothelial cells. The number of amino acids (aa) are shown. ET-1 binds to the G-protein linked receptors, ET-A and ET-B, on the underlying vascular smooth muscle cells and this induces a rise in intracellular calcium which causes a sustained vasoconstriction. ET-1 may also act in an autocrine/paracrine manner on ET-B receptors on the same or adjacent vascular endothelial cells. This stimulates the production of endothelial nitric oxide synthase (eNOS) which converts L-arginine to L-citrulline and nitric oxide (NO). Nitric oxide is a potent vasodilator. It diffuses into the vascular smooth muscle cells, activates soluble guanylate cyclase (sGC) and the rise in cyclic GMP causes muscle relaxation and vasodilatation.

Endothelial cells also produce a number of prostaglandins and PGI_2, like NO, causes vasodilatation. In infections, e.g. sepsis, circulating concentrations of NO can rise as a result of inducible nitric oxide synthase (iNOS) activity. Circulating NO can have the same potent vasodilator effect as that produced locally. Endotoxins and cytokines also stimulate the production of prostaglandins and further vasodilatation can occur as a result of increased production of PGI_2. Sepsis is typically associated with hypotension and if it is sufficiently severe as to compromise perfusion into vital tissues and organs, the condition is known as septic shock.

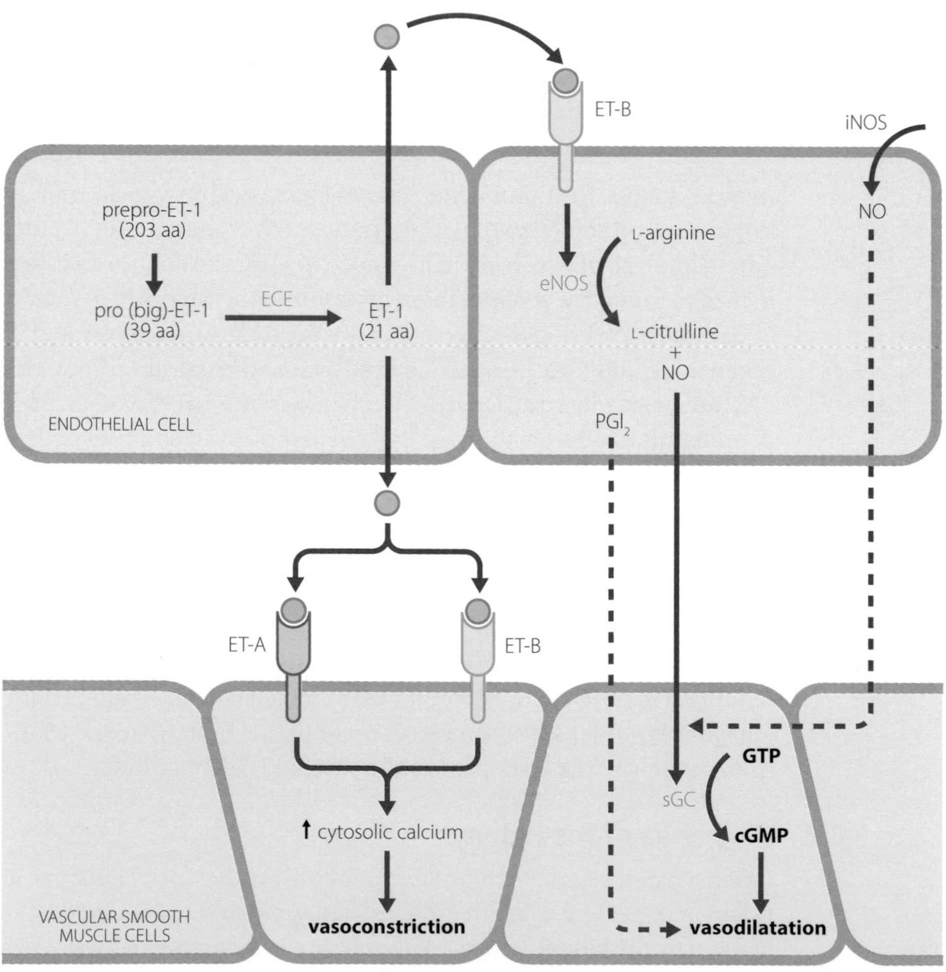

Box figure 8.4. Role of endothelins in vascular homeostasis.

although other sites such as the liver are recognized. Its synthesis is regulated by a feedback loop monitoring the level of blood oxygenation, although its mechanism is poorly understood. There is evidence that transcription factors for EPO known as hypoxia-inducible factors (HIFs) are constitutively synthesized and regulate gene transcription of EPO, but in the presence of oxygen these transcription factors are degraded, limiting EPO gene expression.

Once synthesized, EPO acts on erythrocytes to promote their survival by protecting them from apoptosis and co-operates with growth factors to stimulate production, maturation, and hemoglobin synthesis in progenitor erythrocyte cells in bone marrow. The signaling pathway for EPO, like cytokines, growth hormone, and prolactin, is via the JAK/STAT pathway (see *Section 1.5*).

Factors that increase EPO synthesis include hypoxia of altitude, pulmonary disease (e.g. emphysema), and cardiovascular disease, whilst a decrease in EPO is caused by renal failure and various chronic diseases such as AIDS, malignancy, and chronic inflammatory diseases such as rheumatoid arthritis. Recombinant EPO is used therapeutically to treat anemia resulting from chronic kidney failure, prior to the removal of blood for autologous blood transfusion, and illegally by athletes to improve oxygen carriage and thus performance.

8.6.3 Hormones released from bone

Bone produces two identified hormones: fibroblast growth factor 23, which is involved in phosphate homeostasis (see *Section 4.4*) and osteocalcin (*Figure 8.9*).

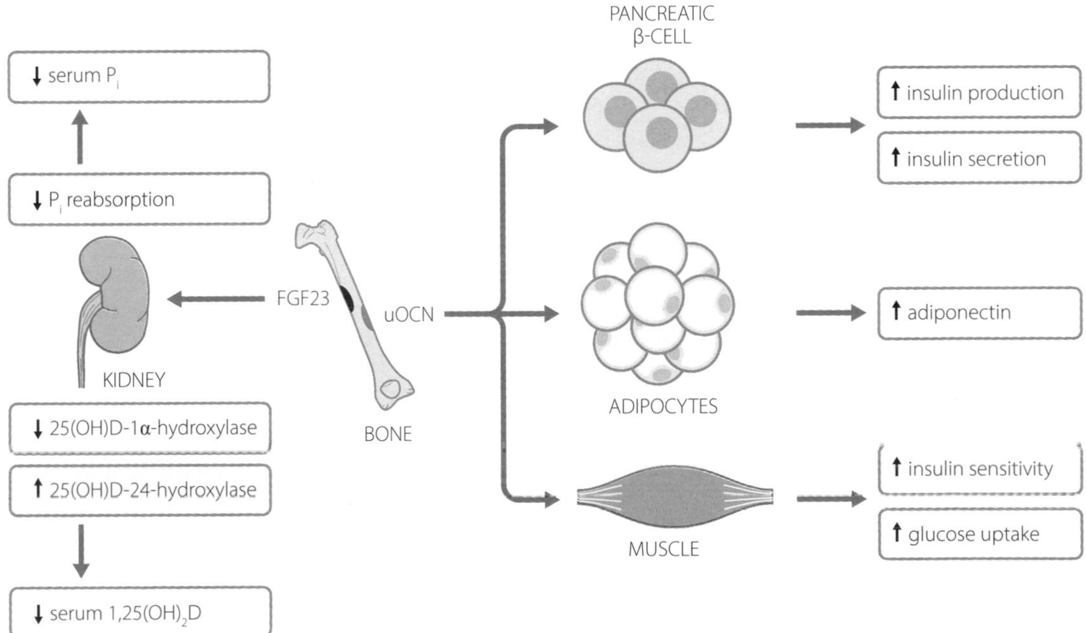

Figure 8.9 Bone as an endocrine organ

In bone, osteocytes produce fibroblast growth factor 23 (FGF23) and osteoblasts produce uncarboxylated osteocalcin (uOCN); each of these circulate as hormones. FGF23 acts on the kidney to decrease activity of 25-hydroxyvitamin-D-1α-hydroxylase (25(OH)D-1α-hydroxylase), to enhance 1,24-hydroxylase expression and to increase excretion of inorganic phosphate (P_i). uOCN acts on pancreatic beta cells to increase insulin production and secretion, on adipocytes to increase adiponectin, and on muscle to increase insulin sensitivity and glucose uptake.

Osteocalcin is secreted solely by osteoblasts (the cells that are responsible for bone formation) and is a positive regulator of insulin secretion. It also increases insulin sensitivity by increasing adiponectin secretion (see *Section 8.3.2*) from adipose tissue. Interestingly, this hormone was identified as a result of the fact that bone remodeling is an energy-demanding process and leptin is a major inhibitor of this process. Thus it was hypothesized that bone cells can regulate energy metabolism through an endocrine mechanism. This led to the identification of osteocalcin which is part of a complex signaling mechanism between bone and organs more classically associated with the regulation of energy homeostasis, such as the pancreas and adipose tissue. The physiology of osteocalcin is still in its infancy, particularly in humans, and also in its relation to human metabolism and pathology.

8.7 Further reading

Bloom SR, Minnion JS, Simpson KA, Shilito JC, and Suzuki K (2010) The role of gut hormones and hypothalamus in appetite regulation. *Endocrine J.* **57:** 359–72.

Bloom SR, Cegla J, and Tan TM (2010) Gut-brain cross-talk in appetite regulation. *Curr. Op. Clin. Nutr. & Metab. Care,* **13:** 588–93.

Clerico A, Giannoni A, Vittorini S and Passino C (2011) Thirty years of the heart as an endocrine organ: physiological role and clinical utility of cardiac natriuretic hormones. *Am. J. Physiol.: Heart & Circ. Physiol.* **301:** H12–20.

Coll AP, Farooqi IS, and O'Rahilly S (2007) The hormonal control of food intake. *Cell,* **129:** 251–62.

Fukumoto S and Martin TJ (2009) Bone as an endocrine organ. *Trends Endocrinol. & Metab.* **5:** 230–6.

Ghevariya V, Malieckal A, Ghevariya N, Mazumder M, and Ananad S (2009) Carcinoid tumors of the gastrointestinal tract. *Southern Med. J.* **102:** 1032–40.

Grimm ER and Steinle NI (2011) Genetics of eating behavior: established and emerging concepts. *Nutrition Rev.* **69:** 52–60.

Lawrence B, Gustafsson Bl, Kidd M, and Modlin IM (2010) New pharmacologic therapies for gastroenteropancreatic neuroendocrine tumors. *Gastro. Clinics N. Am.* **39:** 615–28.

Ouchi N, Parker JL, Lugus JJ, and Walsh K (2011) Adipokines in inflammation and metabolic disease. *Nature Rev. Immunology,* **11:** 85–97.

Pinchot SN, Holen K, Sippel RS, and Chen H (2008) Carcinoid tumors. *The Oncologist,* **13:** 1255–69.

Rehfeld JF (1998) The new biology of gastrointestinal hormones. *Physiological Rev.* **78:** 1087–1100.

Smith BR, Schauer P, and Nguyen NT (2011) Surgical approaches to the treatment of obesity: bariatric surgery. *Med. Clinics N. Am.* **95:** 1009–30 .

Stanley S, Wynne K, McGowan B, and Bloom S (2005) Hormonal regulation of food intake. *Physiol. Rev.* **85:** 1131–58.

Thakker RV (2010) Multiple endocrine neoplasia type 1 (MEN1). *Best Pract. Res. Clin. Endocrinol. Metab.* **24:** 355–70.

Vazquez-Vela MEF, Torres N, and Tovar AR (2008) White adipose tissue as endocrine organ and its role in obesity. *Archives Med. Res.* **39:** 715–28.

Vlassi E, Scacchi M, and Cavagnini F (2008) Neuroendocrine control of food intake. *Nutr. Metab. & Cardio. Dis.* **18:** 158–68.

Wohllk N, Schweizer H, Erlic Z, *et al.* (2010) Multiple endocrine neoplasia type 2. *Best Pract. Res. Clin. Endocrinol. Metab.* **24:** 371–87.

8.8 Self-assessment questions

(1) Which one of the following neurotransmitters stimulates the synthesis and release of melatonin from the pinealocytes?
- (a) Tryptophan
- (b) Nor-epinephrine
- (c) Serotonin
- (d) 5-hydroxytryptophan
- (e) Epinephrine

(2) Which one of the following tumors are associated with MEN-2A and 2B?
- (a) Thyroid tumors
- (b) Carcinoid tumors
- (c) Insulinomas
- (d) Gastrinomas
- (e) Prolactinomas

(3) Which one of the following stimulates the release of atrial natriuretic peptide?
- (a) Raised blood sodium levels
- (b) Hypotension
- (c) Nitric oxide
- (d) B-type natriuretic peptide
- (e) Increased blood volume

(4) In carcinoid syndrome, which one of the following statements is true?
- (a) Carcinoid tumors rarely express somatostatin receptors
- (b) Tumors are very rarely asymptomatic
- (c) Appendicitis may lead to the fortuitous discovery of a carcinoid tumor
- (d) Cardiac carcinoid usually involves the aortic valve
- (e) The prognosis is invariably poor

(5) Which one of the following statements regarding multiple endocrine neoplasia type 1 (MEN-I) is true? It:
- (a) Is associated with mutations in the *RET* proto-oncogene
- (b) Is far more common in women
- (c) Is associated with parathyroid hyperplasia
- (d) Is associated with insulinomas which are the most common enteropancreatic tumors
- (e) Is most frequently associated with pituitary tumors secreting ACTH

(6) The following are commonly associated with obesity with the exception of which one?
- (a) Osteoporosis
- (b) Obstructive sleep apnoea
- (c) Type 2 diabetes mellitus
- (d) Subfertility
- (e) Non-alcoholic steato-hepatitis

(7) Which one of the following statements concerning leptin is true?
   (a) It is an orexigenic hormone
   (b) Deficiency results in increased insulin sensitivity
   (c) Congenital deficiency results in marked obesity
   (d) It is immunosuppressive
   (e) Levels are highest in elderly males

(8) A 56 year old obese man with a BMI of 35 kg/m^2 was prescribed Orlistat (Xenecal) after all other attempts to lose weight had failed. Which one of the following statements best describes how this drug works?
   (a) Stimulation of nor-adrenergic receptors
   (b) Inhibition of leptin receptors
   (c) Activation of gut afferents which signal stomach distension
   (d) Inhibition of serotonin reuptake
   (e) Inhibition of pancreatic lipase

(9) A 44 year old woman was referred to the Endocrine Clinic with weight gain. She described this as 'inexorable' – starting after her first pregnancy some 10 years previously. Prior to this she had never been overweight; at the time of her pregnancy she had weighed 61 kg and now weighed 121 kg for a height of 165 cm (5′5″). She denied eating excessively (in fact insisted that she had a normal appetite), and though not undertaking any formal exercise regime she claimed to walk for at least 30 minutes daily. Initial investigation had revealed a normal fasting blood sugar, normal thyroid function, and a fully suppressible cortisol on dexamethasone suppression testing. There was no family history of note. She had tried Xenecal (Orlistat) but could not tolerate the side-effects and was not prepared to try any other sort of drug intervention.
   (a) What is her BMI?
   (b) Is there likely to be a monogenic cause for her obesity?
   (c) What investigations would lead to a diagnosis of metabolic syndrome?
   (d) What treatment strategies would you recommend?

(10) A 22 year old woman was seen in the Endocrine Clinic due to a lump on her neck which had increased in size over the last year. She was euthyroid. She had no family history of any thyroid problems or of any other endocrinopathies. She underwent a thyroid ultrasound and guided fine needle aspiration which showed a 1 × 3 cm mass and histology confirmed medullary thyroid carcinoma (MTC). She underwent a total thyroidectomy.
   (a) Which cells in the thyroid gland proliferate to cause this particular cancer?
   (b) In a patient diagnosed with MTC, should any further investigations be undertaken and, if so, why?
   (c) Is MEN-2 inherited?

APPENDIX 01 Answers to self-assessment questions

Chapter 1

(1) **b** Vitamin D
(2) **d** About 4–7 minutes
(3) **c** 3β-hydroxysteroid dehydrogenase
(4) **c** Thyroid gland
(5) **d** B cells produce antibodies
(6) **a** Directly proportional to the color change

Chapter 2

(1) **b** Somatotrophs
(2) **a** Prolactin
(3) **a** Octreotide
(4) **d** Measurement of GH levels during a 2 hour glucose tolerance test
(5) **c** Octreotide
(6) **c** Competitively inhibiting GH binding to and activation of the GH receptor
(7) **c** A rise in urine osmolality after DDAVP administration
(8) **d** Craniopharyngioma
(9) (a) A non-functioning macroadenoma with pan-hypopituitarism.
(b) The optic chiasm (OC) lies about 5 mm above the diaphragma sellae and enlargement of the pituitary gland in the sella turcica causes upward extension of the adenoma and compression of the OC resulting in loss of peripheral vision.
(c) Synacthen test, measurement of serum testosterone levels, TFTs, plasma osmolality.
(d) Transsphenoidal surgery or transcranial surgery which is indicated in patients with large invasive tumors and visual impairment. Post-operative radiotherapy may be required in patients with evidence of residual tumor. Many patients will require hormone replacement therapy.
(10) (a) A prolactinoma.
(b) High prolactin levels can suppress the hypothalamic–pituitary–gonadal axis resulting in anovulation and loss of sex steroid hormone secretions.
(c) Dopamine, secreted by hypothalamic neurons, is the predominant hypothalamic regulator of prolactin secretion causing an inhibition of prolactin secretion. Other hypothalamic hormones can stimulate prolactin secretion including thyrotropin releasing hormone (TRH).
(d) These are usually treated medically with the dopamine agonists, bromocryptine or cabergoline. They not only inhibit the synthesis and secretion of prolactin but also reduce the rate of mammotroph cell division and growth of mammotroph cells.

Hyperprolactinemia caused by stalk compression (loss of inhibition by hypothalamic dopamine) as a result of a non-secreting macroadenoma will usually require surgical intervention.

Chapter 3

(1) **e** Primary hypothyroidism
(2) **d** TPO is activated by hydrogen peroxide
(3) **b** Causes heat intolerance
(4) **c** Radioiodine is contraindicated in pregnancy
(5) **c** High dose steroids may be used in the treatment
(6) **c** Anaplastic carcinoma is the commonest type
(7) **a** Hashimoto disease
(8) **d** TSH-secreting adenoma
(9) (a) Graves disease. Auto-antibodies are stimulating TSH receptors with consequent high T_4. Negative feedback effects inhibit TRH/TSH secretion.
(b) Thyroid hormones increase resting metabolic rate and have chronotropic and inotropic effects on the heart. Stimulation of TSH receptors increases thyroid growth and activity of hormone synthesizing follicles. Increased activity leads to increased blood flow and hence bruit.
(c) The severity of eye disease determines the hierarchy of treatment. Thus in the most mild cases the eyes should be kept moist with topical tears, dark glasses should be worn to avoid sunshine and the patient should stop smoking. Moderate cases are treated by non-steroidal anti-inflammatory drugs and in severe cases high doses of oral steroids, local radiotherapy, and finally orbital decompression are required.
(10) (a) The patient has biochemical thyrotoxicosis without family history and with no detectable antibodies. The preceding flu-like illness and acutely tender neck is suggestive of a painful thyroiditis rather than autoimmune thyrotoxicosis.
(b) Nuclear medicine uptake scan will usually show little or no uptake in thyroiditis, whereas uptake in Graves disease will be uniformly increased. The inflammatory markers (Erythrocyte Sedimentation Rate and C-Reactive Protein) are normally elevated in thyroiditis and normal in Graves or other causes of thyrotoxicosis.
(c) In thyroiditis the thyrotoxicosis is usually transient – there is a release of stored thyroid hormone rather than an unregulated increase in *de novo* synthesis of thyroid hormone. Pain relief (with non-steroidal anti-inflammatories) and in more severe cases treatment with relatively high-dose glucocorticoid (e.g. prednisolone 40 mg daily) may help. Monitoring thyroid function tests is important – in the majority these will return to normal but a percentage of patients will develop hypothyroidism. Some advocate symptomatic relief of palpitations and tremor with non-selective β-blockade.

Chapter 4

(1) **b** Raised levels of parathyroid hormone.
(2) **d** Vitamin D deficiency with secondary hyperparathyroidism
(3) **d** Is an important cause of osteoporosis
(4) **d** Vitamin D deficiency
(5) **a** Fluid restriction
(6) **b** Is inhibited by osteoprotogerin
(7) **d** Increased phosphate excretion
(8) **c** Multiple endocrine neoplasia type 1 (MEN-1)
(9) (a) The weight loss and polyuria are symptoms of diabetes, but in this case the patient suffered loss of appetite which contrasts with diabetes type 1 which is usually accompanied by an increased appetite.
(b) Hyperparathyroidism, malignancy, vitamin D intoxication, chronic granulomatous diseases, various drugs.
(c) Measure circulating PTH concentrations and imaging of the parathyroid glands.

(10) (a) Hypoparathyroidism is the most common cause of hypocalcemia in neonates. This may be caused by an abnormality in the fetal development of the parathyroid gland (e.g. DiGeorge syndrome) or some other rare genetic defect. Typically neonatal hypocalcemia is the result of maternal hypercalcemia caused by, for example, hyperparathyroidism, pre-eclampsia, placental insufficiency.
(b) It would be important to measure calcium and phosphate levels in the mother and to measure PTH levels in both mother and baby. The mother was hypercalcemic and hypophosphatemic with PTH levels of 18.5 pmol/L (NR 1.0–6.8) whilst the baby's serum PTH was 4.3 pmol/L.
(c) The high levels of maternal calcium are transferred across the placenta causing hypercalcemia in the fetal circulation. This suppresses fetal PTH secretion. When the baby is born the parathyroid glands, having been suppressed *in utero*, take time to recover. Thus the new-born will rapidly become hypocalcemic with raised levels of phosphate due to insufficient PTH secretion. Serum calcium levels will correct spontaneously over a few weeks so this hypocalcemia is transient and requires no treatment.

Chapter 5

(1) **d** Inhibits glycogenolysis
(2) **b** Promotion of beta oxidation of acetyl CoA
(3) **a** Binding to ATP-dependent potassium channels on beta cell membranes
(4) **a** An elevated fasting venous blood glucose ≥7.0 mmol/L
(5) **d** Postprandial glucose <9 mmol/L
(6) **c** Cortisol excess
(7) **a** Insulinomas
(8) **b** Her age
(9) (a) Most probably type 1 DM due to weight loss (increased lipolysis and proteolysis) and osmotic diuresis due to excess glucose in the glomerular filtrate which cannot be reabsorbed as a result of a tubular maxim for glucose reabsorption.
(b) Diabetes mellitus (both type 1 and 2) is simply confirmed by a fasting blood glucose measurement which is ≥7 mmol/L.
(c) Type 1 DM is caused by an autoimmune destruction of the pancreas and thus the **only** option for treatment is with insulin replacement. This is not the case for type 2 DM. Islet cell or pancreas transplantation is a treatment for type 2 DM but is usually only considered after insulin failure. Immunomodulatory therapy is currently experimental.
(10) (a) In this case the most likely explanation is that she was suffering from hypoglycemia as a result of only having had a small supper, injecting herself with insulin and consuming a considerable amount of alcohol. Indeed on admittance to hospital her blood glucose levels were 0.78 mmol/L.
(b) Alcohol is not taken up by tissues but is metabolized in the liver by hepatic dehydrogenase. This changes the hepatic NAD^+:NADH ratio and this reduces gluconeogenesis, particularly from lactate. Thus the hyperinsulinemic hypoglycemic state could not be corrected. (It should, however, be noted that alcohol can also cause hyperglycemia in people who are well nourished and have a good carbohydrate intake prior to or with alcohol consumption.)
(c) Symptoms of hypoglycemia are caused by lack of glucose to the brain (neuroglycopenia) and increased sympathetic activity. Thus her seizure and collapse would have been due to neuroglycopenia and symptoms of sweatiness and tremor due to sympathetic stimulation.

Chapter 6

(1) **d** Inhibition of insulin signaling in muscle and adipose tissue
(2) **c** The conversion of 17α-progesterone to cortisol and androgens

(3) **a** Steroidal anti-inflammatory drugs
(4) **d** Inhibition of prostaglandin synthesis
(5) **e** Very low basal ACTH levels suggest an adrenal lesion
(6) **d** The aldosterone:renin ratio is useful in the diagnosis
(7) **b** Is most commonly associated with 21-hydroxylase deficiency
(8) **e** Synacthen test
(9) (a) The clinical signs all point to Cushing syndrome in association with an adrenal lesion. The undetectable ACTH level points to an adrenal source of cortisol excess (in pituitary Cushing disease ACTH levels would be higher, and in cases of ectopic ACTH secretion, ACTH levels are usually very high).

(b) In the investigation of presumed cortisol excess the first stage is to prove that excess (unregulated) cortisol secretion is present and the second stage is to localize the source. This can sometimes prove challenging. Screening tests for excess cortisol include salivary cortisol measurements, serum cortisol levels at 09.00h and midnight, 24 hour urinary free cortisol estimations and the dexamethasone suppression test (DST):

- An initial overnight DST using 1 mg of dexamethasone taken at 22.00h with a cortisol estimation at 09.00h the following morning – failure to suppress the cortisol level to (ideally) an undetectable level suggests unregulated cortisol excretion.

If the screening tests are positive further tests are carried out which may include a low and/or high dose DST:

- A formal low dose DST employs 0.5 mg dexamethasone given 6 hourly with a blood test at 48 h. In a high dose DST, 2 mg dexamethasone is given 6 hourly. Many cases of pituitary Cushing disease will fail to suppress on a low dose test but will suppress after a high dose – adrenal Cushing disease or Cushing disease due to ectopic ACTH secretion will generally fail to suppress after a high dose test.
  In this case there is a clear suppression of ACTH and an adrenal lesion visible on CT scanning. In other cases it is often necessary to proceed to further tests (e.g. pituitary MRI, CRH test, inferior petrosal sinus sampling, CT abdomen/chest, etc.) to attempt to localize the source of excess cortisol.

(c) In this case the investigations point to an adrenal source and imaging confirms an adrenal target. The treatment here would be surgical unilateral adrenalectomy (usually laparoscopic). It is likely that the normal adrenal gland would take time to recover function after removal of the unregulated source of cortisol excess, so glucocorticoid support (i.e. hydrocortisone treatment) may need to be instituted post-operatively.

(10) (a) Addison disease.

(b) Excess ACTH acts on melanocyte receptors to stimulate melanin production in the same way as melanocyte stimulating hormone (MSH).

(c) Addison disease is a primary adrenocortical insufficiency resulting in loss of all steroid hormones (i.e. cortisol, aldosterone, and androgens). Loss of cortisol negative feedback would raise ACTH levels.

(d) Replacement hormone therapy with a glucocorticoid and a mineralocorticoid.

Chapter 7

(1) **e** Sertoli cells
(2) **d** Two to four menstrual cycles
(3) **d** A rise in progesterone levels during the luteal phase of the menstrual cycle
(4) **b** Prostate gland
(5) **c** Breast development
(6) **e** Turner syndrome
(7) **c** Insulin resistance
(8) **c** Klinefelter syndrome
(9) (a) Only a small elevation of one adrenal androgen (no indication of premature adrenarche) and growth of the testes.

(b) LH and FSH levels were suppressed as they normally are in young children.
(c) Sertoli cells form the bulk of the testes and the development of the seminiferous tubules is primarily stimulated by FSH. Excess testosterone may stimulate Leydig cell hyperplasia but have less effect on the seminiferous tubules.
(d) An activating mutation of the G-protein coupled LH receptor known as testotoxicosis (gonadotropin-independent pseudo sexual precocity).

(10) (a) Raised LH levels and FSH levels in the low–normal range together with raised testosterone levels and hirsutism indicate polycystic ovary syndrome.
(b) ASRM/ESHRE Consensus Recommendations for the ultrasound diagnosis of polycystic ovaries are:

- 12 or more follicles measuring 2–9 mm in diameter – the presence of a single polycystic ovary is sufficient to make the diagnosis of 'polycystic ovaries'.
  or
- Increased ovarian volume (>10 cm^3); this is diagnosed by a pelvic ultrasound scan. When increased volume is used as the criteria then any scan that shows a follicle >10 mm should be repeated during a period of ovarian quiescence in order to calculate the ovarian volume.

(c) A prolactin secreting adenoma (prolactinoma) can cause amenorrhea due to the suppressive effects of high levels of prolactin on the hypothalamic–pituitary–gonadal axis. Raised levels of 17-hydroxyprogesterone could indicate late-onset congenital adrenal hyperplasia and hence hirsutism.

Chapter 8

(1) **b** Nor-epinephrine
(2) **a** Thyroid tumors
(3) **e** Increased blood volume
(4) **c** Appendicitis may lead to the fortuitous discovery of a carcinoid tumor
(5) **c** Is associated with parathyroid hyperplasia
(6) **a** Osteoporosis
(7) **c** Congenital deficiency results in marked obesity
(8) **e** Inhibition of pancreatic lipase
(9) (a) BMI = weight (in kg)/height^2 (in m). In this case her BMI is 44.4 kg/m^2.
(b) No. Although several monogenic causes of obesity have been described (e.g. deficiencies of POMC, leptin or leptin receptor, prohormone convertase 1 or melanocortin 4 receptor) these have all resulted in childhood obesity with rather specific phenotypes and a significant association with hyperphagia.
(c) The metabolic syndrome is defined by a raised waist circumference (>80 cm in females) with two of:
Raised triglycerides (>1.7 mmol/L)
Reduced HDL cholesterol (<1.29 mmol/L)
Raised BP (>130 mmHg systolic, >85 mmHg diastolic)
Raised fasting sugar (>5.6 mmol/L)
(d) Initially a recommendation for significant lifestyle changes with sensible dieting (in conjunction with dietician input) and increases in aerobic exercise. In the absence of any effective medical interventions, in this case it is likely that the only effective treatment would be bariatric surgery. She should be referred to a multidisciplinary clinic (with nutritional, surgical, endocrine, and psychological input) for further discussion as to the options.

(10) (a) The parafollicular C cells, interspersed between the thyroid follicles, which produce calcitonin. Most patients with MTC have raised concentrations of circulating calcitonin which can provide a good plasma marker.
(b) Yes, because diagnosis of MTC should raise the suspicion of MEN-2 and although MEN-2 is rare, the penetrance of MTC is approximately 100%. Patients should be

screened for overactivity of the adrenal medulla and the parathyroid gland because with MEN-2 penetrance of tumors in these glands is approximately 50% and 30% respectively. Thus urinary catecholamines, calcium, phosphate, and parathyroid levels should be measured. In addition, patients should be tested for mutations in the *RET* gene.

(c) Yes, although spontaneous mutations do occur. The latter is likely in this case, as there was no family history of thyroid cancer, pheochromocytoma or hyperparathyroidism. Screening is important if a family member has a mutation in the *RET* gene because of the very high risk of MTC.

APPENDIX 02 Reference ranges in endocrinology

Analyte	Specimen	Reference range, conventional units	Conversion factor (multiply by)	Reference range, SI units
Adrenocorticotropic hormone (ACTH)	Plasma	<120 pg/mL	0.22	<26 pmol/L
Aldosterone	Serum, plasma	8.1–16.2 ng/dL	27.74	220–450 pmol/l
Androstenedione	Serum			
Male		0.2–3.0 µg/L	3.492	0.5–10.5 nmol/L
Female		0.8–3.0 µg/L	3.492	3–10.5 nmol/L
Angiotensin I	Plasma	<25 pg/mL	0.772	<15 pmol/L
Angiotensin II	Plasma	10–60 pg/mL	0.957	0.96–58 pmol/L
Angiotensin-converting enzyme	Serum	<40 U/L	16.667	<670 nkat/L
Antidiuretic hormone (ADH)	Plasma	1–5 pg/mL	0.923	0.9–4.6 pmol/L
Atrial natriuretic hormone (ANP)	Plasma	20–77 pg/mL	0.325	6.5–25.0 pmol/L
Brain-type natriuretic peptide (BNP)	Plasma	<167 pg/mL	1.0	<167 ng/L
Calcitonin	Plasma	3–26 pg/mL	0.292	0.8–7.6 pmol/L
Calcium				
Ionized	Serum	4.6–5.08 mg/dL	0.25	1.15–1.27 mmol/L
Total	Serum	8.8–10.3 mg/dL	0.25	2.20–2.58 mmol/L
Urinary	Urine	100–300 mg/24h	0.025	2.5–7.5 mmol/L
Cortisol	Serum, plasma	5–25 µg/dL	27.588	140–690 nmol/L
08.00h		4–19 µg/dL	27.588	110–520 nmol/L
16.00h		2–15 µg/dL	27.588	50–410 nmol/L
24.00h		<5 µg/dL	27.588	<140 nmol/L
Cortisol	Urine	1.8–10.9 µg/dL	27.588	50–300 nmol/L
Creatinine	Serum, plasma	0.6–1.2 mg/dL	88.4	53–106 µmol/L

Analyte	Specimen	Reference range, conventional units	Conversion factor (multiply by)	Reference range, SI units
Dehydroepiandrosterone (DHEA)	Serum	1.8-12.5 ng/mL	3.47	6.2-43.3 nmol/L
Dehydroepiandrosterone sulfate (DHEA-S)	Serum	50-450 µg/dL	0.027	1.6-12.2 µmol/L
Deoxycorticosterone	Serum	2-19 ng/dL	30.5	61-576 nmol/L
Epinephrine	Plasma	<60 pg/mL	5.45	<330 pmol/L
Erythropoietin	Serum	5-36 IU/L	1.0	5-36 IU/L
Estradiol (E_2) Female Female peak production Male	Serum	30-400 pg/mL 20-300 pg/mL 200-800 pg/mL <50 pg/mL	3.671 3.671 3.671 3.671	110-1470 pmol/L 70-1100 pmol/L 750-2900 pmol/L <180 pmol/L
Estriol (E_3)	Serum	5-40 ng/mL	3.467	17.4-138.8 nmol/L
Estrogens (total)	Serum	60-400 pg/mL	1.0	60-400 ng/L
Estrone (E_1) Serum, plasma	Serum	1.5-25.0 pg/mL 29-201 pg/ml (depending on stage of cycle)	3.698	5.5-92.5 pmol/L 105-754 pmol/L
Follicle-stimulating hormone (FSH) Luteal phase	Serum, plasma	2-50 mIU/mL 2.6-9.5 mIU/mL	1.0 1.0	2-50 IU/L 2.6-9.5 IU/L
Gastrin	Serum	25-90 pg/mL	0.481	12-45 pmol/L
Glucagon	Plasma	20-100 pg/mL	1.0	20-100 ng/L
Glucose	Serum	60-110 mg/dL	0.0555	3.5-6.1 mmol/L
Growth hormone (GH)	Serum	0-18 ng/mL	3.0	0-54 mIU/L
HbA1c	Serum	4.6-5.6%	NA	20-47 mmol/mol
Homovanillic acid	Urine	1.4-8.8 mg/24h	5.489	8-48 µmol/d
5-Hydroxyindoleacetic acid (5-HIAA)	Urine	2-6 mg/24 h	5.23	10.4-31.2 µmol/d
Insulin	Serum	2.0-20 µIU/mL (mIU/L)	6.945	14-140 pmol/L
Insulin-like growth factor 1*	Serum	130-450 ng/mL	0.131	18-60 nmol/L
(reference ranges for IGF-I should be given as age and sex standardized ranges - those given above are an average)				
Luteinizing hormone (LH) Male Female (luteal) Female (LH surge)	Serum, plasma	 3-12 mIU/mL 0.8-10.4 mIU/mL 20-140 mIU/mL	 1.0 1.0 1.0	 3-12 IU/L 0.8-10.4 IU/L 20-140 IU/L
Melatonin	Serum	10-15 ng/L	4.305	45-66 pmol/L
Metanephrine (total)	Urine	<1.0 mg/24h	5.07	<5 µmol/d
Methyldopa	Plasma	1-5 µg/mL	4.735	5.0-25 µmol/L

Analyte	Specimen	Reference range, conventional units	Conversion factor (multiply by)	Reference range, SI units
Nor-epinephrine	Plasma	110–410 pg/mL	5.911	650–2423 pmol/L
Osmolality	Serum	275–295 mOsm/kg	1.0	275–295 mmol/kg
Osteocalcin	Serum	3.0–13.0 ng/mL	1.0	3.0–13.0 µg/L
Parathyroid hormone	Serum	10–65 pg/mL	0.1053	1.0–6.8 pmol/L
Progesterone	Serum			
Female (follicular phase)		<2 ng/mL	3.18	< 6 nmol/L
Female (luteal phase)		2–20 ng/mL	3.18	6–64 nmol/L
Prolactin	Serum, plasma			
Male		4–20 ng/mL	18	70–360 mIU/L
Female		5.5–30.5 ng/mL	18	100–550 mIU/L
Phosphate	Serum, plasma	2.5–5.0 mg/dL	0.323	0.8–1.5 mol/L
Renin	Plasma	30–40 pg/mL	0.0237	0.7–1.0 pmol/L
Serotonin (5-hydroxytryptamine)	Whole blood	50–200 ng/mL	0.00568	0.28–1.14 µmol/L
Sex hormone binding globulin	Serum	28–150 nmol/L	1.0	28–150 nmol/L
Somatostatin	Plasma	<25 pg/mL	0.6110	<15 pmol/L
Testosterone				
Male	Plasma	4.0–8.0 ng/mL	3.467	14–28 nmol/L
Female	Plasma	0.15–0.8 ng/mL	3.476	0.5–3.0 nmol/L
Thyroid stimulating hormone (TSH)	Serum	0.4–4.2 mIU/L	1.0	0.4–4.2 mIU/L
Thyroxine, free (fT_4)	Serum	0.75–1.55 ng/dL	12.871	10–20 pmol/L
Thyroxine binding globulin	Serum	16.0–24.0 µg/mL	17.094	206–309 nmol/L
Triiodothyronine, free (fT_3)	Serum	0.16–0.4 ng/dL	15.4	2.5–6.2 pmol/L
Vasoactive intestinal polypeptide	Plasma	<50 pg/mL	0.2960	<15 pmol/L
Vasopressin	Plasma	1.5–2.0 pg/mL	0.923	1.0–2.0 pmol/L
Vitamin D	Plasma			
Cholecalciferol		24–40 ng/mL	2.599	60–105 nmol/L
25-hydroxycholecalciferol		18–36 ng/mL	2.496	45–90 nmol/L

These reference ranges are those quoted by our own local laboratory and supra-regional assay services and are those used within the text of each chapter. Reference ranges should always be checked with your local laboratory.

Index

Entries in **bold** represent primary sections pertaining to hormones and endocrine disorders, b indicates boxes, f indicates figures, and t indicates tables.

1-alpha hydroxylase 175, 181
1,25-dihydroxy vitamin D (*see* Vitamin D)
25-hydroxy vitamin D (*see* Vitamin D)

Acarbose 243
Acetoacetic acid/acetoacetate 224, 235
Acetone 224, 235
Acetyl CoA 218
Acromegaly 58, **61**, 66b, 246
Activin 363, 364f, 375f
Adaptive immunity 25f
Adenohypophysis 49
Adenoma 33, 63, 73, 102, 122–123, 131, 285, 317
Adenyl cyclase 16f, 17f, 121, 170f, 231
Adipocyte 405, 406b, 410, 439b
Adipokine 405
Adiponectin 405, 406f, **409**, 439b
Adipose tissue 399, **402**
  development of 405
Adipsia **94**, 95b
Addison disease 283, **306**
  symptoms and signs 308b
Adrenal
  androgens 278–280
  cortex 3, **265**
    steroid synthesis in 268, 278f
  gland **42**, 44, **265**
    embryology 267–268
    fetal 269
  hyperplasia 317
  incidentalomas 300, 305f, 327
  insufficiency **305**, 307b
    diagnosis 309
    treatment 311
  medulla 3, **265**, **324**, 429
Adrenalectomy 295
Adrenaline 3, **324**
Adrenarche **346**, 350, 353
Adrenocortical cancer (ACC) **296**, 317, 427b
  epidemiology 296
  diagnosis 297, 298b, 299n,
  staging 297, 301b
  treatment 300, 301b
Adrenocorticotropic hormone 12, 34, 53t, **84**, **96**, **281**, 310
  resistance 307b
Adrenomedullin 325
Advanced glycation end (AGE) products 251b
Agouti-related peptide 407b
AKT 16f, 17f, 228
Albumin 238b
Amenorrhea 380b, **381**
  causes 391b
Aldose reductase 251b
Aldosterone 12f, **312–316**, 312f
Aldosteronism 316
  causes 317
  diagnosis and management 318
  primary 316
  secondary 318
Allo-tetrahydrocortisol 277
Alpha cells 215, 229, 241
Alprostadil 367
Amenorrhea 57, 362, **379**
Amino acid 220f
Aminoglutethimide 294b
Amiodarone 41, 124b, 131b, 132b, 157b
Androgens
  adrenal 278
  ovarian 385
Androgen insensitivity syndrome **342**
  complete 342, 381
  investigations and management **343**
  partial 342
Andropause 279
Androstenedione 12f, 268f, 346
Angiotensin 314b
  converting enzyme 314b, 315
Angiotensinogen 314b
Annexin 272f, **276b**
Anorexigenic 407b, 409
Anterior pituitary gland **10**, 50f
Antigen 26
Antibody
  inhibition of production by glucocorticoids 273f
  islet cell 234, 247, 272b
Anti-Müllerian hormone **339**, 375f
Antithrombotic control in T1DM 238b
Antral follicle 374f, 375f
Apparent mineralocorticoid excess (AME) 277f
APUD cells 416

Aquaporins 86, 89b
Arachidonic acid 272b, 272f, 275
Arginine vasopressin (*see* Vasopressin)
ATP-sensitive potassium channel 228, 243
Atrial natriuretic peptide 315b, 316, **434**
Autoantibodies, thyroid 127
Autocrine signaling 2f
Autoimmune
 hypothyroidism 142–144
 polyendocrinopathy 390b
 polyglandular syndrome 194b, 392
Autoimmunity and endocrine disorders **24–27**
 Graves disease 123
 hypoparathyroidism 192, 193b
 hypothyroidism 142
 resistin 410
 T1DM 232, 234f
Azoospermia 388

Bariatric surgery 415b, 416f
Baroreceptors 88
Basal lamina 375
Beta cells 215, 233f, 234f, 241
Bicarbonate, in diagnosis of diabetic ketoacidosis 236b, 240
Biguanide 243
Binding globulin 13b, 157b
Bioassay 27,
Bisphosphonates 189b, 191, 205, 206t, 393b
Bitemporal hemianopia 68f, 79b, 428
Blood volume 315b
Body mass index 346, 408b, **411**
Bone 399
 hormones of, **439**
 morphogenic peptide 375f
 remodeling 161, 168b
Brain natriuretic peptide **434**
Breast development 345, 347
Bromocriptine 83
Bruit 108
Bulbourethral gland 360f, 366f

C-type natriuretic peptide **435**
Cabergoline 83
Calbindin 172
Calcidiol (25-hydroxy vitamin D) 173f (*see also* Vitamin D)
Calcimimetic 172, 191
Calcitonin **177**, 189, 206t
Calcitrol (1,25 dihydroxy vitamin D) 173f, 174b (*see also* Vitamin D)
Calcium 161, 162f, **163**
 absorption from gut 172b
 endocrine control of 180b (*see also* Parathyroid hormone *and* Vitamin D)
 transporter (TRPV) 172b, 173
 turnover 163
Calcium-sensing receptor 170f, 171, 183b, 193b, 426
Cancer
 anaplastic 153b
 endocrine-dependent 344b
 follicular 152b
 Hurthle cell 154b
 medulary 153b
 papillary 153b
Cannabinoids 414b
Carbimazole 136
Carcinoid 422b, 427b
 clinical features 420
 diagnosis and treatment 421
 syndrome 420
 tumors **44, 417**
Cardiovascular system 399
 hormones of **342**
Carney complex 62, **290**
Carnitine palmitoyltransferase 220f, 227
Catecholamine(s) 7, 267, 283, 313, **324**, 326b
 receptors 324
Catechol-*O*-methyl transferase (COMT) 325f
Cathepsin 169b
Cell signaling **14**
Cervix 340, 376
Chemical structure of hormones 5b
Chemokines 406f
Cholecalciferol (*see* Vitamin D)
Cholecystokinin 412, 418b
Cholesterol 10, 12f, 55, 269
 side chain cleavage enzyme (P_{450}scc) 10
Chorionic villus sampling 323
Chromaffin cells 283, 313b, 324–325
Chromogranin A 428
Chronic kidney disease 184, 199
Chvostek's sign 195b
Chylomicron 221f, 222f
Cinacalcet 191
Circadian rhythm 281, 283, **400**, 401b
 genetics of 402b, 403b
Climacteric 395
Clitoris 341f
Co-activators 20f
Cocaine and amphetamine-regulated transcript 407b
Congenital
 adrenal hyperplasia 13, 283, **320**, 321b, 353
  causes 320
  signs and symptoms 323b
 GH deficiency 71b
 hypothyroidism 146
Conn syndrome (*see* Aldosteronism, primary)
Contraception 379
Contraceptive
 pill 386, 379b
 coil 392
Corpus
 cavernosum 360f, 366f
 spongiosum 360f, 366f
Co-repressors 20f
Corticotroph 49, 53t
Corticotropic releasing hormone 34f, 50t, **281**
 test 310
Cortisol 12f, **265**, 276, 277f
 receptors 275b
Cortisone 276, 277f
Cryptorchidism 340, 342, 367
CT (*see* Imaging modalities)
Cushing
 disease 246, 284, 285
 syndrome 246, **285**, **313b**
  causes 285–286
  diagnosis 287, 289b, 291b
  endogenous 285
  exogenous 285
  familial 285
  signs and symptoms 288b
  treatment 293–296
Cranial suspensory ligament 339
Craniopharyngioma **55**, 72, 89, 100
Cyclic AMP 11f, **15**, 16f, 87, 121f, 170f, 281
Cyclo-oxygenase (COX) 272b/f
Cyproterone acetate 387
Cytochrome P_{450} enzymes (CYPs) **10**, 11f, 12f, 268f, 269

Dehydroepiandrosterone (DHEA) 12f, 268, 278, 346
Deiodinase 114f, 118, 119f, 137
Delta cells 215
Demeclocycline 94
Dendroaspis natriuretic peptide **432**
Denosumab 205
Deoxyribonucleic acid (DNA) 8f, 19, 21, 162
Desmopressin (DDAVP) 89, 90–91, 95

- DEXA (*see* Imaging modalities)
- Dexamethasone 101, 309, 311, 319, 322
- Diabetes insipidus 57, **88–91**, 182f
  - causes 89b,
  - diagnosis and treatment 88, 100
- Diabetes mellitus 64, **231–254**
  - diagnostic criteria 232b
  - in pregnancy 255b
  - rare forms
    - endocrinopathies 246
    - ketosis prone 247
    - monogenic 247, 248
    - post-transplant 247, 248
  - type 1 (T1DM) 213, **232,** 239b
    - etiology 232, 234b
    - metabolic disturbances 234
    - treatment and management 237
  - type 2 (T2DM) 22, 213, 230b, **241**, 346
    - etiology 241
    - metabolic disturbances 241
    - treatment and management 241
- Diabetic
  - complications
    - etiology 250b
    - macrovascular 249
    - microvascular 252
  - emergencies
    - diabetic ketoacidosis 236b
    - hyperosmolar hyperglycemic state 242b
- Diacyl glycerol 17f, 121f, 170f,
- DIDMOAD 89b
- Diet 243
- DiGeorge syndrome 194b
- Dihydrotestosterone 342f, 343
- Di-iodotyrosine 116
- Dipeptidyl peptidase-4 230b
  - inhibitors 230b, 245
- Dominant follicle 374f
- Dopamine 50t, 69, 77f, 78, 325b
- Dynamic test of endocrine function 32f, 33

- Ejaculation **365**, 366f
- Embryology
  - of adrenal gland 267
  - of gonads 338
  - of pancreas 215
  - of parathyroid gland **109**, 165
  - of pituitary gland **53**
  - of thyroid gland **109**
- Emission phase 365
- Endocrine
  - function of the pancreas 213
  - glands 4b
  - hypertension 313b
- Endometriosis 344b
- Endoplasmic reticulum 9f
  - rough 8
  - smooth 269
- Endothelin **437**, 438b
  - receptors 437
- Enterochromaffin cells 416
- Enteropancreatic tumors 427b
- Enzyme-linked immunosorbent assay 29b, **30**
- Epididymis 361f
- [illegible]
- Epithelial Na⁺ channel (ENaC) 312
- Eplerenone 319
- Equilibrium constant 13b
- Erectile dysfunction 365
- Erection 365, 366f
- Erythropoietin **437**
- Esterification 227
- Estradiol 373, 377f
- Estrogen 101, 202, 206t
- Estrone 373
- Euvolemic 95b
- Exenatide 230b, 245
- Exercise 239b
- Exocrine function of pancreas 213
- Exon 8, 225f, 229f, 273
- External genitalia **341**

- F cells 215
- Fallopian tubes 340, 360f
- Familial
  - hypocalciuric hypercalcemia 183b
  - medullary thyroid carcinoma 430
- Fasting blood glucose 231, 232b
- Fatty acid 7, 218f, 220f, **221**
- Fetus 271, 343
- Fludrocortisone 293–295, 311
  - suppression test 318
- Flutamide 387
- Fibroblast growth factor 23 (FGF23) 167f, 173, **176**, **439**
- Finasteride 387
- Fine needle aspiration cytology **36**, **150**, 151f, 298
- Follicle stimulating hormone (FSH) 13, 53t, **84**, 335, 363, 363f, 373f, 377f, 389
- Folliculogenesis 336, **374**
- Follistatin 363f, 364f
- Free fatty acids 221, 270f, 418t

- Galactosemia 258b, 390b
- Gastrin 412, 418b
- Gastric inhibitory peptide 230b, 418b
- Gastrinoma 423b
- Gastroenteropancreatic
  - tract 415
  - tumors 419
- Gastrointestinal tract 399, 407b
  - endocrinology **412**
  - tumors 419b
- GDF-9 375f
- G-protein coupled receptors (GPCRs) **14**, 87, 120, 121f, 170f, 231, 281, 336
- Genes
  - *Bmal1* 402b
  - *Clock* 402b
  - *CRY* 402b
  - *CYP* **10**, 173, 175, 320
  - *DAX-1* 337
  - *Db/db* 406
  - *GH1* 60
  - *GH2* 60
  - *GNAS1* 195, 196b
  - *HESX1* 72, 100
  - *KAL* 356
  - *Lhx3* 55, 77, 100
  - *MEN* 426
  - *Ob/ob* 406
  - *OXY* 85
  - *PER* 402b
  - *Pit-1* 55, 72, 100
  - *POU1F1* 54
  - *PROP1* 55, 72, 100
  - *RET* 426, 429–430, 432f
  - *REV ERB* 402b
  - *ROR* 402b
  - *RSPO* 337
  - *SF 1* 337
  - *SRY* 337
  - *THR* 115
  - *TPIT 100*
  - *TR*a/*TR*b 115f, 144
  - *WNT4* 337
- Genetic control of sex determination 337b

Genital tubercle 341f
Genitalia 341
Genomic effects 21f, 275f
GEP-NETS 421, 422b (*see also* Carcinoid tumors *and* Pancreatic/islet cell neuroendocrine tumors)
  treatment of 422
Germ cells 340f
Ghrelin 60, 407b, 418b
Ghrelinoma 424b
Glucagon 215, 217, **223**, **229**, 241, 270, 418b
  actions 231, **270**
  receptors 273
  resistance 307
  stimulation test 67,73
  synthesis and release 229
  transport/metabolism 276
Glucagon-like peptide 229f, 230b, 243, 418b
  agonists 243
Glucagon-related polypeptide 229f
Glucagonomas 423b, 428
Glucocorticoids **270**, 272b/f, 273b
  anti-inflammatory actions 272
  metabolic effects 270
  receptors 273, 274f
Gluconeogenesis 217f, 218, 235
Glucosamine 251b
Glucose **217**
  tolerance 64
    test 32f, 65,67b, 232b
  transporters (GLUTs), 217f, 218f, 219b, 226f, 227
Glucose-6-phosphate 217f, 231
Glucose-6-phosphatase 231
Glutathionine 251b
Glycation 251b, 252b
Glycemic control 237, 238b, 242
Glycentin 229
Glycogen **217**
  synthase 227, 228f
Glycogenesis 217f
Glycogenolysis 217f
Glycolysis 217f,
Glycoprotein hormone **84**, 120
Glycosylated hemoglobin (HbA1c) 230b, 237, 241, 242f, 243, 245
Glycosylation 10
Golgi apparatus 10
Gonadotroph 49, 53t
Goiter 123b, 124b, 132, 142b,
Gonadarche 347
Gonadotropin **97**, 344b
  releasing hormone 50t, 335, 344b, 349f
    agonist 344b, 352b
    antagonist 344b, 387
Gonads 3, 335
  development **336–343**
  steroid production **343**
GPR54 348
Granulocyte macrophage colony stimulating factor 167f, 179f
Granulomatous disease 95b, 189
Granulosa cells 374
Graves disease 24, 27, **123**
  cause 123,
  diagnosis 125,
  in pregnancy 135, 138b
  signs and symptoms 124f, 125b
  treatment 136
Growth hormone 23f, **32**, 53t, **58**, **59b**, 61f, 63f
  actions 59–60
  deficiency **71**
    causes, adult 73, childhood 71
    investigations 67b, 73, 75
    symptoms and signs 74b
  excess 61–70 (*see also* Acromegaly)
  releasing hormone 50t, **60**
  synthesis and secretion 60
Growth spurt 345
Gubernaculum 339
Gynecomastia 369

Hashimoto disease 27, 123b, 143
Heat shock proteins 19
Hematopoietic stem cell 169
Hepatic portal vein 214f, 215
Hexosamine pathway 251b, 252b
High density lipoproteins 222f
Hirsutism 279b, 320
  Ferriman and Gallwey system 280f
  treatment of 387
Histamine 418b
Histone 12f
Homeostasis **23**
Hormones
  chemical classification 3–7, 5b
  measuring levels 27–30
  synthesis and secretion 7–13
Hormone replacement therapy 205, 392, 393b
Human
  chorionic gonadotropin 138b, 343
  glucocorticoid receptor (α and β) **273**, 274f
  leucocyte antigen 25, 233, 234f
Hungry bone syndrome 192,
Hydrocortisone 101, 311
Hydroxybutyric acid/hydroxybutarate 224, 235
Hydroxylase (21) 268, 321b, 323b
Hydroxysteroid dehydrogenase
  3b 11, 12f, 268
  11b-1 and 11b-2 268, 277, 313b
Hyperaldosteronism 313b
Hyperandrogenism 382
Hypercalcemia 172, **181** (*see also* Hyperparathyroidism)
  causes 181b, 182, 186
  signs and symptoms 182
  treatment 188
Hypercalciuria 172, 187
Hyperglycemia 235b, 236b, 237, 241
Hypergonoadotropic hypogonadism 18, 356, 368,
Hyperkalemia 236b, 317
Hyperinsulinism 258, 362
Hyperosmolar
  hyperglycemic state 241, 242b
  non-ketotic coma (HONK) 241
Hyperparathyroidism 182, 427, 430 (*see also* Hypercalcemia)
  primary 182
  secondary 184
  symptoms and signs of 183b
  tertiary 184
  treatment 188
Hyperprolactinemia **77**
  causes 78b, 381
Hyperthyroidism 18, 27, 31, **110–140**
  causes of 124 (*see also* Graves disease, Thyroiditis, Nodular thyroid disease)
  in pregnancy **134**, 138b
  investigation and diagnosis of 125
Hypervolemic 92b
  treatment **136**, 138b
Hypervitaminosis D 200
Hypoadrenalism 307b
Hypocalcemia 172, 180f, **191** (*see also* Hypoparathyroidism, Vitamin D deficiency)
  causes 193b
  diagnosis and treatment 192
  signs and symptoms 192f, 193, 195b
Hypocalciuria 172
Hypoglycemia **254**
  autoimmune 259b

causes 257, 258b, 259b
symptoms 257b
Hypogonadism 13, 63, 356
Hypogonadotropic hypogonadism 353, 368
Hypokalemia 236b, 278
Hyponatremia **91**
classification 92t
clinical features and management 93
symptoms and signs 94b
Hypoparathyroidism 13, **192**
clinical features 193
diagnosis and treatment 193
genetic syndromes causing 194b
Hypophyseal
artery 50f,
portal vein 50f
Hypopituitarism 73, **95**, **368**
causes 74b, **97**
symptoms 96b
treatment **101**
Hypospadias 341, 342
Hypothalamic-pituitary axis **23**, 31, 50f, 51f, 61f
Hypothyroidism 31, 107, 139b, **141**
autoimmune 142–143
causes 141b
central (secondary) 144
fetal, neonatal and childhood 146–148
signs and symptoms 142f, 145
treatment 146
Hypovolemic 92b
Hypoxia inducible factor 439

Imaging modalities 34–46
computed tomography (CT) 38, 55, 184, 299
dual-energy X-ray absorptiometry (DEXA) 203, 204b
magnetic resonance imaging (MRI) 39–40, 40f, 55, 76, 80, 91f, 98f, 184, 429f
positron emission tomography (PET) scans 45, 45ff
scintigraphy 40–44, 42f, 43f
ultrasound 36
Immunity
adaptive 25f
auto 24, 26f
innate 25f
Immunoassays 28b, 29b
Immunosuppressant 272b
In vitro fertilization 344b, 394
Incretins 239b
Infertility
female 385b, **386**
male **367**, 368b
Inflammatory
pathogenesis of T1DM 233, 234f
process 99b
response 25f, 271, 272b
Infiltrative disease 97
Inhibin 363, 364f, 375f
Innate immunity 25f,
Insulin 215, 217, **223**, **225**, 439
actions 227
infusion 239
receptor substrate 227, 228f
replacement 237f
resistance 65, 241, 382, 385, 406
secretagogues 218
sensitizers 243
stress test 32f, 67b, 73, 310
synthesis and release 225, 226f
Insulin-like
growth factor-1 **59**, 61f, 74
hormone-3 339
Insulinoma 259b, 423b
localization of 259b
treatment 260b
Insulinopenia 241
Interleukin 405, 406f, 410
Intermediate lobe **49**
Intracrine signaling 2f
Intracytoplamic sperm injection 370
Intrauterine insemination 370
Intron 8, 225f
Iodine 41, **115**, 131b, 137, 139, 144, 157
Iodine-metaiodobenzylguanidine 42, 43f
Irradiation 97, 100
Islet cell antibodies 247
Islets of Langerhans 214, 232, 258b
Isotonic saline test 318

JAK/STAT signaling pathway 16f, 17f, 60, 76, 409
Jod-Basedow effect 131b
Juxtaglomerular cells 314b

Kallman syndrome 356, 357b, 382
Keto acids 218f, **224f**
Ketoacidosis 235, 236, 247
Ketoconazole 294b
Ketogenesis 218f, **224**
Ketosis-prone diabetes 247
Kidney 166f, 167f, 399, **437**
hormones of the **437–438**
stone (nephrolithiasis) 182f, 183, 189
Kisspeptin 348, 349f, 375
KIT 374, 375f
ligand 375f
Klinefelter syndrome 338, 367, **368**, 369b, 370f
clinical manifestations 369b

Labia 341f
Labioscrotal swelling 341f
Labor 85
Lactation 85
Lactotroph 49, 53t
Lanreotide 62b, 69, 424
Leptin 22, 348, 405, 406f, **406**, 407b
functions of 409
Leucotrienes 272b, 272f, 275
Leydig cells 338, 343, 360, 362f
Libido 367
Lipid 238
Lipogenesis 217f
Lipolysis 217f, 235
Lipoprotein lipase 220f, 221f
Liraglutide 230b, 245
Lithium 89b, 188
Looser zones 200f
Low density lipoproteins 222f
Lymphocyte 24,
Lymphocytic hypophysitis 98b
Luteinizing hormone (LH) 53t, **84**, 335, 347f, 367f, 373f, 377f
Luteolysis 376

Macroadenoma 63, 68b, 70, 428
Macula densa 314b
Magnesium 193b
Magnocellular neuron 50f
Major histocompatability complex **25**
Major proglucagon fragment 229f
Malignancy 107, 109
Mammillary bodies **52**
McCune-Albright syndrome 19, 62, 207, 350
Meglitinides 243, 257
Meiosis 365f
MEK/ERK signaling pathway 16f, 17f
Melanocyte
receptors 282b
stimulating hormone 49, 282

Melatonin 401, **402**
secretion 403f
synthesis 400f
Menarche 348
Menopause 278, 374, **395**
symptoms 391
Menorrhagia 379
Menstrual cycle **376–379**
disorders 379–381
Metabolic
acidosis 240
syndrome 238b
Metabolism
in adipose tissue 221f
in liver 218f, 220f, 223
in muscle 220f
in T1DM 235f
of amino acids 221
of fatty acids 221
of glucagon **223**
of glucose 217
of insulin **223**
Metanephrine 325d,
Metformin 242b, 243, 386
Methimazole 136
Metyrapone 294b
Microadenomas 83
Micropenis 342
Milk-alkali syndrome 188
Mitochondria 269
Mitosis 338, 365f
Mitotane 294b, 301b
Monoamine oxidase 325b
Monogenic diabetes 247
Mononuclear cell 169
Mono-iodotyrosine 116
Motilin 418b
MRI (*see* Imaging modalities)
Müllerian ducts **338**, 339f, 381
Multiple endocrine neoplasia (MEN) 62, 181, 182, 285, 329, **426**
type 1 **426**, 427b
type 2 **429**, 430b
Mutation 13, 15, 131, 172, 193, 192, 320, 375, 390b
Myoinositol 251b

Natriuretic peptides **432**, 433f
therapeutic aspects of 435
Negative feedback **23**, 61f, 77f, 120f, 122f, 286f, 363f,
Nelson syndrome 295b
Nesidioblastosis 259b
Neuroendocrine tumors 417
Neurofibromatosis 329
Neuroglycopenia 254
Neurohypophysis 49, 86
Neuropeptide Y 407b, 418b
Neurophysin 85, 86
Nitric oxide 365, 367, 428b
synthase 438b
Nodular thyroid disease 131 (*see also* Hyperthyroidism)
Non-esterified fatty acids (*see* Free fatty acids)
Nor-adrenaline 3, **324**, 325b
Nor-epinephrine 3, **324**, 325b
Nuclear factor-kB 167f, 170, 275
Nuclear medicine
radionucleotides 34
scan 128f, 184

Obesity 22, 405, **410**
genetics 408b
management 413b
Octreotide 33, 44, 46, 62b, 69, 424
Oligospermia 379b
Oocyte 338, 372
cryopreservation 394
Oogenesis **374**
Oogonia 338, 340
Optic chiasm 52, 68
Oral salt loading 318
Orchidectomy 343
Orchidometer 355b
Orchitis 367
Orexigenic 407b, 409
Orlistat 414b
Osmolality 87, 315b, 316
Osmoreceptors 87, 315b
Osmotic diuresis 236
Osteoblast 167, 168b, 202
Osteocalcin 439b
Osteoclast 167, 168b, 202
Osteoid 168b, 169f
Osteomalacia 199
Osteopetrosis 201
Osteoporosis 182b, 188, **202**
causes 203
diagnosis and treatment 202b, 203, 204b, 206b
signs and symptoms 203
Osteoprotogenin 167f
Ovary **371** (*see also* Menstrual cycle, Polycystic ovary syndrome)
anatomy 371
functions 372–373
Ovulation **376**
Oxaloacetate 218f
Oxyntomodulin 229f, 418b
Oxytocin 49, 53t, **85**, 85f

Paget disease 201, **205**
causes 207
clinical features 208
diagnosis and treatment 208
Pancreas 23f, 30, **214**, 407b
anatomy 214
embryology 215–216
Pancreatic/islet cell neuroendocrine tumors 418b, 419, **421**
Pancreatic
polypeptide 215, 418b
polypeptidoma (PPoma) 424b
Paracrine signaling 2f
Parafollicular C cells 152, 177
Parasympathetic nerves 215
Parathyroid
gland 23f, 30, **41**, 108, 164f, 429
anatomy 164
embryology 165
hormone 13, 3, 162, 173, 178f
actions **166**
synthesis **171**
hormone-related peptide **177**, 179f, 187
Parathyroidectomy 189, 193b
Paraventricular nucleus 85, 86
Parvicellular neuron 50f
Pasireotide 69
Pegvisomant 70f
Penis 360f
Peptide and protein hormones 6f, 7, 9, 14
Peroxisome proliferator-activated receptors 244b, 241, 242b
Persistent Müllerian duct system 340
PET scans (*see* Imaging modalities)
Pheochromocytoma 246, **324**, 427, 430
causes 327, 329b
clinical features 327
diagnosis and management 328
Phosphate
endocrine control of 162, **163**
excretion from kidney 439f
turnover 163

Phosphatidylinositol 16f, 17f, 87, 121f, 170f
Phosphoenolpyruvate 218f, 231
  carboxykinase 231
Phospholipase
  A_2 272f, 275
  C 16f, 17f, 121, 231
Pilosebaceous units 279f
  sebaceous 279f
  vellus 279f
Pineal gland 3, **400**
  tumors of 404
Pituitary
  apoplexy 96, 99
  function test 34f
  gland **49**, 52f
    anatomy 51–2
    embryology 53–5
  incidentalomas 81b, 82b
  infarction 99
Polydipsia 88, 182f, 236b
Polycystic ovary syndrome (PCOS) 361, 381, **382**
  causes 383
  diagnosis 385, 386b
  Rotterdam criteria for 383b
Polyol pathway 251b, 252b
Polyuria 88, 182f, 188, 236b
Post-absorptive state 223
Posterior pituitary gland **49**
Potassium 226f, 240
Prader–Willi syndrome 408b
Preantral follicle 375f
Prednisolone 101
Pregnancy
  and hyperthyroidism 134
  test 27
  treatment of thyroid dysfunction during 138b
Pregnenolone 11f, 12f
Premature ovarian failure **388**
  causes 388, 390b
  diagnosis 389
  treatment 391
Pre-prohormone 9, 10
Primary follicle 374, 375f
Primordial follicle 371, 374, 375f
Progesterone 11, 12f, 101, 379, 377f
Proglucagon 229
Prohormone, 9, 10
Prolactin 23, 53t, 63, **75**
  deficiency 96b, 97
  receptor 76
  synthesis 76
Prolactinomas 77, **79**, 427
  clinical features 79b
  diagnosis and treatment 79
Pro-opiomelanocortin 282b, 407b
Propylthiouracil 136
Prostaglandins 272b, 272f, 275
Prostate 360
Post-partum thyroiditis 130
Protein kinase
  A 12, 16f, 17f, 121f, 170f
  C 16f, 17f, 170f, 252b
Proteolysis 235
Pseudohypoparathyroidism 18, 193, **195**
  GNAS1 gene [illegible]
Pubarche [illegible]
Puberty 56, **345**, 369
  consonance 348
  delayed **353**, 354b
  hormonal changes during 346–347
  onset 348
  precocious 320, 344b, 348, **350**, 351b
  Tanner stages of 346f, 350f

Pyruvate 218f

Radioimmunoassay 28b
RANK
  ligand 167
  receptor 170
Rathke's pouch 54f
Rearranged during transfection (RET) receptor 426, 432b
Receptor 7, **14**, **22**
Reifenstein syndrome 342
Renin 314b, 315
Resistin 405, 406f, **410**
RET (*see* Rearranged during transfection receptor, Gene)
Rete testis 361f
Retinol binding protein 405, 406f, **410**
Reverse T_3 **112**
Ribonucleic acid (RNA) 8f, 21, 162
Rickets **198**
Rotterdam criteria (*see* Polycystic ovary syndrome)

Salt and water balance 315b, 316
Scintigraphy (*see* Imaging modalities)
Scrotum 341
Secondary sexual characteristics 350f
Secretin 412
Selective estrogen receptor modulators (SERMS) 205, 206b, 393b
Sella turcica 50f, 55
Seminal fluid 366
Seminferous tubules 360, 361f
Serotonin 417, 418b
Sertoli cells 340, 338, 362f, 365f
Serum glucocorticoid-activated kinase (SGK-1) 312f, 313
Sestamibi 41, 42f, 185b, 190f,
Set point **23**
Sex
  determination **336**, 337b
  hormone binding globulin 278
Sexual differentiation **336**, 339f
Sheehan syndrome 89b, 99
Sibutramine 414b
Signal sequence 9f
Signal transduction 15, 70f
  in glucocorticoid and androgen production 281
  in MEN-2 429
Signaling mechanisms in endocrine system 2f
SNARE proteins 10, 228f
Sodium-dependent glucose transporters 219b
Sodium iodide transporter 117f, 121f, 143
Somatostatin 50t, 60, 62b, 69, 215, 217, 418b
  analogs 69, 424b
  receptors 44, 60
Somatostatinomas 423b
Somatotroph 49, 53t
Sorbitol 251b
SOX-9 339
Sperm 366
Spermatic cord 361f
Spermatid 365f
Spermatocyte **364**, 365f
Spermatogenesis 336, 361, **364**, 365f
Spermatogonia 338, **364**
Spironolactone 315, 319, 387
Stalk compression 102
STAT 275
Sterilization 375
Steroidogenic acute regulatory protein (StAR) 10, 11f, 269
Steroid
  hormones 6f, **10**, 23f,
  receptors **19**,
  synthesis **10**, 268, 362f, 373f
Structural thyroid disease 131, 146 (*see also* Hyperthyroidism)
Succinate dehydrogenase mutations 329b
Sulfonylureas 242f, 243, 257

Suprachiasmatic nucleus 401b
Supraoptic nucleus 85, 86
SUR protein 226f, 243
Sympathetic
  nerves 215
  nervous system 254, 267
Synacthen test 309
Syndrome of inappropriate ADH secretion 88, **92**, 100
  causes 93b
  clinical features 93
  diagnosis and management 93

Tamoxifen 393b
Tanner stages of puberty 346f, 350f
Technetium pertechnetate **41**
Teriparatide 205, 206t
Testicular failure 367
Testis **359**, 360f, 361f
  anatomy 359
  functions 361-365
Testosterone 101, 339, 342f, 261
Testotoxicosis 18, 350
Tetrahydrocortisol 277
Tetrahydrocortisone 277
Theca cells 374
Thelarche 350, 353
Thiazide diuretics 187
Thiazolidinediones 243
Thionamide 117f, **136**, 141, 157
Third ventricle 52
Thromboxanes 272b
Thyroglobulin 117f, 143
Thyroid
  cancer 138b, **151**, 429 (*see also* Cancer)
  eye disease 125b
  function tests **125**, 136, 145, **154**, 156b, 157b
  gland 3, 27, **41**, **108**
    anatomy 108
    embryology 109
  hormone 23f,
    actions 111
    receptors **19**, **113**, 115b
    synthesis 115
    resistance **144**, 147b
    transporters 114b
  hormone releasing hormone 33, 50t, 66
  investigation 149, 149b, 150b
  nodule 131, **148** (*see also* Thyroid cancer)
  peroxidase 116, 117f, 143
  stimulating hormone (TSH) 13, 31, 24, 53t, **84**, **97**, 117, **119**
    receptor 120, 121f
Thyroidectomy 140, 193
Thyroiditis 124b, **127**, 144 (*see also* Hyperthyroidism)
  de Quervain's 124b, **127**
  painful 129
  painless 129
Thyrotoxicosis 27, 107, **131**, 247
Thyrotroph 49, 53t
Thyroxine (T_4) 101, 107, **111**, 146,
  binding globulin 118
Tibolone 393
Transcortin (cortisol binding globulin) 276
Transcription 7-8
  factor 21, 54, 55f, 113
Transforming growth factor β 375b, 376
Translation 7
Transsphenoidal surgery 58f
Transthyretin 118
Triacylglycerides 220f, 221f
Triacylglycerol 218
Tri-carboxylic acid (TCA) cycle 217f, 218
Triiodothyronine (T3) **107**, **112**
Trousseau's sign 195b
Tryptophan 7
TSH (*see* Thyroid stimulating hormone)
Tuberculosis 310
Tumor necrosis factor-α 405, 410
Turner syndrome 143, 338, **356**, 358b, 390b
Tyrosine 6, **115**
  kinase **15**, 16f, 17f, 227

Ultrasound **34**, 133, 184, 384
Urethra 360f, 365
Urodilatin 433f
Urogenital
  fold 341f
  sinus 341f
Uterus 340, 377f

Vagina 340, 342
Vanillylmandelic acid 325f
Vaptans 94
Vas deferens 361f, 365
Vasa efferentia 360f
Vasoactive
  intestinal polypeptide 418b
    tumors (VIPomas) 423, 423
Vasopressin 9f, 49, 53t, **86**, 87f, 281, 316
  deficiency 97 (*see also* Diabetes insipidus)
  disorders of vasopressin secretion and action 88, 97, 188
  receptors **86**
Very low density lipoproteins 221f, 222f
Viagra 367
Visfatin 405, 406f
Visual field defects 63, 68b
Vitamin D 162, 171, **172**, 179, 180b, 186, 209, 439
  actions 172, 174b, 180b
  assay 175
  binding protein 173
  deficiency 175, 180f, 192, **197**
  receptors 172, 174b
  synthesis 173
Volume receptors 87b, 88, 315b
Von Hippel-Lindau disease 329b

Water deprivation test 88, 90f
Wolff-Chaikoff effect 117, 131b, 144
Wolffian ducts 338f, **339**
Wolfram syndrome 89

X-ray **35-37** (*see also* Imaging modalities)
  for bone age 36f, 351b, 355b
  for confirmation of clinical signs 36f, 37f

Y chromosome **336**

Zinc fingers 19
Zollinger-Ellison syndrome 428
Zona
  fasiculata 266
  glomerulosa 266
  reticularis 266